Clinical Genitourinary Pathology

Andreas C. Lazaris
Editor

Clinical Genitourinary Pathology

A Case-Based Learning Approach

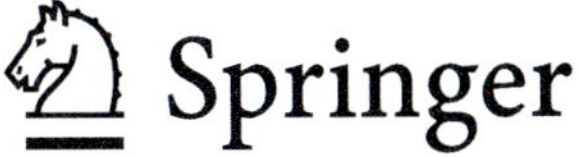

Editor
Andreas C. Lazaris
First Department of Pathology
School of Medicine
National and Kapodistrian University of Athens
Athens, Greece

ISBN 978-3-319-72193-4 ISBN 978-3-319-72194-1 (eBook)
https://doi.org/10.1007/978-3-319-72194-1

Library of Congress Control Number: 2018946222

This Springer imprint is published by Springer Nature, under the registered company Springer International Publishing AG
The registered company address is: Gewerbestrasse 11, 6330 Cham, Switzerland

To those colleagues who enjoy their studies and their work

Foreword: Case-Based Learning: An Important Tool for Pathology Education

Pathologists use many sources of information to come to a diagnosis, in the center of which remains the morphology of a process as seen in a tissue slide. To become a reliable pathologist, one has to have a broad knowledge base on disease processes and their features and the ability to integrate the various forms of information into a diagnosis that needs to be communicated to the clinician. Basic knowledge can be found in textbooks and images of processes in atlases. These provide therefore a sound basis that each trainee can use to acquire most of the skills that are needed. But the most important qualities a pathologist needs to have, integration and communication, can only be achieved through experience with real cases/patients. It is often stated that only in routine practice after the traineeship the reliable pathologist is created. It therefore makes sense that case-based learning is used to improve the process by which a person becomes the pathologist who is such an important person for many patients. As an experienced medical oncologist once said to me, I can only be as good as my pathologist. Many experienced pathologists know this quite well (although trainees often think that formal education is more important), which explains why slide seminars and video microscope sessions at congresses are so popular. I am convinced already for many years that only through experiencing many cases one can become an expert.

Therefore, I am so pleased that Prof. Andreas C. Lazaris took up the challenge to create a book fully based on case-based learning. This book is a timely and welcome addition to the possibilities there are to learn pathology. Such a book can only be made by a person who has exceptional teaching qualities, great experience in routine practice, and the stamina to do the work that is needed. I therefore congratulate him with the completion of this work. Not only Prof. A. C. Lazaris should be congratulated, but also the reader and user of the book. He or she will find a wealth of information presented in a way that is different from textbooks and atlases, and using this thoroughly will largely increase the speed by which a young pathologist becomes the reliable partner in the clinic. So, in the end, the patient who will benefit from the increased quality of the pathologist through this book can be congratulated, too.

Han van Krieken
Department of Pathology,
Radboud University Medical Centre,
Nijmegen, The Netherlands
han.vankrieken@radboudumc.nl
15.7.2017

Preface

This book aims to present basic clinicopathological insights into common genitourinary diseases, especially those of neoplastic nature, and to introduce experiential learning based on case presentations (case-based learning). One of the tasks that trainees face is converting the extensive amount of data available in classical medical textbooks into medical experience. A beginner pathologist often does not know where to start his/her study under the microscope and what exactly he/she should first assess. By using successive microscopic images within an educational rationale, the book gradually and analytically presents diagnostic procedures for lesions of the genitourinary system (kidney, urinary bladder, prostate gland, and testis). Characteristic real cases from my personal archive of the past 20 years, closely related to day-to-day medical practice, are presented for each organ, each case ending with a clinical commentary and key points/messages. This practical form of presentation helps readers acquire the valuable skill of effective diagnostic thinking, focusing their attention on the essential microscopic findings and disregarding insubstantial findings. A number of images have been deliberately kept showing some artifacts of the respective slides in order to achieve simulation with the daily operating conditions of a pathology laboratory.

Although clinical applications are frequently based on pathologic findings which therefore need to be clearly described and recorded, the importance of this in everyday medical practice is often ignored by medical students and downplayed by clinicians. Demonstrating how knowledge can be practically applied and how pathological-report data determine clinicians' decision-making, this book aims to be a valuable resource mainly for residents in pathology, urology, and oncology but also for medical students with a special interest in histopathology.

The pathology part of this book was developed by me personally, and it was based on classical genitourinary pathology textbooks which are cited as references. I attempted to record my medical experience in common diagnostic practical issues of genitourinary pathology for the benefit of trainees in pathology, urology, and oncology, interested clinicians, and medical students, in order that learners gain practical insight of the theoretical background they are traditionally taught, recognize basic patterns of tissue injury, and correlate pathologic findings with clinical data. The acquisition of my diagnostic experience in the field of genitourinary pathology was made possible by the fruitful discussions of the presented cases – and many more cases – in the last 20 years, with the following colleague pathologists whom I warmly thank: Prof. Agapitos E, Baliou E, Bobos M, Assoc. Prof. Goutas N, Koniaris E, Liakea A, Liapis G, Masaoutis C, Michaelides C, Assoc. Prof. Nonni A, Prof. Pavlakis K, Perdiki M, Pouloudi D, Sarlanis H, Assist. Prof. Thymara E, Assoc. Prof. Vlachodimitropoulos D, and Xirou P.

The contribution of the graduates of the School of Medicine of the National and Kapodistrian University of Athens Drs. Dimitrios Drekolias and Ilias Nikolakopoulos to the final configuration and clarification of the texts of this book is greatly appreciated.

Andreas C. Lazaris
Athens, Greece

Introduction: Implementing Case-Based Learning in Pathology

> There is an intimate and necessary relation between the process of actual experience and education.
> *John Dewey,* 1938

It is indisputable that nowadays one of the hardest and most important tasks in medicine and especially in medical education is the conversion of the extensive amount of available data into medical experience, after a proper analysis and systematization of what constitutes basic knowledge. Medical students are required to learn and retain vast amounts of knowledge on the path to becoming physicians (Yang et al. 2014). It is a common idea that achieving excellence in students once they enter clinical medicine practice poses a challenge in education. In recent years, innovative tools have been developed to supplement traditional materials and are being progressively included into medical education (Kim et al. 2011, Worm and Jensen 2013) due to their teaching potential; the relevant educational methods, in which students are no longer requested to be passive recipients of knowledge (Alur et al. 2002), have been shown to be associated with increased learning outcomes, with regard to various areas of health and medical education (Cook et al. 2010, Lakshmanan et al. 2014).

Pathology represents a major diagnostic field in modern medicine; it is linked with a number of distinct but interrelated medical specialties which diagnose diseases mostly through the analysis of biological samples. Through the analysis of tissue samples, i.e., biopsies and surgical resections, it allows medical doctors to exclude or confirm a suspected clinical diagnosis, such as cancer, and even to identify the presence of unsuspected concurrent diseases. The role that pathologists have in patient care is indeed crucial, since they are responsible for documenting fully the diagnostic evidence tissue samples can provide, in order that a correct final diagnosis is established. For example, the pathologist's interpretation of a tumor specimen is critical to establish the diagnosis of a benign or a malignant tumor, to distinguish between distinct histogenetic types of neoplasia, as well as to estimate the grade and the stage of the malignant neoplastic disease. In everyday working life, pathologists must be able to interpret a biopsy in order to make a final diagnosis, the accuracy of which is crucial for patients. All information provided by pathologists determines patients' prognosis and efficient treatment selection. The pathological examination of specimens under the microscope may be supported by further, tissue-based laboratory tests such as those making use of molecular biology techniques. A high level of competence in recognizing patterns of injury when tissue specimens are approached and in correlating the essential pathological data with other clinical-laboratory information is of vital importance to ensure that the correct diagnosis is made.

In the immense field of modern pathology, an extensive amount of data is available; as many practical skills as possible are requested to be developed by future or present medical professionals. It takes a considerable amount of time and real devotion to acquire professional experience in the field of pathology; actually, it may take over 14 years to become a fully qualified pathologist. Being part of fundamental medical knowledge, pathology is currently taught, firstly on a theoretical basis, from the undergraduate level of medical studies. Medical students are requested to retain an extensive amount of knowledge. Attending lectures and taking advantage of textbooks and atlases, students are supposed to learn how to recognize the state of disease and describe main patterns of tissue injury. In their professional life, pathologists are requested to evaluate microscopic diagnostic features in patients' tissue sections so that a definite diagnosis is set. Too often, trainees/residents in pathology misunderstand the significance of their microscopic findings and cannot distinguish, even after 2 or 3 years of professional experience in the field, the most helpful ones for the correct diagnosis; it takes a considerable amount of time and real devotion to obtain this capacity and become "experienced," though mistakes in the beginning of a pathologist's career can cost time, money, or deterioration of human health.

Teaching is an activity which is helping the student in learning. Teaching and learning are being modified due to innovations in education. Teachers have to understand the modern trends in teaching-learning process and make learning more interesting and interactive, so that students may be motivated to learn and learn better, after having personally experienced the value of a subject (Ambrose et al. 2010, Bass 2012, Boud et al. 1993, Ewert and Sibthorp 2009, Kolb 1984, Lave and Wenger 1991, Linn et al. 2004, Moore 2010, Qualters 2010, Schon 1983, Wurdinger and Carlson 2010). Conventional medical textbooks follow an encyclopedic-type formula citing single diagnostic features of specific diseases. In terms of pathology training, the "encyclopedic" knowledge of pathology is of secondary importance by comparison to the "experiential" one. Today's global educational environment is rapidly changing. The dominant perspective with regard to the future of medical education is experiential learning. Learning authentically implies that learners, simulating their present or future professional practice, gain medical experience in the process of diagnosing human diseases (Herrington and Kervin 2007).

After discussing and implementing teaching strategies in pathology and evaluating students' learning, teachers have been developing new-style pathology courses (Marshall et al. 2004). The main characteristics of the modern pathology module consist of pathology images combined with delivery of compact and guided learning courses (Hamilton et al. 2012, Lam et al. 2005). It is indisputable that simulation with everyday practice is a promising pedagogical tool in medicine (Carron et al. 2011). In this context, case-based learning is a newer modality of teaching healthcare. Case-based learning is a teaching tool used in a variety of medical fields using human cases to impart relevance and aid in *connecting theory to practice*. The impact of case-based learning can reach from simple knowledge gains to changing patient care outcomes (McLean 2016, Nair et al. 2013). The application of experiential learning principles in the field of pathology aims at the integration of theory and practice in pathology, and this is directly linked with case-based learning (Lazaris et al. 2015, Riccioni et al. 2015). One of the major challenges for the medical student approaching the subject of pathology, the resident in pathology starting his/her diagnostic practice, and the future professional in general is to acquire the *basic knowledge* deriving from the huge amount of available information and be able to transform it to medical experience, essential for daily pathology practice. The introduction of experiential learning based on real, common cases helps the learner notice the connections between basic theory and experience. The prospect to record basic professional experience is intimately associated with the presentation of selected, common case studies; in this way, as many practical skills as possible can be developed by medical professionals. A new teaching approach based on case studies and discussions/commentaries has already been considered successful in medical teaching (Van Dijiken et al. 2008). The motivation *to learn* is greatly improved by the *study of cases* (Dacre and Fox 2000); the latter makes pathology *easier to understand*, and, furthermore, in this way, students can relate knowledge to a *real-world context* and their future profession (Weurlander et al. 2009). Cases should of course be carefully chosen for their learning potential. Through selected educational case studies, the learner is assisted to gain *practical insight* of the theoretical background he is traditionally taught, recognize and consolidate patterns of injury in basic pathologic lesions, and correlate them with clinical data and decisions.

Andreas C. Lazaris

References

Alur P, Fatima K, Joseph R (2002) Medical teaching websites: do they reflect the learning paradigm? Med Teach 24(4):422–424

Ambrose SA, Bridges MW, Di Pietro M, Lovett MC, Norman MK Mayer RE (2010) How learning works: seven research-based principles for smart teaching. Jossey–Bass, Wiley, San Francisco, CA

Bass R (2012) Disrupting ourselves: The problem of learning in higher education. EDUCAUSE Review, 47(2). Available via http://er.educause.edu/articles/2012/3/disrupting-ourselves-the-problem-of-learning-in-higher-education

Boud D, Cohen R, Walker D (eds) (1993) Using experience for learning. Open University Press, McGraw-Hill Education, Bristol

Carron PN, Trueb L, Yersin B (2011) High-fidelity simulation in the nonmedical domain: practices and potential transferable competencies for the medical field. Adv Med Educ Pract 2:149–155

Cook D, Levinson AJ, Garside S, Dupras DM, Erwin PJ, Montori VM (2010) Instructional design variations in internet-based learning for health professions education: a systemic review and meta-analysis. Acad Med 85(5):909–922

Dacre JE, Fox RA (2000) How should we be teaching our undergraduates? Ann Rheum Dis 59(9):662–627

Ewert A, Sibthorp J (2009) Creating outcomes through experiential education. New directions for teaching and experiential education: the challenge of confounding variables. J Exp Educ 31(3):376–389

Hamilton PW, Wang Y, McCullough SJ (2012) Virtual microscopy and digital pathology in training and education. APMIS 120(4):305–315

Herrington J, Kervin L (2007) Authentic learning supported by technology: 10 suggestions and cases of integration in classrooms. EMI Educ Media Int 44(3):219–236

Kim S, Song SM, Yoon YI (2011) Smart learning services based on smart cloud computing. Sensors, Basel, 11(8):7835–7850

Kolb DA (1984) Experiential learning: experience as the source of learning and development, 1st edn. Prentice-Hall, Englewood Cliffs

Lakshmanan A, Leeman KT, Brodsky D et al (2014) Evaluation of a web-based portal to improve resident education by neonatology fellows. Med Educ Online 19:24403

Lam AK, Veitch J, Hays R (2005) Resuscitating the teaching of anatomical pathology in undergraduate medical education: web-based innovative clinicopathological cases. Pathology 37:360–363

Lave J, Wenger E (1991) Situated learning: legitimate peripheral participation. Cambridge University, New York

Lazaris AC, Riccioni O, Solomou M et al (2015) Implementation of Experiential Learning in Pathology: impact of Hipon Project Concept and Attainment. Int Arch Med 8(211):1–7

Linn PL, Howard A, Miller E (eds) (2004) The handbook for research in cooperative education and internships. Lawrence Erlbaum Associates, Mahwah

Marshall R, Cartwright N, Mattick K (2004) Teaching and learning Pathology: a critical review of the English literature. Med Educ 38(3):302–313

McLean SF (2016) Case-based learning and its application in medical and health-care fields: a review of worldwide literature. J Med Educ Curric Dev 3:39–49

Moore DT (2010) Forms and issues in experiential learning. In: Qualters DM (ed) New directions for teaching and learning, Wiley, New York, p 3–13

Nair SP, Shah T, Seth S et al (2013) Case Based Learning: a method for better understanding of biochemistry in medical students. J Clin Diagn Res 7(8):1576–1578

Qualters DM (2010) Bringing the outside in: assessing experiential education. Special Issue 124: Experiential Education: Making the Most of Learning Outside the Classroom, p 55–62

Riccioni O, Vrasidas C, Brcic L et al (2015) Acquiring experience in pathology predominantly from what you see, not from what you read: the HIPON e-learning platform. Adv Med Educ Pract 8(6):439–45

Schon D (1983) The reflective practitioner: how professionals think in action. Basic books, New York

Wurdinger DD, Carlson JA (2010) Teaching for experiential learning: five approaches that work. Rowman & Littlefield Education, Lanham

Van Dijiken PC, Thevoz S, Jucker-Kupper P et al (2008) Evaluation of a case-based interactive approach to teaching pathophysiology. Med Teach 30(5):e131–e136

Weurlander M, Masiello I, Soderberg M et al (2009) Meaningful learning: students' perceptions of a new form of case seminar in pathology. Med Teach 31(6):248–253

Worm BS, Jensen K (2013) Does peer learning or higher levels of e-learning improve learning abilities? A randomized controlled trial. Med Educ Online 18:21877

Yang A, Goel H, Bryan M et al (2014) The Picmonic(®) Learning System: enhancing memory retention of medical sciences, using an audiovisual mnemonic Web-based learning platform. Adv Med Educ Pract 5:125–332

Contents

Contributors

George Agrogiannis
First Department of Pathology
School of Medicine, National and
Kapodistrian University of Athens
Athens, Greece
agrojohn@med.uoa.gr

Christos Alamanis
First University Urology Clinic
"Laikon" General Hospital, School of
Medicine, National and Kapodistrian
Univerisy of Athens
Athens, Greece
alamanis@otenet.gr

Konstantinos Charitopoulos
West Middlesex University
Hospital, NHS Trust Middx
London, UK
konstantinos.charitopoulos@wmuh.nhs.uk

Danai Daliani
Oncology Department
Euroclinic of Athens
Athens, Greece
ddaliani@euroclinic.gr

Maria Gkotzamanidou
Alexandra Hospital, National University
Athens, Greece
mgkotzamanidou@yahoo.com

Eleni A. Karatrasoglou
First Department of Pathology, School
of Medicine
National and Kapodistrian
University of Athens
Athens, Greece
elina_karat@hotmail.com

Georgios Kousournas
First University Urology Clinic
"Laikon" General Hospital, School of
Medicine, National and Kapodistrian
Univerisy of Athens
Athens, Greece
giorgoskousournas@gmail.com

Andreas C. Lazaris
First Department of Pathology
School of Medicine, National and
Kapodistrian Univeristy
School of Athens
Athens, Greece
alazaris@med.uoa.gr

Argyris Siatelis
Department of Urology
Attikon General Hospital, School of
Medicine, National and Kapodistrian
University of Athens
Athens, Greece
argysiat@yahoo.gr

Vasileios Spapis
Department of Urology
Hippokrateion General Hospital
of Athens
Athens, Greece
vspapis@hotmail.com

Nikolaos Spetsieris
Internal Medicine Department, Athens
General Hospital "Elpis"
Athens, Greece
nick1989_2004@msn.com

Georgia-Eleni Thomopoulou
Department of Diagnostic Cytopathology
Attikon General Hospital, School of
Medicine, National and Kapodistrian
University of Athens
Athens, Greece
gthomop@med.uoa.gr

Popi Tsagaraki
Radiology Laboratory
Heraklion
Crete, Greece
tsagapo@otenet.gr

Dionysia N. Zouki
First Department of Pathology, School
of Medicine
National and Kapodistrian
University of Athens
Athens, Greece
denisezouk@hotmail.com

Adult Kidney Neoplastic Pathology

Eleni A. Karatrasoglou, Andreas C. Lazaris, Vasileios Spapis, and Dionysia N. Zouki

A. C. Lazaris (ed.), *Clinical Genitourinary Pathology*,
https://doi.org/10.1007/978-3-319-72194-1_1

A pathologic report for renal tubular cancer nephrectomy specimens should include the following information: type of procedure, specimen laterality, tumor site, tumor size (largest tumor, if multiple), tumor focality, macroscopic extent of tumor, histologic subtype, sarcomatoid features, tumor necrosis (any amount), WHO/ISUP nucleolar/nuclear grade, microscopic tumor extension, margins, lymph-vascular invasion (in addition to invasion of renal vein and its segmental branches and inferior vena cava), pathologic staging (pTNM), pathologic findings in nonneoplastic kidney, and other tumors or tumorlike lesions (such as cysts, papillary adenomas).

A pathologic report for renal tubular cancer biopsy specimens should include the following information: type of procedure, specimen laterality, histologic subtype, sarcomatoid features, and WHO/ISUP nucleolar/nuclear grade.

Four major common renal cell tumor subtypes can be distinguished based on morphologic and genetic characteristics [i.e., clear cell renal cell carcinoma (RCC), papillary RCC, chromophobe RCC, and oncocytoma]; WHO/ISUP nucleolar/nuclear grading system is implemented in the first two of the above subtypes.

Based on clinicopathologic findings (such as histologic tumor type, bilateral tumor location, and tumor multifocality), hereditary syndromes (i.e., Birt-Hogg-Dubé, hereditary leiomyomatosis renal cell carcinoma, hereditary papillary renal carcinoma, tuberous sclerosis, and von Hippel-Lindau syndrome) can be suspected and relevant investigation can be proposed. Cytogenetic analysis can confirm the diagnosis of MiTF/TFE family translocation-associated carcinoma.

1.1 Introduction to Adult Kidney Neoplastic Pathology

Dionysia N. Zouki, Eleni A. Karatrasoglou, Vasileios Spapis, and Andreas C. Lazaris

The two bean-shaped kidneys are attached to the posterior abdominal wall, one on each side of the vertebral column. The kidneys have a tough fibrous capsule (irregular dense connective tissue) for protection. The kidney has a granular cortex (outer region) and a medullar inner region which has a more striated appearance. The kidney is organized into many lobes, in a pyramidal structure, where the outer portion is made up of the cortex and the inner portion is made up of the medulla. The kidney contains about one million functional units called nephrons, which are continuous with a system of tubules. The nephron consists of the renal corpuscle and the renal tubule. After leaving the renal corpuscle, the filtrate passes through the renal tubule in the following order: proximal convoluted tubule (found in the renal cortex), loop of Henle (mostly in the medulla), distal convoluted tubule (found in the renal cortex), collecting tubule (in the medulla), and collecting duct (in the medulla).

Renal cell carcinoma (RCC) accounts for about 3% of all adult cancers and approximately 85% of all malignant renal tumors. The incidence of RCC seems to have an upward trend during the last decades (Hock et al. 2002; Levi et al. 2008). It is estimated that about 30% of the patients die of their disease. There is a clear predominance of males over females with a 3:2 male to female ratio. It appears usually between the age of 60 and 70 (Ljungberg 2016). Black men are known to have the highest incidence of RCC, while Asian men the lowest (Miller et al. 2006). Smoking, obesity, hypertension, acetaminophen, and exposure to asbestos and cadmium are other known risk factors. Having a first-degree relative with kidney cancer also increases the risk of RCC (Clague et al. 2009).

RCC can be either sporadic or inherited. Von Hippel-Lindau disease is the best known familial cancer syndrome involving RCC. Patients tend to develop tumors in multiple organs including cerebellar hemangioblastomas, retinal angiomata, and bilateral clear cell RCC. Hereditary papillary renal carcinoma is another familial syndrome characterized by a tendency to develop multiple bilateral renal tumors of the papillary RCC subtype. Acquired cystic disease (ACD) is a well-described entity of multiple bilateral renal cysts. Patients with ACD undergoing dialysis are 30 times more likely to develop RCC (Konety et al. 2013).

About 50% of RCCs are asymptomatic and are diagnosed incidentally. The classic triad of flank pain, palpable mass, and hematuria is now rarely seen (<10%). Symptoms, when they are present, include hematuria, dyspnea, cough, and bone pain; the latter three are typical symptoms secondary to metastases (Konety et al. 2013). Moreover, RCC is associated with a wide number of paraneoplastic syndromes including erythrocytosis, hypercalcemia, hypertension, and Stauffer syndrome (nonmetastatic hepatic dysfunction).

As said before, most renal masses are diagnosed incidentally by abdominal computed tomography (CT) or ultrasound (US) performed for other medical reasons. Traditionally US, CT, and magnetic resonance imaging (MRI) are used for detecting and characterizing renal masses. Most cases are diagnosed accurately by imaging alone (Campbell and Lane 2012). When there is a suspicion that renal function could be impaired, an isotope renogram and total renal function evaluation should be considered to optimize treatment decision-making. The value of positron-emission tomography (PET) in the diagnosis and follow-up of RCC remains to be determined, and PET is not currently recommended (Ljungberg 2016).

Traditionally, radical nephrectomy (RN) was the treatment of choice for all localized renal cancers. The last two decades, however, Nephron Sparing Surgery (NSS) has been the treatment of choice instead, especially for T1-T2a tumors in a favorable position (Ljungberg 2016). NSS offers similar cancer-specific survival and a better quality of life when compared to RN (Poulakis et al. 2003).

Macroscopically, RCCs are usually yellow to orange, unencapsulated masses, even though pseudocapsules made of compressed renal tissue and inflammatory alterations could be present. Histologically, the most common subtypes are the clear cell carcinoma, papillary (types I and II), chromophobe, collecting duct, and unclassified (Campbell and Lane 2012).

Renal cell carcinoma (RCC) in adult patients comprises a heterogeneous group of neoplasms with clinical outcomes that range from indolent to overtly malignant. Soft tissue (perinephric or sinus fat) and vascular spread beyond the kidney are recognized as major adverse prognostic parameters. WHO/ISUP nucleolar/nuclear grading system is prognostically useful in clear cell RCC, the commonest type of renal cancer, and some other cortical carcinomas; its utility remains ambiguous in chromophobe RCC. Established prognostic factors in RCC include primary tumor stage, size (< or = 4 cm, > 4 but < or = 7 cm, > 7 but < or = 10 cm and >10 cm, in greatest dimension), distant/nodal metastases, histologic subtype, nucleolar/nuclear grade, sarcomatoid features, and tumor necrosis (Algaba et al. 2011; Murphy et al. 2004; Zhou and Magi-Galluzzi 2007). Overlapping features among the histologic subtypes of RCCs and benign entities are frequent; so the most characteristic findings of each common (or relatively common) tumor type must be highlighted (Magi-Galluzzi and Zhou 2010; Ross et al. 2012).

With regard to immunohistochemistry, CD10 and RCC antigen (marker) are sensitive to renal cell neoplasms derived from proximal tubules, including clear cell and papillary RCC, whereas kidney-specific cadherin (Ksp-cadherin), parvalbumin, claudin-7, and claudin-8 are, among others, sensitive markers for renal neoplasms from the distal portions of the nephron including chromophobe RCC and oncocytoma (Algaba 2013; Truong and Shen 2011).

Clear cell RCC shows various architectural patterns and is composed of cells with optically transparent, clear cytoplasm with abundant, fine fibrovascular network, often admixed with cells with eosinophilic (acidophilic)/granular cytoplasm. Clear cytoplasm in clear cell RCC is due to rich cytoplasmic glycogen and lipid contents. Cystic changes may be extensive in clear cell RCC. Carbonic anhydrase IX (CAIX) and CD10 membranous immunoreactivity are consistent with clear cell RCC subtype.

Papillary RCC exhibits a papillary, tubulopapillary or even solid growth, foamy macrophages within fibrovascular cores, psammoma bodies, and possibly mucin. Similar neoplasms measuring 15 mm or less are considered benign and called "papillary adenomas." Based primarily on cytologic features, papillary RCCs have been divided into type 1 and type 2, the latter displaying cells with prominent eosinophilic cytoplasm on papillary cores, nuclear pseudostratification, prominent nucleoli, higher nuclear grade, and a quite variable immunophenotype, which, in contrast to type 1, sometimes includes both CAIX positivity and cytokeratin 7 negativity. An "oncocytic" type of papillary RCC has been described.

Chromophobe RCC is a pseudo-encapsulated tumor characterized by solid sheets of cells separated by long, curvilinear vessels; large cells with voluminous, optically translucent, pale (not clear), reticulated cytoplasm are often mixed with smaller cells with eosinophilic/granular cytoplasm. Cancerous cells of chromophobe RCC display nuclear wrinkling, perinuclear haloes, frequent binucleation, and prominent cell membranes. A diffuse cytoplasmic staining reaction with Hale's iron colloid stain is characteristic.

Oncocytomas are the most common benign renal neoplasms and share similar morphology and immunoprofile with chromophobe RCC, eosinophilic variant. Hybrid tumors do exist (Hes et al. 2013).

In contrast to chromophobe RCC and to oncocytoma, clear cell RCC and papillary RCC are usually immunonegative for KIT (CD117), k-sp cadherin, and parvalbumin. Chromophobe RCC and oncocytoma are usually immunonegative for vimentin, CAIX, and AMACR; oncocytoma is also negative for RCC antigen (marker) (Wang and Mills 2005).

Collecting duct carcinoma, characteristically involving kidney central region, displays various patterns and consists of often highly atypical cells within prominent desmoplastic stroma and associated, adjacent tubular epithelial dysplasia. In order to exclude other subtypes of RCC, we look for lectins PNA and UEA positivity in combination with RCC antigen (marker), CD10, AMACR, and k-sp cadherin immunonegativity. In order to exclude invasive *urothelial carcinoma of the pelvis*, we should consider that the latter displays immunopositivity for thrombomodulin, uroplakin III, GATA3, and S100P (placental), especially when of low to intermediate grade. High-grade urothelial carcinoma must also be distinguished from RCC; the former is typically immunonegative for the common markers for RCC, such as RCC antigen (marker), CD10, and, most importantly, PAX2 and PAX8; the latter two exhibit nuclear immunopositivity in RCC.

Renal tumors with high-grade spindle cells include all RCC subtypes with sarcomatoid transformation; these RCC subtypes should be carefully searched with thorough sampling before a diagnosis of a sarcoma is made.

In the handling of small round cell tumors of the kidney, valuable immunomarkers include cytokeratin, leukocyte common antigen, S100, WT1, vimentin, desmin, CD99, CD56, chromogranin, and synaptophysin.

In *angiomyolipoma* (AML), a benign, usually triphasic tumor, the identification of myoid cells, fat tissue, and perivascular tumor cell cuffing is the rule. However, in unusual cases, cellular areas of spindle or polygonal cells predominate (myoid-rich or epithelioid AML, respectively). In epithelioid AML, clear cells frequently show dispersed, irregular, intracytoplasmic, often perinuclear granularity; marked cytologic atypia of cells with abundant eosinophilic cytoplasm may resemble high-grade RCC. Neoplastic cells' desmin, smooth muscle actin, and melanocytic markers' immunopositivity in conjunction with negativity to S100 protein, epithelial markers (i.e., keratins, EMA), CD10, and RCC antigen (marker) confirm the diagnosis of angiomyolipoma, when necessary.

From the *oncologist's view*, RCC patients with metastatic disease divide into three risk categories using International Metastatic Renal Cell Carcinoma Database Consortium criteria (IMDC) (Kantarjian and Wolff 2010). The prognostic criteria are the following (Heng et al. 2009; Heng et al. 2013):

- Karnofsky performance status (PS) <80%
- Hemoglobin <lower limit of normal
- Time from diagnosis to treatment of <1 year
- Corrected calcium above the upper limit of normal
- Platelets greater than the upper limit of normal
- Neutrophils greater than the upper limit of normal

Patients with none of the previously mentioned risk factors have favorable prognosis [first-line median overall survival (OS) 43.2 months and second-line median OS 35.3 months]. One or two risk factors change the prognosis to intermediate with statistically significant decrease in OS [first-line median OS 22.5 months, second-line median OS 16.6 months]. Finally, the prognosis deteriorates and becomes poor, when the total number of risk factors is more than three [maximum 6]. In this case, the first-line median OS is 7.8 months and the second-line median OS is 5.4 months. The International Metastatic Renal Cell Carcinoma Database Consortium prognostic model has an improved prognostic performance and is very useful and applicable in everyday clinical routine.

Management of Local/Locoregional Disease

Currently, there is no evidence from randomized phase III trials that adjuvant therapy is of survival benefit or prolongs disease-free survival (DFS). Several randomized control trials (RCTs) of adjuvant sunitinib, sorafenib, pazopanib, axitinib, and everolimus are ongoing. Data from a large adjuvant trial of sunitinib versus sorafenib versus placebo were reported in 2015 (ASSURE). Results demonstrated no significant differences in DFS or overall survival (OS) between the experimental arms and placebo. As for the neoadjuvant approaches, they are experimental and should not be proposed outside clinical trials. Furthermore, the attempt to downsize venous tumor thrombi with systemic targeted therapy cannot yet be recommended.

Systemic Treatment

Recommendations mainly relate to *clear cell* histology, since most of the pivotal trials have been done in this common histological subtype (Escudier et al. 2016). In addition, recommendations will differ according to risk stratification (see above). The time to start systemic therapy is not well defined because some RCCs have a very indolent course; a period of observation before starting treatment should be considered, especially in patients with limited tumor burden and few symptoms. The safety of observation has also been suggested by retrospective and prospective studies.

First-Line Treatment of Patients with Favorable or Intermediate Prognosis

- Three treatments have demonstrated efficacy in pivotal phase III trials: bevacizumab (combined with interferon), sunitinib, and pazopanib (Escudier et al. 2007b; Motzer et al. 2007; Sternberg et al. 2010). All three drugs have been registered based on the improvement of progression-free survival (PFS) over either interferon or placebo. More recently, pazopanib has been shown not to be inferior to sunitinib in a large phase III trial (Motzer et al. 2013). These two tyrosine kinase inhibitors (TKIs) are currently the most commonly used treatments.
- Sorafenib, high-dose interleukin-2, and low-dose interferon combined with bevacizumab are alternative options.
- Single-agent interferon-alpha should no longer be regarded as a standard option.
- Interestingly, very recently, cabozantinib has been reported to be superior to sunitinib in a randomized phase II trial. If these results are confirmed, the role of cabozantinib in the first-line setting will have to be assessed.

First-Line Treatment of Patients with Poor Prognosis

- Temsirolimus is currently the only drug tested in a phase III study, demonstrating evidence of activity in this patient population (Hudes et al. 2007). This pivotal trial demonstrated improvement of OS compared with interferon or the combination of temsirolimus and interferon.
- Sunitinib, sorafenib, as well as pazopanib are other possible alternatives.
- It is clear that, for some poor prognosis patients, best supportive care remains the only suitable treatment option.

Second-Line Treatment

- Recent clinical trials showed that tyrosine kinase inhibitors (TKIs) are active after first-line treatment with cytokines. Sorafenib, pazopanib, and, recently, axitinib can be used (Escudier et al. 2007a; Rini et al. 2011; Sternberg et al. 2010). Sunitinib also has activity in this setting.
- After first-line treatment with VEGF-targeted therapy, both axitinib and everolimus are active (Motzer et al. 2008; Rini et al. 2011). Both drugs have shown significantly improved progression-free survival (PFS). Sorafenib can also be used as an option.
- However, two large trials showed improvement in OS with nivolumab [an anti-programmed death 1(PD-1) inhibitor] and cabozantinib (Choueiri et al. 2015; Choueiri et al. 2016; Motzer et al. 2015) over everolimus (PFS was improved only in the cabozantinib trial). In both trials, patients could be treated after either one or two TKIs.

Third-Line Treatment

Beyond second-line treatment, enrolment into clinical trials is recommended where possible. Recent trials showed that nivolumab or cabozantinib are the standard options for these patients. If neither of these drugs is available, everolimus or axitinib can be used. In addition, sorafenib has shown activity in patients previously treated with anti-

VEGF-targeted therapy and an mTOR inhibitor (Motzer et al. 2014b). Finally, another TKI or rechallenge with the same TKI is considered as an option.

Medical Treatment of Metastatic Disease of *Non-clear Cell* Histology

In small prospective trials for this group of patients (Motzer et al. 2014a; Armstrong et al. 2016; Tannir et al. 2016), sunitinib and everolimus have been compared, and in every trial, there is a trend in favor of sunitinib. In addition, patients with non-clear cell histology may benefit from treatment with everolimus, sorafenib, pazopanib, or temsirolimus. However, in most of these studies, only patients with papillary and chromophobe RCCs were enrolled. In the absence of prospective data, genetic considerations may influence treatment decisions: in papillary type 1 tumors, activation of the c-MET pathway has commonly been reported. Novel agents inhibiting the cMET receptor are currently under investigation. However, as the c-MET receptor and VEGF-receptor were shown to cooperate, VEGF-inhibiting agents may be a reasonable choice. Similarly, there is no evidence for the optimal treatment of papillary type 2, which is characterized by inactivation of the fumarate hydratase gene, fumarate accumulation, and HIF upregulation. Again, VEGF inhibitors may be considered in this context. Patients with chromophobe RCC may benefit from mTOR inhibitors since mutation on chromosome 7 was shown to lead to a loss of the folliculin gene with upregulation of mTOR. Finally, collecting duct carcinomas (and also medullary carcinomas) were reported to behave more like aggressive urothelial tumors rather than RCCs and may, therefore, be considered for chemotherapy. None of these "genetic" recommendations can be graded, as data are limited and no clear treatment recommendation can be made for these subgroups with distinct biology (Junker et al. 2012).

Medical Treatment of Renal Cell Carcinoma with Sarcomatoid Features

Approximately 5% of all patients with renal cell carcinoma will demonstrate sarcomatoid transformation/dedifferentiation in their tumors. Presence of sarcomatoid features consists a poor prognostic factor (the median survival for these patients is 9 months). A retrospective analysis of an empirical regimen, which is based on the combination of gemcitabine, capecitabine, and bevacizumab, showed a median PFS of 5.9 months and a median OS of 10.4 months. This observation formed the basis for more studies using this combination of drugs in this group of patients.

1.2 Case 1.1 Clear Cell Renal Cell Carcinoma

Case Study

Data Prior to Microscopy

A 65-year-old obese male smoker is being investigated for hematuria.

A large, solitary, rounded cortical mass of the upper pole of the right kidney, measuring *9 cm* in its maximum diameter and protruding from the cortical surface, is found and surgically resected.

Macroscopically, it is well-circumscribed, bosselated, and lobulated, with a predominant bright, golden-yellow cut surface; focally, the cut surface becomes either brown or tannish gray. Focal cystic change and hemorrhage are noticed.

1.2.1 Microscopic Evaluation of the Radical Nephrectomy Specimen

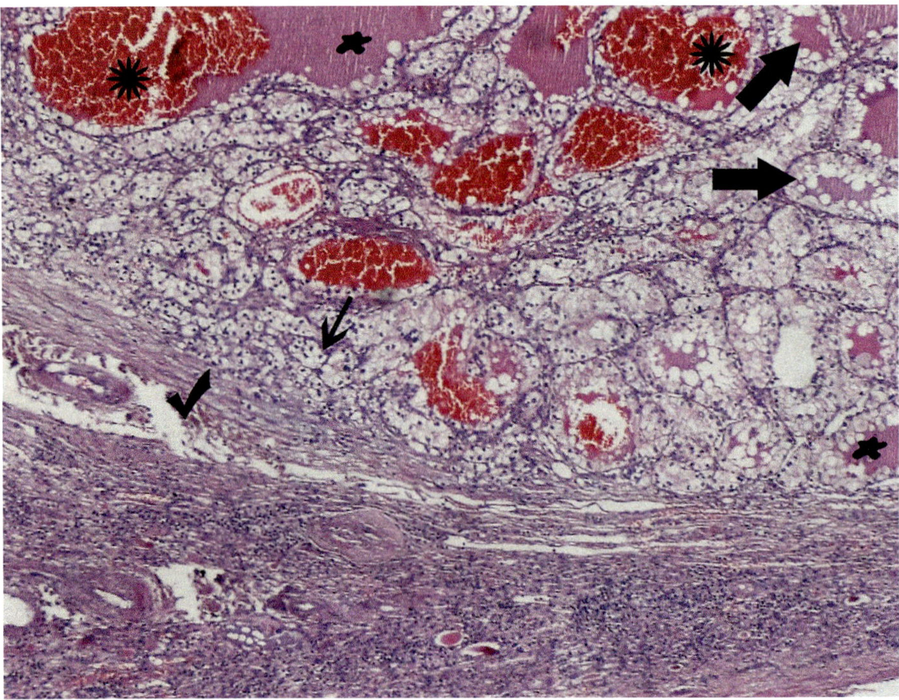

Fig. 1.1 (H-E, ×50) Tumor "pushing" margin – expansile growth. Well- demarcated tumor from adjacent uninvolved kidney with a pseudocapsule (*tick*). *Solid alveolar nests* of clear cells interspersed by a fibrovascular network (*thin arrow*). Fresh hemorrhage (*asterisks*) or eosinophilic amorphous, proteinaceous fluid (*blobs*) into rounded pseudoglandular/microcystic spaces – *acinar arrangement* (*thick arrows*) The solid alveolar and the acinar patterns are the most common patterns of *clear cell renal cell carcinoma (clear cell RCC)*

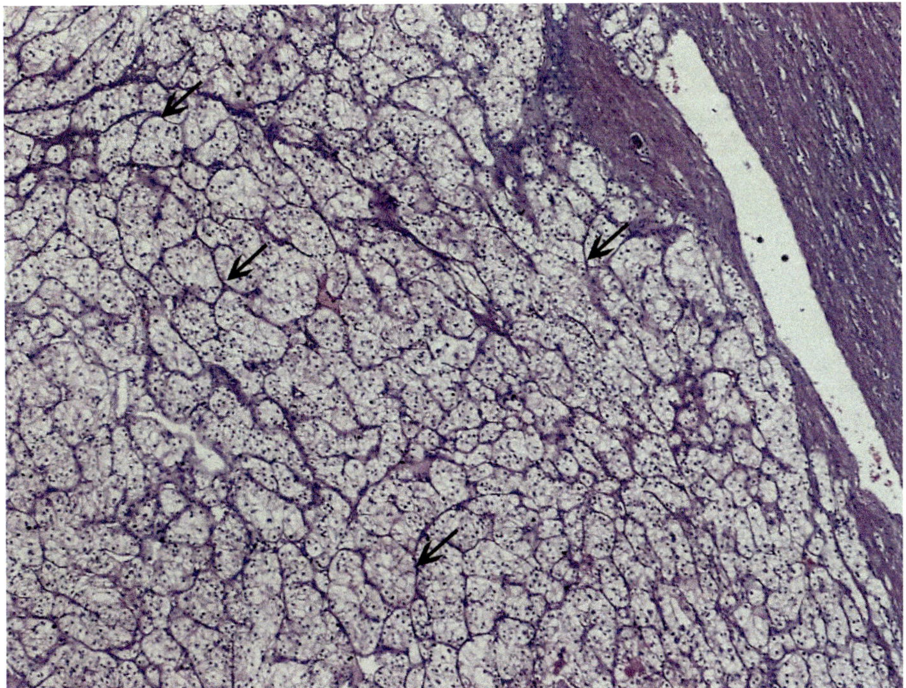

Fig. 1.2 (H-E, ×50) Clear cell RCC. Characteristic regular fibrous network of sinusoidal, small, "chicken wire" vasculature (*arrows*).

Clear cell RCC is the most common histologic variant of RCC, accounting for approximately 70% of the cases

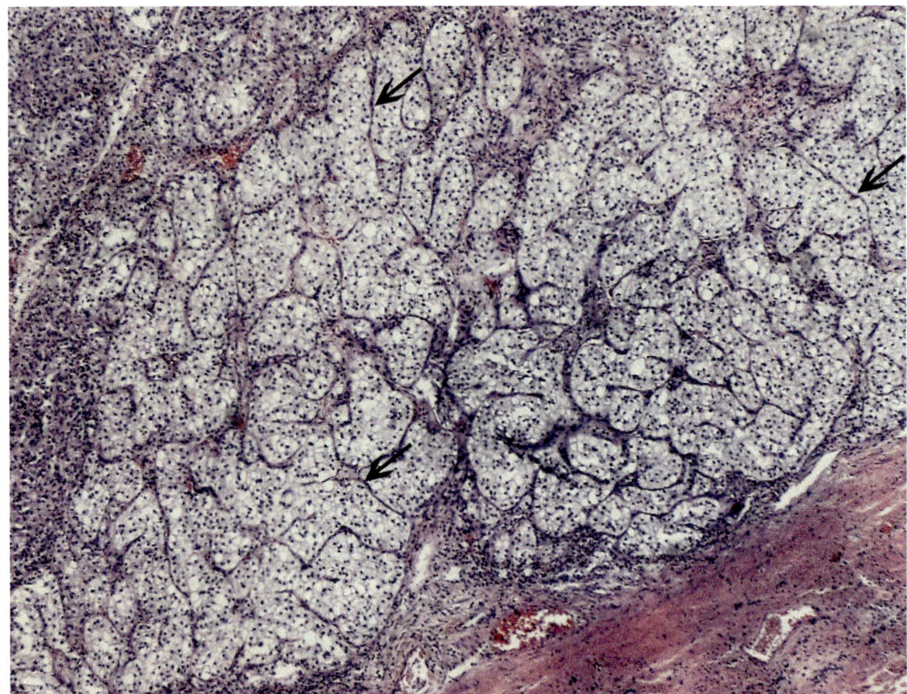

Fig. 1.3 (H-E, ×50) Tumor solid nests surrounded by complete, delicate fibrovascular septa with abundant thin-walled vessels (*arrows*)

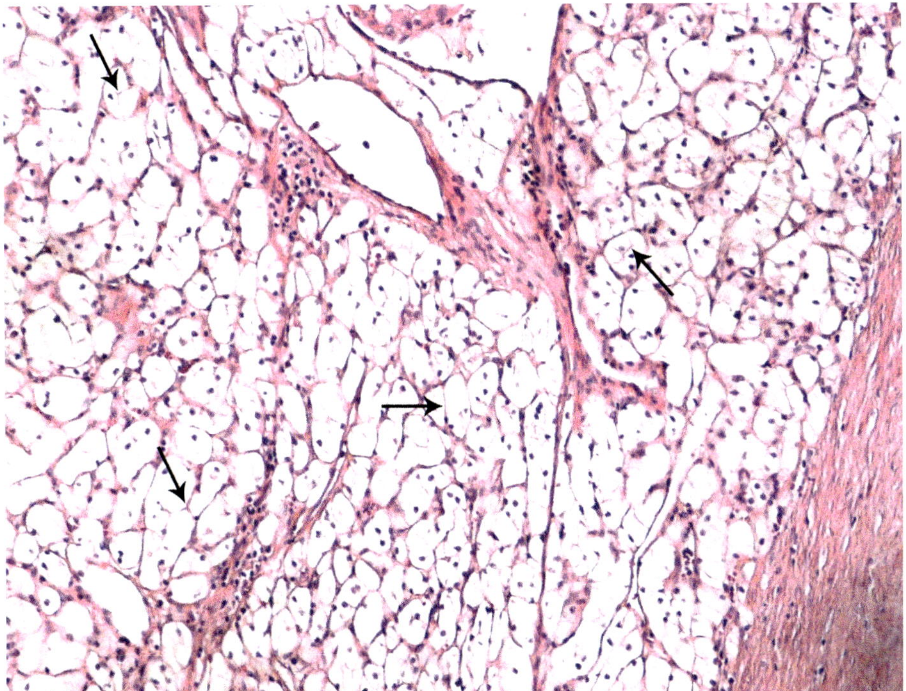

Fig. 1.4 (H-E, ×100) Typical, water-clear cytoplasm of tumor cell nests due to loss of their rich cytoplasmic glycogen and lipid contents during histologic processing. Rounded polygonal tumor cells with frequently quite distinct, but not prominent, cell membranes (*arrows*). Small, round and uniform, low-grade nuclei, resembling those of lymphocytes, dense chromatin, nucleoli absent or inconspicuous and basophilic at ×400 magnification [World Health Organization/International Society of Urological Pathology (WHO/ISUP) grade 1]. Lower-grade areas usually exhibit this clear cell (optically transparent) cytology. Clear cell RCC cell cytoplasm is generally more water-clear than microvesicular, although the latter can be seen.

In contrast, adrenal cortical tumor clear cells are characterized by "bubbly" appearance. In suspicious cases, correlation with imaging findings is crucial; immunohistochemistry is also helpful (in contrast to clear cell RCCs, adrenal cortical tumors are EMA and cytokeratin negative and inhibin- and Melan-A-positive)

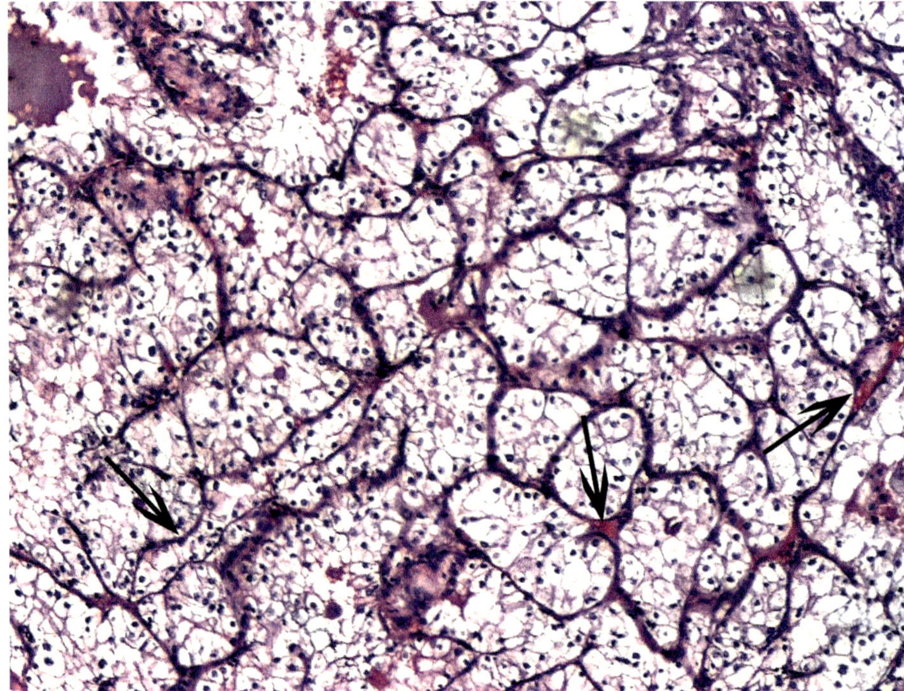

Fig. 1.5 (H-E, ×100) Thin and *complete*, intricately branching fibrovascular septations that surround the tumor cell nests and solid alveoli (*arrows*) are diagnostically the *most important characteristic of clear cell RCC*. Irregular outlines in some nuclei but still low grade of malignancy with no prominent nucleoli at this magnification (WHO/ISUP grade 2).

WHO/ISUP grading system based on nucleolar/nuclear parameters correlates with the clinical course and should always be applied to clear cell, papillary, and unclassified RCCs as well as to multilocular cystic renal neoplasms of low malignant potential

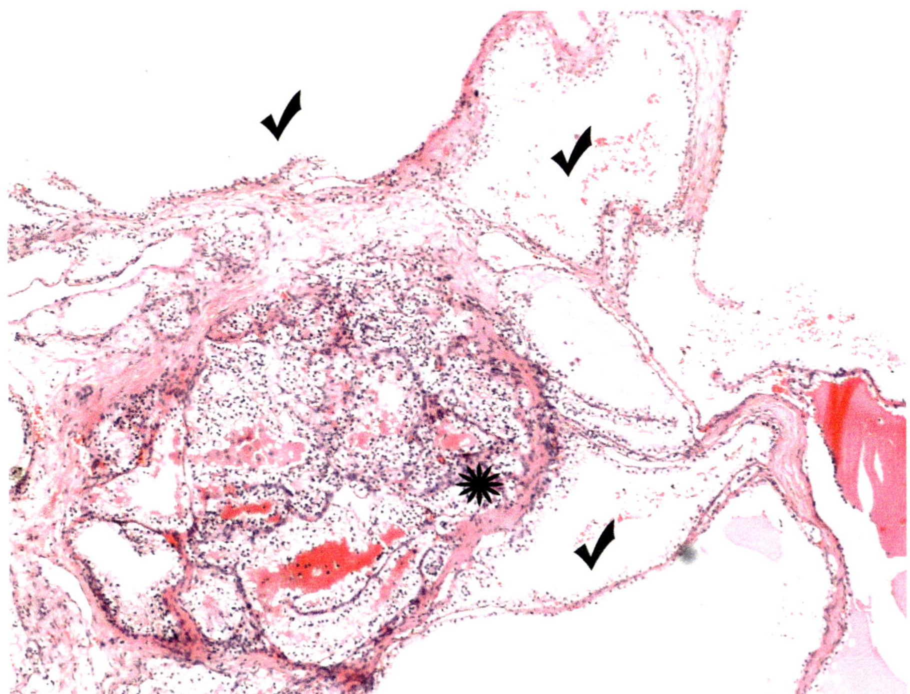

Fig. 1.6 (H-E, ×50) Focal cystic change within the clear cell RCC parenchyma. In clear cell RCC, cystic change may vary from focal to extensive. Cysts may represent an intrinsic component of the tumor (as above) or result from extensive tumor necrosis (see Fig. 1.10.). A solid, expansile tumor nodule (*asterisk*) in an area of evident cystic change (*ticks*) is noted in this clear cell RCC.

The extensive cystic change that occurs in some renal neoplasms may render the differentiation between malignant and benign cystic lesions problematic, on radiologic and gross examination, in particular. Multiple sections of the cyst wall are needed to reveal a more solid nodular neoplastic component which will permit the diagnosis of RCC. An extensively cystic/necrotic tumor may still exhibit malignant behavior even with only rare identifiable tumor cells. Extensively cystic RCCs are not classified as separate pathologic entities. As mentioned before, they may present diagnostic challenges; as a general rule, malignancy should be suspected when any cystic mass in the kidney contains hemorrhagic or necrotic material, and extensive sampling is warranted if necessary, since identifiable tumor may be scant

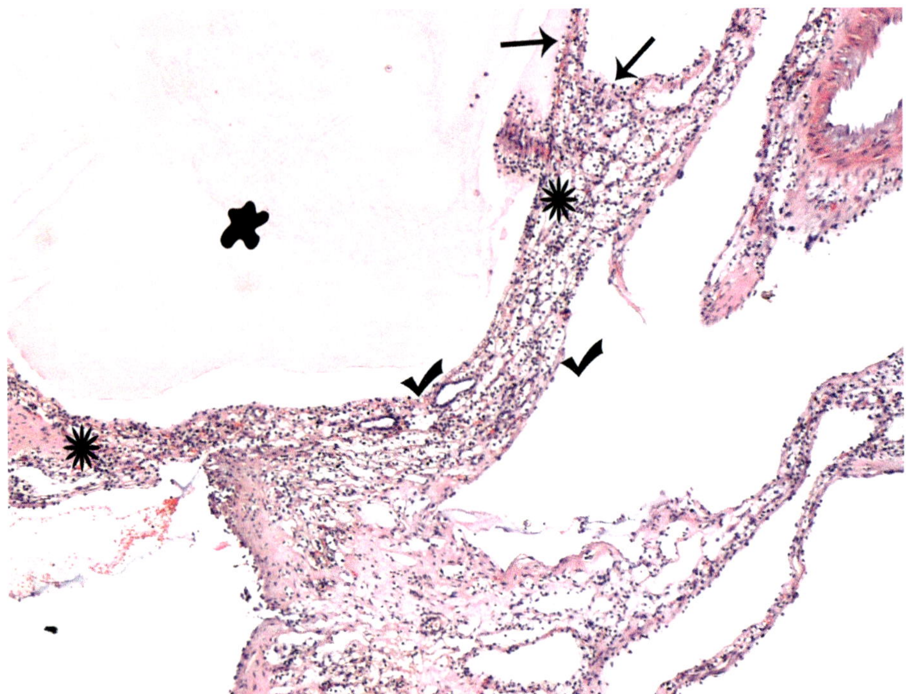

Fig. 1.7 (H-E, ×50) Here is a case with some features indicative of a *multilocular cystic renal neoplasm of low malignant potential*, formerly known as multilocular cystic "RCC." This is a separate, rare entity with an excellent prognosis, being cured by surgical resection. It is a unilateral, well-circumscribed, *entirely* cystic solitary mass. Numerous, variably sized, noncommunicating cysts filled with serous (*blob*) or hemorrhagic fluid may be lined by a single layer of attenuated, low nucleolar grade (WHO/ISUP grade 1 or 2) clear to pale cells (*arrows*); small collections of clear, low-grade epithelial cells closely resembling those lining the cysts and accompanied by increased vascularity should be noted *within fibrous septa/walls of the cysts* (*asterisks*) or *in adjacent pseudocapsule, without expansile growth*; clear cells should not alter the smooth profiles of the septa (*ticks*), but, as a rule, septa should be thinner than those in the image above. The septal clear cells are often difficult to distinguish from histiocytes or lymphocytes with surrounding retraction artifact. In difficult cases, the epithelial nature of the tumor cell clusters can be confirmed immunohistochemically; immunohistochemical findings are identical to clear cell variant of RCC. Solid or expansile tumor nodules of any size should be completely absent in order that a multilocular cystic renal neoplasm of low malignant potential is diagnosed. RCCs with cystic change have expansile clear cell nodules in their cyst walls (see Fig. 1.6) or papillary excrescences covered by clear cells, no matter how extensive the cystic change. Necrosis, vascular invasion, and sarcomatoid dedifferentiation are incompatible with the diagnosis of multilocular cystic renal neoplasm of low malignant potential.

To sum up, the definition of a multilocular cystic renal neoplasm of low malignant potential, as it is called from now on, is as follows:

Neoplasm with a fibrous pseudocapsule and composed entirely of numerous cysts, the septa of which are thin and contain individual or groups of clear cells without expansile growth; clear cells have low-grade nuclei; briefly, a multicystic growth with no expansile growth/solid nodules (Moch et al. 2016)

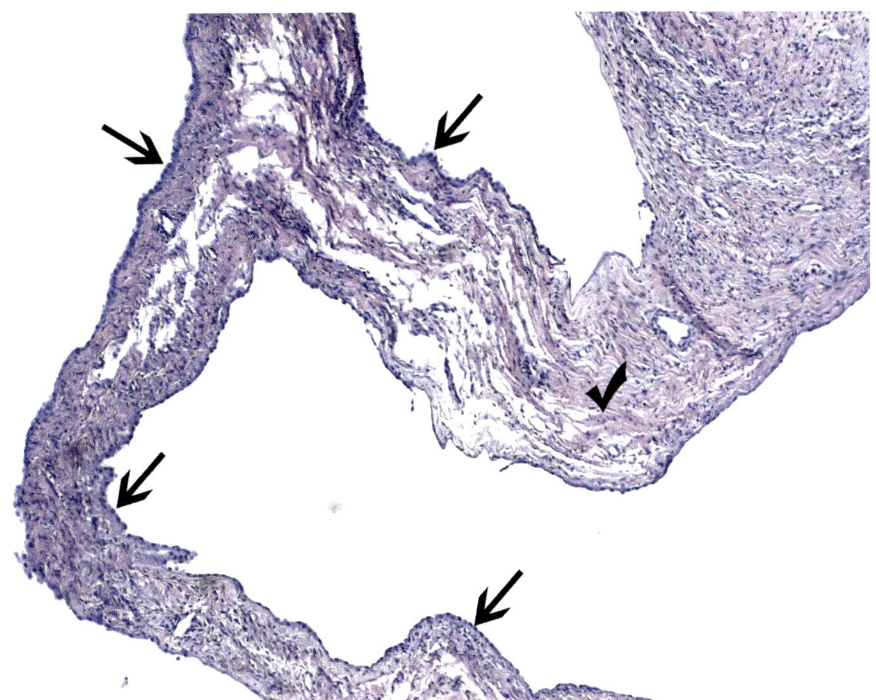

Fig. 1.8 (H-E, ×50) This is a case of an *adult cystic nephroma* in a middle-aged woman. Cystic nephroma in adults is a close differential diagnostic consideration for multilocular cystic neoplasm of low malignant potential. Cystic nephromas are typically sharply demarcated from the adjacent renal parenchyma; they are unilateral, benign, *biphasic* renal tumors with epithelial and stromal elements, within the spectrum of tumors that fall under the heading "renal epithelial and stromal tumors" which includes mixed epithelial and stromal tumors. They are seen mainly in middle-aged females. *No* renal parenchyma (present in polycystic disease) or blastema/embryonal elements (present in cystic partially differentiated nephroblastoma) or nests of malignant cells (seen in clear cell neoplasms) are present within the cyst septa.

This is a solitary, thin-walled, multiloculated, encapsulated, well-circumscribed cystic lesion with a simple epithelial lining (*arrows*), with acidophilic cytoplasm (clear cell cytology is rare). *No* clear cells should be found within fibrous septa; the latter frequently are quite thin, correspond to the smooth outlines of the cysts, and often have cellular spindle cell histology. In the present case, the stroma is densely collagenous/fibrous (*tick*). The cysts in this kind of tumor are discrete, without any apparent interconnections. Of course, expansile nodules of solid growth are not encountered in cystic nephromas

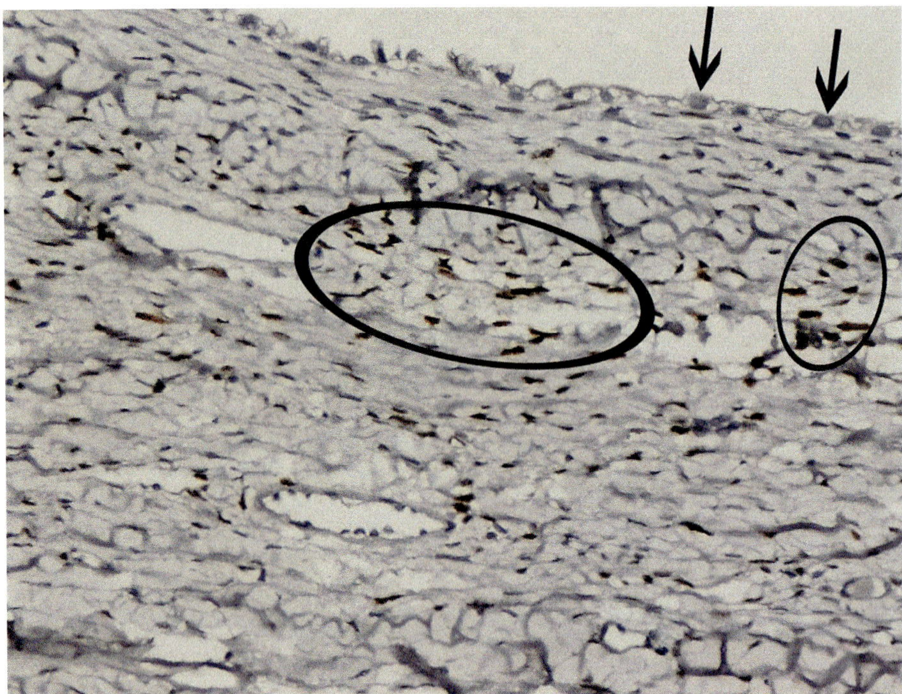

Fig. 1.9 (Immunoperoxidase stain for PR, X 200) Nuclear PR immunoreactivity in the stroma of an adult cystic nephroma (*ellipses*). The simple, here flattened or cuboidal (*arrows*), epithelial lining of the cystic nephroma of the previous figure is noticeable in this magnification. The cellular stroma of a cystic nephroma is reactive to estrogen and progesterone receptors (ER and PR, respectively) and to inhibin.

Other differential diagnostic considerations:

- Tubulocystic RCC, an uncommon malignancy of WHO/ISUP low grade (never higher than grade 3) constitutes a renal epithelial malignancy of indolent behavior, composed of small- to intermediate-sized *tubules* admixed with larger cysts; its cytoplasmic features include abundant, oncocytoma-like aspects.
- Simple renal cysts represent the most common cystic lesion in the kidney. In multiple simple cortical cysts, the cysts are widely separated and do *not* congregate in a single region. These nonneoplastic renal cortical cysts may be multiloculated and are lined with flattened to cuboidal, usually non-clear cells or have no lining at all. In contrast to the multilocular cystic renal neoplasm of low malignant potential, in nonneoplastic multilocular cysts, no clear cell nests are found within septa or within the cyst wall. The presence of clear cells lining the cystic spaces, a feature possibly found in both entities, is not sufficient for an interpretation of neoplasm, and thus it is not a reliable feature to separate a nonneoplastic, multilocular renal cyst from a multilocular cystic renal neoplasm.
- In acquired cystic disease, multiple, *bilateral* cysts are typically located in the cortex, and, as a rule, patients are on dialysis for quite a long time before cysts develop; so, the history of end-stage kidney disease is crucial. The patient's chronic renal failure cannot be attributed to a hereditary cystic disease. In such patients, computed tomography is recommended to periodically evaluate cysts and look for development of suspicious masses.
- In adult (autosomal dominant) polycystic kidney disease, *both* kidneys are markedly enlarged and show numerous, irregularly clustered small cysts in the cortex *and* medulla with *intervening* fibrotic, atrophic renal *parenchyma*. Family history and extrarenal manifestations are often present. A *unilateral* and *segmental* form of cystic disease that histologically resembles dominant polycystic kidney disease but lacks the progression, extrarenal complications, and familial nature, has been reported in the literature

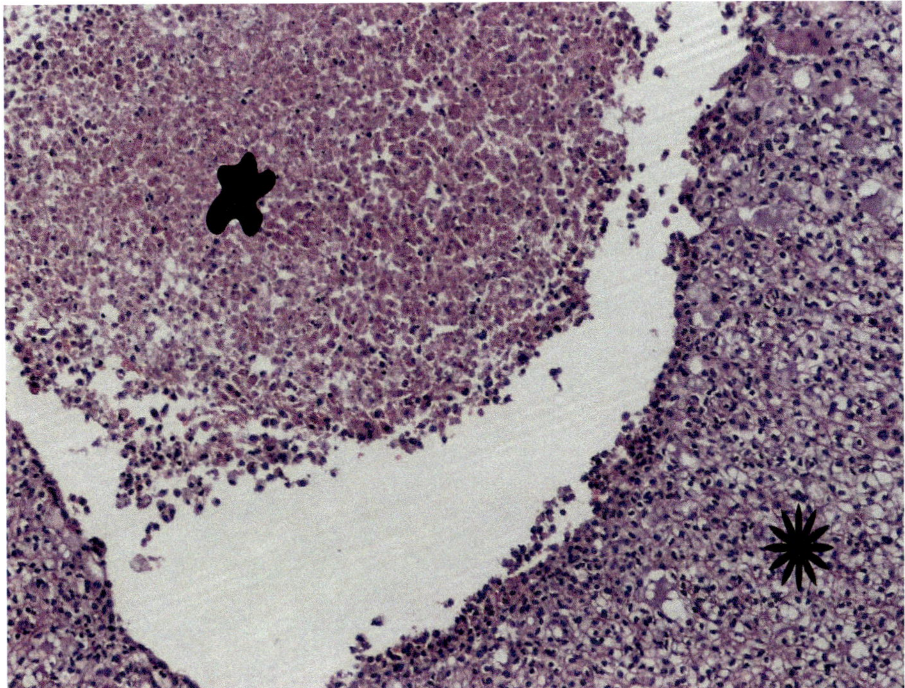

Fig. 1.10 (H-E, ×100) Transition of a sheet of clear cells (*asterisk*) to a necrotic area (*blob*). *Micro*-scopically detected, coagulative tumor necrosis is an ominous prognostic parameter, frequently associated with aggressiveness, and has an independent prognostic significance, especially for *clear cell* RCC (and for chromophobe RCC). In general, "geographical," microscopically detected tumor necrosis accounting for >10% of the total tumor volume is associated with a less favorable outcome

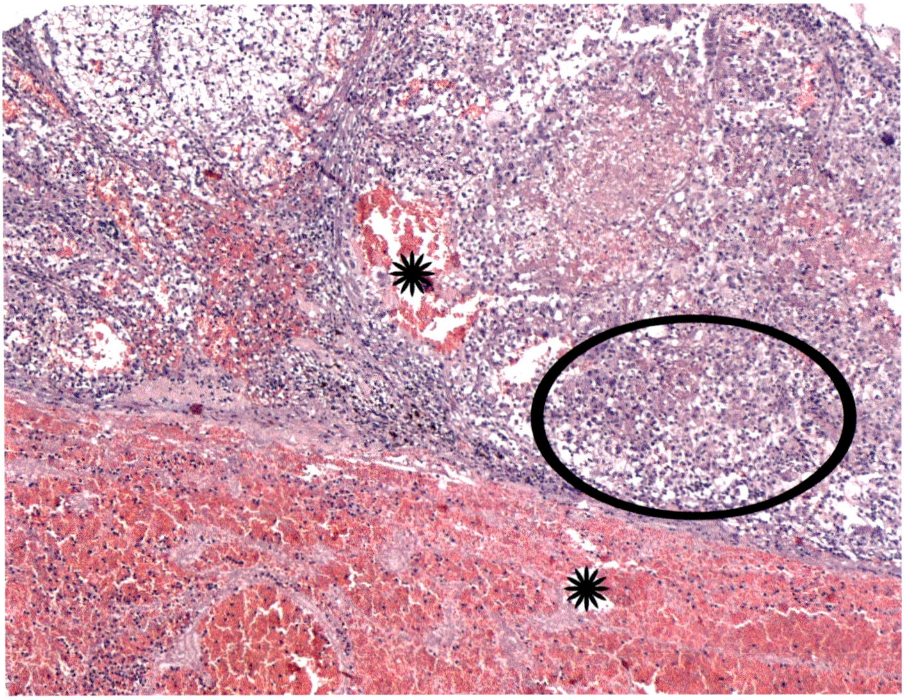

Fig. 1.11 (H-E, ×50) Some cases of clear cell RCC display varying numbers of cells with granular/eosinophilic cytoplasm (*ellipse*); such cells are more often seen in high-grade cancer or near areas of hemorrhage (*asterisks*) or necrosis. Most clear cell RCCs are associated with little or no inflammatory response

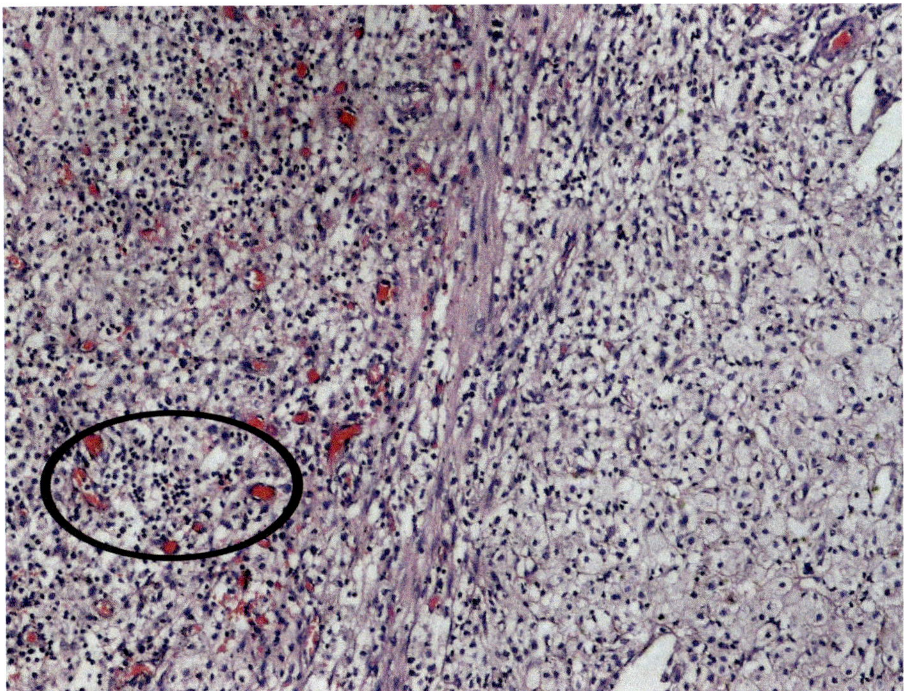

Fig. 1.12 (H-E, ×50) A case of xanthogranulomatous pyelonephritis; the space-occupying mass lesions of this uncommon entity, which mainly affects women in the fourth to sixth decade of life, may clinically, radiologically, and pathologically mimic RCC. The presence of a large calculus and xanthomatous thickening of the pelvis mucosa should suggest the correct diagnosis. A central nidus of necrotic debris and neutrophils is rimmed by foam cells (macrophages/histiocytes) and a fibroblastic response. Note the interstitial accumulation of abundant, lipid-laden foamy macrophages (more evident at the *right part of the image*), resembling clear cell RCC cells, in a background of inflammatory granulation tissue with newly formed, thin-walled vessels and inflammatory cells (*ellipse*). A fibroblastic response is evident in the middle. This fibroblastic response can resemble a spindle cell neoplasm. The bubbly microvesicular fat of the foamy cells contrasts with the cleared-out cytoplasm that is characteristic of clear cell RCC. Intricately branching vascular septations which are prominent in low-grade clear cell RCCs are absent here. Clear cell RCC lacks inflammatory component; in contrast to foamy macrophages, *neoplastic clear cells* are immunohistochemically positive for vimentin (attention to the expression of this particular marker in neoplastic cells themselves), pan-cytokeratin, and CAIX and negative for CD68

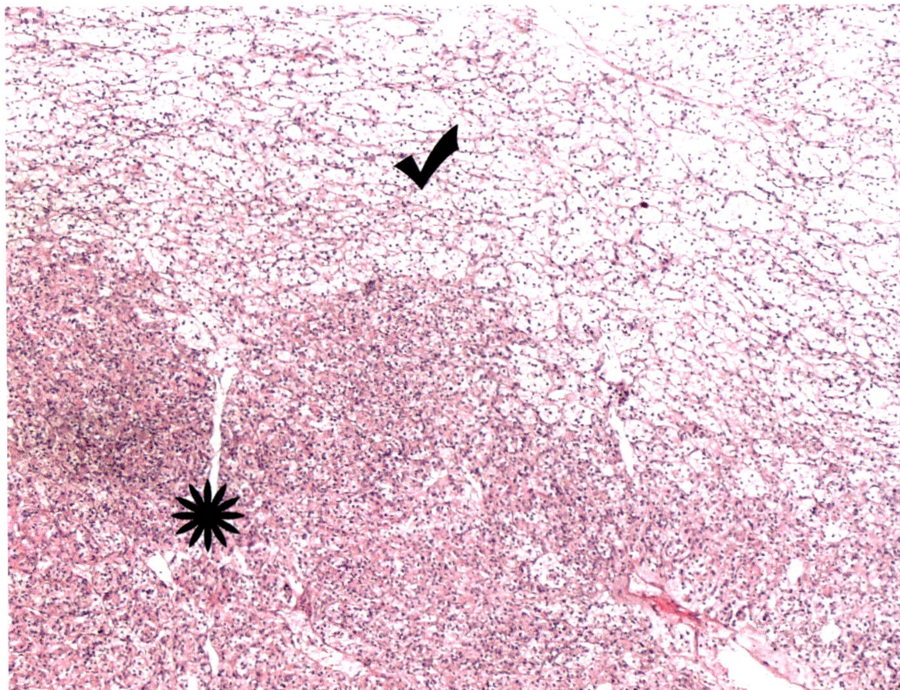

Fig. 1.13 (H-E, ×50) Many clear cell RCCs show a combination of cells with clear (*tick*) and granular/eosinophilic (*asterisk*) cytoplasm, either intimately admixed or as separate discrete foci, the latter, macroscopically, brown in color. This is not a distinct subtype of RCC but belongs to the conventional, "clear cell" subtype.

Clear cell RCC is a morphologically heterogeneous group of malignant neoplasms composed of cells with clear *or* granular/eosinophilic cytoplasm

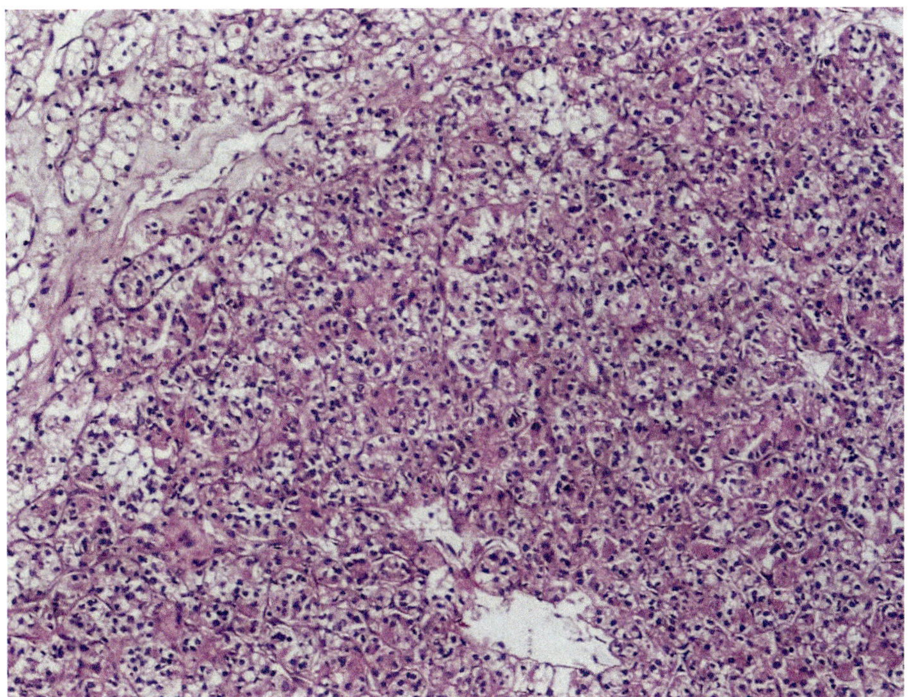

Fig. 1.14 (H-E, ×100) A predominance of granular/eosinophilic cells in this tumor area.
More than 50% granular eosinophilic features may predict poor response to IL-2 therapy. Clear cell RCCs with >40% eosinophilic component may have worse clinical outcome.
In contrast to the eosinophilic variant of chromophobe subtype of RCC, the eosinophilic component of conventional "clear cell" subtype of RCC lacks KIT (CD117) immunoreactivity

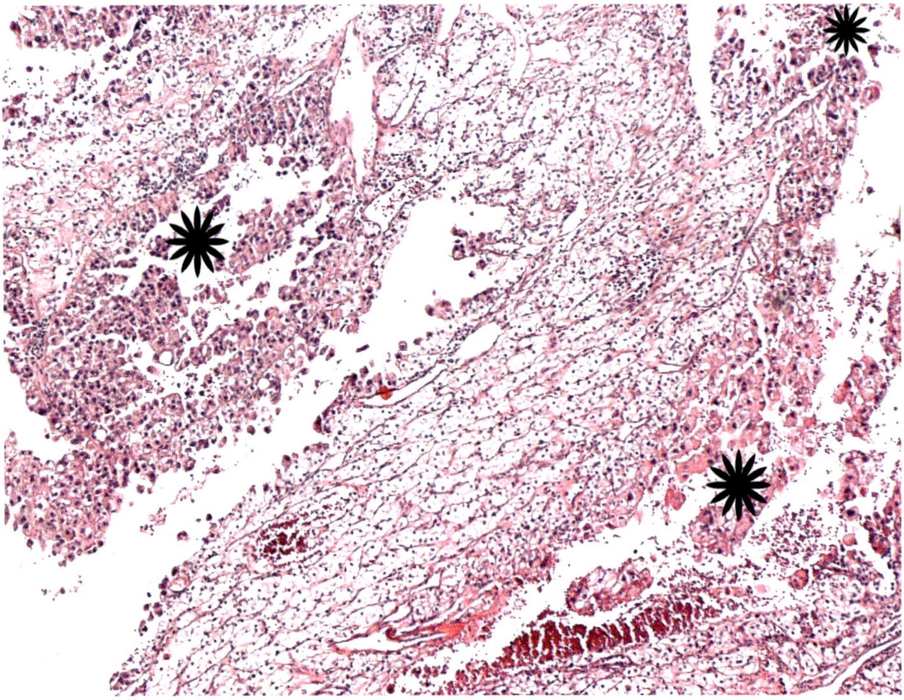

Fig. 1.15 (H-E, ×50) Areas with granular/eosinophilic cytoplasm (*asterisks*) are usually of higher grade. It is the nucleolar/nuclear grade rather than the type of cell cytoplasm that represents the more important prognostic discriminator.

Nucleolar/nuclear grade is assigned according to *highest* grade in tumor, even if focal. Grading should be based on the worst areas, not counting scattered cells

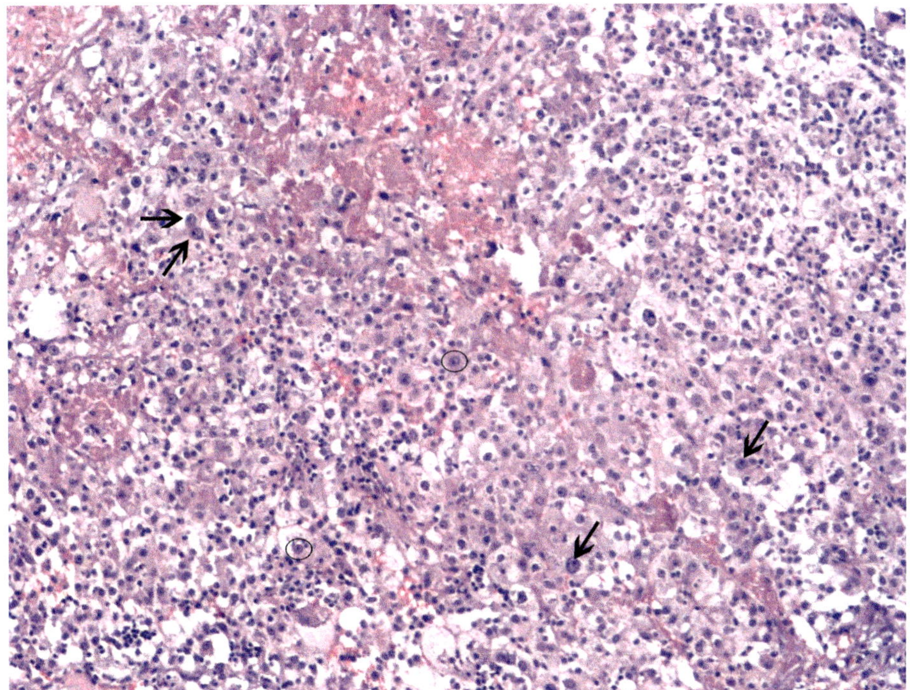

Fig. 1.16 (H-E, ×100) A tumor area composed of cells with granular/eosinophilic cytoplasm and irregular nuclei, at least 20 μm and larger. Nucleoli conspicuous at ×100 magnification (*arrows*) and often eosinophilic (*circles*) indicate a high grade of malignancy (WHO/ISUP grade 3). The typical interconnecting vascular framework of clear cell RCC is not retained in high-grade areas.

For grade 1–3 tumors, the World Health Organization/International Society of Urological Pathology (WHO/ISUP) grading system is based on *nucleolar* prominence (also see Figs. 1.4 and 1.5) (Moch et al. 2016)

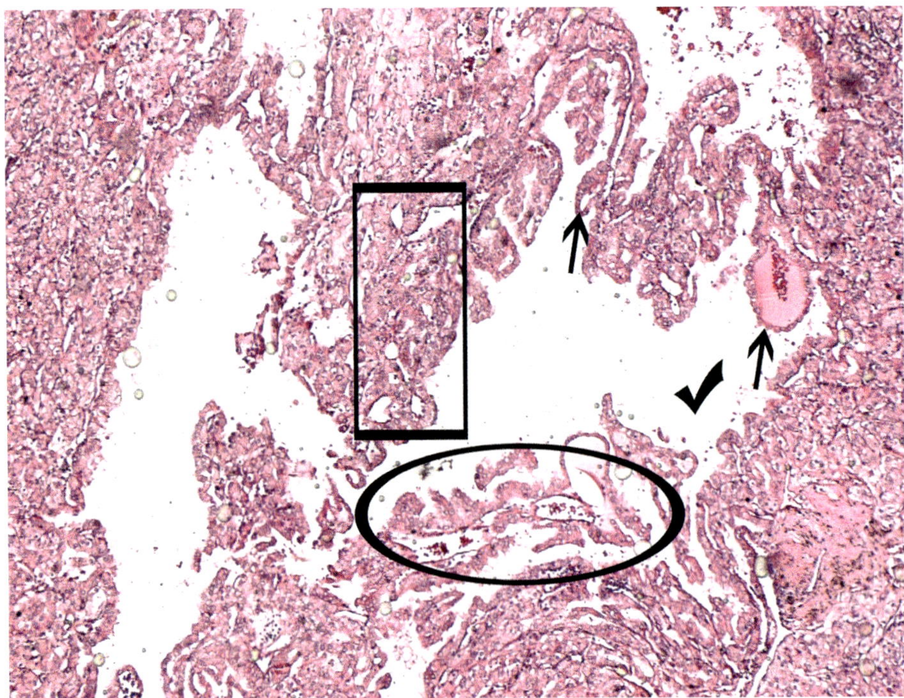

Fig. 1.17 (H-E, ×50) A pseudopapillary (*ellipse*) and tubular (*square frame*) pattern of tumor cell growth is possible in clear cell RCCs. Granular cell cytology is noted throughout this area. Tumor cell dropout sparing the cells at the periphery of blood vessels (*arrows*) and pseudopapillary architecture with lack of fibrovascular cores at the papillary-like structures (*ellipse*) can be observed in clear cell RCC. Papillary and papillary-like structures extend into the cystic area (*tick*). Papillary structures should be small and account for an insignificant proportion of the overall architecture of a clear cell RCC. Focal true papillations are rare in clear cell RCC; when prominent, the possibility of alternative diagnoses including translocation-associated, clear cell papillary, papillary, or unclassified RCC should be considered.

Unclassified RCCs include, among others, those with a combination of features of more than one recognized subtypes.

Unlike papillary RCC, histiocytes and intracellular hemosiderin are usually absent from the rare papillae of a clear cell RCC, and classical clear cell foci are usually evident elsewhere.

Furthermore, we should remember that clear cell cytology may not be present in all cases of clear cell RCC. The term "conventional" RCC had previously been proposed as a synonym for granular/eosinophilic variant of "clear cell" RCC subtype; the latter, however, should currently be reported as mere "clear cell RCC"

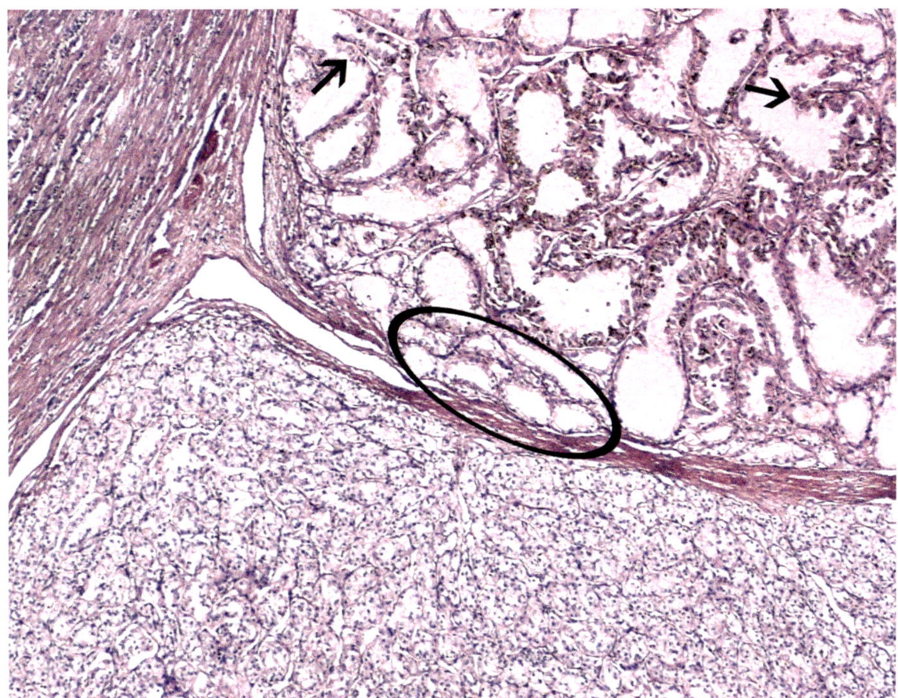

Fig. 1.18 (H-E, ×50) A diverse combination of growth patterns is often identified in clear cell RCCs when multiple sections from any given tumor are examined. The typical tumor component with the alveolar nests (lower image half) is neighboring a tubulopapillary tumor component (upper image half, *arrows* and *ellipse* for papillary and tubular patterns, respectively).

As previously mentioned, histologic features that would fit into more than one RCC subtype (e.g., separate areas of clear cell RCC and of papillary RCC) might lead to a diagnosis of an unclassified subtype of RCC

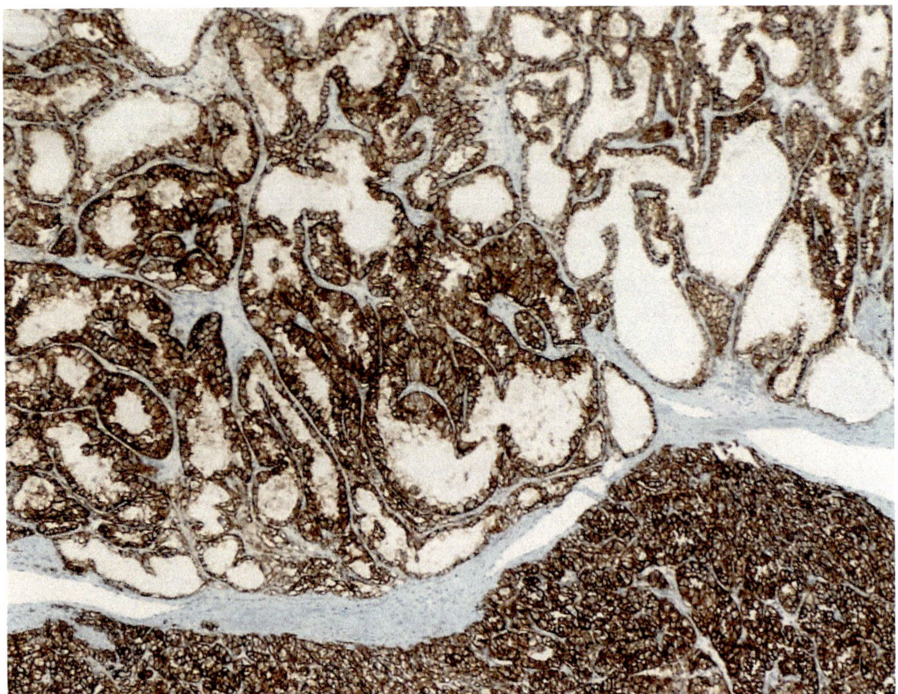

Fig. 1.19 (Immunoperoxidase stain for CAIX, ×50). *Both* tumor components of the previous image (i.e., the alveolar and the tubulopapillary one) diffusely overexpress carbonic anhydrase IX (CAIX) in the cytoplasm and on the membranes of tumor cells, by means of immunohistochemistry; this complete cytoplasmic membrane CAIX staining pattern confirms that this is a (pure) clear cell RCC.

Diffuse membrane-predominant immunostaining for CAIX is present in up to 100% of clear cell RCCs; nevertheless, high-grade clear cell RCCs may exhibit reduced CAIX immunoexpression.

In papillary RCCs, CAIX is negative to focally perinecrotic/papillary tip-positive.

CAIX is also negative in chromophobe RCCs which, like clear cell RCC, may exhibit two cell populations (eosinophilic and clear cells), with characteristic nuclear features, though.

In addition to CAIX, clear cell RCC is immunopositive for CD10 (a proximal tubule membranous marker), vimentin (more intensely positive in high-grade areas), RCC antigen (cytoplasmic/membranous immunomarker which, however, may be positive in other renal tumor types and nonrenal neoplasms), EMA, and pancytokeratin. Cytokeratin 7 expression is rare and limited in clear cell RCCs.

PAX8 is the more useful indicator to confirm the diagnosis especially of metastatic clear cell RCC and other renal epithelial neoplasms

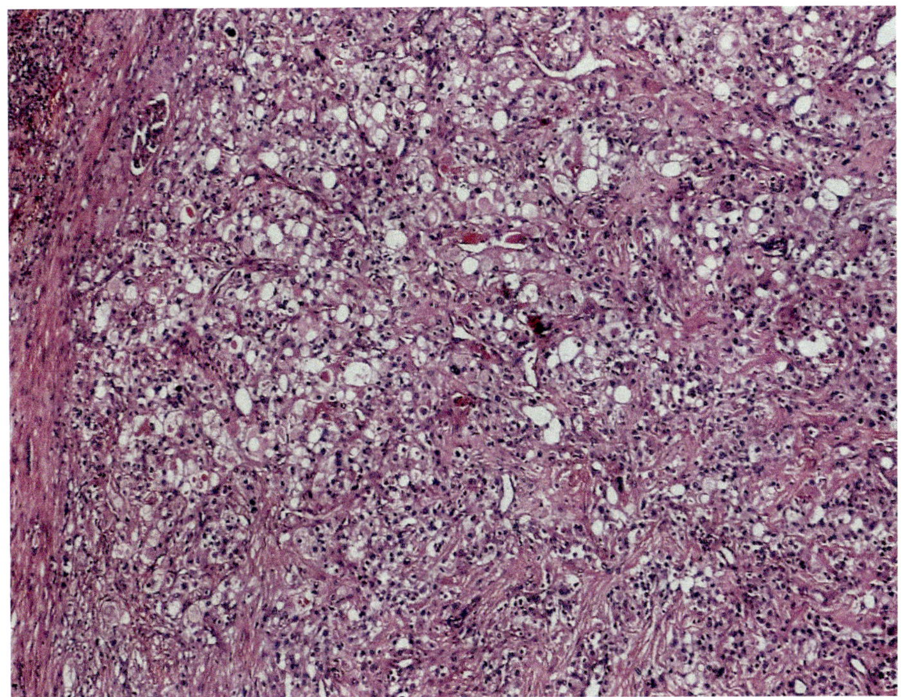

Fig. 1.20 (H-E, ×100) A high-grade tumor area with clear and granular/eosinophilic cells which warrants closer inspection

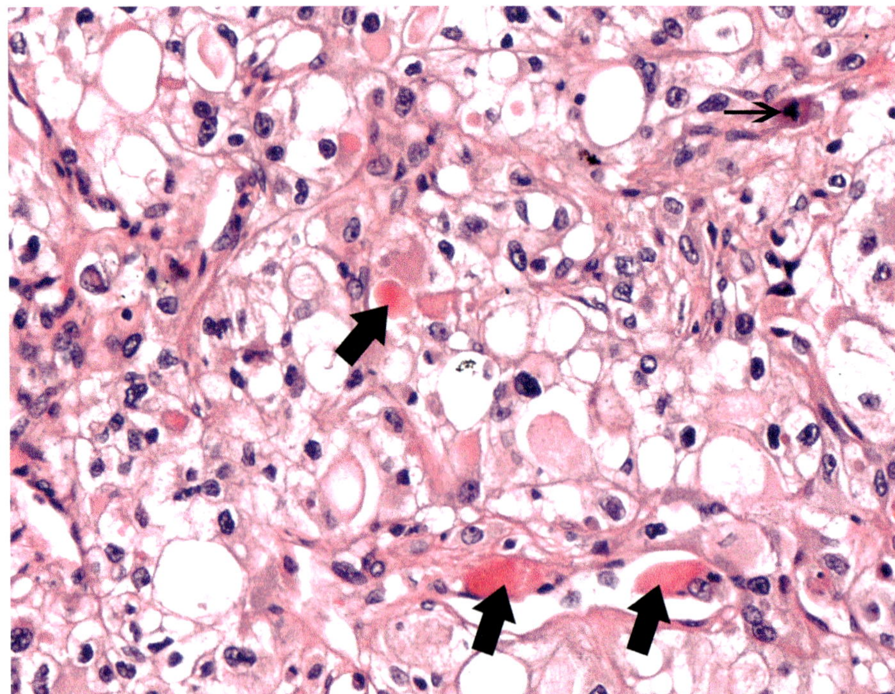

Fig. 1.21 (H-E, ×200) Irregular, high-grade nuclei, mitotic activity (*thin arrow*) and focal rhabdoid cytology (*thick arrows*) in this tumor area. Discohesive rhabdoid cells with densely acidophilic, globular cytoplasm (*thick arrows*), not to be confused with rhabdoid tumors of the kidney. Similarly to coexistent conventional clear cell component, rhabdoid cells of RCC express CAIX and EMA, coexpress cytokeratin and vimentin, and are negative for desmin and smooth muscle actin.

RCC with rhabdoid dedifferentiation has increased risk of death (hazard ratio 5.25) when compared with RCC without rhabdoid dedifferentiation, independent of non-rhabdoid component grade, tumor stage, and presence of necrosis (Przybycin et al. 2014). Approximately 25% of tumors with a rhabdoid morphology also have a sarcomatoid component

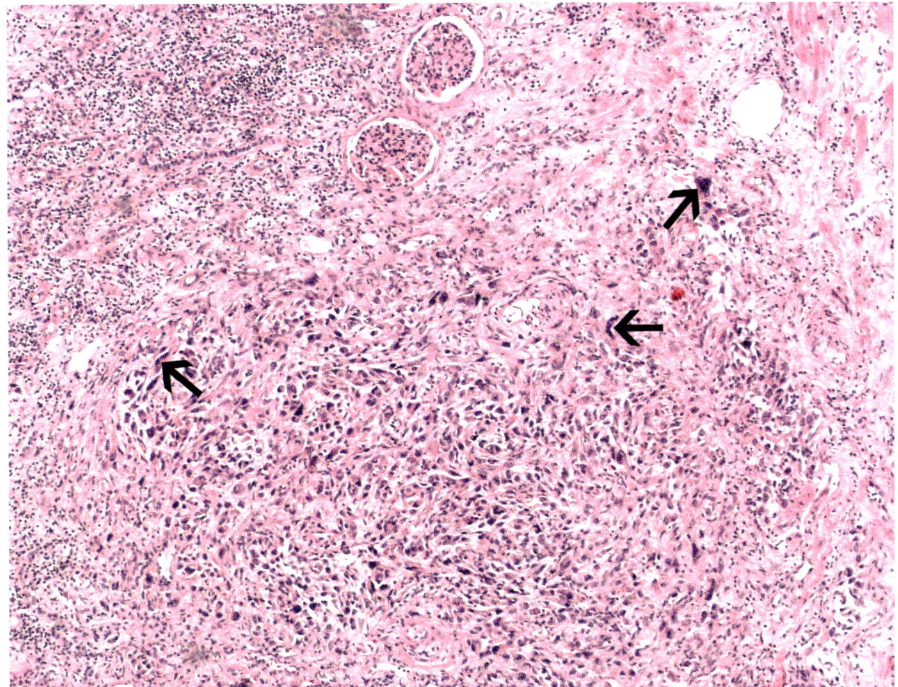

Fig. 1.22 (H-E, ×50) Sarcomatoid morphology with whorled bundles of spindle cells with bizarre and multilobulated, high-grade nuclei (*arrows*), associated with the clear cell RCC presented in the previous images. This is an area of sarcomatoid dedifferentiation of the clear cell RCC, reported herein.

Sarcomatoid and rhabdoid dedifferentiation have higher rates of tumor recurrence and metastasis and should be reported when observed within a RCC parenchyma. Even a focal sarcomatoid component is associated with a poorer prognosis; generous sampling is therefore needed. The area of sarcomatoid histology required for diagnosis of a sarcomatoid component usually comprises at least one low-power field; there is, however, no minimum percentage required for the diagnosis of a sarcomatoid component. The greater the proportion of the sarcomatoid component, the worse the prognosis.

Pure sarcomatoid morphology *without* elsewhere identifiable epithelial RCC component (not the present case) places this high-grade tumor to the *unclassified subtype of RCCs*; in such cases, the sarcomatoid component has probably overgrown the original antecedent element to such a degree that the latter becomes unrecognizable. Most purely spindle cell malignant renal neoplasms are sarcomatoid unclassified RCCs rather than purely mesenchymal tumors, i.e., sarcomas. Sarcomas of the kidney are rare; in order to be diagnosed, no epithelial component after careful sampling should be detected either by morphology or by immunohistochemistry. Immunohistochemistry is necessary for sarcomas' distinction from sarcomatoid, unclassified RCCs; the latter are expected to express CAIX, Pax8, RCC marker, and CD10. Sarcomatoid RCC is not recognized as a distinct histologic subtype, but the common pathway of transformation of all different subtypes of renal cell carcinoma, probably of the clear cell, and, perhaps more often, of the chromophobe subtype of RCC; therefore, the latter subtypes, if identifiable, should constitute the main histologic diagnosis. In order that sarcomatoid unclassified carcinomas are reported as such, there should be no morphologically identifiable epithelial element of a recognized RCC subtype; the diagnosis is based on immunohistochemical evidence of renal epithelial derivation

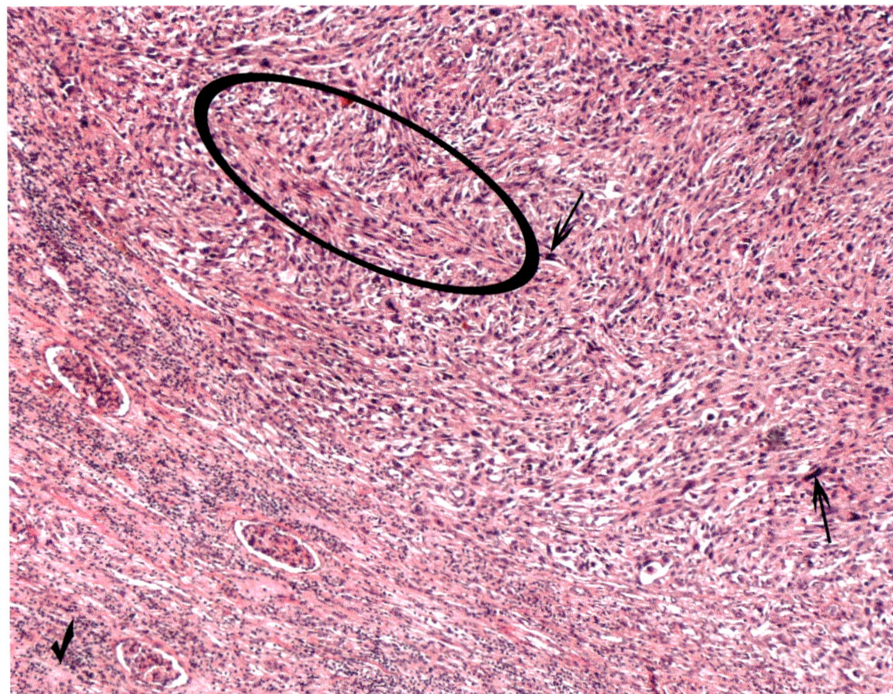

Fig. 1.23 (H-E, ×50) Interlacing bundles of malignant spindle cells (*ellipse*) with marked nuclear pleomorphism and hyperchromasia (*arrows*), corresponding to the macroscopically recognized tannish-gray areas. Lymphocytic aggregates in tumor- adjacent kidney cortex (*tick*). RCCs with sarcomatoid areas are assigned grade 4 (i.e., the highest grade of malignancy). WHO/ISUP grade 4 is defined by the presence of pronounced nuclear pleomorphism, tumor giant cells, and/or rhabdoid and/or sarcomatoid dedifferentiation. So, the reported clear cell RCC finally belongs to the grade 4 group, due to its sarcomatoid component.

WHO/ISUP four-tier grading system has been validated as an indicator of prognosis for clear cell RCC and papillary RCC

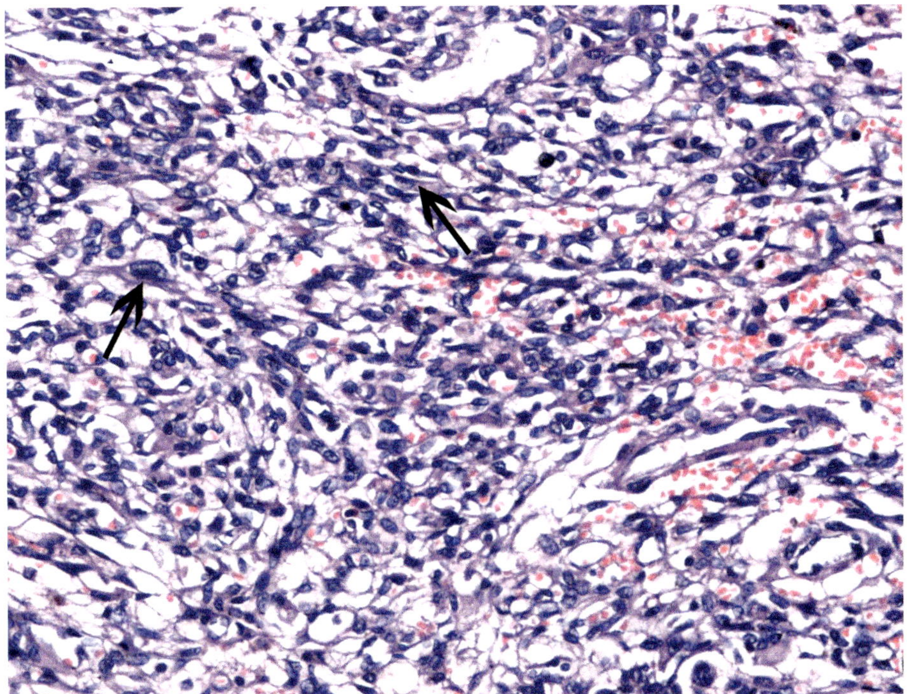

Fig. 1.24 (H-E, ×200) Sarcomatoid dedifferentiation of the clear cell RCC, here in the form of spindle tumor cells (*arrows*) simulating a malignant fibro/histiocytic lesion. Renal histogenesis can be immunohistochemically supported by expression of PAX8, CAIX, RCC marker, and CD10

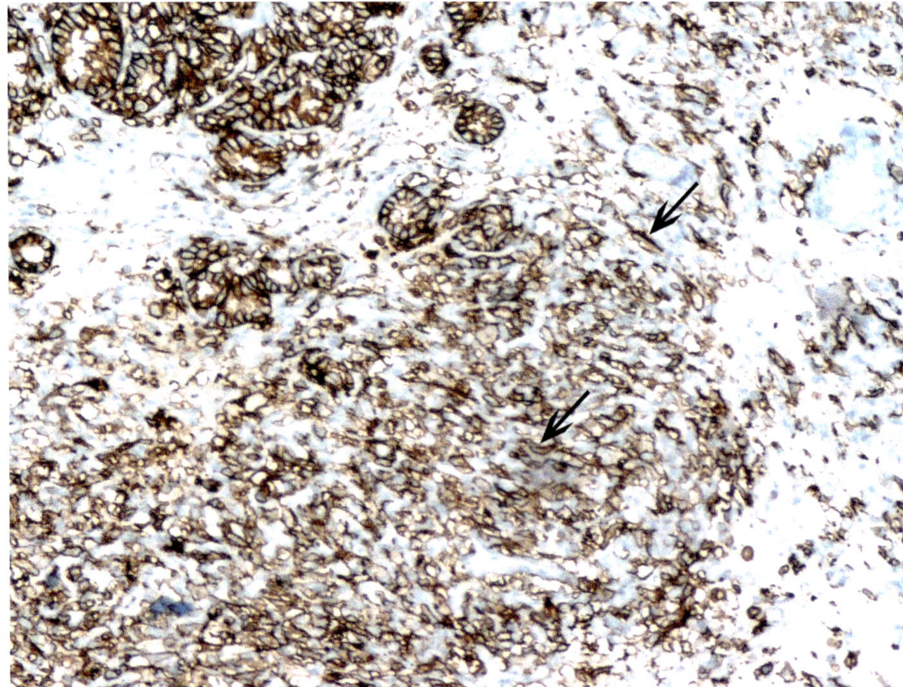

Fig. 1.25 (Immunoperoxidase stain for CAIX, ×100) Unlike most other clear cell RCC antibodies, CAIX is often positive with a diffuse, membranous pattern even in high-grade and sarcomatoid areas of clear cell RCCs (*arrows*); some reduction in CAIX staining may be expected in high-grade tumors

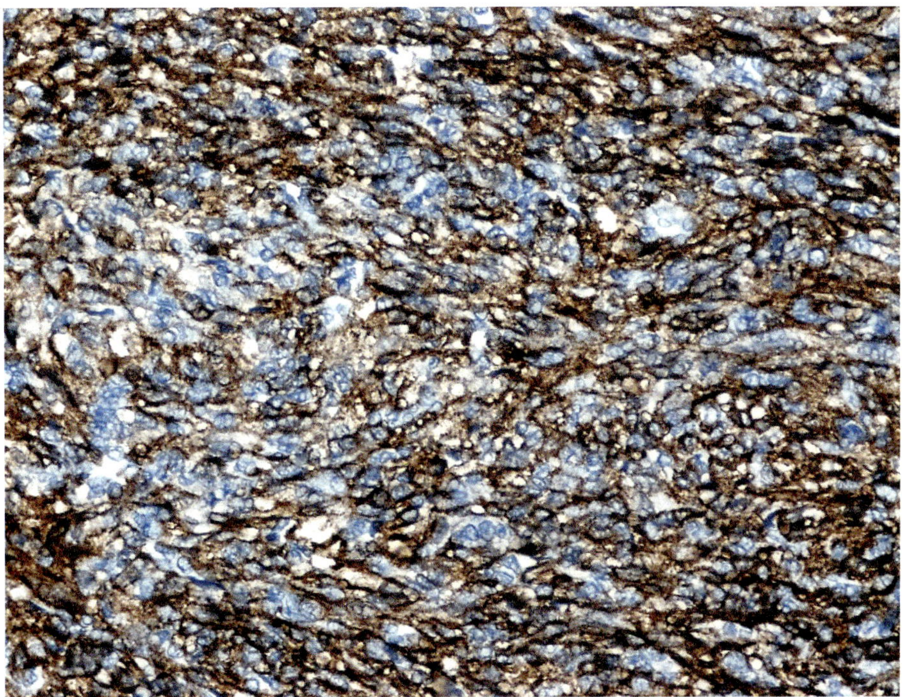

Fig. 1.26 (Immunoperoxidase stain for CD10, ×200) Retained membranous CD10 immunoreactivity of sarcomatoid cells. CD10 positivity may, however, become weaker in high-grade areas of clear cell RCCs

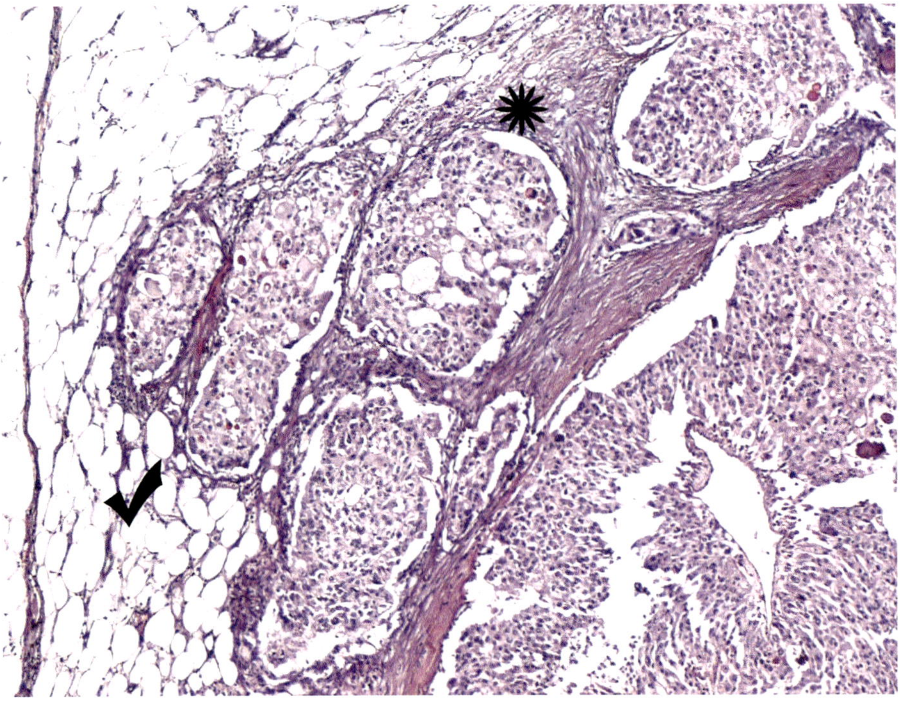

Fig. 1.27 (H-E, ×50) As RCCs enlarge, perinephric fat (*tick*) may become effaced by tumor, and tumor cell collections may appear encapsulated by reactive, desmoplastic fibrous tissue (*asterisk*). This RCC shows multiple extensions into the extrarenal fat compatible with perinephric fat invasion (pT3a). Perinephric fat invasion is defined as follows: either the tumor directly touches the fat or extends as irregular tongues into the perinephric tissue, with or without desmoplasia

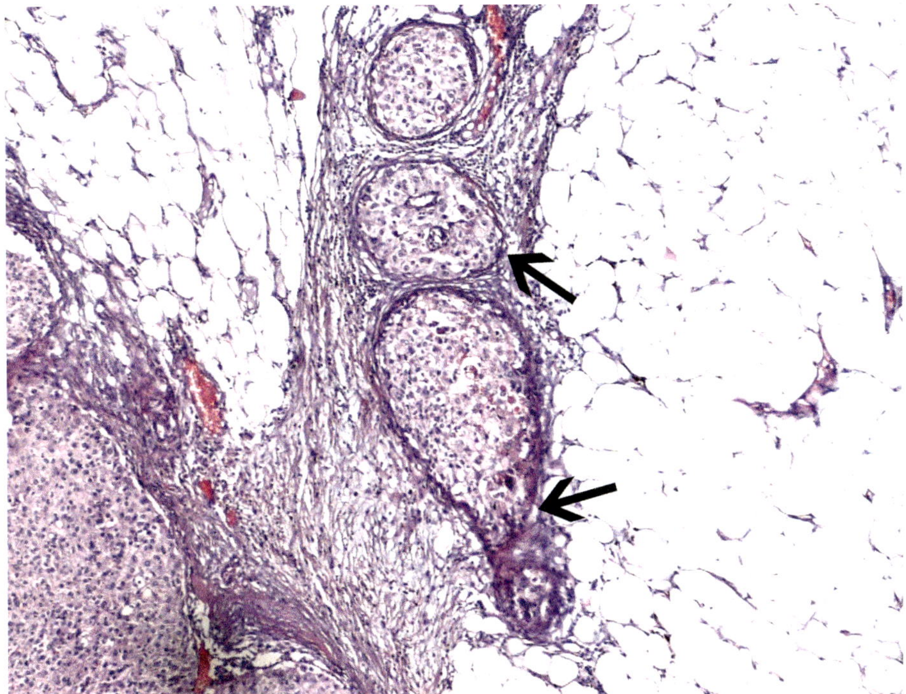

Fig. 1.28 (H-E, ×50) RCC extracapsular/perinephric fat invasion (pT3a) is defined as either tumor irregular satellite extensions (evident here, *arrows*) or extensions with incomplete pseudocapsules or single cells invading fat

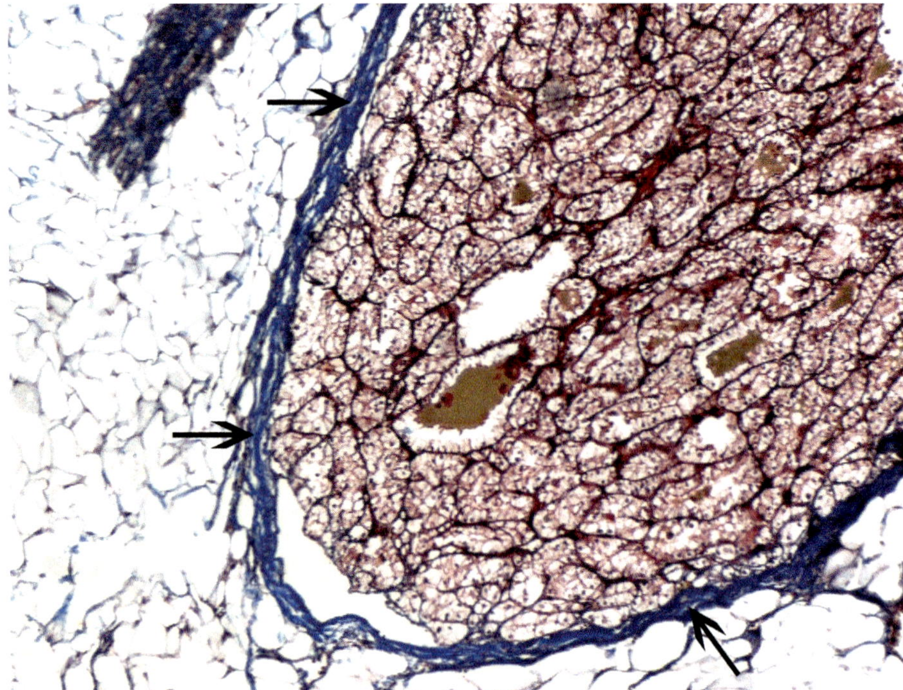

Fig. 1.29 (Trichrome Masson, ×50) Clear cell RCCs are typically globular tumors protruding from the renal cortex. This *solitary*, exophytic RCC component *smoothly* protrudes into extrarenal fat and is capped by well-defined smooth continuous fibrous capsule (*arrows*); this should *not* be regarded as pT3a

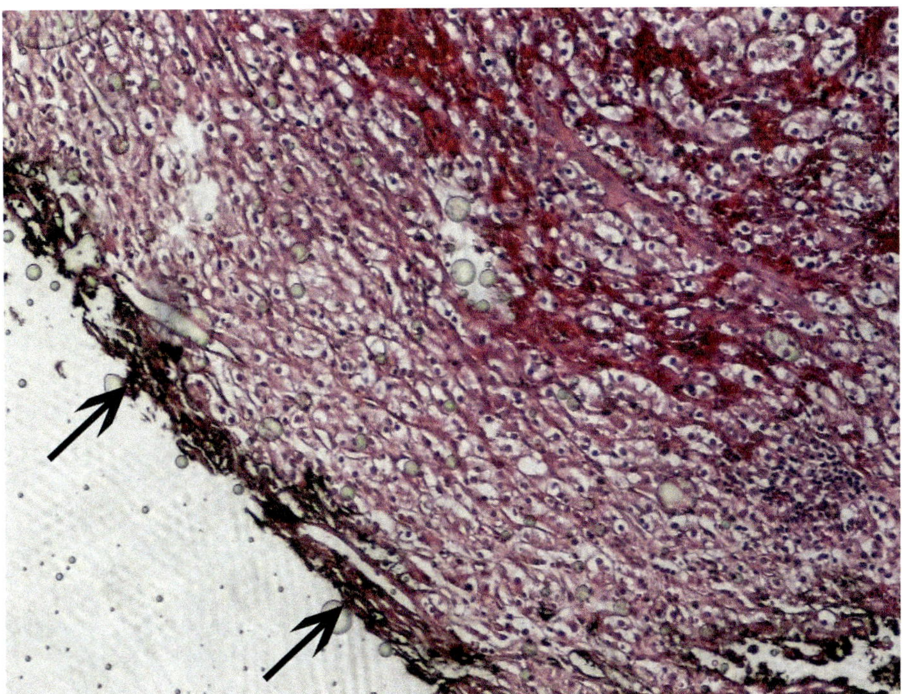

Fig. 1.30 (H-E, ×100) Another case of clear cell RCC. Intraoperative frozen section evaluation may be asked in order to determine whether the tumor is a renal cortical neoplasm or a urothelial carcinoma of pelvicalyceal system or in order to evaluate surgical margins. Positive "frozen section" margins, particularly in partial nephrectomies, often lead to additional surgical resection for cortical tumors. Inking of parenchymal resection margin (*arrows*) is a must in the evaluation of the surgical resection margin.

Surgeons typically remove the kidney along with its Gerota fascia. In case the above image corresponds to the perinephric adipose tissue surgical margin, invasion beyond Gerota fascia is detected and the tumor is staged as pT4 (distant spread). Microscopically, Gerota fascia does not have any distinctive features, other than ill-defined, somewhat compressed connective tissue. pT4 category also includes *direct* extension into the adrenal gland (hematogenous spread within the adrenal gland is staged as pM1)

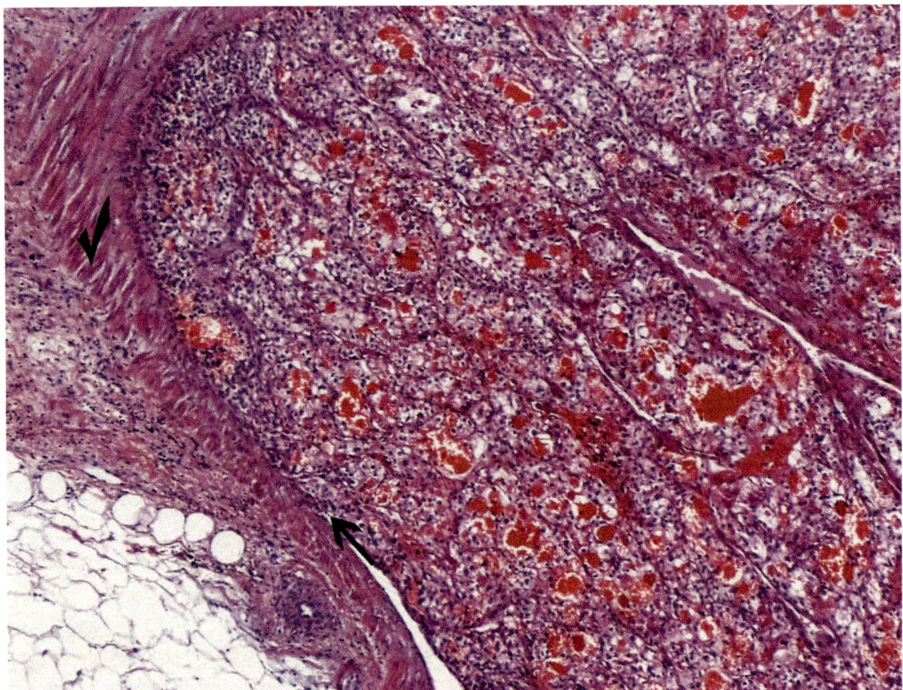

Fig. 1.31 (H-E, ×50) Renal sinus constitutes extrarenal soft tissue lateral to imaginary vertical line joining medial aspects of upper and lower renal poles. Unlike that in the rest of the organ, the kidney lacks a renal capsule in its sinus. Invasion of sinus fat (based on criteria similar to those of perinephric fat invasion) or invasion of sinus muscle-containing veins (*tick*) may occur around the pelvis or deep within the portion of sinus-surrounding calyces. Invasion of either muscle-containing or non muscle-containing branches of renal vein in renal sinus and main renal vein invasion are both defined as of the same pT stage (i.e., pT3a). Apparent attachment of the tumor to the intima (*arrow*) or tumor filling and stretching the vascular lumen is equivalent to vein invasion.

Renal sinus invasion is defined as follows:

- When the tumor is in direct contact with the sinus fat (direct tumor extension into fat)
- Extends to the loose connective tissue of the sinus, clearly beyond the renal parenchyma
- Involves any endothelium-lined space within the renal sinus and either penetrates through its wall or not

In all the above cases, pT3a is assigned. Meticulous examination of at least two to three blocks from tumor-renal sinus interface reveals sinus fat or vein invasion in the vast majority of tumors exceeding 7 cm in diameter. Regional spread of RCC (pT3, according to 2010 TNM staging system) is recognized as major prognostic factor

1.2.1.1 Clinical Commentary

Vasileios Spapis

This is a case of a high-grade clear cell RCC with regional spread. Focal cystic change, necrotic activity, a considerable proportion of granular/eosinophilic tumor cells, and presence of rhabdoid cells and of a sarcomatoid component were microscopically noted.

Clear cell RCC is the most common subtype of RCC, accounting for more than 70% of all RCCs (Rini et al. 2009; Campbell and Lane 2012). Clear cell RCCs are highly vascular tumors, typically yellow in color. Two to five percent of clear cell RCCs demonstrate sarcomatoid features. However, sarcomatoid changes can be found in all RCC subtypes and are always equivalent to high-grade, highly aggressive tumors (Campbell and Lane 2012). Moreover, clear cell RCCS are very likely to demonstrate venous tumor extension which is another risk factor for poor patients' prognosis. In all RCC subtypes, prognosis worsens with stage and histopathological grade (the latter wherever applicable, of course). Clear cell RCCs have a worse prognosis when compared to chromophobe and papillary RCCs (Ljungberg 2016). It should be mentioned though that of the responders to immunotherapy, the majority is diagnosed with clear cell RCC (Campbell and Lane 2012). There is also an indolent variant of clear cell RCC, multilocular cystic neoplasm of low malignant potential, which accounts for about 4% of all clear cell RCCs and has excellent prognosis (Ljungberg 2016).

Due to their location in the retroperitoneum, all renal masses can remain unsymptomatic for a long time. About 50% of them are diagnosed incidentally (Novara et al. 2010; Sheth et al. 2001; Jayson and Sanders 1998). Extensive use of the ultrasound (US) contributed to the early diagnosis of renal tumors, even the ones smaller than 2 cm. Another factor that contributes to early diagnosis is the screening of populations with specific characteristics such as patients with end-stage renal disease, patients with von Hippel-Lindau syndrome or tuberous sclerosis. Further investigation of suspicious lesions usually includes CT scanning (Ljungberg 2016). Symptoms, when they exist, are caused by local tumor growth, hemorrhage, paraneoplastic syndromes (hypertension, anemia, cachexia, pyrexia, etc.), or metastatic disease.

Treatment for RCC is primarily surgical. During the last 20 years, nephron sparing surgery (NSS) is the treatment of choice for all T1 tumors. For T2 RCCs (tumor diameter > 7 cm) though, radical nephrectomy (RN) remains the most popular solution. Adrenalectomy is not recommended unless there is evidence of invasion of the adrenal gland (Ljungberg 2016 and Van Poppel H 2011). The presence of venous tumor thrombus in the renal vein and the muscle-containing branches of renal vein in renal sinus is a significant adverse prognostic factor and classifies the tumor as T3a.

When it comes to metastatic disease, the last decade is the era of the targeted therapies in RCC. Most published trials have selected clear cell RCC subtype; thus, no robust evidence-based recommendations can be given for non-clear cell RCC subtypes. Tyrosine kinase inhibitors (TKIs), anti-VEGF antibodies, and mTor inhibitors are agents in use today (Ljungberg 2016). When sarcomatoid changes are present, multimodal approaches should be considered based on the extremely poor prognosis with surgery alone. Selected reports demonstrated modestly improved response rates in patients receiving IL-2-based immunotherapy, chemotherapy, or targeted molecular therapy after surgery (Rini et al. 2009).

Key Messages

- Clear cell cytology is not absolutely necessary for the diagnosis of a clear cell RCC. Some clear cell RCCs have predominately or even exclusively granular cytoplasmic acidophilia.
- Presence of brisk inflammatory infiltrate intimately admixed with sheets of clear cells should raise possibility of xanthogranulomatous pyelonephritis over clear cell RCC.
- When necrotic activity is microscopically noticed in a clear cell RCC, its amount should be reported as a percentage of the total tumor volume.
- Renal sinus fat or extrarenal fat invasion are both defined as pT3a. Invasion of segmental branches of renal vein in renal sinus and main renal vein invasion are both also defined as pT3a.

1.3 Case 1.2 Papillary Renal Cell Carcinoma

Case Study

Data Prior to Microscopy

A 60-year-old man with spontaneous hemorrhage of a kidney tumor with no prior symptoms.

A well-circumscribed tumor, 6.4 cm in diameter, eccentrically situated within the renal cortex, with a prominent pseudocapsule, dark brown in color due to intratumoral hemorrhage and friable consistency.

Apart from the main tumor mass, a much smaller (8 mm in diameter), wedge-shaped, yellow-gray lesion, with its base at the cortical surface, was noticed.

1.3.1 Microscopic Evaluation of the Total Nephrectomy Specimen

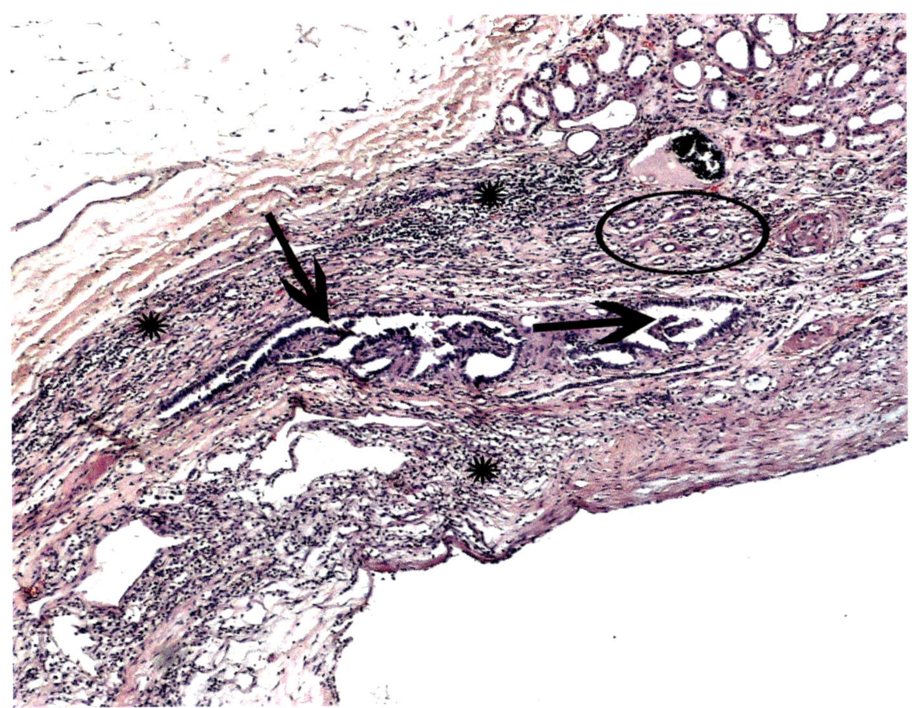

Fig. 1.32 (H-E, ×50) Focal tubular hyperplasia with papillary projections extending into lumen of tubular space (*arrows*), incidentally found within the renal cortex, away from the main tumor. Chronic inflammatory (*asterisks*) and tubular atrophic (*ellipse*) changes at the renal cortex are evident

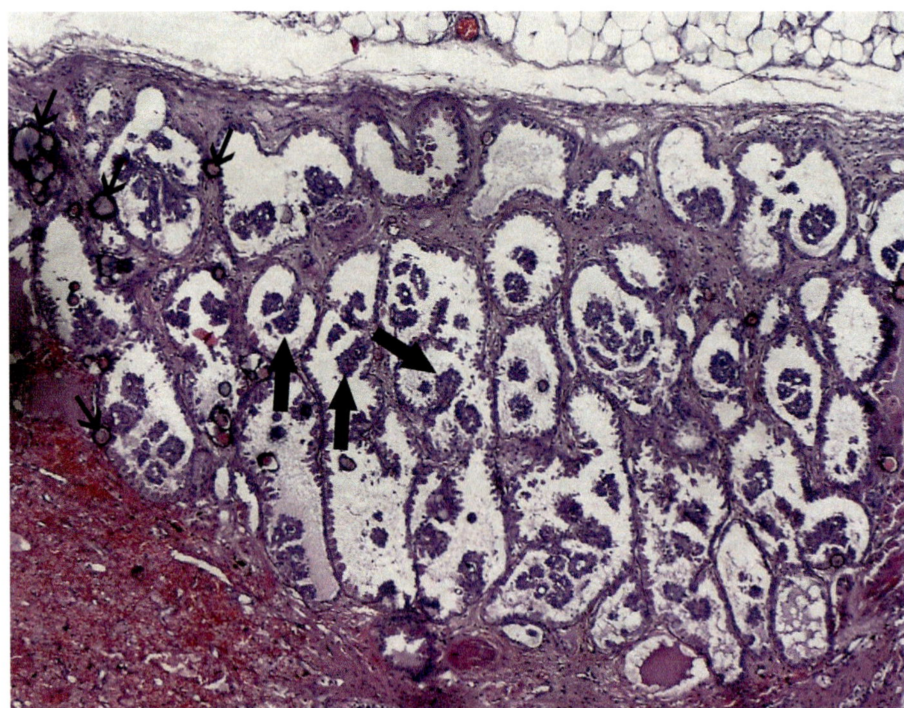

Fig. 1.33 (H-E, ×50) Papillary adenoma of the kidney is the most common tumor of renal tubular epithelium. A subcapsular papillary adenoma, macroscopically noticed as a small lesion away from the main tumor mass, and bearing a striking resemblance to tubular epithelial hyperplasia. *Papillary adenomas* are defined as unencapsulated tumors of the renal cortex with papillary or tubular architecture of *low* WHO/ISUP *grade* and a diameter of *less than 15 mm* (Moch et al. 2016). Papillary architecture (*thick arrows*), psammoma bodies (*thin arrows*), scanty cytoplasm of low-grade, regular cuboidal neoplastic cells. No areas of clear cell differentiation. Mitotic figures are absent or very rare. Pushing, noninfiltrative border. Papillary adenomas are more common in kidneys bearing papillary renal cell carcinomas (RCCs).

In instances of multiple and/or bilateral papillary renal cell tumors, hereditary papillary RCC-associated syndromes should be considered

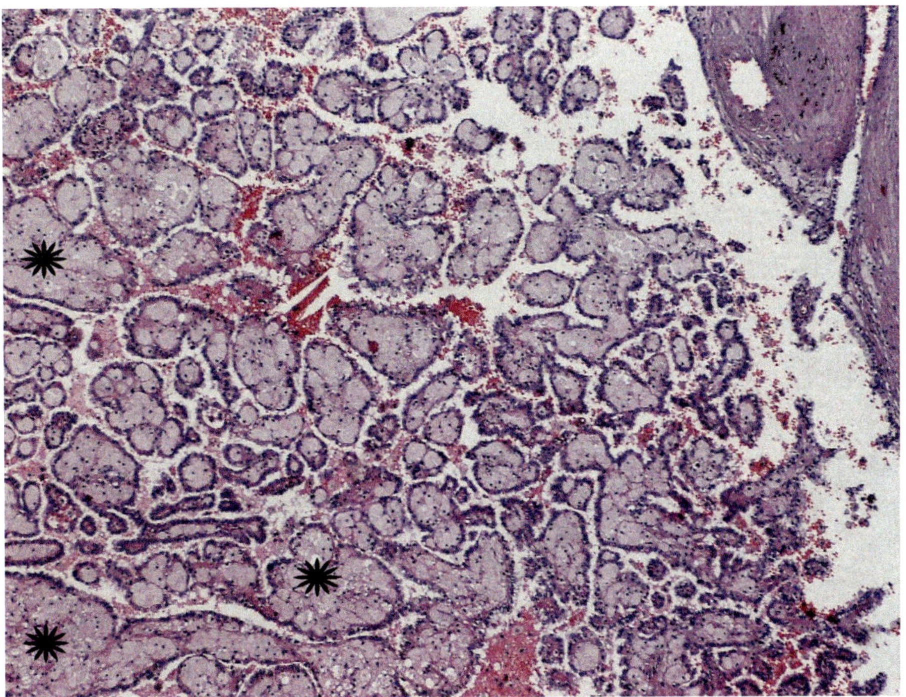

Fig. 1.34 (H-E, ×50) The main tumor mass of the resected kidney, easily identified as a papillary RCC due to discrete papillary fronds. Papillae formed by true fibrovascular cores containing foamy macrophages (*asterisks*). Collections of foamy, lipid-laden macrophages *expanding papillary cores* are characteristic for *papillary* RCC. Predominant areas of foam cells *in the interstitium* may raise concern for a *clear cell* RCC

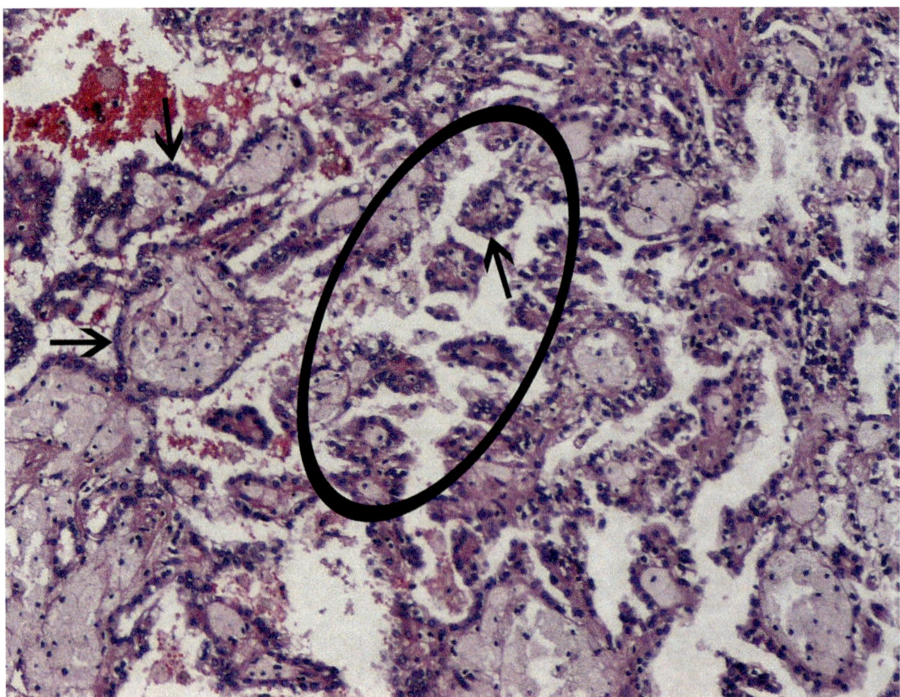

Fig. 1.35 (H-E, ×100) Delicate fibrovascular cores (*ellipse*). Papillae in type 1 papillary RCCs are covered by columnar/cuboidal cells with amphophilic or pale, finely granular, often scanty cytoplasm, usually low-grade nuclei, with longitudinal nuclear grooves, lying at the basal aspect, in a *single* layer on the papillary cores (*arrows*). These cells often look blue due to their scant basophilic cytoplasm and hyperchromatic nuclei

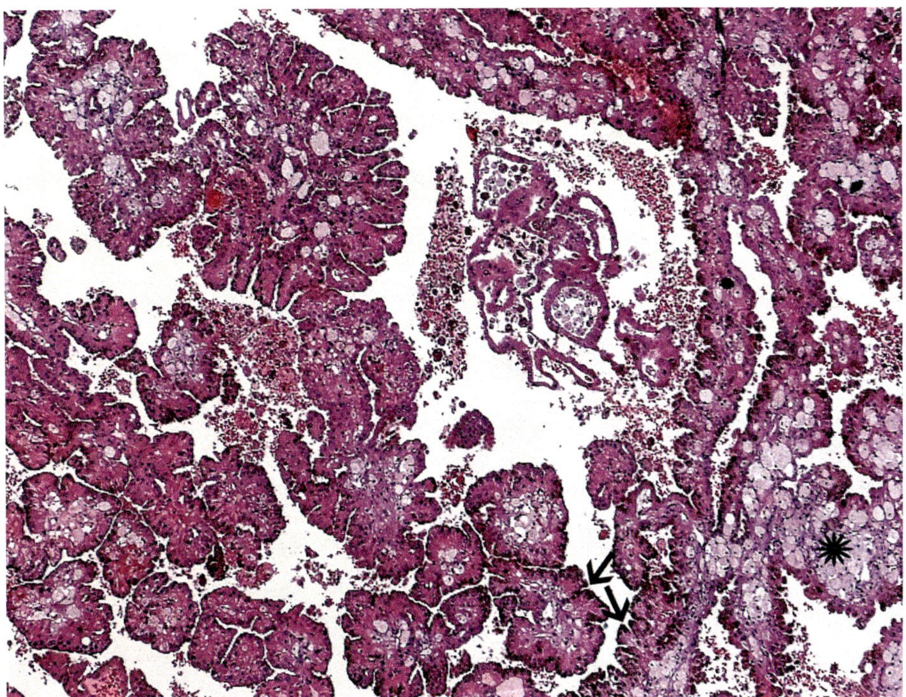

Fig. 1.36 (H-E, ×50) Identification of true fibrovascular cores is the key to the diagnosis of a papillary RCC, because other subtypes of RCC may contain "pseudopapillary" areas. Foamy macrophages expand the fibrovascular cores (*asterisk*). Intracellular hemosiderin, as indicated here (*arrows*), also favors the diagnosis of papillary RCC

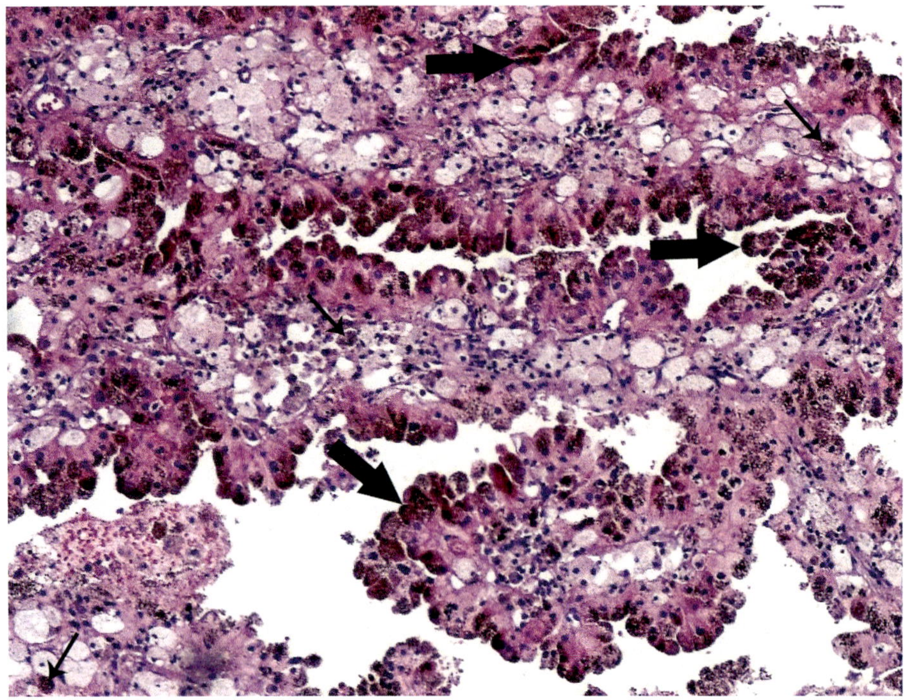

Fig. 1.37 (H-E, ×100) Hemosiderin granules (*thick arrows*) are frequently present in tumor cell cytoplasm, particularly in type 1 papillary RCCs, and also in macrophages (*thin arrows*). The connective tissue stalks show the presence of large numbers of lipid-laden macrophages (xanthoma or foam cells)

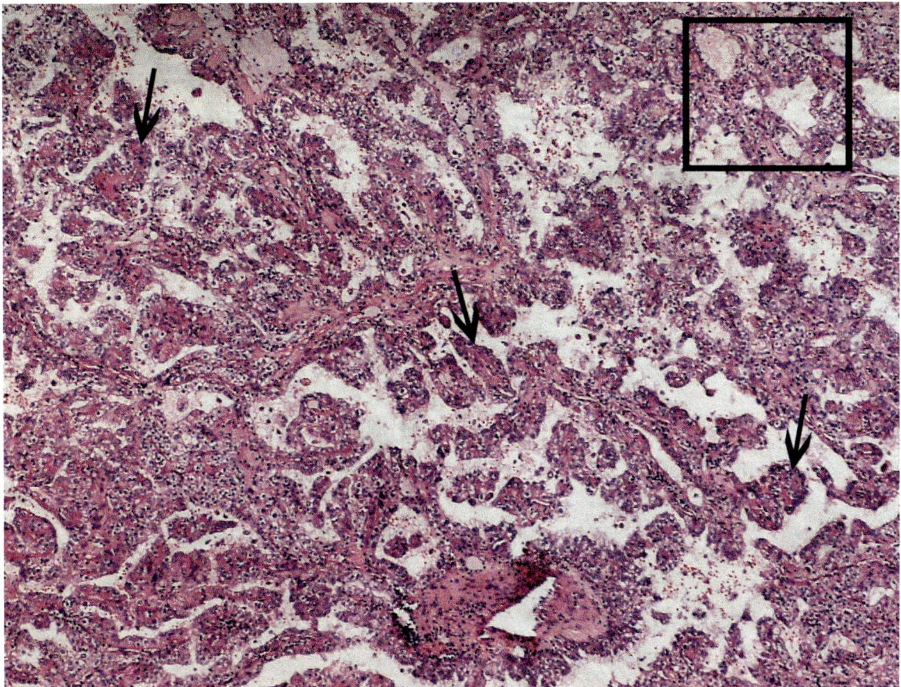

Fig. 1.38 (H-E, ×50) A papillary RCC has papillary or tubulopapillary architecture [tubular structures (*square frame*), papillae (*arrows*)]. Because papillary structures are also seen in collecting duct carcinoma, and as papillary RCC can exhibit extensive tubule formation and even solid areas, the term "papillary" is neither specific for, nor entirely descriptive of this neoplasm

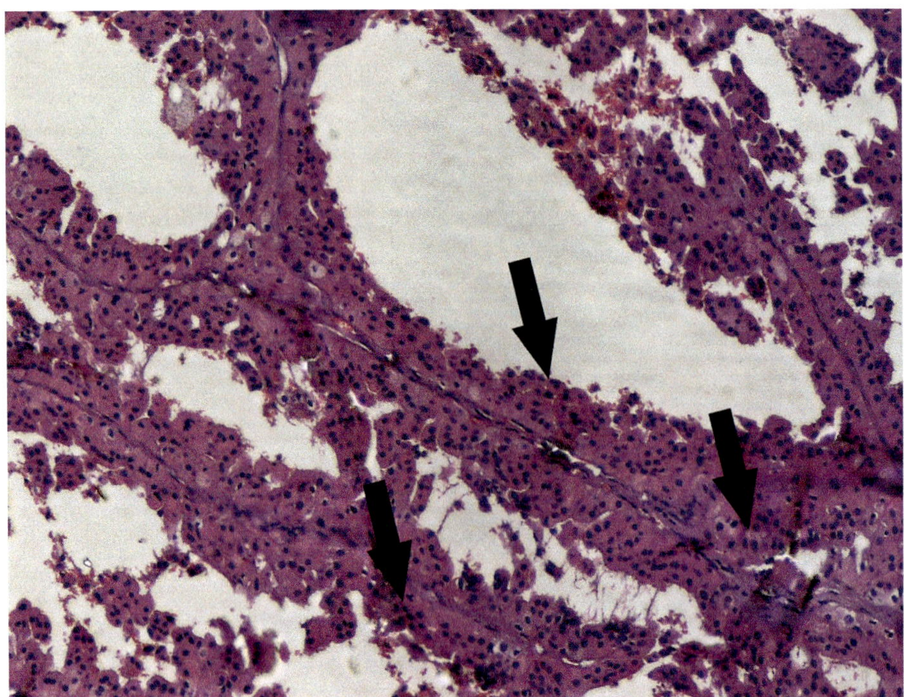

Fig. 1.39 (H-E, ×100) Type 2 papillary RCCs characteristically exhibit nuclear pseudostratification (*arrows*) in the single layers covering the papillae; cells are larger and contain abundant, eosinophilic cytoplasm. Type 2 papillary RCC usually shows a paucity of foamy macrophages.

Type 1 and type 2 histology can coexist in a papillary RCC; their distinction is of prognostic significance. Tumor classification should be based on the predominant component. The WHO/ISUP nucleolar/nuclear grading system appears to stratify papillary RCC; type 2 papillary RCCs tend to be of higher grade with a relevant effect on their prognosis. With regard to the above tumor, it exhibits nuclear features typical of type 1 but cytoplasmic features typical of type 2. Biological behavior is based on nuclear/nucleolar grade

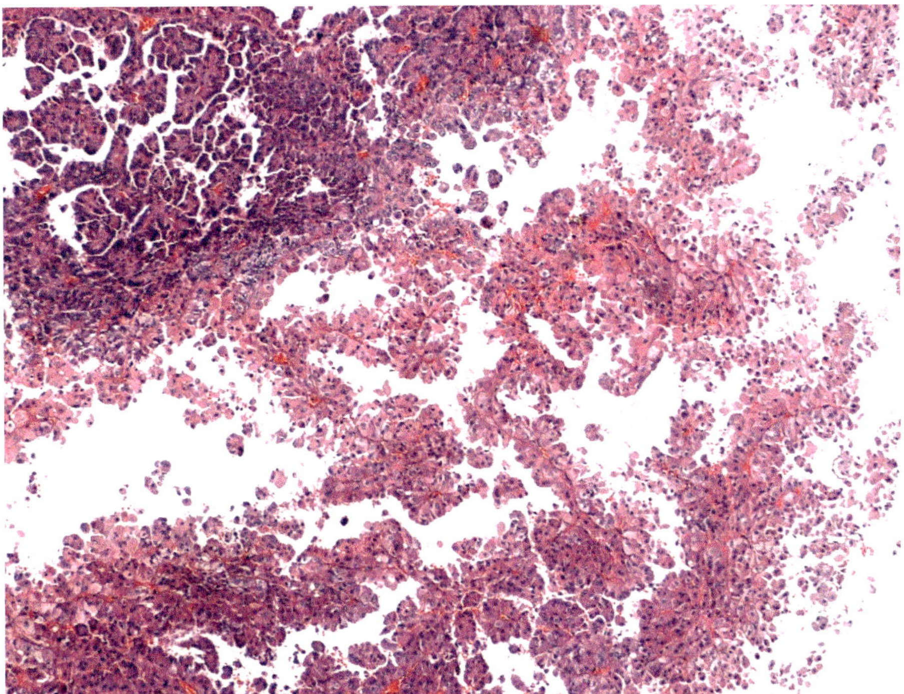

Fig. 1.40 (H-E, ×50) In type 2 papillary RCC category, an oncocytic variant has been described. More abundant, in comparison to type 1, the typically eosinophilic cytoplasm of type 2 area (*upper left part*) transits to even more abundant, voluminous, oncocyte-type cytoplasm (*remaining part of the image*)

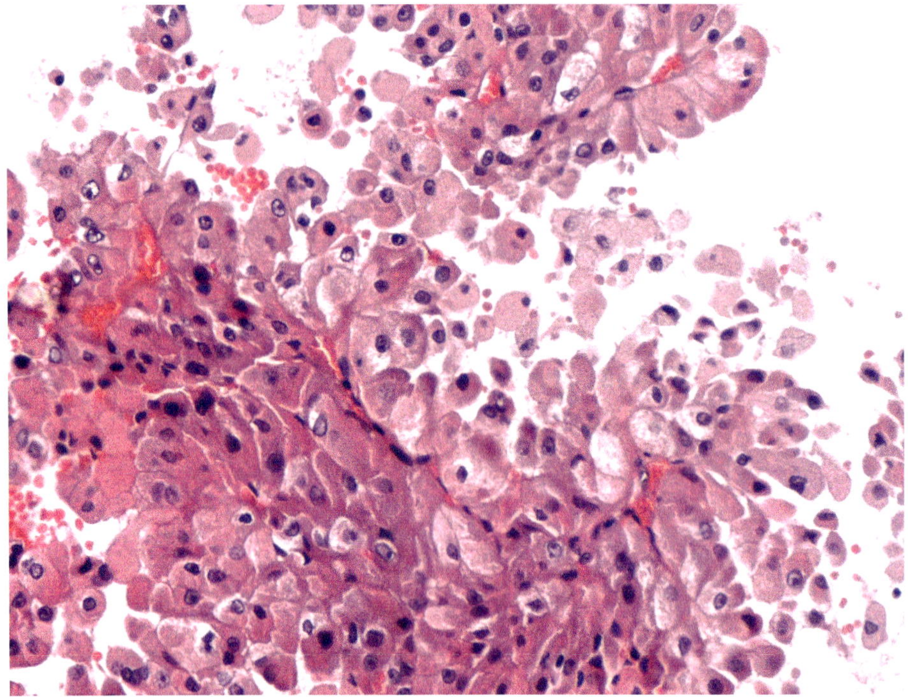

Fig. 1.41 (H-E, ×200) Oncocytic papillary RCC. Voluminous, finely granular, evenly distributed eosinophilic cytoplasm and oncocytoma-like, *non*overlapping nuclei. These tumors show CK7 immunopositivity and biological behavior similar to type 1 papillary RCC, the latter particularly when the nuclei are of low WHO/ISUP grade

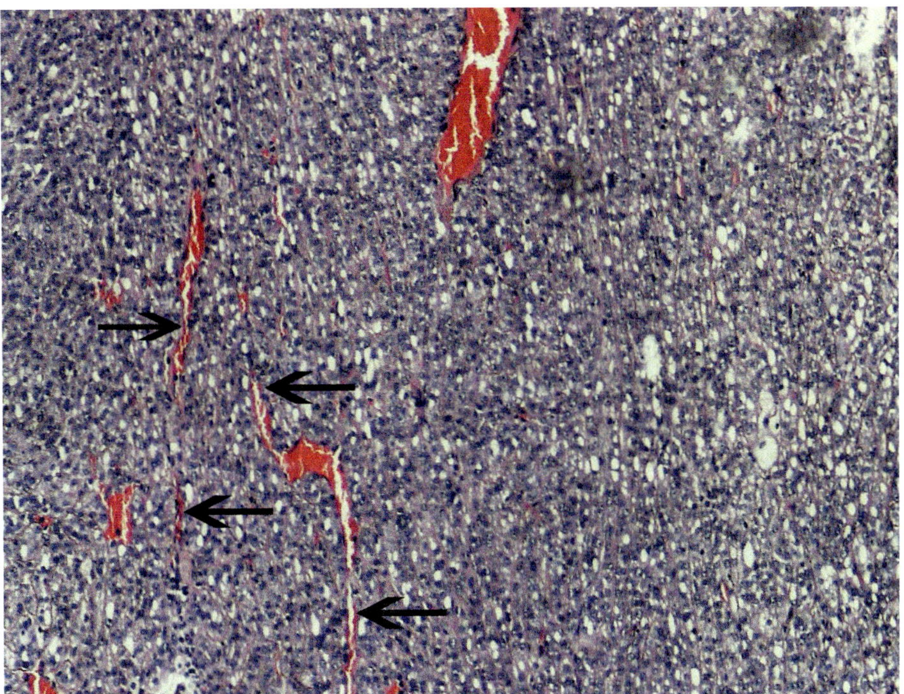

Fig. 1.42 (H-E, ×100) Tightly packed, compact papillae imparting a solid tumor appearance. The compressed vessels (*arrows*) probably correspond to compressed fibrovascular stalks/cores of the papillae. Less than 50% of the tumor parenchyma exhibits true papillae, but, otherwise, these tumors are similar to classic papillary RCCs

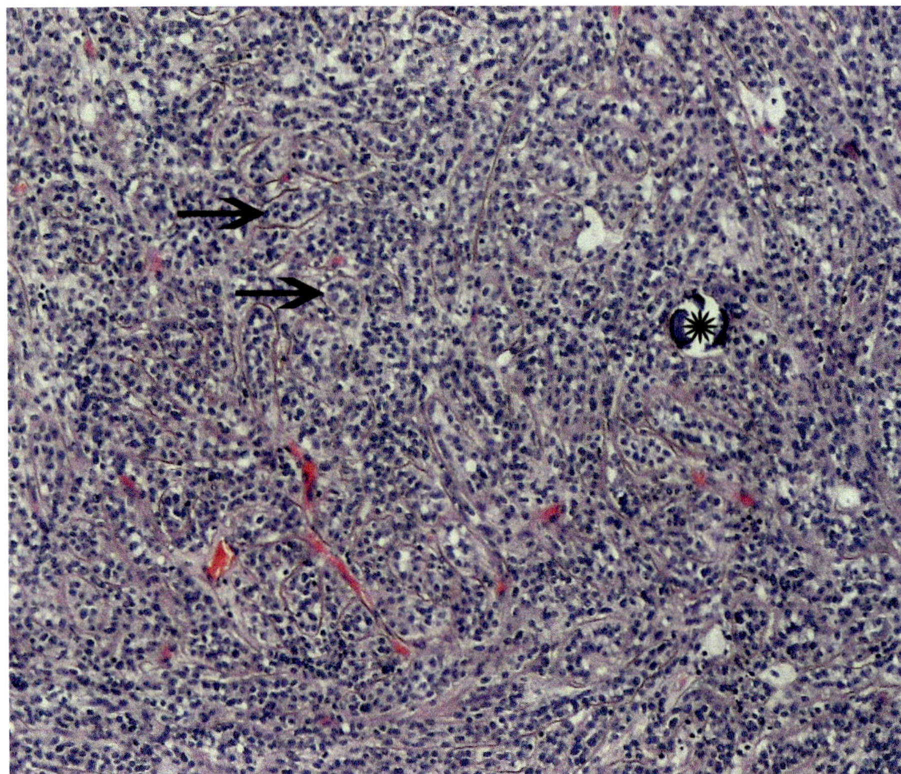

Fig. 1.43 (H-E, ×100) Collapse of the papillae and tubules; solid sheets of cells. Distinct micronodules (*arrows*) resembling abortive papillae. Many of the tubules represent cross-sectional profiles of papillae. Psammomatous calcification (*asterisk*) is common in papillary RCC.

Papillae may be arranged in long parallel arrays, creating a trabecular appearance

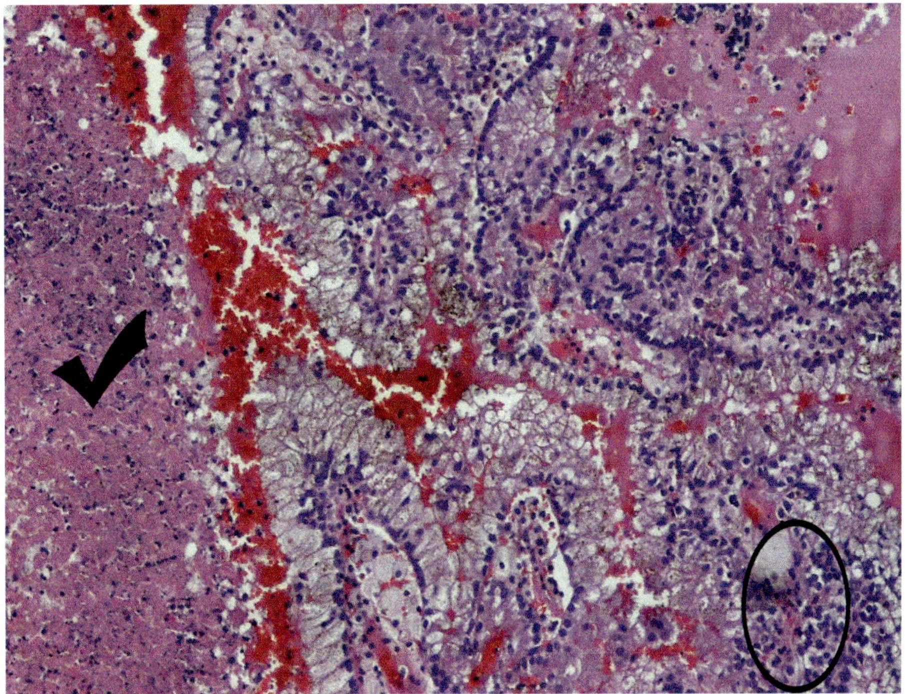

Fig. 1.44 (H-E, ×200) Papillary RCCs tend to undergo a much greater degree of necrosis (*tick*) than is usually seen in RCCs but have a better prognosis, probably because they tend to spread more slowly. Tumor-associated acute and chronic inflammation can also be observed (*ellipse*). Clear-appearing cells often contain finely granular hemosiderin (*image center*)

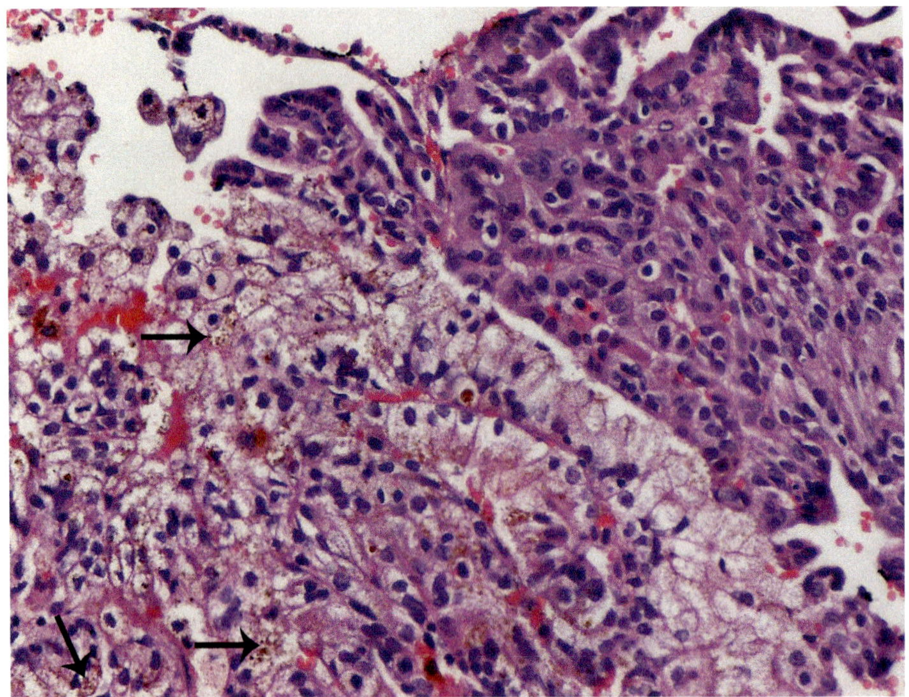

Fig. 1.45 (H-E, ×200) Focally clear cell areas may be present in papillary RCCs; clear-appearing cells usually exhibit variable granularity and often fine hemosiderin (*arrows*). Clear cell carcinoma is much less likely to exhibit cytoplasmic hemosiderin than papillary RCC (the same is true with regard to calcification)

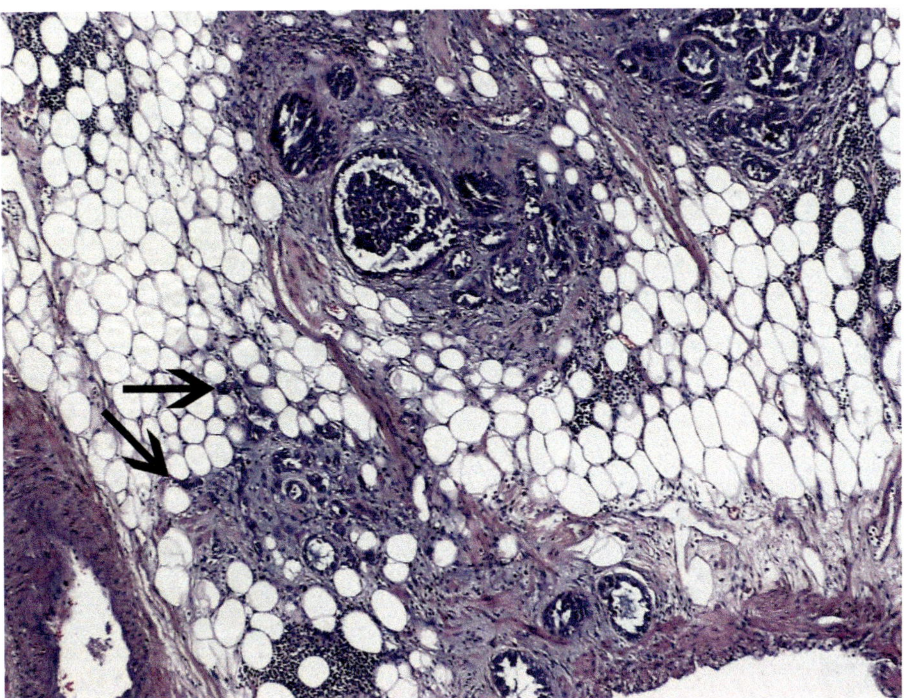

Fig. 1.46 (H-E, ×50) Another papillary RCC with retroperitoneal spread after perirenal fat infiltration, evident here (*arrows*).

Like clear cell RCCs, papillary RCCs also show vascular spread and, more commonly than the former, lymphatic spread to the nodes of the renal hilum

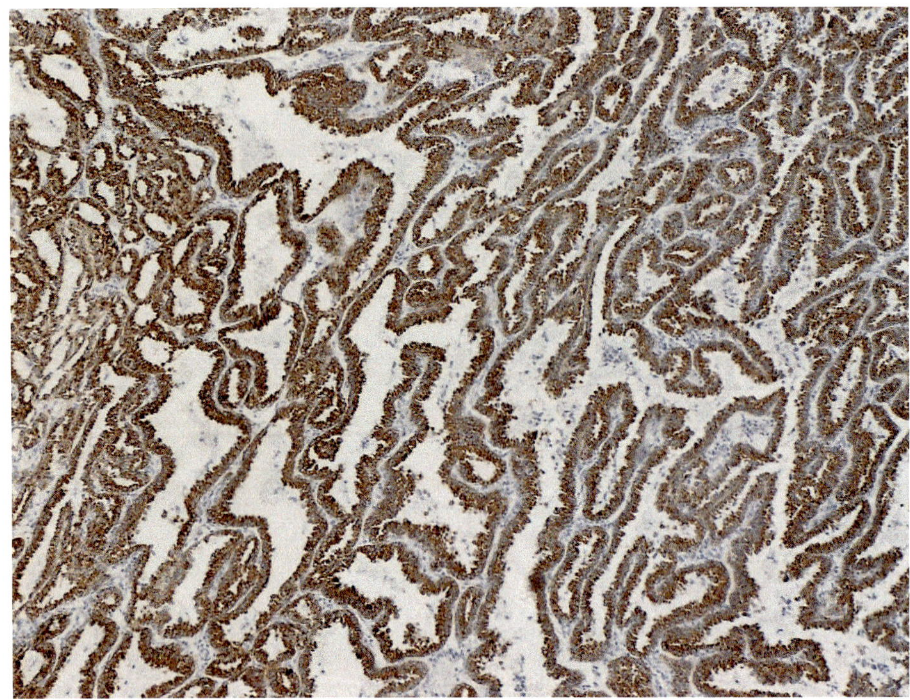

Fig. 1.47 (AMACR (racemase) immunohistochemistry, ×50). Diffuse and strong cytoplasmic granular staining of α-methyl-acylCoA racemase (AMACR)

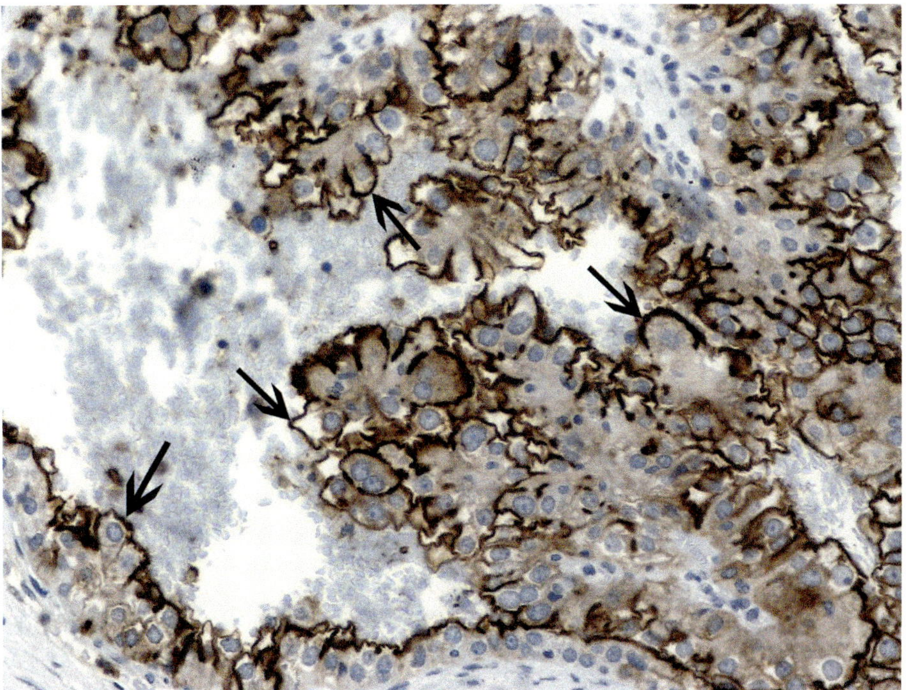

Fig. 1.48 (CD10 immunohistochemistry, ×200) Luminal membranous staining (*arrows*).The same polarized immunoexpression has been reported with regard to MUC1 antibody.

In clear cell RCCs, CD10 is expressed in all cell membranes, in a box-like fashion.

In addition to the above two immunohistochemical markers, papillary RCCs express pancytokeratin, CK19, vimentin (rather inconsistently), pax-2, CD15, and RCC antigen. CAIX is either negative or its focal positivity is limited to papillary tips or perinecrotic areas.

In contrast to collecting duct carcinoma, papillary RCC only rarely reacts with antibodies to high molecular weight cytokeratins (HMWCKs)

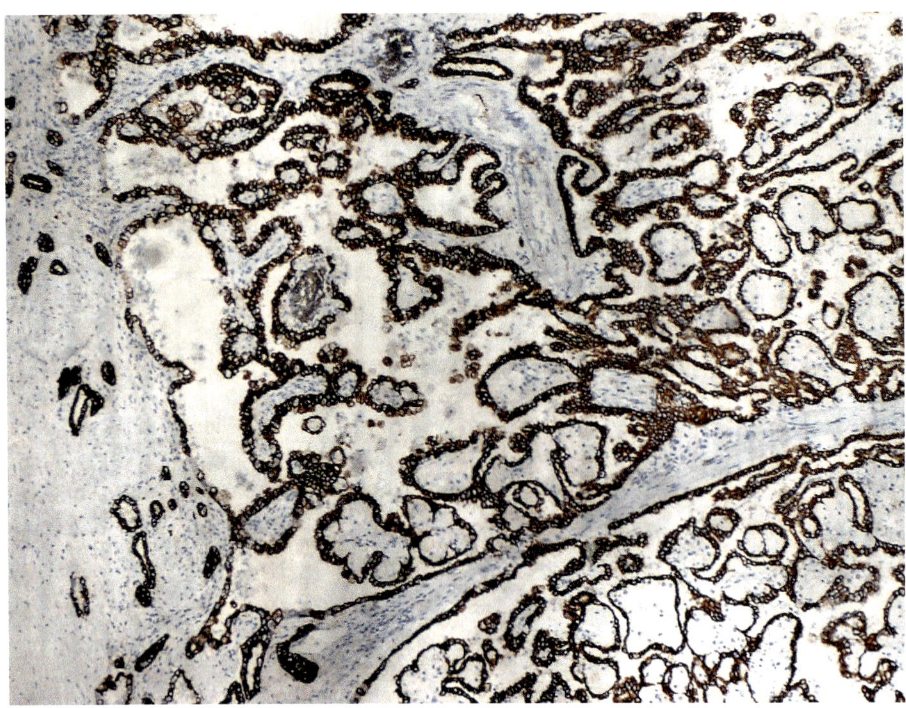

Fig. 1.49 (Cytokeratin 7 immunohistochemistry, ×50) Diffuse, cytoplasmic, and membranous positivity. Cytokeratin 7 (CK7) expression is more common in type 1 papillary RCCs (87% of cases) than in type 2 (20% of cases). Oncocytic papillary RCC is CK7 immunopositive, like type 1 papillary RCC. CK7 is virtually lacking in clear cell RCC. Coexpression of CK7 and AMACR is supportive of a papillary RCC diagnosis over other tumors with a papillary architecture

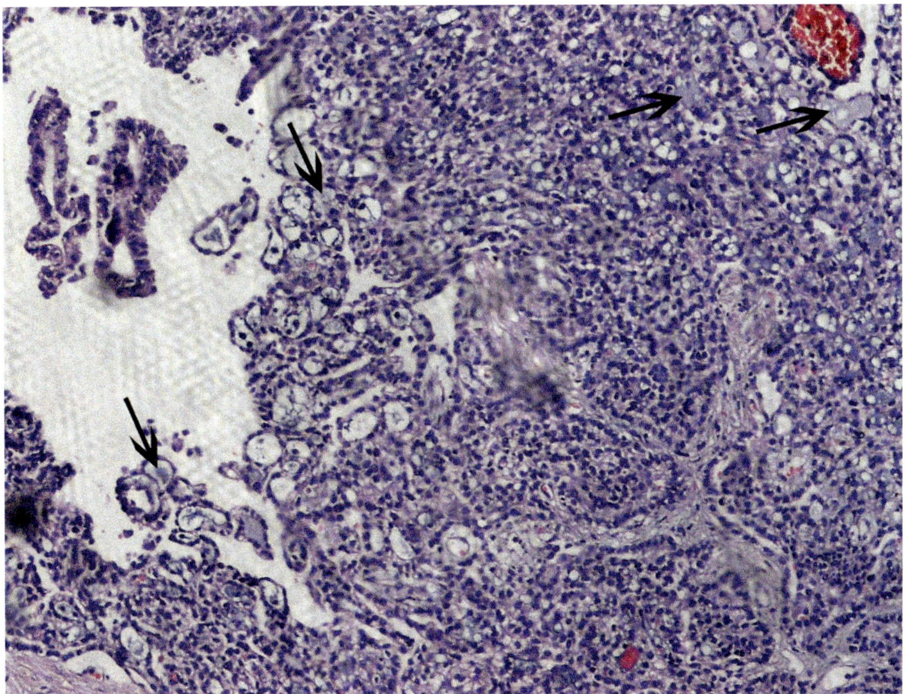

Fig. 1.50 (H-E, ×100) Differential diagnosis of papillary RCC:

- Mucinous tubular and spindle cell carcinoma. Most such tumors have an indolent course. In them you may note anastomosing tubular or cord-like formations merging with bland spindle cells, regular and smooth spindle cells, regular and smooth luminal surfaces, irregular luminal outlines, and myxoid or mucinous stroma with a bubbly appearance (*arrows*). Solid papillary RCCs may have compact areas of low-grade spindle cells lining thin, angulated tubules resembling mucinous tubular and spindle cell carcinoma, but no mucinous stroma.
- Collecting duct carcinoma with papillary features can be distinguished from papillary RCC by the central, medullary location in the kidney of the main portion of the tumor, prominent multinodular growth pattern, sheet-like areas infiltrating tubules and border, high-grade, typically hobnail features, intracytoplasmic and luminal mucin, pronounced desmoplastic stroma, associated epithelial dysplasia in collecting ducts adjacent to the tumor, and CEA and HMWCK immunoreactivity.
- RCC associated with Mit family translocation. This tumor often affects children and young adults. Often papillary architecture with intermingled solid or nested areas can be found, as well as both clear and eosinophilic cells showing voluminous cytoplasm. Unlike most RCCs, Mit family translocation RCCs lack or underexpress epithelial immunohistochemical markers such as pancytokeratin; antibodies for specific gene fusions are necessary for the diagnosis of Mit family translocation RCCs

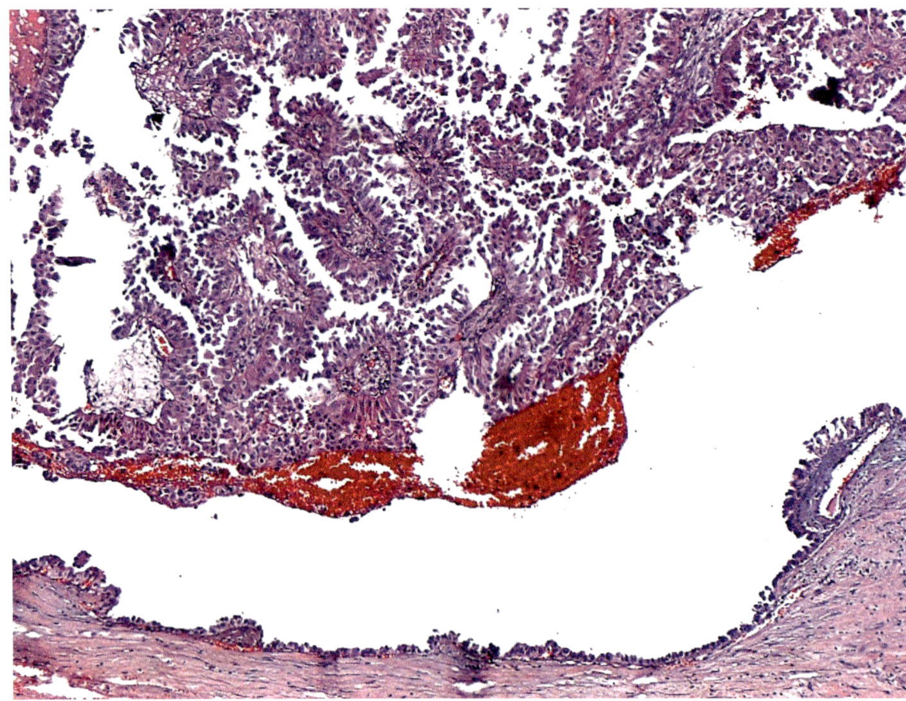

Fig. 1.51 (H-E, ×50) Differential diagnosis of papillary RCC: Hereditary leiomyomatosis and renal cell carcinoma-associated renal cell carcinoma with papillary features. Often prominent papillary architecture. Rare multifocality. Thick papillae covered by large cells with eosinophilic cytoplasm in a single unilateral cystic renal mass with solid enhancing components

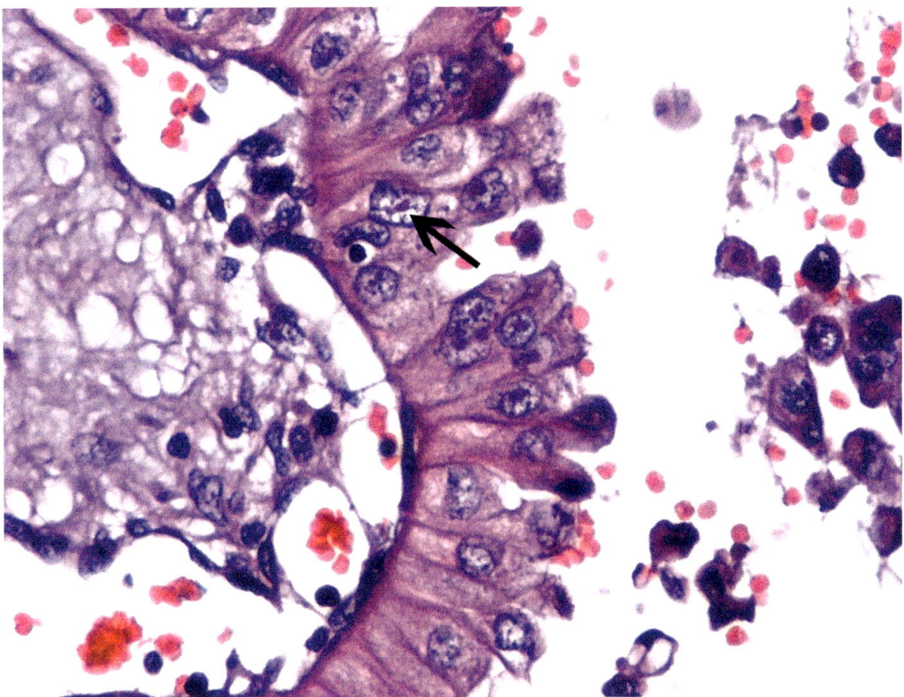

Fig. 1.52 (H-E, ×400) Abundant eosinophilic cytoplasm. Nuclei contain inclusion-like nucleoli with characteristic perinucleolar clearing (*arrow*)

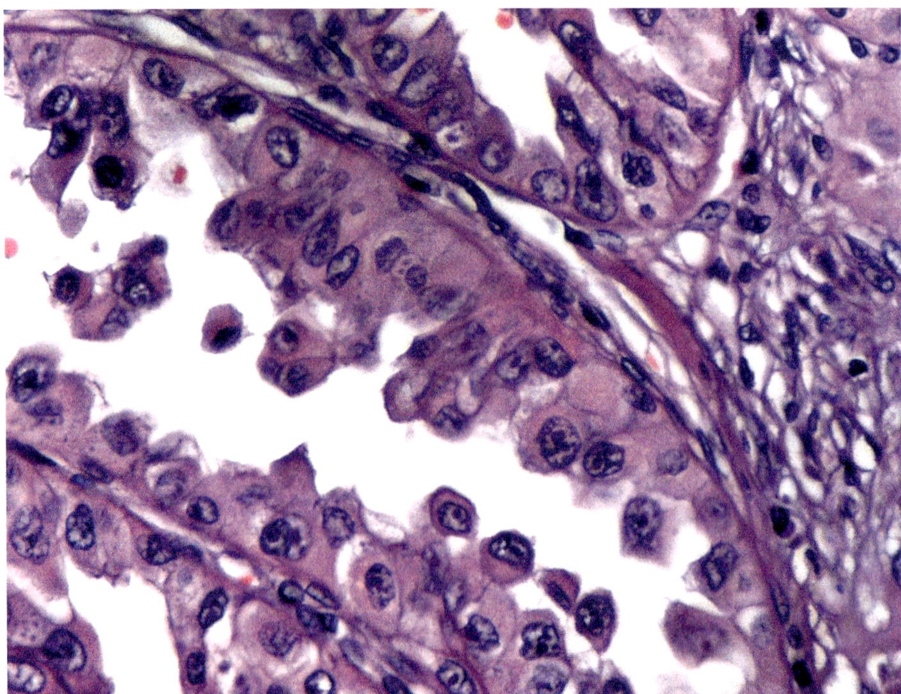

Fig. 1.53 (H-E, ×400) When morphology is indicative, germline mutations in the gene encoding fumarate hydratase should be searched so that the diagnosis of hereditary leiomyomatosis and renal cell carcinoma-associated renal cell carcinoma is confirmed. Clinical correlation with leiomyomas of the skin and uterus is also important

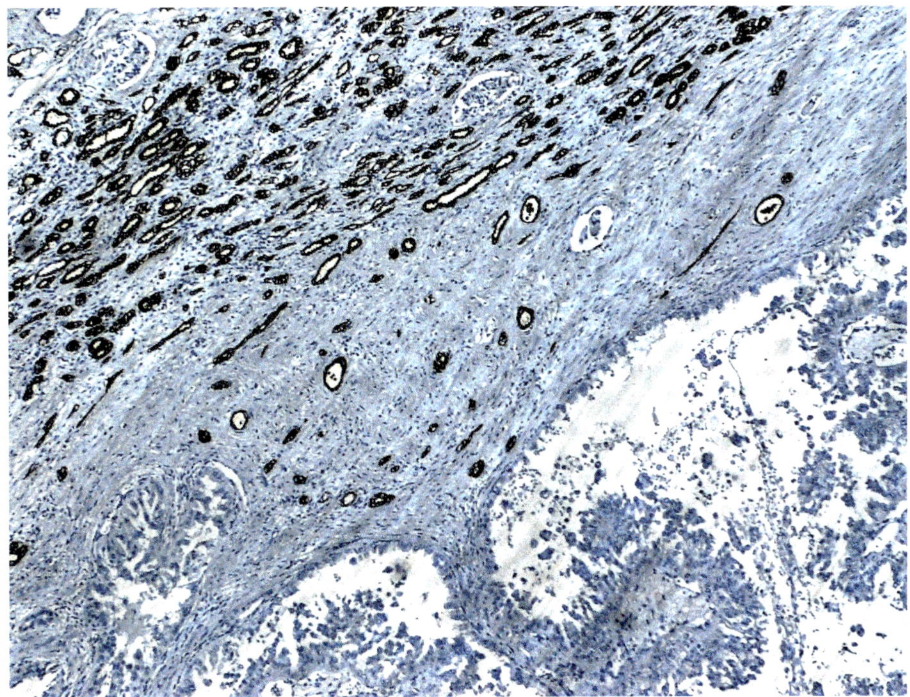

Fig. 1.54 (Cytokeratin 7 immunohistochemistry, ×50) The usual CK7 negativity (*lower part*) in this kind of papillary RCC associated with hereditary leiomyomatosis. Urinary tubules (*upper part*) serve as an internal positive control

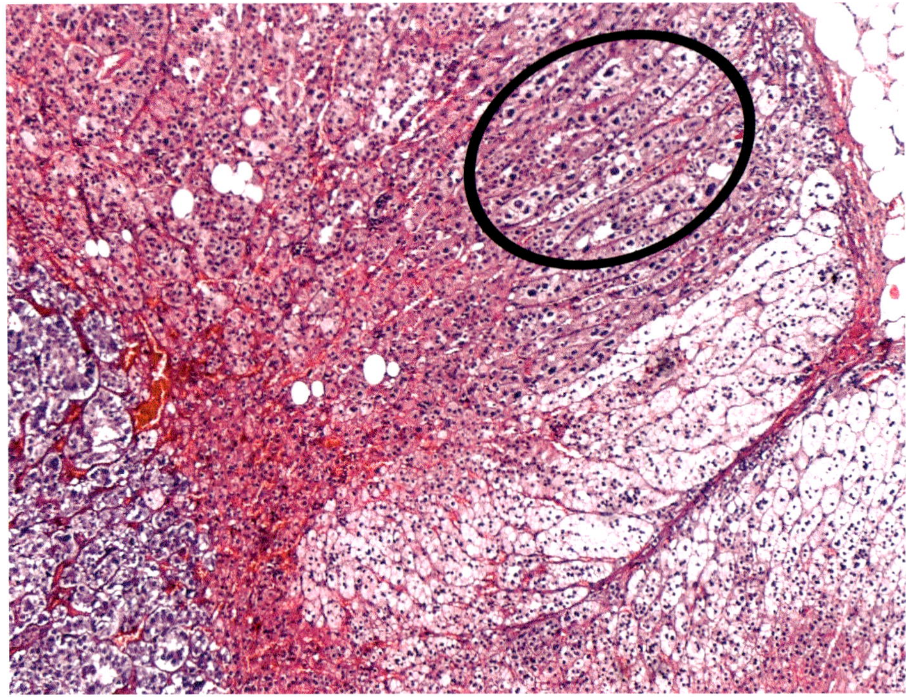

Fig. 1.55 (H-E, ×100) Hypertrophic (*ellipse*), proliferating eosinophilic adrenal cortical cells in the previous patient (Figs 1.51–1.54). Adrenal nodular hyperplasia of cortical cells has been observed in a subset of patients with hereditary leiomyomatosis and RCC

1.3.1.1 Clinical Commentary

Vasileios Spapis

This is a case of papillary RCC of low grade, limited within the renal cortex. Concomitant presence of a papillary adenoma and foci of papillary hyperplasia.

Papillary RCC is considered to be the second most common histologic subtype of RCC, representing about 10–15% of all RCCs (Störkel et al. 1997). It has also been referred to as "chromophilic" RCC, especially in earlier classification systems. It is usually found in patients with acquired renal cystic disease and end-stage renal failure, although its most unique feature is multicentricity which reaches almost 40%. Macroscopically, it is usually seen as a well-circumscribed mass with a pseudocapsule and brown or yellow color (Campbell and Lane 2012).

At least two variants of papillary RCC have been described: type 1 and type 2. Some authors describe the presence of a third type, the oncocytic type. Type 1 has a better prognosis and sometimes corresponds to hereditary papillary RCC syndrome, while type 2 seems to be more aggressive and was initially thought to be connected to hereditary leiomyomatosis and RCC syndrome (Pignot et al. 2007). Extensive necrosis is not unusual, causing the tumor to be fragile and resulting in spontaneous rupture and retroperitoneal bleeding, even though a well-developed pseudocapsule in type 1 carcinomas probably prevents these tumors from rupturing. Oncocytic papillary carcinomas have no pseudocapsule or massive necrosis and are considered to be of low malignant potential (Sukow et al. 2012).

Like any other RCC, most of the tumors are diagnosed incidentally, by noninvasive imaging, used to investigate nonspecific symptoms or coexisting diseases (Ljungberg 2016). In post-contrast CT scanning, the typical necrosis of papillary RCC is seen as a hypodense central area of the tumor. Vital tumor tissue surrounds this area which is seen as a contrast-enhancing margin (Urge et al. 2010).

The prognosis of papillary RCC remains controversial. For years it was considered to have a tendency towards an indolent, low-grade disease. In any case, papillary RCC (especially type 1) appears to carry a better prognosis than clear cell RCC when compared grade for grade and stage for stage (Campbell and Lane 2012). It is noteworthy that the prognosis of the hereditary leiomyomatosis and RCC-associated RCC is much poorer than that of papillary RCC and, actually, poorer than that of clear cell RCC (Moch et al. 2016).

Papillary adenomas are benign neoplasms and resemble papillary RCC under the microscope. They are small (by definition <15 mm), often well encapsulated and low grade. They are of no clinical significance and are commonly found at autopsy. Interestingly though, they possess many of the same genetic alterations that are found in larger, papillary RCCs.

Key Messages

- Papillary RCC is the second most common RCC subtype with a significantly better prognosis than clear cell RCC. Type 1 papillary RCCs have a better prognosis than do those with type 2 morphology.
- Papillary RCC is also more likely to be multifocal and necrotic than other common RCC subtypes.
- A solid pattern due to the tight compact growth of papillae is possible.

1.4 Case 1.3 Clear Cell Papillary Renal Cell Carcinoma

Case Study

Data Prior to Microscopy

A middle-aged patient with an incidentally detected, unicentric, focally cystic, tumor within the renal parenchyma (stage pT1), with a maximum diameter of 2.5 cm (stage pT1a), and a prominent capsule.

Due to size and nonaggressive radiologic appearance, partial nephrectomy was performed.

Absence of recurrence and of lymph node or other metastases, after partial nephrectomy (28 months follow-up).

1.4.1 Microscopic Evaluation of the Partial Nephrectomy Specimen

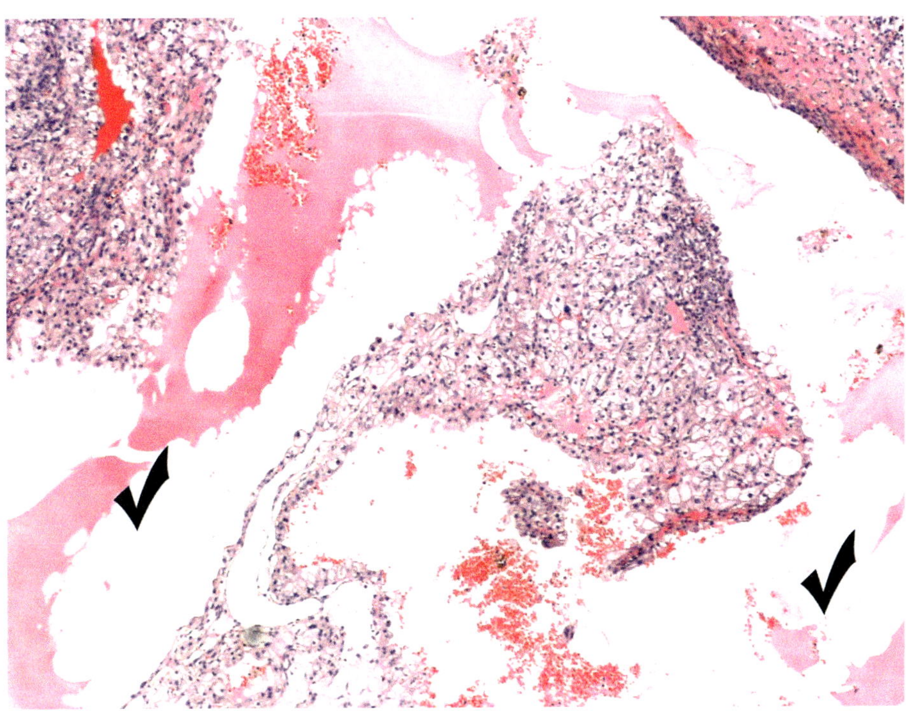

Fig. 1.56 (H-E, ×50) In the first image of this case, a cystic area of the tumor is shown (*ticks*). Clear cell papillary RCCs are usually cystic, at least focally

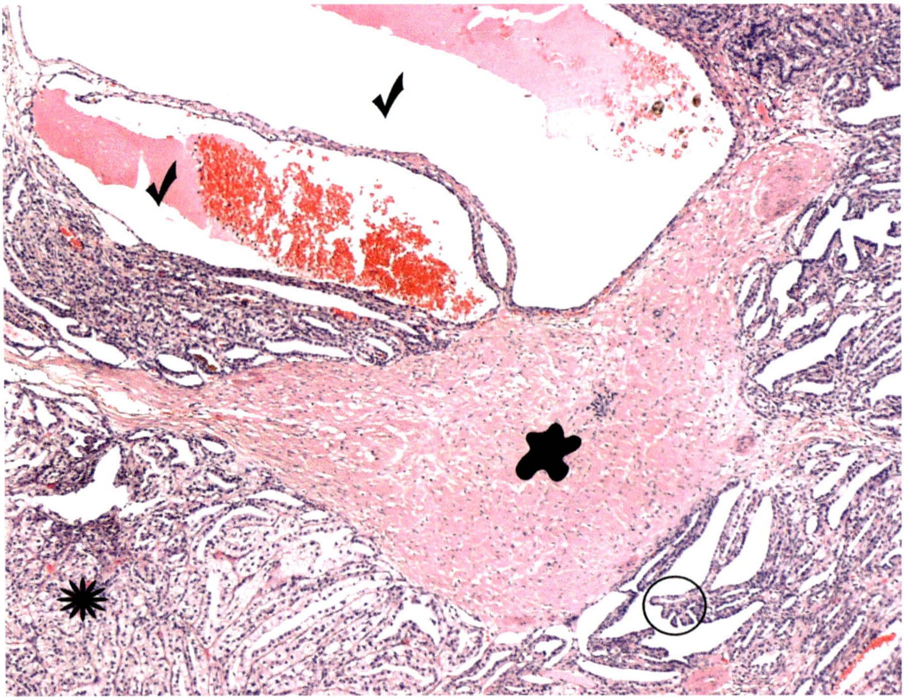

Fig. 1.57 (H-E, ×50) Cystic areas (*ticks*), a solid area (*asterisk*), and papillary proliferations (*circle*) are noticed. The stroma demonstrates smooth muscle metaplasia (*blob*), a finding consistent with the diagnosis of clear cell papillary RCC

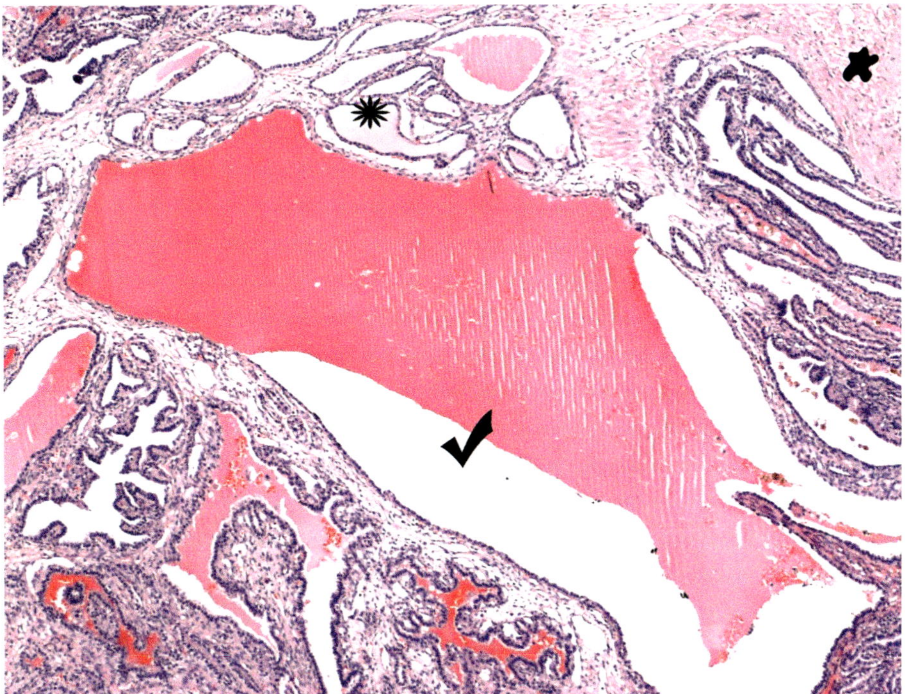

Fig. 1.58 (H-E, ×50) Elongated tubules (*asterisk*) and a prominent cystic component (*tick*). The characteristic prominent capsule may occasionally be quite thick, as also seen in other slow-growing renal tumors, and may show myoid metaplasia (*blob*)

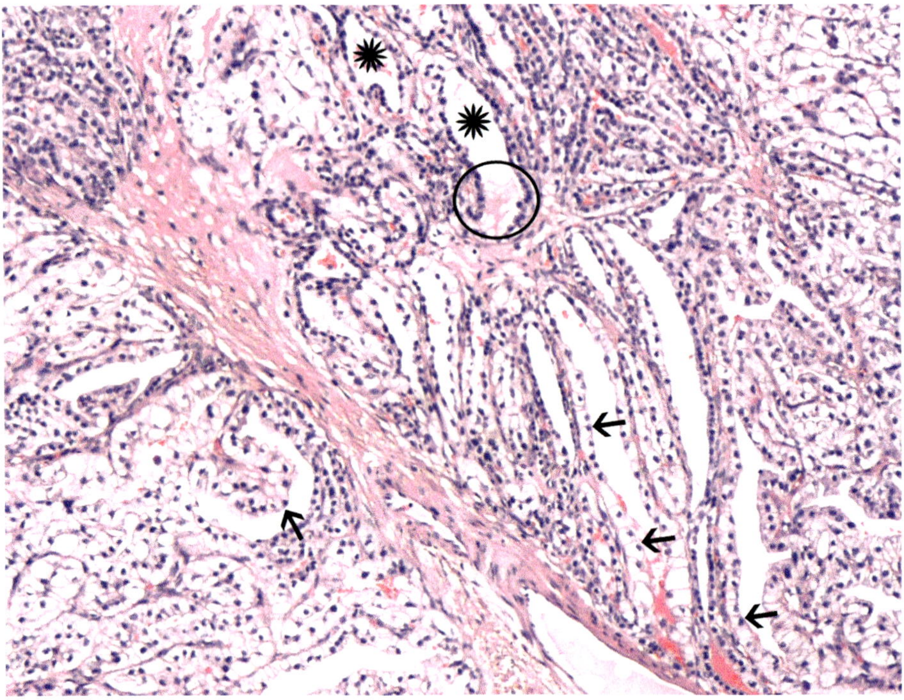

Fig. 1.59 (H-E, ×100) Papillary-type structures/fronds (*arrows*) and tubules (*asterisks*) – the latter, often closely packed or in an acinar configuration (*lower left part*) – are lined by cells with clear cytoplasm (*arrows*) and nuclei with inconspicuous nucleoli (low WHO/ISUP grade). In this image the scanty cytoplasm of a considerable number of cells makes them appear somewhat amphophilic (*ellipse*). In general, the nuclei are characteristically in linear arrangement, and they are typically polarized away from the basal aspect, usually in the center of cytoplasm or more apical, often creating a subnuclear vacuole (*arrows*)

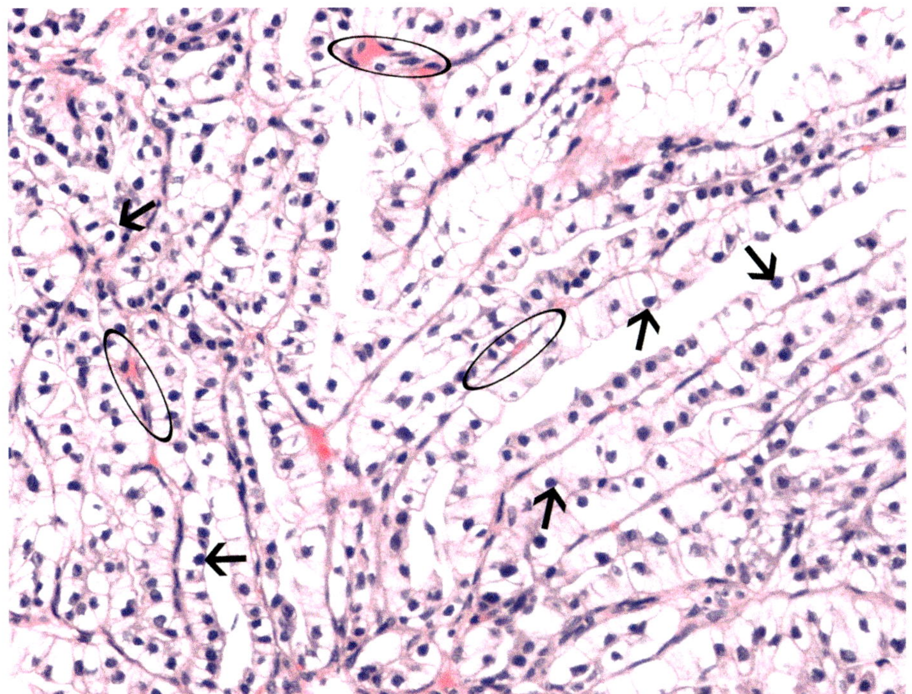

Fig. 1.60 (H-E, ×200) Tightly packed papillae. The presence of true papillae with thin fibrovascular cores is implied (*ellipses*). The distinction of delicate fibrovascular cores of papillae in papillary RCCs from vascular septa of (conventional) clear cell RCCs can be quite difficult when the tumor configuration appears solid. The presence of prominent clear cell cytology distinguishes this tumor from a papillary RCC.

In this case, tightly packed, small, collapsed tubules/acini often give the tumor a solid, occasionally sheet-like in other areas, appearance. All cells have sufficient, clear cytoplasm in this image; interestingly, their nuclei are polarized away from the basal aspect (*arrows*), a finding consistent with the diagnosis of clear cell papillary RCC. Whether cystic, solid, or papillary, the most characteristic feature is the linear alignment of the nuclei away from the basal aspects of the cells. Although the nuclear arrangement in a linear array and away of the basilar aspect is typical, there may be foci in otherwise typical tumors in which the nuclei, particularly in some tubular areas, may not be aligned in a linear manner

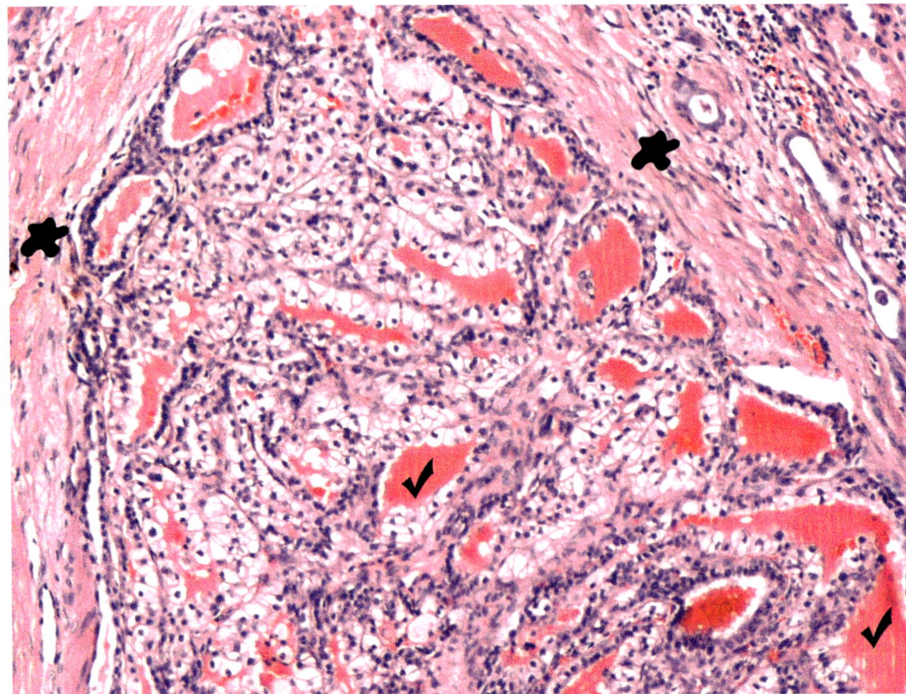

Fig. 1.61 (H-E, ×200) Fibrous capsule and variable amounts of hyalinized or sclerotic stroma (*blobs*) that may separate tumor into nodules. Branching tubules, often with clear cells, are noticed. Intraluminal proteinaceous, eosinophilic secretions (*ticks*) and hemorrhage are often present in clear cell papillary RCC. Distinct delicate vasculature, typical of clear cell RCC, is absent here

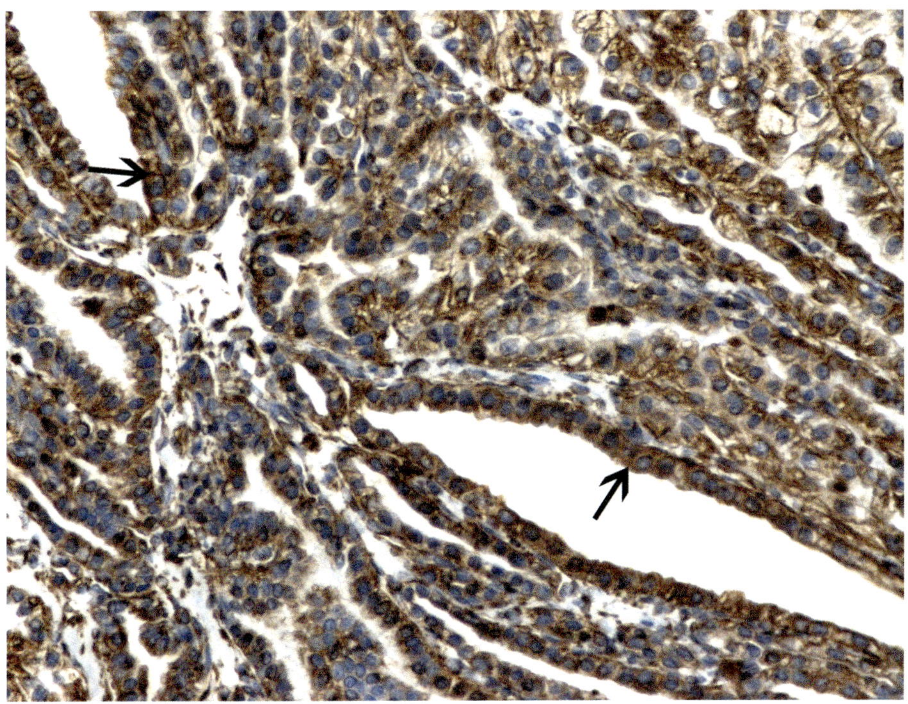

Fig. 1.62 (Vimentin immunohistochemical stain, ×200) Tumor cells (*arrows*) are vimentin-immunopositive

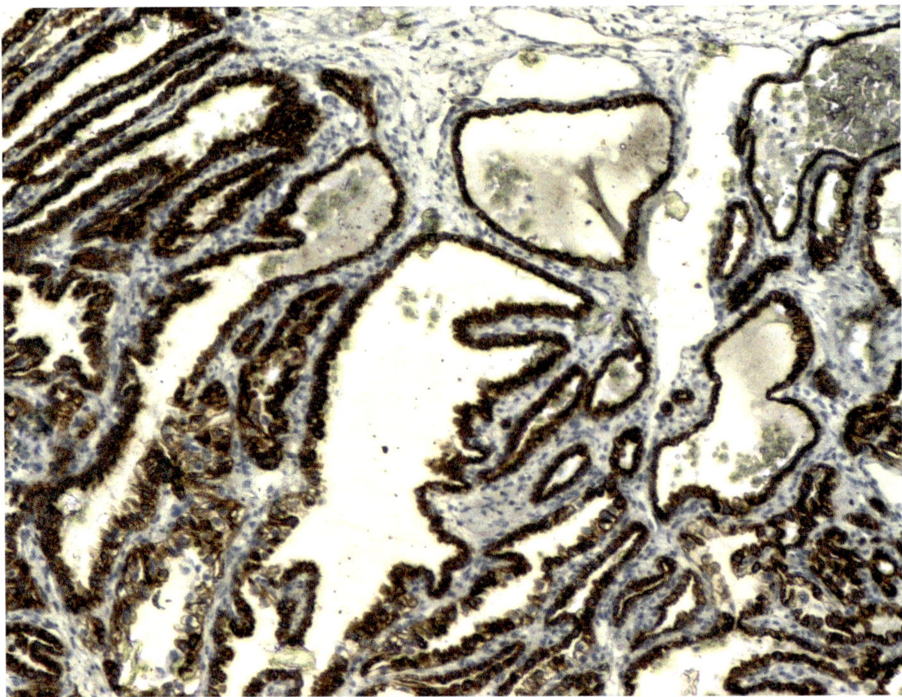

Fig. 1.63 (High Molecular Weight Cytokeratin 34βE12 immunohistochemical stain, ×100) In general, expression of this marker is limited in the more common subtypes of RCC. Clear cell papillary RCCs (as above) and collecting duct carcinomas are notable exceptions

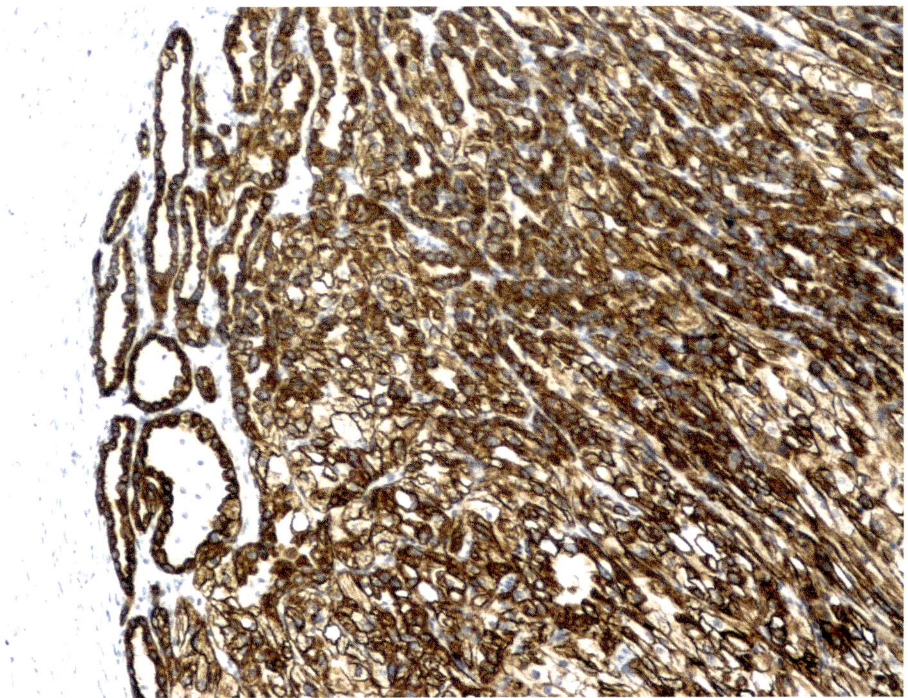

Fig. 1.64 (Cytokeratin 7 immunohistochemical stain, ×100) Diffuse and intense positivity for cytokeratin 7 in tubular and tightly packed areas of the clear cell papillary RCC. A common finding in papillary RCC

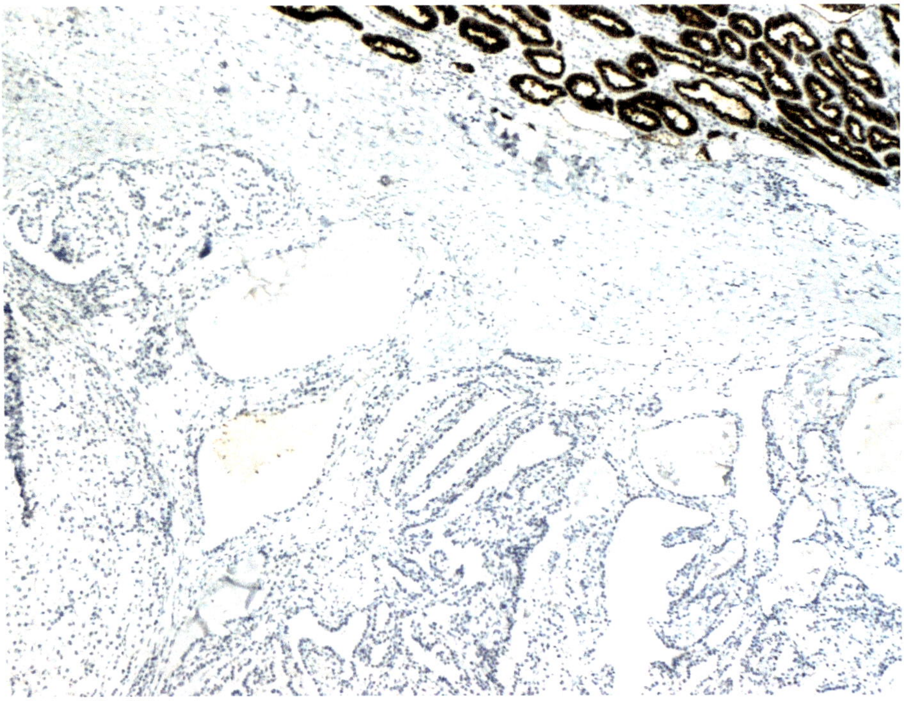

Fig. 1.65 (AMACR immunohistochemical stain, ×50) Unlike papillary RCC, clear cell papillary RCC (*lower part of the image*) is negative for AMACR

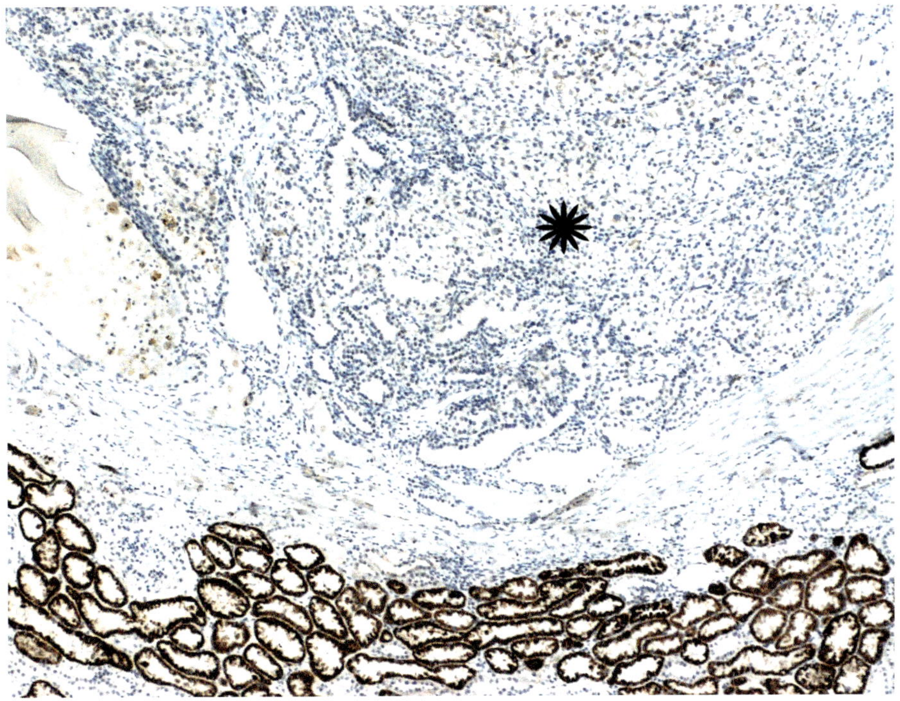

Fig. 1.66 (CD10 immunohistochemical stain, ×50) In clear cell papillary RCC, CD10 is typically negative (*asterisk*) or focally positive

- To sum up, clear cell papillary RCC is an indolent renal epithelial neoplasm composed of bland clear cells of low nuclear grade, variable papillary, tubular/acinar and cystic architecture, and at least a predominant, characteristic linear arrangement of nuclei away from the basal aspect of cells. No foamy macrophages, no vascular invasion, no oxalate crystals, no necrosis, and no perirenal invasion.
  1. Typical distinctive immunohistochemical profile: coexpression of CK7/CAIX and negative CD10/AMACR expression.

Differential Diagnosis (Algaba et al. 2011; Magi-Galluzzi and Zhou 2010; Ross et al. 2012)

- (Conventional) clear cell RCC is characterized by hypervascular septa intimately associated with cancerous cells, the latter with optically transparent cytoplasm and random nuclear arrangement in it; papillary areas are uncommon. Alveolar nests and sheets of clear cells are interspersed by delicate vascular network. Sometimes focal subnuclear clearing causing linear arrangement of nuclei may be observed, but extensive papillary structures are absent. In contrast to the present case, immunohistochemical features supporting the diagnosis of clear cell RCC are:
  1. Diffuse, strong, *complete* membranous CAIX staining. CAIX also marks clear cell papillary RCC in a diffuse staining pattern but usually shows characteristic "cup-shaped" basolateral distribution, with absence of staining along luminal aspect
  2. Diffuse strong membranous CD10 immunoreactivity
  3. Absence of CK7 staining

Chromosome arm 3p loss by genetics is compatible with the diagnosis of clear cell RCC

- In papillary RCC, one may occasionally see clear cell changes; clear cells, if present; are finely bubbly, granular, and focal. Fine, pigmented cytoplasmic reticulations, representing hemosiderin are a diagnostic clue for papillary RCC. In contrast to papillary clear cell RCC, foamy macrophages expanding papillary cores, psammoma bodies and areas of necrosis are common in papillary RCC. The diagnosis of papillary RCC is supported by strong, diffuse CK7 immunoreactivity, AMACR (racemase) positivity (the latter, absent in clear cell papillary RCC), and negative or only focal CA IX expression. Cytogenetically, papillary RCCs are characterized by trisomy of chromosomes 7 and 17, as well as loss of the Y chromosome.
- MiT family translocation-associated RCCs share similar diversity of architectural features (papillary, tubular, cystic, and solid-collapsed acinar) with clear cell papillary RCC. In XP11 translocation carcinoma, predominantly clear cell histology is rare and a nested pattern made up of cells with eosinophilic cytoplasm is easily observed; a papillary structure lined with cells with voluminous clear cytoplasm is indeed characteristic, but, in contrast to the present tumor, the patients are young, nuclear grade is usually high, and stromal psammomatous calcifications and hyalinized fibrovascular cores are noticed. Cytokeratins are underexpressed immunohistochemically, and a concomitant immunopositivity of CD10, cathepsin K, and TFE confirms the diagnosis. TFE gene rearrangements by fluorescence in situ hybridization (FISH) are detectable.

1.4.1.1 Clinical Commentary

Vasileios Spapis

This is a case of an indolent, incidentally detected renal tumor treated with partial nephrectomy. Clear cell papillary RCC is a relatively new entity described during the last decade. It has also been reported under the term renal angiomyomatous tumor (RAT) (Ljungberg 2016). It is considered to be a rather low-grade renal tumor with low malignant potential (Srigley et al. 2013) and an excellent prognosis; therefore, nephron sparing surgery (NSS) is the treatment of choice, when technically feasible. Disease recurrence and distant metastases are extremely rare (Moch et al. 2016). Clear cell papillary RCC is thought to be found in less than 4% of all resected renal tumors (Zhou and Magi-Galluzzi 2007). It carries both papillary and clear cell features, but its rare incidence and short history of existence compel the need for further investigation of its imaging characteristics and biologic behavior.

For decades, radical nephrectomy (RN) was the treatment of choice for all renal tumors. However, later studies proved that localized renal cancer is better treated with partial nephrectomy (PN) in terms of oncological and quality of life (QoL) outcomes. Even when analyzing RCCs of 4–7 cm (stage T1b), no differences in cancer-specific survival (CSS) were observed (Crépel et al. 2010). Moreover, patients who underwent PN reported better scores in most aspects of QoL (Poulakis et al. 2003). So, unless the tumor is locally advanced, partial resection is not feasible due to tumor location, or the patient's health has deteriorated, PN (open/laparoscopic/robotic assisted) is currently the treatment of choice (Ljungberg 2016).

Key Messages

- In renal tumors with clear cell morphology, nuclear polarity should be evaluated.
- Clear cell papillary RCCs (along with multilocular cystic renal neoplasm of low malignant potential) constitutes the best prognostic group of nonbenign renal cell tumors.

1.5 Case 1.4 Renal Oncocytoma

Case Study

Data Prior to Microscopy

Partial nephrectomy was performed in a 62-year-old male patient with an incidentally diagnosed, rounded, well-circumscribed mass within the renal cortex, protruding with a "pushing margin," with a maximum diameter of 4.5 cm, and a tan – mahogany brown, relatively homogeneous cut surface. An area of central irregular scarring was observable (this feature is seen in slow-growing renal tumors that have reached a considerable size).

Absence of recurrence and of lymph node or other metastases, after partial nephrectomy (5-year follow-up).

1.5.1 Microscopic Evaluation of the Partial Nephrectomy Specimen

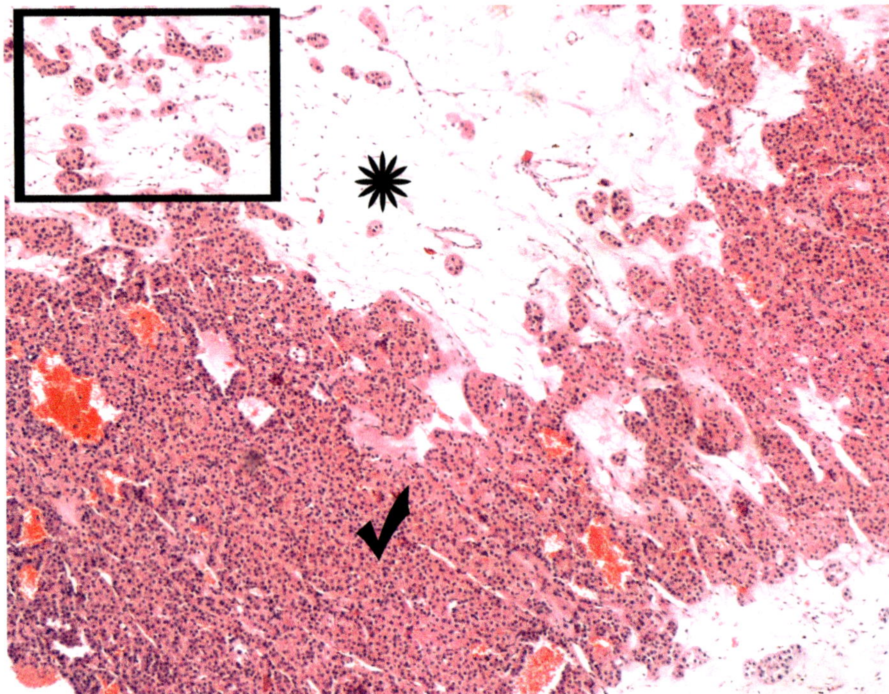

Fig. 1.67 (H-E, ×50) Renal oncocytoma. Prominent nested, organoid architecture of tumor cells (classic pattern). Small islands of oncocytic cells (*square frame*) within loose, hypocellular connective tissue (*asterisk*) corresponding to the grossly noted scar; surrounding closely packed nests of oncocytes (*tick*). The typical well-defined solid *nests* (alveoli) are packed at the tumor periphery and more separated centrally. When closely packed, tumor nests impart a solid appearance (*tick*); a *pure* sheet-like arrangement of cells is *not* a feature of renal oncocytoma

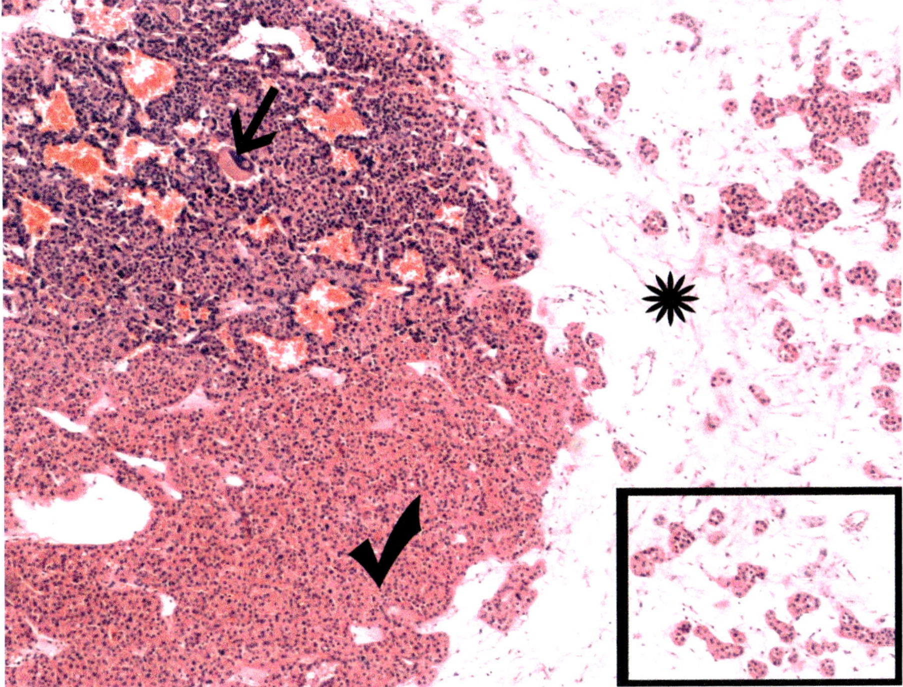

Fig. 1.68 (H-E, ×50) Solid nests/alveoli and tubules. Small islands of oncocytic cells (*square frame*), again within edematous stroma (*asterisk*). Confluent tumor nests (*tick*) can be seen at the periphery of the lesion; they should be outlined by interlacing framework of thin fibrous septa (and they should not form compact sheets like those of the eosinophilic variant of chromophobe RCC).

Aggregate of cells with pronounced nuclear degenerative-appearing pleomorphism, high nuclear/cytoplasmic ratio, and hyperchromatic smudged nuclei (*upper left part, arrow*); this atypia, however, should *not* be associated with the presence of mitotic figures. Oncocytomas having these bizarre cells are biologically benign, and the term atypical should not be applied to them. Generally, in oncocytomas very rare mitoses may occur

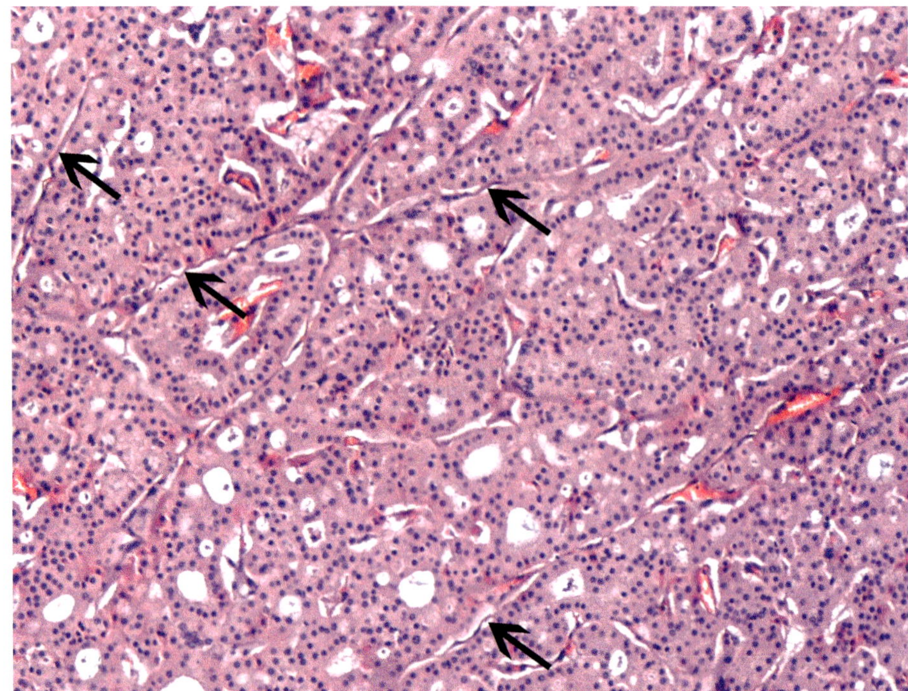

Fig. 1.69 (H-E, ×100) An alternative tumor architectural configuration for renal oncocytoma: the tubulocystic pattern. Variably sized luminal structures lined by cells indistinguishable from those of the classic pattern. Spaces often contain secretion. Lack of stroma but a delicate reticulum framework (*arrows*) separates the tumor structures

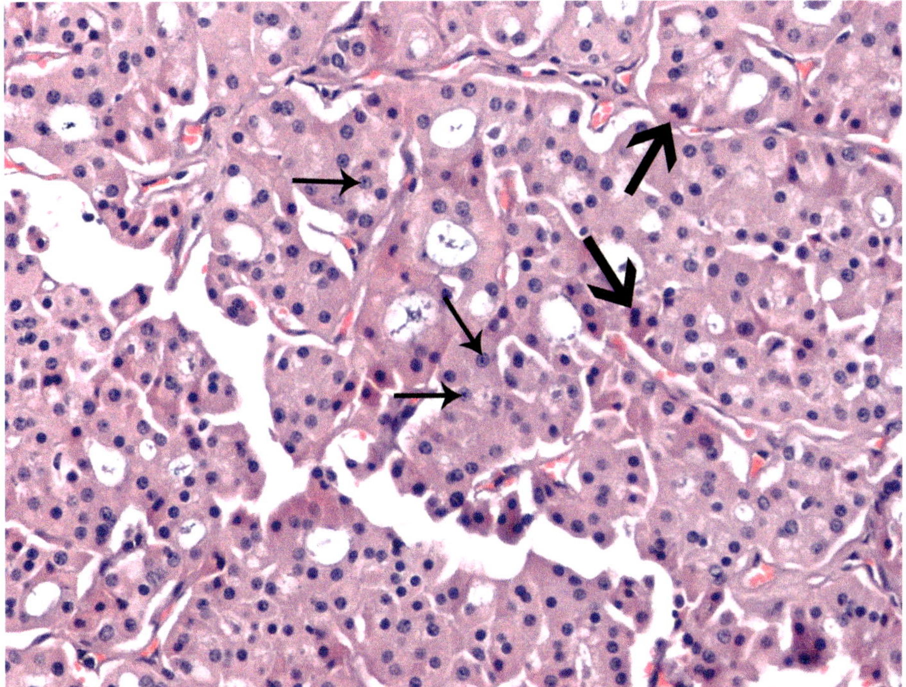

Fig. 1.70 (H-E, ×200) Morphology of oncocytes. Large, round to polygonal cells with abundant, homogeneous, densely granular (due to the presence of many mitochondria) intensely eosinophilic cytoplasm and generally *uniform*, *round*, *and regular*, *benign-appearing*, central nuclei under this medium magnification, with smoothly dispersed chromatin and a central, often inconspicuous nucleolus (*thin arrows*). Scattered few binucleate cells (*thick arrows*). With regard to the architectural pattern, tubules of oncocytes predominate in this tumor area

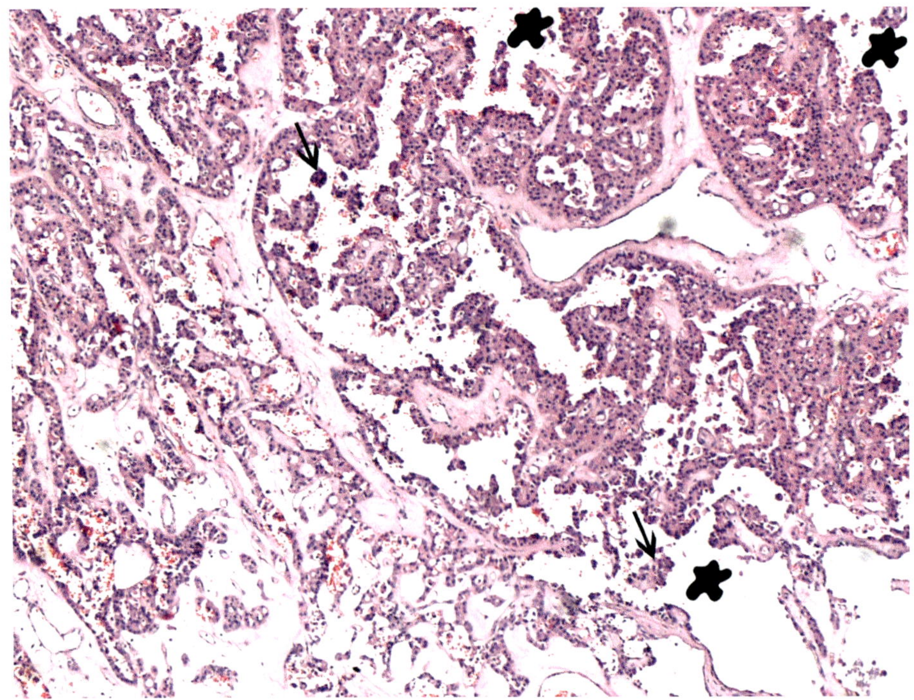

Fig. 1.71 (H-E, ×50) Tumor cell dropout (*arrows*) and pseudopapillary architecture (small papillary-like fronds without fibrovascular stalks protruding in cystic areas, *blobs*). True papillary architecture should be absent in oncocytomas

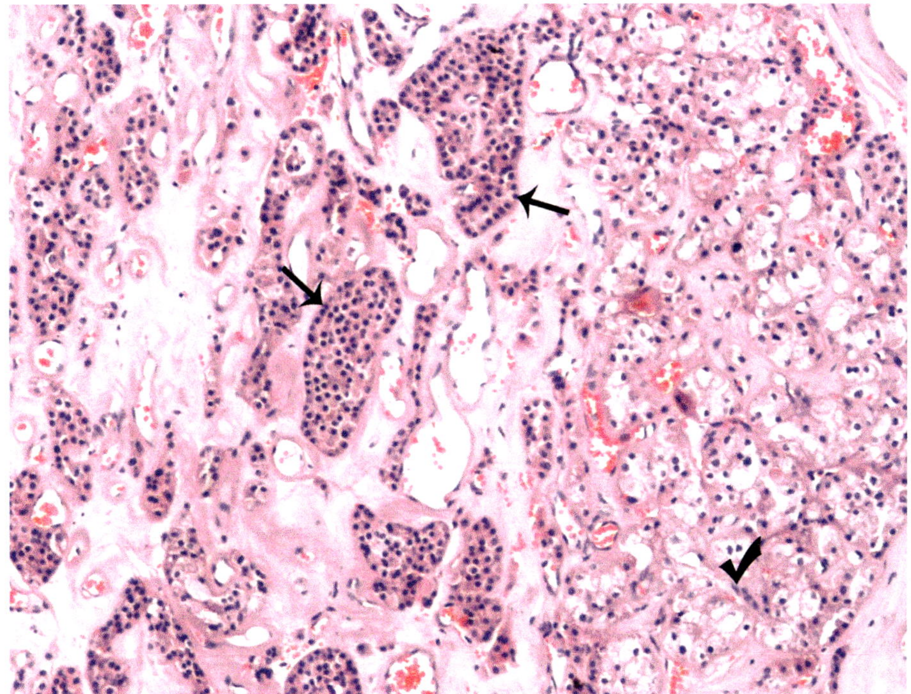

Fig. 1.72 (H-E, ×50) A population of small cells with rather scanty cytoplasm is usually present around the tumor's scar, at the edge of the epithelial islands (*arrows*).

In this field, cells with optically translucent, slightly reticulated cytoplasm are also noticed (*right part of the image*). Vacuolation of the tumor cell cytoplasm produces a focal clear cell appearance (*tick*). Such clusters, when small, are considered permissible in an otherwise typical oncocytoma. Cytoplasmic clearing is rarely encountered in oncocytomas and, when encountered, it is usually restricted to scarred areas.

Rarely, upon *microscopic* evaluation, the cells of some oncocytomas extend into the perirenal or renal sinus fat or within vessels. In order that a diagnosis of oncocytoma is safely established, perirenal invasion, renal vein invasion, or necrosis should *not* be *macroscopically* identifiable.

Findings that are considered *impermissible* for a diagnosis of oncocytoma include areas of clear cell RCC, spindle cell or sarcomatoid areas, prominent papillary architecture, macroscopic or conspicuous microscopic necrosis, and significant mitotic activity, possibly including atypical mitotic figures. *Adequate sampling* of the tumor is *mandatory* in order that such features are not overlooked

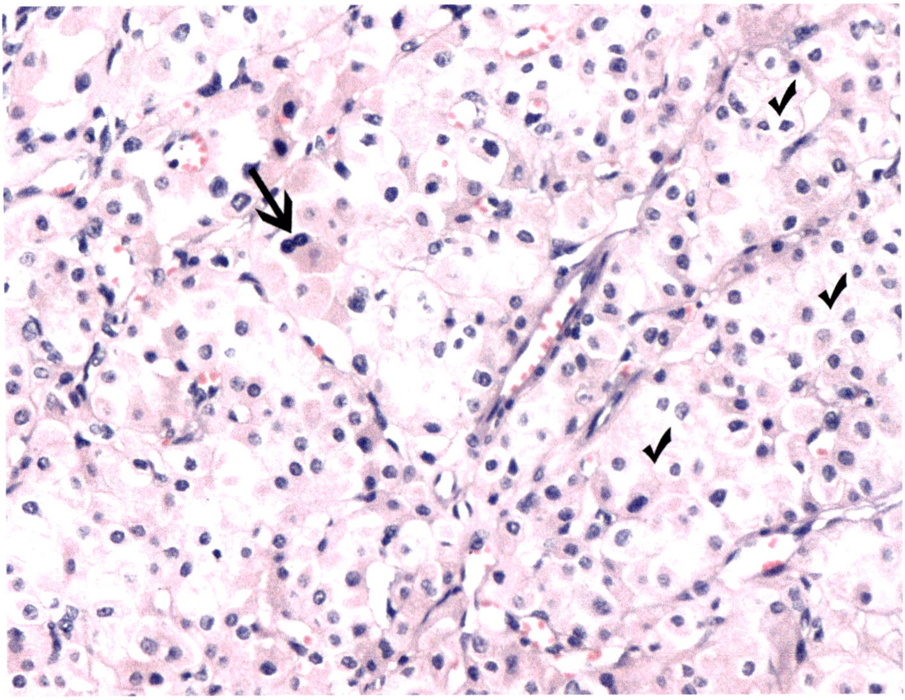

Fig. 1.73 (H-E, ×200) Oncocytes among cells with optically translucent, slightly reticulated cytoplasm (*tick*), all separated by fine, delicate fibrous bands and rather inconspicuous vasculature. Few binucleated cells are noticed (*arrow*)

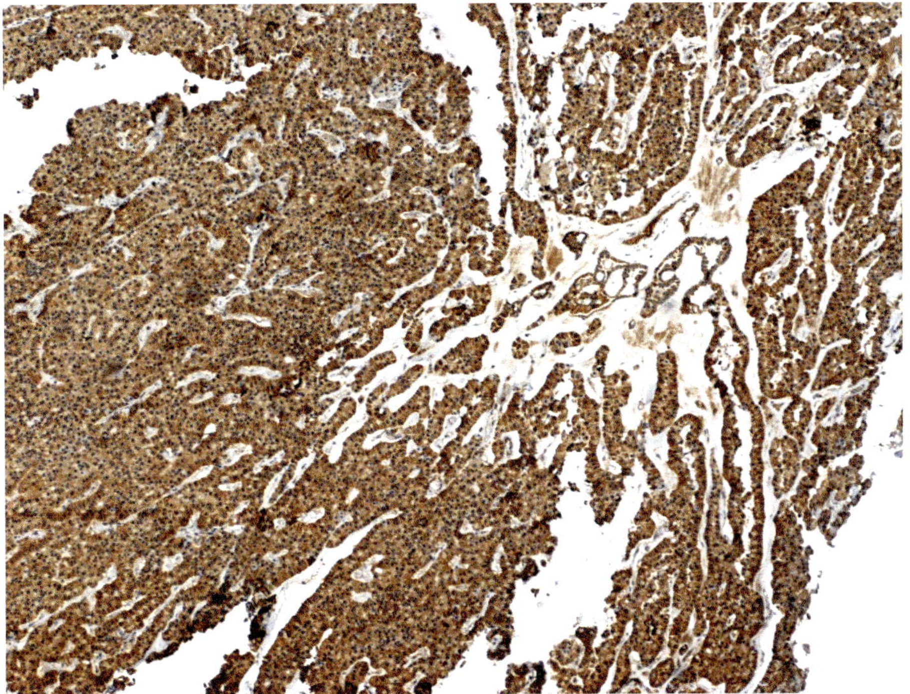

Fig. 1.74 (KIT immunohistochemistry, ×50) KIT (CD117) and Ksp-cadherin are expressed both in oncocytomas and chromophobe RCCs, possibly due to the common origin of these two tumors from the collecting ducts' intercalating cells.

There is also strong positivity for cytokeratin 14 in oncocytomas, a finding also present in chromophobe RCC, but not in clear cell RCC.

In oncocytomas, low molecular weight cytokeratins and S100A are positive. E-cadherin is expressed with a mixed, granular cytoplasmic and membranous pattern. Cytokeratin 20 and CD15 are *focally expressed* in oncocytomas. Cytokeratin 7 is usually negative and occasionally focally positive, decorating scattered, strongly positive single cells or small clusters. Ki67 labeling index is low in oncocytomas.

Renal oncocytomas are supposed to show negative immunostaining for vimentin; however, focal strong vimentin positivity in oncocytes can be present, often at the edge of their central scar, within the stroma, in small cells with scanty cytoplasm or in small clusters scattered throughout the tumor. CD10, CAIX, and renal cell carcinoma marker are frequently negative in oncocytomas

▪ Differential Diagnosis

Primary renal cell neoplasms which may be predominantly or even entirely composed of cells with granular, eosinophilic (acidophilic) cytoplasm, pose a diagnostic challenge for practicing pathologists.

- Oncocytomas are benign, well-circumscribed, nonencapsulated, renal epithelial cells, frequently with a central stellate scar. Tumor architecture is solid, solid-nested, or (rarely) cystic. They are almost entirely composed of cells with uniform, round to oval, central nuclei, abundant granular, mitochondria-rich, eosinophilic cytoplasm (oncocytes) with evenly dispersed, finely granular chromatin, often small nucleoli and very rare, never atypical, mitoses. The neoplastic cells frequently grow in solid nests with inconspicuous vasculature, often on the background of an edematous, hypocellular stroma. Occasionally, scattered cells with scanty granular cytoplasm, binucleated forms, dark hyperchromatic nuclei and high nuclear/cytoplasmic ratio are *focally* present. Hale's colloidal iron stain is negative, but it may occasionally be positive in neoplastic cells' luminal aspect in tubular areas and not in neoplastic cells themselves; the latter occurs in chromophobe RCC. As a rule, CD10, RCC marker, CAIX, and vimentin are negative; CK7 reactivity may only be focal. S100A is positive with a coarse cytoplasmic pattern; KIT (CD117) and Ksp-cadherin are positive. *Thorough sampling* is mandatory before a diagnosis of oncocytoma can be made. Histologically, any foci of clear cells, papillae, pure sheet-like growth, "plant-like" cells with distinct, thickened cell borders, or more than rare mitoses exclude the interpretation of oncocytoma.
  - (Conventional) *clear cell RCC, rich in granular/eosinophilic cells*, with a compact alveolar growth pattern, is composed predominantly of eosinophilic (acidophilic) cells, more often of *high grade*, particularly near areas of hemorrhage or necrosis. However, cells with optically transparent, water-clear, PAS-positive cytoplasm have to be detected elsewhere, after thorough sampling. Focal pseudopapillary configuration related to tumor cell dropout or even papillary architecture (the latter limited and in rare cases) is acceptable in (conventional) clear cell RCC. Furthermore, several clear cell RCCs exhibit large areas of plain stroma (devoid of tumor cells) with degenerative changes (e.g., hyalinization) or, occasionally, prominent smooth muscle. Similarly to classic clear cell RCC, the rich in eosinophilic/granular cells clear cell RCC is characterized by fine, hypervascular *septa intimately associated with cancerous cells*. Alveolar nests and sheets of cells are interspersed by a prominent delicate vascular network; this *arborizing vascularity* is surely less intricate in oncocytoma. Mitotic activity is readily identifiable in clear cell RCC rich in eosinophilic/granular cells. Immunohistochemical features supporting the diagnosis of clear cell RCC are diffuse, strong, complete membranous CAIX staining, vimentin immunoreactivity of tumor cells, diffuse strong membranous CD10 immunoreactivity, and, as a rule, RCC marker immunopositivity and absence of CK7 staining. Chromosome arm 3p loss by genetics is compatible with the diagnosis of clear cell RCC.
  - In the *eosinophilic variant of chromophobe RCC, nuclear irregularities*, with *perinuclear haloes* are detected, at least focally. In contrast to oncocytomas, even seemingly pure eosinophilic variants of the chromophobe type of RCC have a sheet-like pattern (or, rarely, a densely packed nested pattern but without

intervening fibrous stroma), strong blue cytoplasmic staining with Hale's colloidal iron, wrinkled, raisinoid nuclei and perinuclear haloes; in addition, many have adequate mitotic activity (if mitotic figures are detected in more than one 20× field, the oncocytic tumor should be classified as eosinophilic chromophobe carcinoma) and at least very small foci of typical *plant-like cells* due to distinct, thickened cell borders, which exclude the interpretation of oncocytoma. *CK7* is often *diffusely positive* (in more than 90% of tumor cells) or positive in at least 5% of tumor cells but with concomitant CK20 and CD15 immunonegativity. E-cadherin is arguably expressed with a purely membranous pattern in the eosinophilic variant of chromophobe RCC.
"Oncocytic neoplasm of uncertain malignant potential" is a term proposed for *hybrid* oncocytic tumors with *predominant* features of *oncocytoma* and some areas with definite "chromophobe" features [i.e., solid, sheet-like growth pattern, prominent, sharply outlined cell membranes (plant-like cells) irregular, raisinoid nuclei, perinuclear haloes, Hale's colloidal iron diffuse cytoplasmic staining] ("hybrid tumors"). [In case of the contrary (i.e., a chromophobe RCC with some areas of oncocytoma), a diagnosis of chromophobe RCC should be made.] Hybrid oncocytic tumors with features of both oncocytoma and chromophobe RCC may occur sporadically but can also be seen in patients with Birt-Hogg-Dubé syndrome. The latter syndrome is characterized by multiple tumors (mean 5.3), mean patients' age 51 years at first renal tumor diagnosis, usually bilateral chromophobe carcinomas, oncocytomas or hybrids; patients may also have oncocytosis.

- Unclassified RCC, as mentioned in the first case of this chapter, comprises a heterogeneous group of tumors with little in common which do not entirely and readily fit into one of the other RCC categories; these RCCs (approximately 5% of RCCs) share no defined clinical, morphologic, immunohistochemical, ultrastructural, or genetic characteristics. By definition, this category does not include only high-grade, aggressive tumors such as those with pure sarcomatoid morphology, but some low-grade, indolent tumors are also part of this category. In the latter encapsulated tumors, there is coarsely granular distribution of chromatin and moderate nuclear pleomorphism not just in isolated cells or groups of cells but *throughout* the tumor, as evidenced under high magnification; furthermore, there are *more than rare* (although less than frequent) *mitoses* in neoplastic cells. Tumor vasculature is quite prominent. No edematous stroma is found. *Unclassified renal cell carcinoma, low grade, oncocytic (oncocytoma-like)* usually shows solid nests/alveoli with oncocytoma-like architecture; tumor necrosis may rarely and only focally be present. These tumors have cytoarchitectural features resembling renal oncocytoma, under low or medium magnification. Nevertheless, under *high* magnification, in unclassified renal cell carcinoma, low-grade, oncocytic (oncocytoma-like), nuclear pleomorphism is *diffuse* and mitoses are identifiable with an index beyond that acceptable for oncocytoma and with atypical morphology in some cases. This tumor does not show nuclear wrinkling and perinuclear haloes as seen in chromophobe RCC. There is no consistent immunohistochemical phenotype for these tumors; in most reported cases, CD10, CAIX, vimentin, and CK7 are diffusely positive in neoplastic cells, while KIT (CD117), Ksp-cadherin, and S100A are negative.

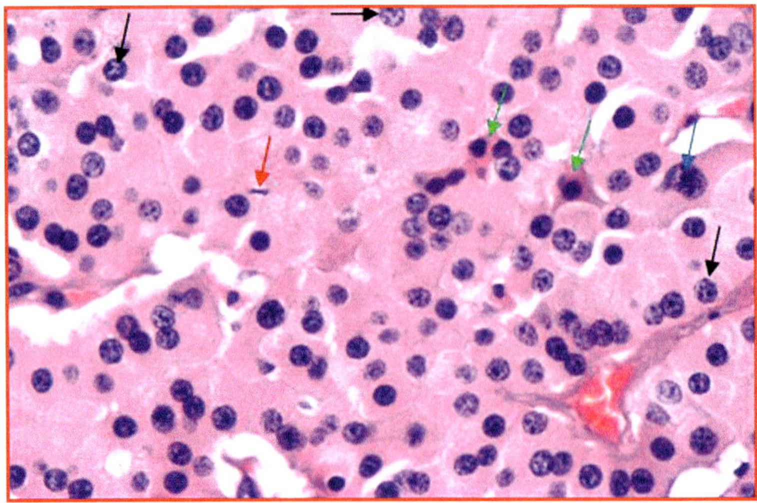

Figs. 1.75 (H-E, ×400) Features indicative of unclassified renal cell carcinoma, low grade, oncocytic (oncocytoma-like), when diffusely observed throughout the tumor parenchyma. Coarsely granular chromatin (*thin black arrows*), mitotic activity (*thin red arrows*), pleomorphic nuclei (either hyperchromatic and/or with increased nuclear cytoplasmic ratio, *blue thin arrow*) in oncocytes. Occasional presence of cells with scanty granular cytoplasm and hyperchromatic nuclei (*thin green arrows*)

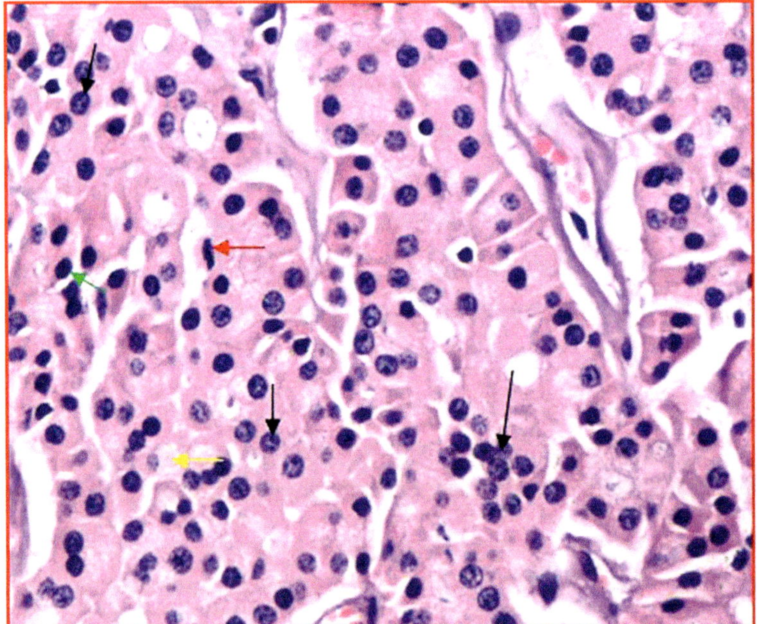

Figs. 1.76 (H-E, ×400) Features indicative of unclassified renal cell carcinoma, low grade, oncocytic (oncocytoma-like), when diffusely observed throughout the tumor parenchyma. Coarsely granular chromatin (*thin black arrows*), mitotic activity (*thin red arrows*), pleomorphic nuclei in oncocytes. Occasional presence of cells with scanty granular cytoplasm and hyperchromatic nuclei (*thin green arrows*) and of cells with optically translucent, slightly reticulated cytoplasm (*thin yellow arrow*)

- Oncocytoma-like angiomyolipomas are rare tumors consisting of a homogeneous population of polygonal cells with strongly eosinophilic cytoplasm; the presence of dysmorphic vessels, sclerosing areas, adipocytes, and nuclear variability point toward the diagnosis of oncocytoma-like angiomyolipoma. It is noteworthy that such tumors may coexist with oncocytomas in the same kidney. Oncocytoma cells are usually arranged in nests and solid alveoli, nuclei are uniform, and, immunohistochemically, in contrast to angiomyolipomas, there is positivity for epithelial markers and negativity for melanocytic markers in oncocytomas.

Key Messages

- Many renal neoplasms contain oncocytic cells, but only oncocytomas are composed entirely of oncocytes.
- The designation "oncocytoma" should confirm the presence of a *benign* renal neoplasm. Considering that renal tumors commonly have intralesional heterogeneity, confirmation of their nature usually requires evaluation of thoroughly sampled, well-preserved tissue. Sections frozen at the time of a rapid intraoperative consultation do not meet this standard and an unequivocal interpretation of oncocytoma is discouraged.

1.5.1.1 Clinical Commentary

Vasileios Spapis

This is a case of a pathologically diagnosed renal oncocytoma, which is believed to be a benign tumor. Malignant behavior has been reported but is extremely rare and could represent cases of malignant degeneration or pseudometastases (Paner et al. 2005; Oxley et al. 2007). Oncocytoma is the most common benign kidney tumor and accounts roughly for 3–5% of all renal neoplasms (Romis et al. 2004). Just like RCC, men are affected more often than women. It derives from the distant renal tubules (like chromophobe RCC).

Oncocytomas are usually well-circumscribed with a pseudocapsule and a central stellate scar. Their color is tan or light brown and necrosis is normally absent. They are mainly solitary and unilateral, although several cases of bilateral or multiple oncocytomas have been reported. Oncocytomas have also been associated with benign neoplasms of hair follicles, polyps of the colon, and pulmonary cysts as part of the Birt-Hogg-Dubé syndrome (Toro et al. 1999). A familial form of renal oncocytomas (oncocytomatosis) has been described. Chromosomal abnormalities seen in RCC are not seen in renal oncocytomas, thus reinforcing the idea that these tumors are genotypically distinct from RCC. However, histologically, the greatest difficulty is distinguishing chromophobe and clear cell RCC with eosinophilic characteristics from oncocytoma (Margulis et al. 2012).

It is practically impossible to safely differentiate between renal oncocytoma and RCC on clinical or radiographic testing alone (Ljungberg 2016); so the role of pathology is crucial. Most oncocytomas are asymptomatic, and hematuria or flank pain occurs in less than 20% of the patients (Konety et al. 2013). There are no characteristic US or CT findings. On angiography, the most typical feature is the spoke-wheel appearance and the lucent rim sign of the capsule, but these patterns are suggestive and not definitive findings (Ljungberg 2016). This means that diagnosis is predominantly pathological. The role of fine needle aspiration and renal biopsy remains controversial but the combination of these two has increased the diagnostic accuracy (Ljungberg 2016). Even frozen section analysis is usually not sensitive enough and cannot be used to guide surgical strategy. So when oncocytoma is suspected, a NSS (nephron sparing surgery) approach should be preferred (Ljungberg 2016).

1.6 Case 1.5 Chromophobe Renal Cell Carcinoma

Case Study

Data Prior to Microscopy

A 58-year-old male patient from the Middle East complains of flank pain due to a tumor of the lower pole of his kidney. Radical nephrectomy is performed.

Well-circumscribed, solitary spherical tumor, 8 cm in greatest dimension, confined to the kidney, with homogeneous, beige cut surface.

1.6.1 Microscopic Evaluation of the Radical Nephrectomy Specimen

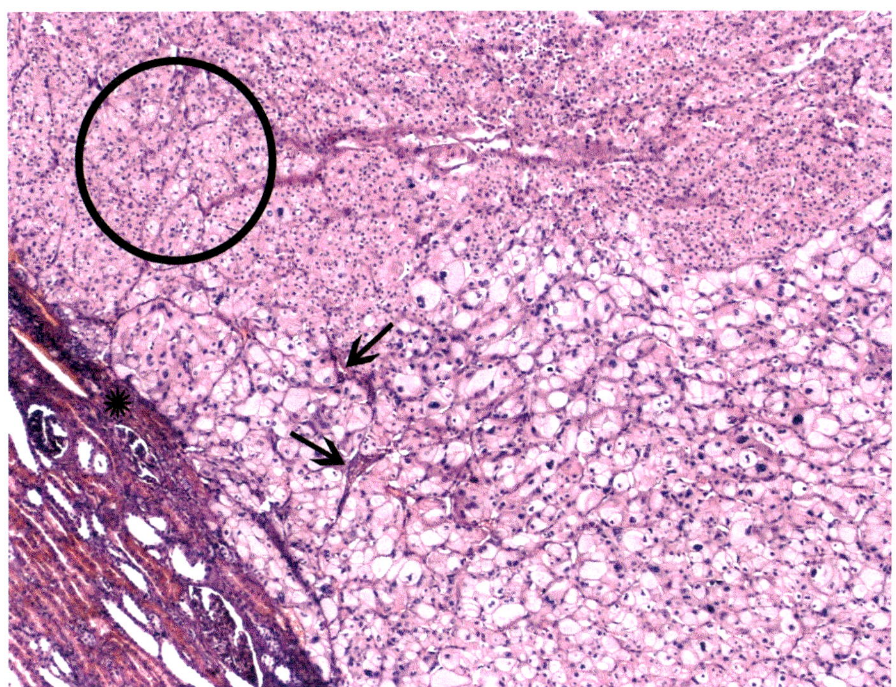

Fig. 1.77 (H-E, ×50) Chromophobe RCC margin: well-circumscribed tumor (*asterisk*) but not truly encapsulated. Predominant solid, sheet-like pattern of growth; proliferation of compact cells typically arranged in solid sheets.

Tubulocystic architecture with focal papillations is rare in chromophobe RCC.

In the classic type of chromophobe RCC (lower half of the image), the large polygonal tumor cells with abundant, *almost* transparent and slightly flocculent, pale cytoplasm and prominent membranes are arranged in broad trabeculae, along ill-defined septa with interspersed, rather thick-walled blood vessels of medium caliber (*arrows*). Chromophobe RCC with "clear" cells is more likely to show sheet-like architecture than clear cell RCC, which typically exhibits a solid-acinar growth pattern.

In the eosinophilic variant of chromophobe RCC (upper half of the image), the nested/alveolar pattern predominates; the tumor cells are smaller, with less abundant granular and eosinophilic cytoplasm, arranged in small nests (*circle*) or in solid sheets.

The two cell types are often admixed in typical chromophobe RCCs

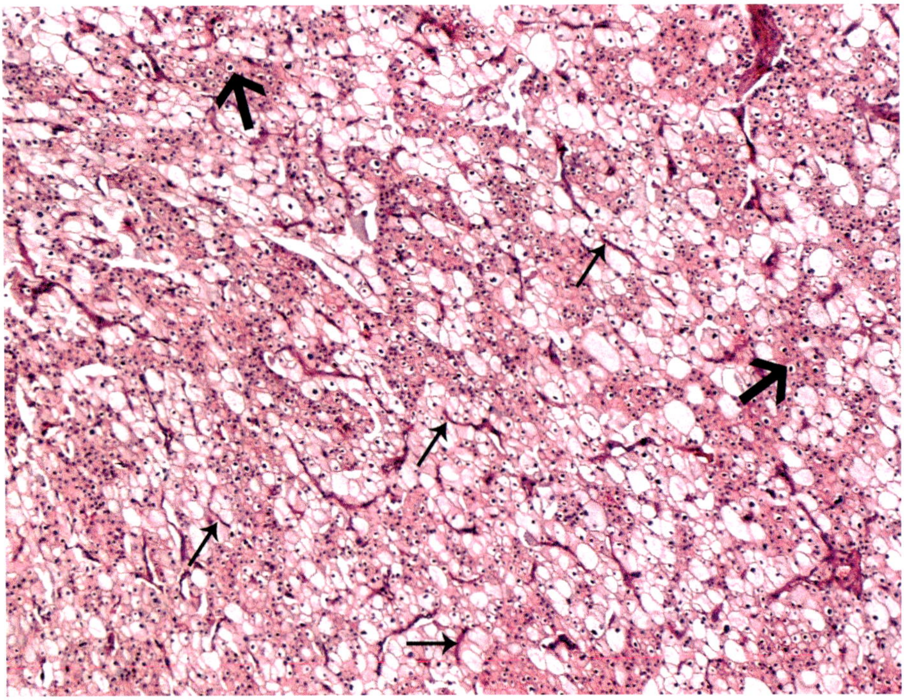

Fig. 1.78 (H-E, ×50) As in the majority of chromophobe RCCs, this tumor shows a mixture of the classic, plant-like cells and the smaller, eosinophilic-type cells with fine oxyphilic granularity. Perinuclear haloes are observed in eosinophilic cells (*thick arrows*). Eosinophilic cells tend to be located in the center, distal to septations, while clear cells at periphery of the sheets or nests. Thin, *incomplete* hyalinized fibrovascular septa are observed in chromophobe RCC (*thin arrows*) (in contrast, clear cell RCC shows intricate, branching vasculature and complete septa, at least focally)

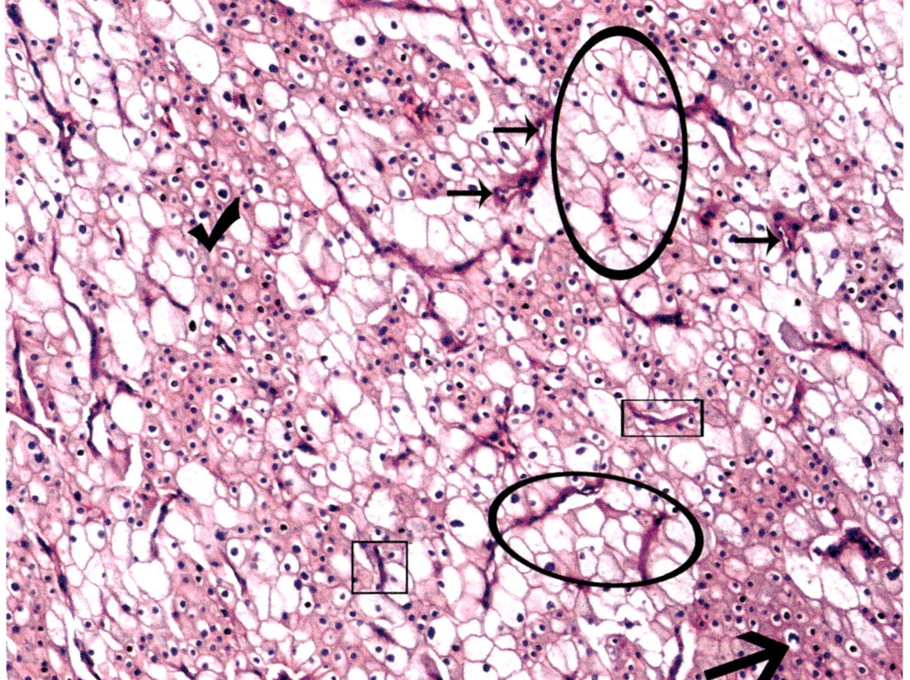

Fig. 1.79 (H-E, ×100) Incomplete septa (*square frames*) that do not completely surround cell nests or alveoli. Unlike clear cell RCC, the blood vessels in chromophobe RCC are often thick-walled and hyalinized (*small arrows*).

A mixture of the two cell types of chromophobe RCC, as often occurs.

In the classic type, the neoplastic cells have abundant, finely reticular, vesicular cytoplasm with a more intense peripheral acidophilia, giving the cell borders a distinctive thick, "plant-like" appearance (*ellipses*). The cytoplasmic membranes appear prominent due to the concentration of cell organelles at the peripheral portion of the cytoplasm.

The smaller cells with eosinophilic granular cytoplasm (eosinophilic type) are essentially oncocytes, but have prominent perinuclear haloes due to microvesicles concentration around the nuclei. When the tumor is entirely composed of eosinophilic cells, it is diagnosed as the eosinophilic variant of chromophobe RCC (which may closely resemble oncocytoma).

The nuclei of both cell types are typically hyperchromatic and often wrinkled (*thick arrow*); this koilocytic-type atypia due to raisinoid nuclei is detected in both cell types. Nuclear contours may also be spherical and slightly pleomorphic (*tick*).

There are no clinical differences between the classic and eosinophilic variants of chromophobe RCC

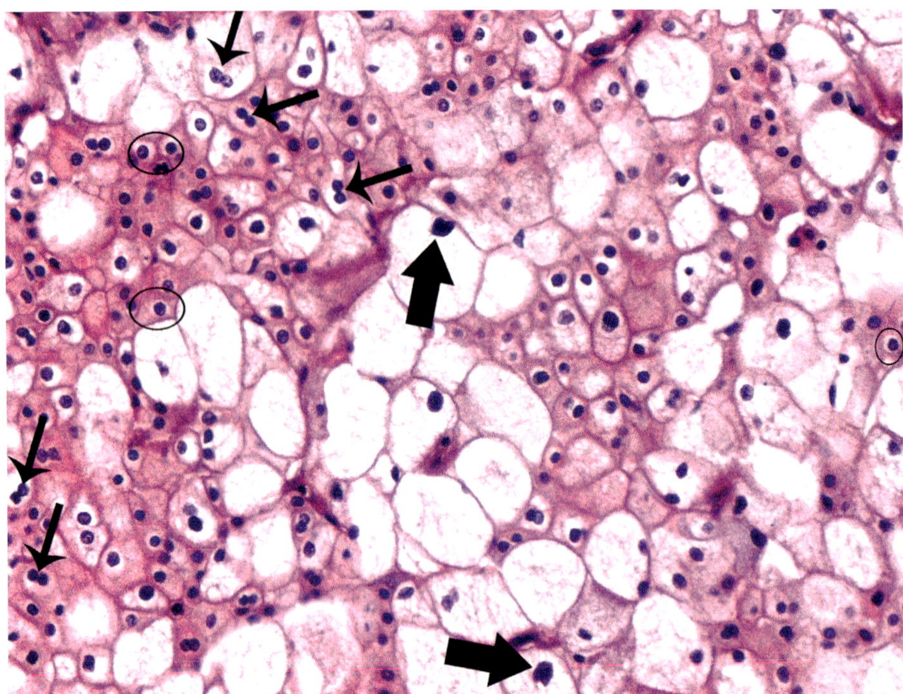

Fig. 1.80 (H-E, ×200) Binucleation (*thin arrows*) is common in chromophobe RCC. Wrinkled nuclear outlines are more prevalent in cells of the classic type (see ballooned-out "clear" cells, *thick arrows*). Unlike clear cell RCC, cytoplasm is not optically entirely clear but somewhat translucent and finely reticulated or irregularly granulated.

Perinuclear clarity (*haloes, ellipses*) are frequently present in the more eosinophilic cells; this feature can be of considerable diagnostic importance in their distinction from tumor cells of oncocytomas

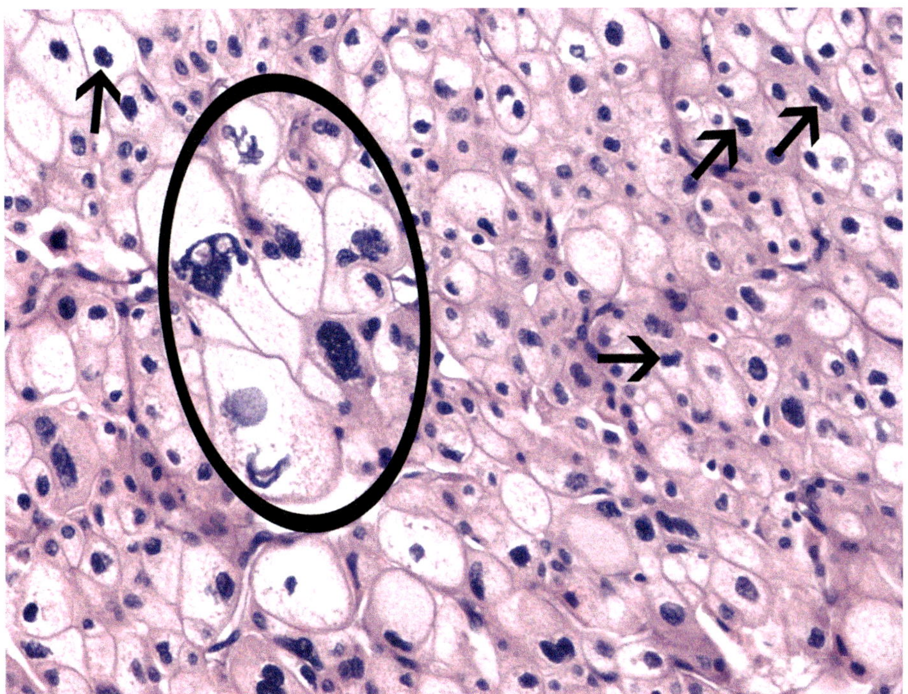

Fig. 1.81 (H-E, ×200) A focus with bizarre nuclei (*ellipse*).

Such foci of "degenerative" nuclear atypia with pleomorphism can be seen in 20% of oncocytomas (see Case 1.4. Fig. 1.68) but are rarely prominent in chromophobe RCCs.

Apart from this, sharply outlined plant-like cell membranes, voluminous, reticular, translucent to pale acidophilic cytoplasm and "raisinoid" nuclei (*arrows*) with perinuclear haloes, favor the diagnosis of chromophobe RCC. The nuclei of both classic and eosinophilic types of chromophobe RCC tend to be similar

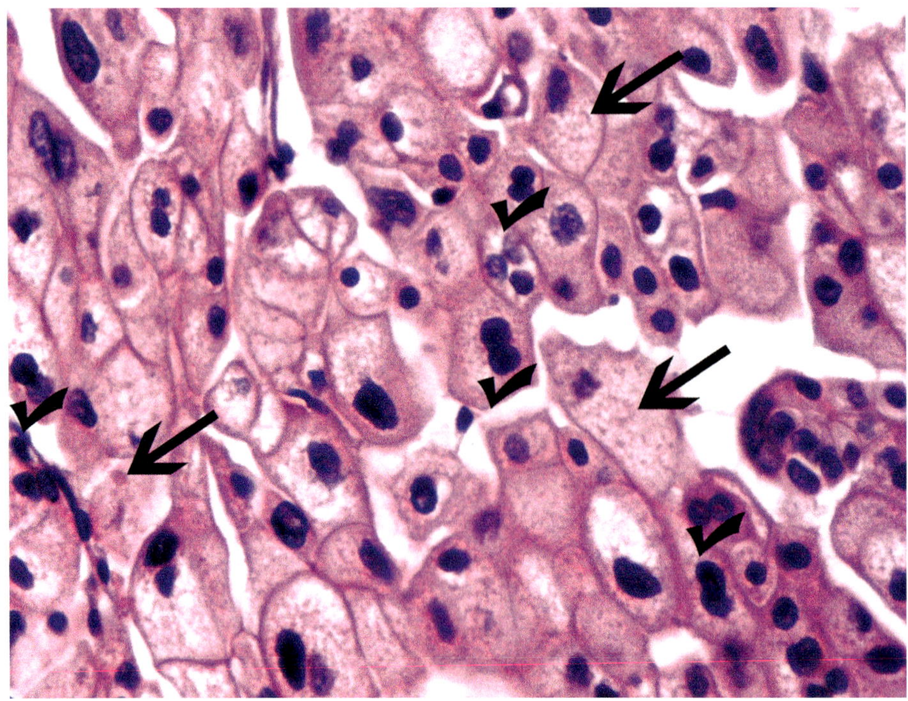

Fig. 1.82 (H-E, ×400) Thick cell walls resembling plant cells. Abundant, flocculent cytoplasm with frequent clumps of pink material in it (*arrows*). The "raisinoid" wrinkled appearance of many of the nuclei is a consistent feature of both cell types (classic and eosinophilic) of chromophobe RCC (mainly of the classic type, though). The WHO/ISUP nuclear/nucleolar grading is not appropriate for chromophobe RCC.

Binucleate cells are often seen (*ticks*), a feature that is rather rare in oncocytomas. Multinucleated cells are also more common in chromophobe RCC than in oncocytoma

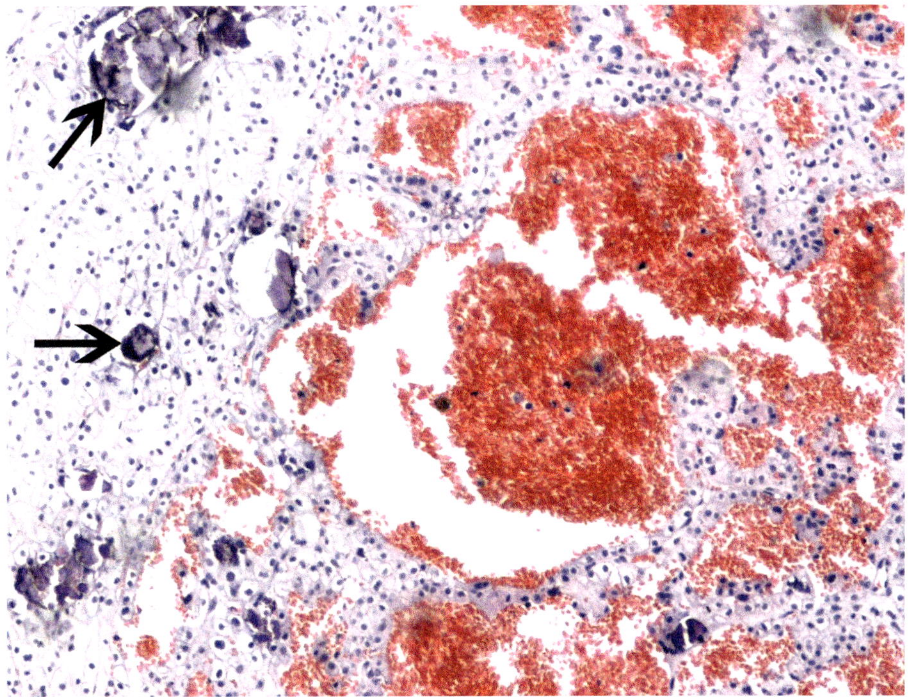

Fig. 1.83 (H-E, ×100) Calcification [small numbers of psammoma bodies (*arrows*) or irregular aggregates of finely granular calcium deposits] and small areas of hemorrhage (*image center*) may be present in chromophobe RC, but are not typical for this RCC subtype

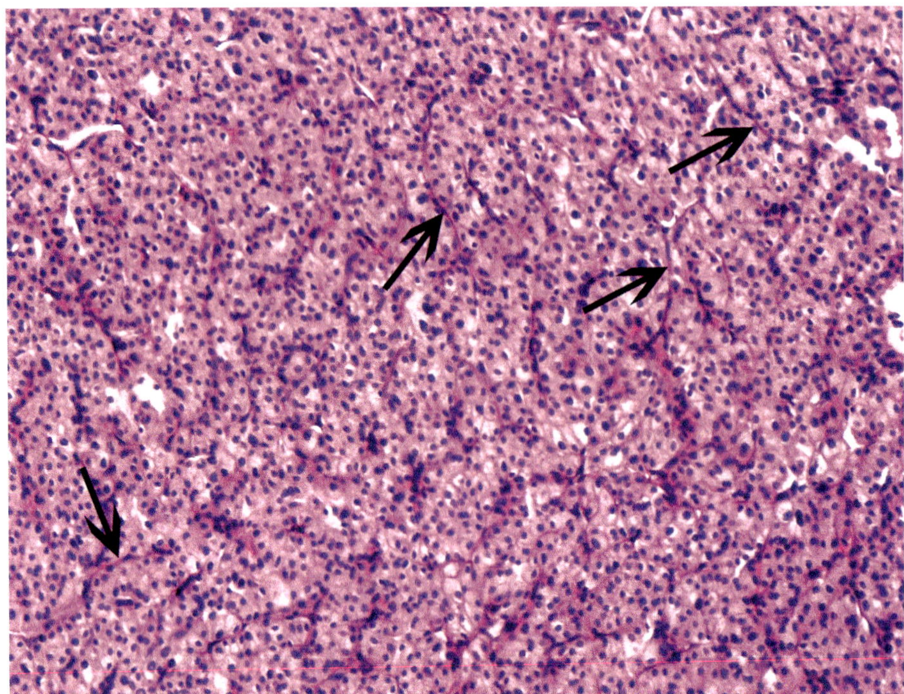

Fig. 1.84 (H-E, ×100) The cells of this eosinophilic area are essentially small oncocytes and have many of the features expected in an oncocytoma. Fibrous septa are observable in this field (*arrows*); thin and incomplete vascular septations *do not* completely encircle cell nests in chromophobe RCC

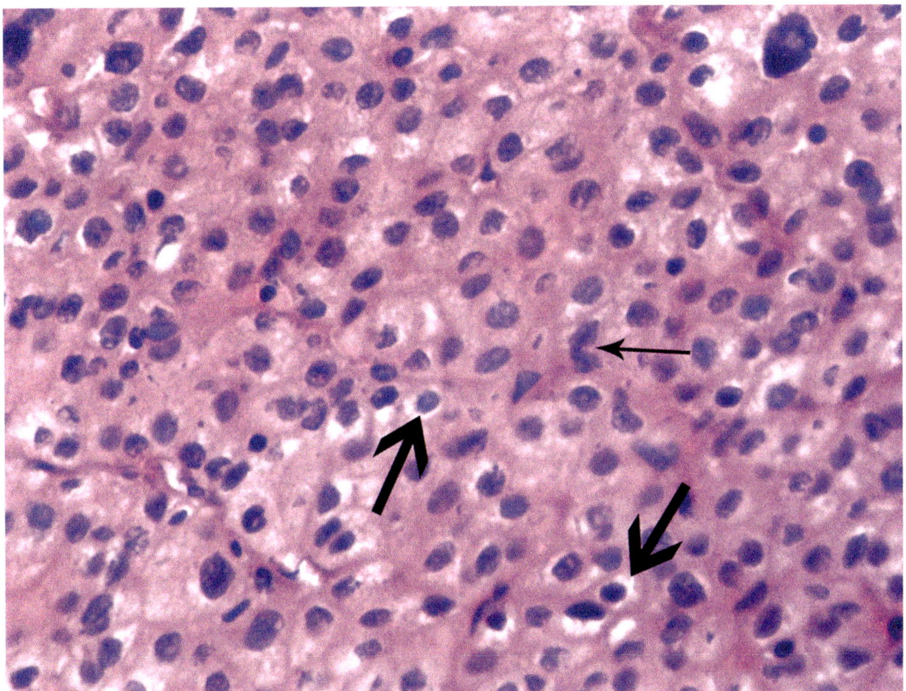

Fig. 1.85 (H-E, ×200) Sheet of predominantly eosinophilic, granular tumor cells intersected by delicate fibrous septa. Cell borders are not as hard as in the classic variant. Nuclei with irregular shape and focal perinuclear haloes (*thick arrows*) favor the diagnosis of the eosinophilic variant of chromophobe RCC; careful search in such areas is required. With regard to cellular morphology, most useful in distinguishing the eosinophilic variant of chromophobe RCC from an oncocytoma is the former's variation in nuclear size and irregularity in nuclear outline (*thin arrow*) as well as its diffusely positive immunostaining for cytokeratin 7. Nuclei in renal oncocytoma are round and uniform without koilocytic atypia; perinuclear haloes (and prominent cell membranes) are absent in oncocytoma.

Three types of cells can be encountered in chromophobe RCC, with the first two referring mostly to the eosinophilic variant and the last referring to the classic variant.

- Type 1 cells: small cells with solid, slightly granular eosinophilic cytoplasm
- Type 2 cells: perinuclear halo or translucent zone
- Type 3 cells: large, polygonal cells with hard cell borders, abundant cytoplasm with reticular pattern

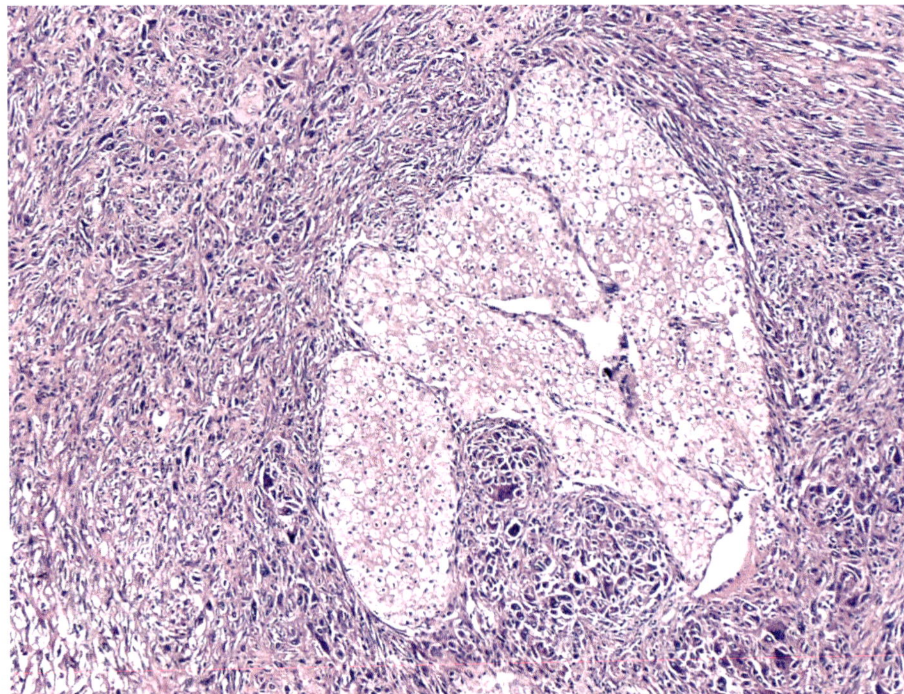

Fig. 1.86 (H-E, ×50) Another case, in which a focus of chromophobe RCC is surrounded by sarcomatoid elements. Chromophobe RCC is the subtype of RCC which, arguably, more often exhibits sarcomatoid dedifferentiation by comparison to other RCC subtypes; this feature considerably worsens the patient's prognosis (also see Case 1.1)

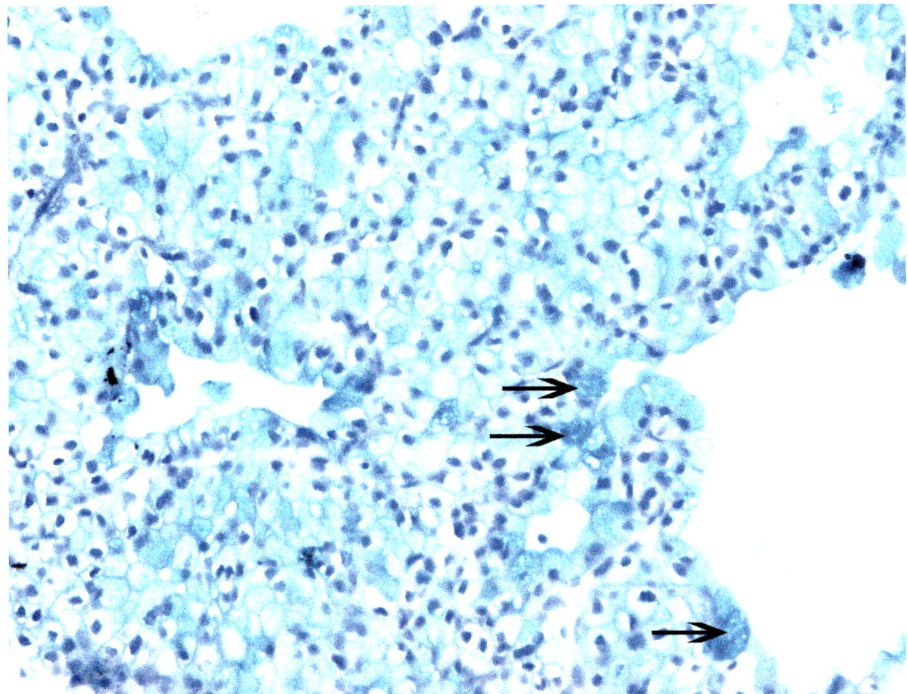

Fig. 1.87 (Hale's colloidal iron stain, ×100) Hale's colloidal iron stain stains acid mucopolysaccharides in microvesicles. *Variable* granular or reticular cytoplasmic staining is observed; an internal positive and negative control (i.e., glomeruli and renal tubules, respectively) is necessary in order to assess the staining reliably. *Cytoplasmic* positivity in several (not all) neoplastic cells of the classic variant of chromophobe RCC is observed here (*arrows*).

When successful, staining should be diffuse, intense, and reticular in character.

Hale's colloidal iron stain of the eosinophilic variant of chromophobe RCC usually shows cytoplasmic staining of weaker intensity.

Hale's colloidal iron staining results must always be used in conjunction with other findings in finalizing a diagnosis

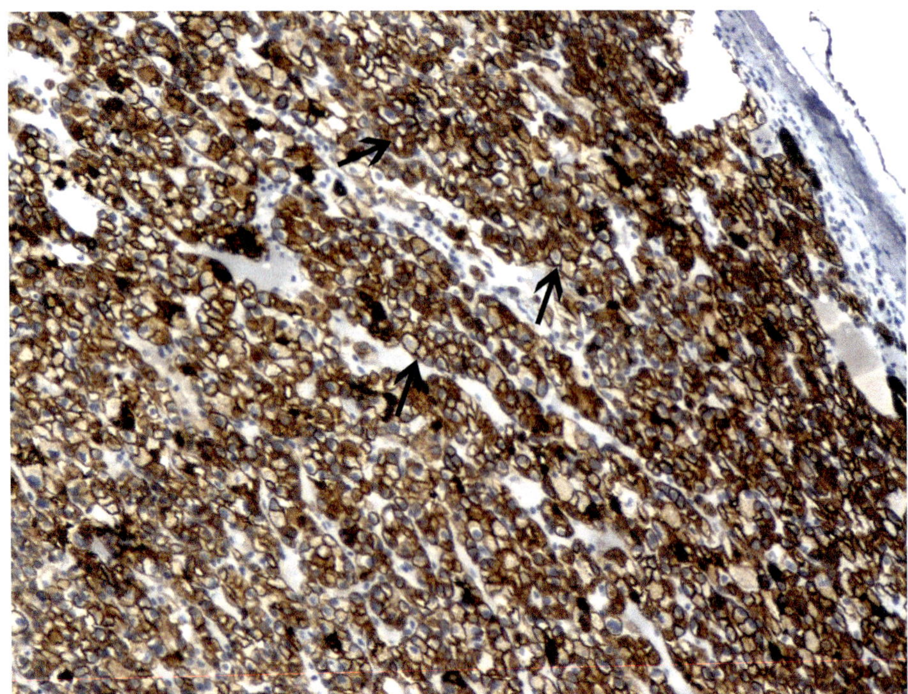

Fig. 1.88 (Cytokeratin 7 immunohistochemistry, ×50) *Diffuse, intense* immunoreactivity for cytokeratin 7 (CK7) is potentially helpful in distinguishing chromophobe RCC from oncocytoma; as such immunoreactivity is observed in >75% of chromophobe RCCs; in the eosinophilic variant, however, CK7 positivity is often less diffuse. The distinctive pseudomembrane-like pattern of accentuation (*arrows*) is due to compression of intermediate filaments toward the periphery of the cytoplasm.

Ksp-cadherin is also diffusely positive in the majority of chromophobe RCCs.

In contrast to low molecular weight cytokeratin, high molecular weight cytokeratins, S100A, and CAIX are not generally expressed in chromophobe RCC. Ki67 labeling index is low.

The most useful, suggested markers in distinguishing between chromophobe and clear cell RCC are CK7, KIT (CD117), parvalbumin, E-cadherin, RCC antigen, CD10, and vimentin; the former four are expected to be positive in chromophobe RCC and negative in clear cell RCC, while the latter three, vice versa. RCC antigen may be variably positive in chromophobe RCC, though. As always, the role of immunohistochemistry is complementary to morphology. Clear cell RCC has no koilocytic nuclear atypia or prominent cell membranes.

Apart from oncocytoma and clear cell carcinoma, chromophobe RCC should be distinguished from succinate dehydrogenase-deficient RCC, a rare tumor composed of vacuolated eosinophilic to clear cells, with flocculent cytoplasmic vacuoles with a pale eosinophilic, wispy or bubbly appearance and low grade nuclei (at least focally), and defined by the loss of immunohistochemical expression of SDHB – a marker of dysfunction of mitochondrial complex II (Moch et al. 2016)

1.6.1.1 Clinical Commentary

Vasileios Spapis

This is a case of chromophobe RCC, the third most common subtype of renal cancer accounting for about 2–5% of all RCC cases. This subtype of RCC appears to derive from the collecting ducts and is typically associated with loss of chromosomes 2, 10, 13, 17, and 21 (Vera-Badillo et al. 2012). The WHO/ISUP nuclear/nucleolar grading system does not apply to chromophobe RCC due to its innate nuclear atypia. A special histopathological grading system has been proposed, instead (Paner et al. 2010; Cheville et al. 2012).

Chromophobe RCC is considered to be a subtype with favorable prognosis compared to clear cell RCC (Volpe et al. 2012). Patients tend to present at a lower stage of the disease. Tumors seem to remain localized despite growth to large size. There is also predominance of "low-grade" disease, according to the proposed grading systems. There's one great exception though: presence of sarcomatoid features or metastasis suggests poor prognosis for this subset of patients (Campbell and Lane 2012).

Only 16.9% of patients with chromophobe RCC present with advanced disease at diagnosis (T3–4,M+,N+). These cases seem to have poor response to IL-2, and only mTor inhibitors seem to have some effectiveness. It should be mentioned though that most published trials have selected the clear cell RCC subtype, thus no robust evidence-based recommendations can be given for non-clear cell RCC subtypes (Ljungberg 2016). For the patients with locally confined disease, cancer-specific survival remains well above 90%, 5 years after undergoing surgery (Cindolo et al. 2005).

Key Messages

- Separation between chromophobe and clear cell RCC is essential because of relatively indolent clinical behavior and significantly better prognosis of chromophobe RCC.
- It is important to look for foci with perinuclear haloes to make diagnosis of chromophobe RCC.
- Chromophobe RCCs and oncocytomas share some common features; the difference in the appearance of the nuclei is important for their distinction.
- Chromophobe RCC cannot be graded according to the WHO/ISUP system, because of its innate nuclear atypia.

1.7 Case 1.6 Renal Angiomyolipoma

Case Study

Data Prior to Microscopy

Female patient, 54 years old, with hematuria and acute flank pain due to a palpable renal mass and with signs of acute retroperitoneal hemorrhage. By computerized tomography, the lesion was diagnosed an angiomyolipoma, the most common mesenchymal tumor of the kidney with benign clinical behavior in the overwhelming majority of cases. Conservative surgery was under consideration, but the tumor size and complication rendered it impossible.

Macroscopically, the tumor arose in the kidney cortex as an isolated, lobular, well-demarcated but nonencapsulated mass, bulging into the perirenal fat, with a maximum diameter of 9.4 cm and a pinkish tan and focally yellow cut surface, when not hemorrhagic.

1.7.1 Microscopic Evaluation of the Total Nephrectomy Specimen

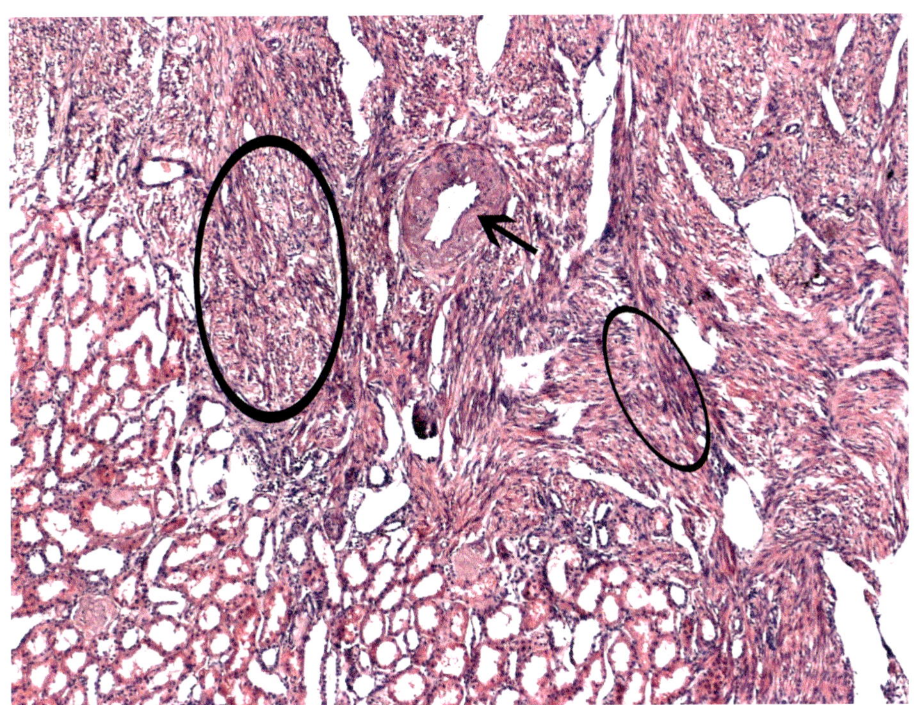

Fig. 1.89 (H-E, ×50) A rather sharp, pushing tumor border. A minimal intermingling of tumor and native renal tubules is implied. Smooth muscle predominance with fascicle arrangement (*ellipses*).

Some angiomyolipomas resemble leiomyomas as they are composed almost entirely of smooth muscle cells; when thin-walled vessels coexist, hemangiopericytoma-like architecture can be observed. The characteristic thick-walled vessel (*arrow*) favors the diagnosis of angiomyolipoma which can be confirmed by immunohistochemistry (HMB45 immunopositivity; see below).

Primary smooth muscle tumors of the kidney are extremely rare; immunohistochemical staining for melanocytic markers is thus a reasonable approach in order to rule out a smooth muscle-predominant angiomyolipoma

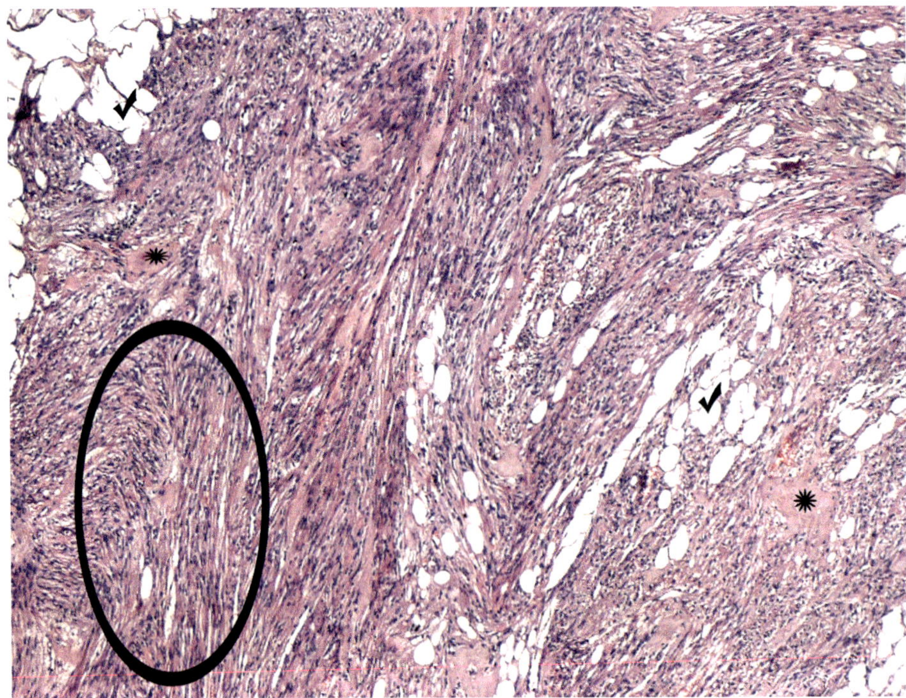

Fig. 1.90 (H-E, ×50) The predominant muscular tissue is fully differentiated, here rather hypercellular, and arranged in interlacing fascicles of spindle cells (*ellipse*); the latter can be replaced by dense fibrous connective tissue (*asterisks*) of irregular thickness. The angiomyolipoma lipomatous component can be focal and typically consists of mature adipose tissue (*ticks*)

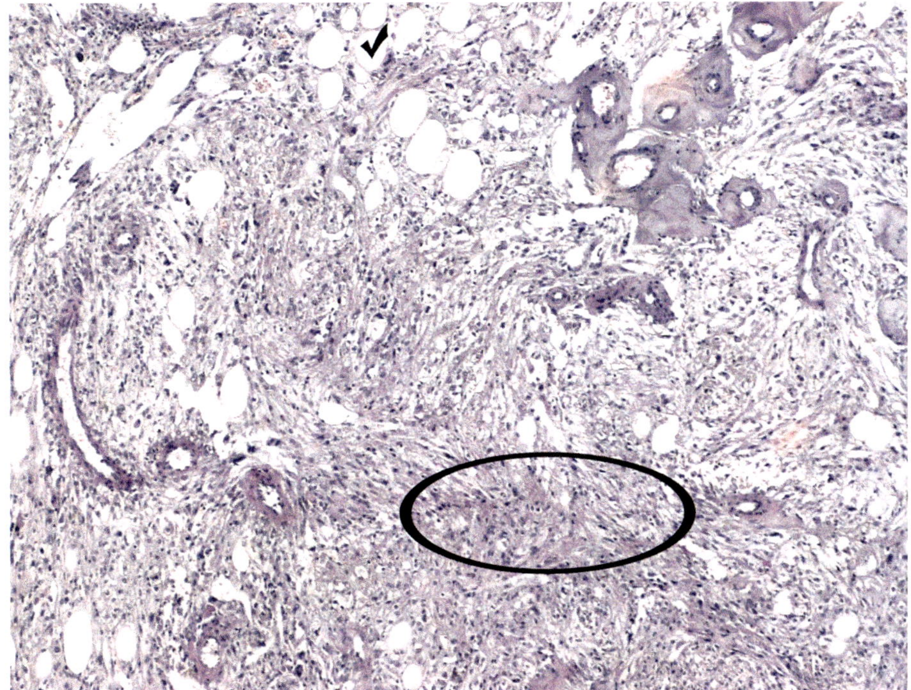

Fig. 1.91 (H-E, ×50) The classic *triphasic* histology of angiomyolipoma: mature *fat* (*tick*), thick-walled, poorly organized *blood vessels* with eccentric lumina and devoid of elastic laminae (*upper right part of the image*) and *smooth muscle* (*ellipse*), in varying proportion. The dysmorphic blood vessels of angiomyolipoma lack the normal internal elastic laminae of arteries and, when such blood vessels are prominent, they may resemble a vascular malformation (arterialized veins)

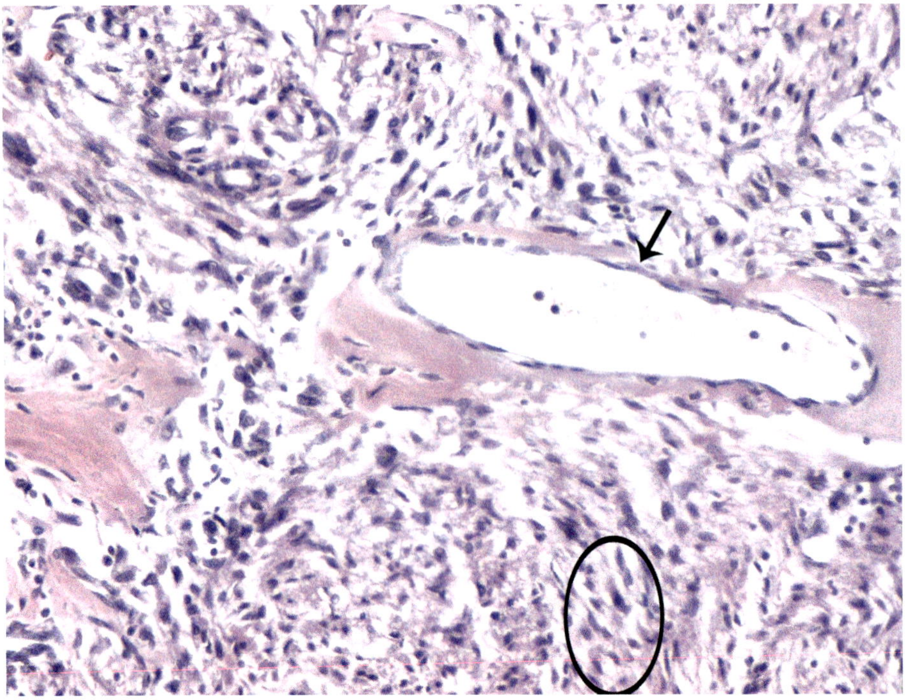

Fig. 1.92 (H-E, ×200) Blood vessel wall, focally thinned (*arrow*) and lacking muscular tissue. The surrounding myoid cells are spindle (*ellipse*), as most commonly occurs in angiomyolipomas, and appear to originate from vessel walls

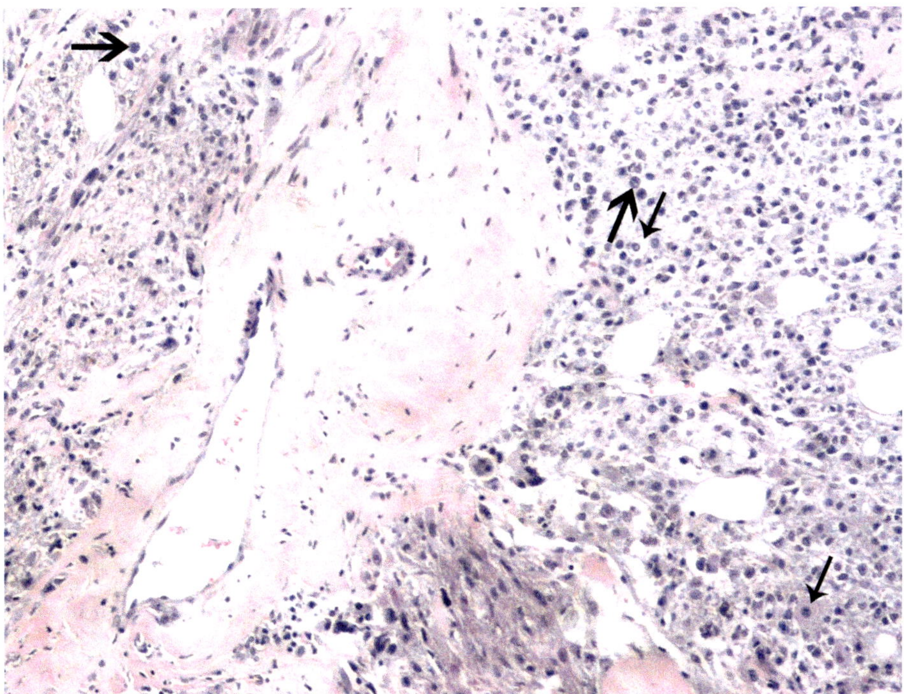

Fig. 1.93 (H-E, ×100) Angiomyolipoma belongs to a family of lesions called perivascular epithelioid cell tumors (PEComas), which are characterized by the proliferation of perivascular *epithelioid* cells. The perivascular epithelioid cell is thought to be the cell of origin of angiomyolipomas.

The smooth muscle cells appear to emanate from the dystrophic blood vessel's thick, hyalinized wall, possibly in a radial pattern or as a collar. A sheet of *epithelioid* smooth muscle cells is formed, with cells having abundant eosinophilic or clear cytoplasm (*thin arrows*) and large nuclei (*thick arrows*)

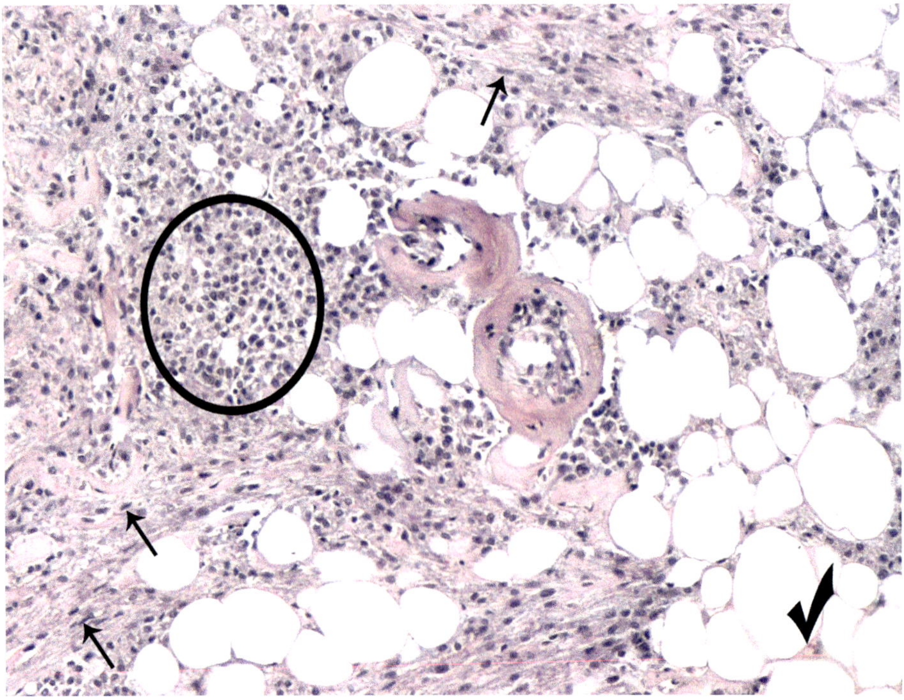

Fig. 1.94 (H-E, ×100) In addition to spindle-shaped smooth muscle cells, the smooth muscle cells of the angiomyolipoma can focally be rounded epithelioid cells (*ellipse*), occasionally simulating clear cell RCC, rich in granular/eosinophilic cells. Melanocytic markers' immunostaining is helpful for the correct diagnosis. A distinct adipocytic component in the form of islands of mature adipose tissue (*tick*) also favors the diagnosis of angiomyolipoma. Angiomyolipomas predominantly composed of adipose tissue may be confused with well-differentiated liposarcoma or other lipomatous tumors. The presence of even rare, dysmorphic, thick-walled blood vessels (image center) and focal spindle cells (*arrows*) is an important clue to the diagnosis of angiomyolipoma; in addition, careful evaluation for even focal melanocytic markers' immunostaining is imperative. With regard to a predominant fatty tissue component of an angiomyolipoma, the pathologist must recognize that fatty tissue is part of the lesion, and not interpret it as invasion into perirenal adipose tissue

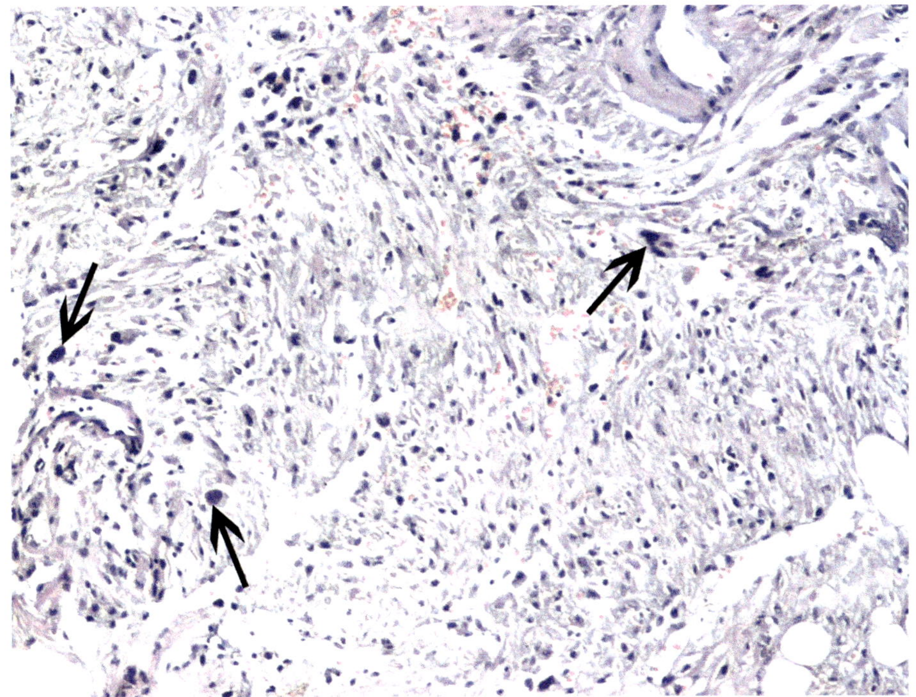

Fig. 1.95 (H-E, ×100) Some degree of nuclear atypia (*arrows*) is not uncommonly observed in scattered cells of the smooth muscle component of an angiomyolipoma. Paucity of mitotic figures, despite cytologic atypia, distinguishes angiomyolipoma from malignant spindle cell neoplasms, e.g., RCC with sarcomatoid dedifferentiation and sarcoma. Angiomyolipoma typically lacks the degree of anaplasia and mitotic figures seen in the latter tumors, which, furthermore, unlike angiomyolipoma, lack triphasic appearance, are poorly circumscribed with clearly infiltrative borders, and do not express melanocytic markers, immunohistochemically. Nevertheless, the pathologist must sample angiomyolipomas extensively to rule out the presence of a *coexisting* RCC. Striking degrees of nuclear atypia, when seen in *epithelioid* muscle cells, raise the possibility of malignancy in an angiomyolipoma. Angiomyolipomas composed of highly pleomorphic cells that show high mitotic activity and numerous foci of necrosis should be considered potentially malignant.

On the other hand, interestingly, invasion of muscular veins has no adverse influence on prognosis, if the tumor is an otherwise typical angiomyolipoma. The same applies to regional lymph nodes which occasionally contain classic angiomyolipomas due to tumor multicentricity and consequential possible extrarenal involvement without any aggressive behavior. Multifocality and bilaterality are rather common in angiomyolipomas; the presence of multiple angiomyolipomas is strong evidence that the patient has tuberous sclerosis.

Epithelioid angiomyolipoma is a potentially malignant mesenchymal neoplasm capable of invasion and metastasis, characterized by proliferation of predominantly epithelioid cells with clear or eosinophilic cytoplasm; the latter often shows fine vacuolization. Epithelioid angiomyolipoma is closely related to the triphasic (classic) angiomyolipoma (composed of a variable proportion of adipose tissue, spindle and epithelioid smooth muscle cells, and abnormal, thick-walled blood vessels); therefore, epithelioid angiomyolipoma expresses *melanocytic markers* [e.g., HMB45, Melan-A, (but not S100 protein, in most cases, including those of metastatic epithelioid angiomyolipoma)] with variable coexpression of smooth muscle markers, while epithelial markers are expectedly negative. It is noteworthy that when epithelioid angiomyolipoma recurs, HMB45 may be negative due to dedifferentiation. *Severe* (not moderate) *nuclear pleomorphism* with enlarged vesicular nuclei, often with prominent nucleoli, is usually detected in eosinophilic cells of *epithelioid* angiomyolipoma; such tumors were thus initially misdiagnosed as high-grade carcinomas, particularly in frozen sections. Angiomyolipomas with *epithelioid* features must be distinguished from RCC and melanoma; the immunopositivity of RCCs for epithelial markers and the immunopositivity of melanomas for S100 protein provide important diagnostic assistance

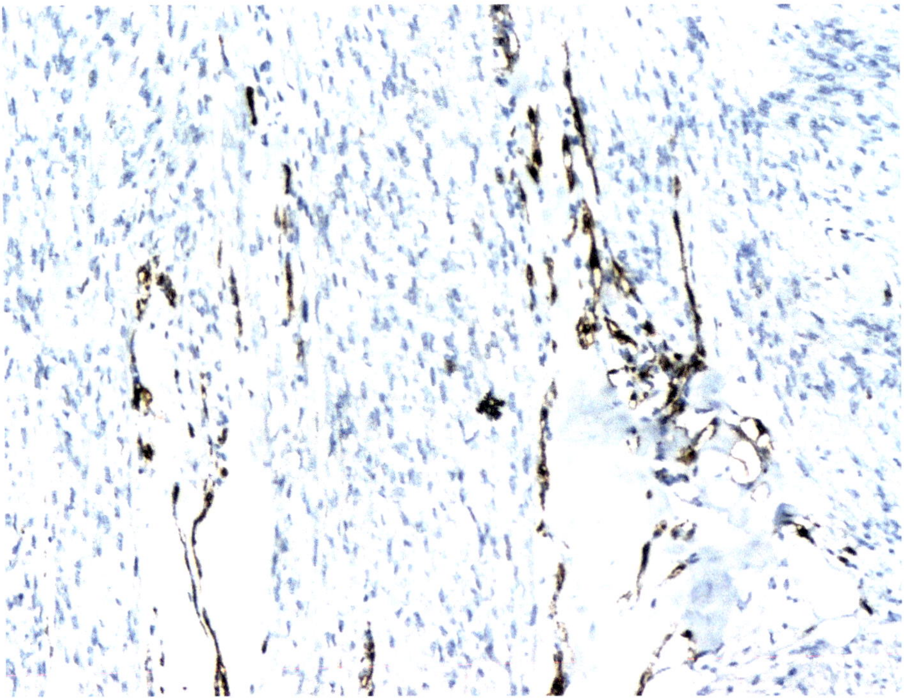

Fig. 1.96 (HMB45 immunohistochemistry, ×100) Focal immunopositivity. Angiomyolipoma cells are invariably positive for melanocytic markers except for S100 protein; in particular, those cells of epithelioid morphology show stronger melanocytic markers' expression. HMB45 and Melan-A can be positive in fat, smooth muscle and blood vessel components, often with only very focal positivity

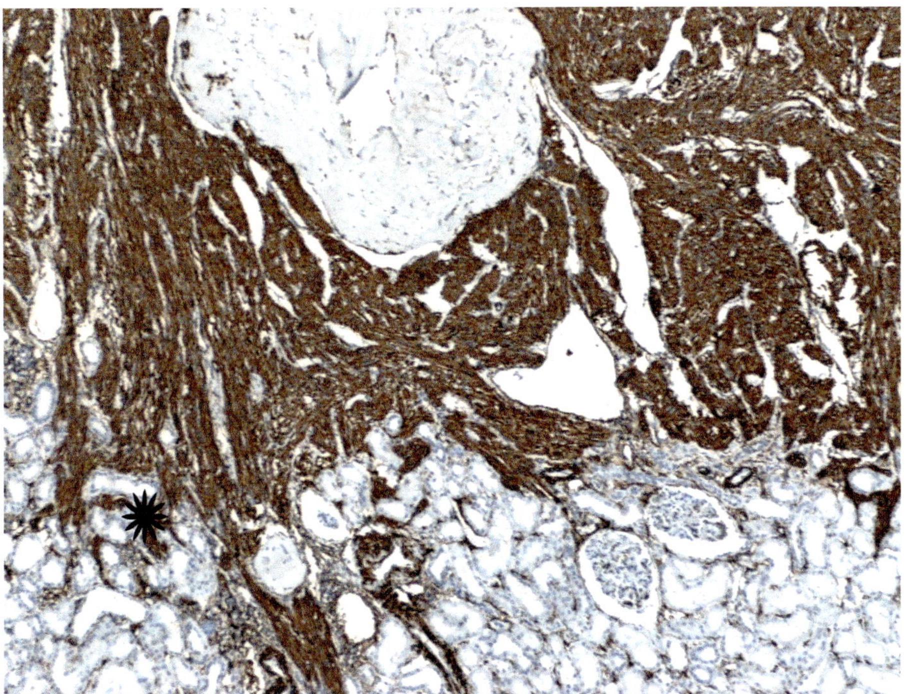

Fig. 1.97 [Smooth muscle actin (SMA) immunohistochemistry, ×50] Diffuse, SMA-immunopositive smooth muscle tumor elements.

Some renal tubules (*asterisk*) appear to be entrapped at the periphery of this angiomyolipoma.

Angiomyolipomas are characterized by *coexpression of melanocytic markers* [HMB45, Melan-A (MART-1), tyrosinase, and microphthalmia transcription factor (MiTF)] *and smooth muscle markers* (actins, desmin, h-caldesmon, and calponin). KIT and vimentin positivity have also been described. *Epithelial markers* including cytokeratins and epithelial membrane antigen are *negative*, except in areas with coexistent epithelial cysts, which may occasionally be encountered in angiomyolipomas. RCC antigen and CD10 are also negative in angiomyolipoma; CD10 as well as progesterone receptors may be positive in the stroma around the before mentioned epithelial cysts, but not in the other angiomyolipoma components

1.7.1.1 Clinical Commentary

Vasileios Spapis

This is a case of renal angiomyolipoma (AML) complicated with bleeding. AML is a benign mesenchymal tumor. It accounts for less than 10% of all renal tumors and about 1% of surgically removed tumors (Eble 1998, Ljungberg 2016). It is more often seen in women and the women/men ratio is about 4:1. It can occur sporadically or within the context of tuberous sclerosis (TS). In patients without TS, angiomyolipomas tend to be unilateral and larger than those associated with TS. AMLs are found in approximately 45–80% of patients with TS, where typically they are bilateral and asymptomatic (Konety et al. 2013); they also present at a younger age (mean age 30 years) and have less female to male predominance (2:1) (Margulis et al. 2012). TS is a familial inherited disorder which presents with the classic triad of adenoma sebaceum, mental retardation, and epilepsy.

AMLs are usually unencapsulated, yellow/gray tumors, mostly round, that push the renal capsule giving the impression of a bulging smooth mass. They are typically asymptomatic, with a slow and consistent growth rate, and minimal morbidity. There is though a 25% of cases that present with spontaneous rupture and bleeding in the retroperitoneum or into the urinary collection system, and sometimes this can be life-threatening (Ramon et al. 2009). Renal insufficiency can be another complication, when AMLs are large and multiple.

Like RCC, AMLs are usually diagnosed incidentally. AML is the only benign renal tumor that is confidently diagnosed on cross-sectional imaging. The presence of fat cells in a renal tumor is considered diagnostic. Ultrasonography and CT scanning seem to be the most helpful examinations. Despite its characteristic radiographic appearance, diagnosis can sometimes be difficult and confusing in cases of liposarcoma, fat-containing RCC, and fat-poor angiomyolipoma resembling a RCC (Margulis et al. 2012).

Active surveillance (AS) is the first approach of AMLs (Mues et al. 2010, Ouzaid et al. 2014). Tumor size >4 cm and presence of symptoms are considered risk factors for delayed intervention (Ouzaid et al. 2014). Selective arterial embolization is the first option when AS is discontinued; it can control the loss of blood during bleeding and reduces tumor size but has limited long-term efficacy (Murray et al. 2015). When surgery is decided, most AMLs can be treated with nephron sparing surgery (NSS) although sometimes tumor size and location require complete removal of the kidney. Using mTor inhibitors could be a promising alternative to surgery and a phase II trial is showing 81% response to everolimus by week 96 (Bissler et al. 2016).

Key Messages

- Angiomyolipoma is a significant tumor that can predispose to life-threatening complications, the most significant being hemorrhage, especially as far as large tumors are concerned.
- Classic angiomyolipoma is occasionally seen in the renal vein or in regional lymph nodes, but this is not a sign of malignant transformation.

References

Algaba F (2013) Immunohistochemistry in renal cell carcinoma. What's new?-What's new in uropathology? Handout. Working group symposium. 25th European Congress of Pathology. ESP

Algaba F, Akaza H, Lopez-Beltran A, Martignoni G et al (2011) Current pathologic keys of renal cell Carcinoma. Eur Urol 60(4):634–643

Armstrong AJ, Halabi S, Eisen T et al (2016) Everolimus versus sunitinib for patients with metastatic non-clear cell renal cell carcinoma (ASPEN): a multicentre, open-label, randomised phase 2 trial. Lancet Oncol 17:378–388

Bissler JJ, Kingswood JC, Radzikowska E et al (2016) Everolimus for renal angiomyolipoma in patients with tuberous sclerosis complex or sporadic lymphangioleiomyomatosis: extension of a randomized controlled trial. Nephrol Dial Transplant 31(1):111–119

Campbell S, Lane B (2012) Malignant renal tumors. In: Kavoussi L, Novick A, Partin A, Peters C (eds) Campbell-Walsh urology, 10th edn. Saunders, Philadelphia, pp 1413–1474

Cheville JC, Lohse CM, Sukov WR et al (2012) Chromophobe renal cell carcinoma: the impact of tumor grade on outcome. Am J Surg Pathol 36:851–856

Choueiri TK, Escudier B, Powles T et al (2015) Cabozantinib versus everolimus in advanced renal-cell carcinoma. N Engl J Med 373:1814–1823

Choueiri TK, Escudier B, Powles T et al (2016) Cabozantinib versus everolimus in advanced renal cell carcinoma (METEOR): final results from a randomised, open label, phase 3 trial. Lancet Oncol 17:917–927

Cindolo L, de la Taille A, Schips L et al (2005) Chromophobe renal cell carcinoma: comprehensive analysis of 104 cases from multicenter European database. Urology 65(4):681–686

Clague J, Lin J, Cassidy A et al (2009) Family history and risk of renal cell carcinoma: results from a case-control study and systematic meta-analysis. Cancer Epidemiol Biomark Prev 18(3):801–807

Crépel M, Jeldres C, Perrotte P et al (2010) Nephron-sparing surgery is equally effective to radical nephrectomy for T1BN0M0 renal cell carcinoma: a population-based assessment. Urology 75: 271–275

Eble JN (1998) Angiomyolipoma of kidney. Semin Diagn Pathol 15(1):21–40

Escudier B, Eisen T, Stadler WM et al (2007a) Sorafenib in advanced clear-cell renal-cell carcinoma. N Engl J Med 356:125–134

Escudier B, Pluzanska A, Koralewski P et al (2007b) Bevacizumab plus interferon alfa-2a for treatment of metastatic renal cell carcinoma: a randomised, double-blind phase III trial. Lancet 370:2103–2111

Escudier B, Porta C, Schmidinger M et al (2016) Renal cell carcinoma: ESMO clinical practice guidelines for diagnosis, treatment and follow up. Ann Oncol 27(Suppl.5):v58–v68

Heng DY, Xie W, Regan MM et al (2009) Prognostic factors for overall survival in patients with metastatic renal cell carcinoma treated with vascular endothelial growth factor-targeted agents: results from a large, multicenter study. J Clin Oncol 27:5794–5799

Heng DY, Xie W, Regan MM et al (2013) External validation and comparison with other models of the International Metastatic Renal- Cell Carcinoma Database Consortium prognostic model: a population-based study. Lancet Oncol 14:141–148

Hes O, Petersson F, Kuroda N et al (2013) Renal hybrid oncocytic/chromophobe tumors- A review. Histol Histopathol 28:1257–1264

Hock LM, Lynch J, Balaji KC (2002) Increasing incidence of all stages of kidney cancer in the last 2 decades in the United States: an analysis of surveillance, epidemiology and end results program data. J Urol 167(1):57–60

Hudes G, Carducci M, Tomczak P et al (2007) Temsirolimus, interferon alfa, or both for advanced renal-cell carcinoma. N Engl J Med 356:2271–2281

Jayson M, Sanders H (1998) Increased incidence of serendipitously discovered renal cell carcinoma. Urology 51:203–205

Junker K, Ficarra V, Kwon ED et al (2012) Potential role of genetic markers in the management of kidney cancer. Eur Urol 63(2):333–340

Kantarjian HM, Wolff RA (eds) (2010) The MD Anderson manual of medical oncology Chapter 35, 3rd edn. McGraw-Hill Medical, New York, p 916

Konety B, Vaena D, Williams R (2013) Renal parenchymal neoplasms. In: McAninch J, Lue T (eds) Smith and Tanagho's general urology, 18th edn. McGraw-Hill, New York, pp 330–340

Levi F, Ferlay J, Galeone C et al (2008) The changing pattern of kidney cancer incidence and mortality in Europe. BJU Int 101(8):949–958

Ljungberg B (2016) Renal cell carcinoma. In: European Association of Urology Guidelines. European Association of Urology. Available via https://uroweb.org/guideline/renal-cell-carcinoma. Accessed 26 Feb 2017

Magi-Galluzzi C, Zhou M (2010) Ureter, urinary bladder and kidney chapter 10. In: Gattuso P, Reddy VB, David O, Spitz DJ, Haber MH (eds) Differential diagnosis in surgical pathology, 2nd edn. Saunders, Elsevier, Philadelphia, pp 487–538

Margulis V, Matin S, Wood C (2012) Benign renal tumors. In: Kavoussi L, Novick A, Partin A, Peters C (eds) Campbell-Walsh urology, 10th edn. Saunders, Philadelphia, pp 1496–1501

Miller BA, Scoppa SM, Feuer EJ (2006) Racial/ethnic patterns in lifetime and age-conditional risk estimates for selected cancers. Cancer 106(3):670–682

Moch H, Humphrey PA, Ulbright TM, Reuter VE (eds) (2016) WHO classification of tumours of the urinary system and male genital organs. IARC, Lyon

Motzer RJ, Hutson TE, Tomczak P et al (2007) Sunitinib versus interferon alfa in metastatic renal-cell carcinoma. N Engl J Med 356:115–124

Motzer RJ, Escudier B, Oudard S et al (2008) Efficacy of everolimus in advanced renal cell carcinoma: a double-blind, randomised, placebo-controlled phase III trial. Lancet 372:449–456

Motzer RJ, Hutson TE, Cella D et al (2013) Pazopanib versus sunitinib in metastatic renal cell carcinoma. N Engl J Med 369:722–731

Motzer RJ, Barrios CH, Kim TM et al (2014a) Phase II randomized trial comparing sequential first-line everolimus and second-line sunitinib versus first-line sunitinib and second-line everolimus in patients with metastatic renal cell carcinoma. J Clin Oncol 32:2765–2772

Motzer RJ, Porta C, Vogelzang NJ et al (2014b) Dovitinib versus sorafenib for third-line targeted treatment of patients with metastatic renal cell carcinoma: an open-label, randomised phase 3 trial. Lancet Oncol 15:286–296

Motzer RJ, Escudier B, McDermott DF et al (2015) Nivolumab versus everolimus in advanced renal-cell carcinoma. N Engl J Med 373:1803–1813

Mues AC, Palacios JM, Haramis G et al (2010) Contemporary experience in the management of angiomyolipoma. J Endourol 24(11):1883–1886

Murphy WM, Grignon DJ, Perlman EJ (2004) Tumors of the kidney, bladder and related urinary structures AFIP Atlas of Tumor Pathology Series 4, Washington

Murray TE, Doyle F, Lee M (2015) Transarterial embolization of angiomyolipoma: a systematic review. J Urol 194(3):635–639

Novara G, Ficarra V, Antonelli A et al (2010) Validation of the 2009 TNM version in a large multi-institutional cohort of patients treated for renal cell carcinoma: are further improvements needed? Eur Urol 58:588–595

Ouzaid I, Autorino R, Fatica R et al (2014) Active surveillance for renal angiomyolipoma: outcomes and factors predictive of delayed intervention. BJU Int 114(3):412–417

Oxley JD, Sullivan J, Mitchelmore A et al (2007) Metastatic renal oncocytoma. J Clin Pathol 60(6):720–722

Paner GP, Turk TM, Clark JI, Lindgren V, Picken MM (2005) Passive seeding in metanephric adenoma: a review of pseudometastatic lesions in perinephric lymph nodes. Arch Pathol Lab Med 129(10):1317–1321

Paner GP, Amin MB, Alvarado-Cabrero I et al (2010) A novel tumor grading scheme for chromophobe renal cell carcinoma: prognostic utility and comparison with Fuhrman nuclear grade. Am J Surg Pathol 34:1233–1240

Pignot G, Elie C, Conquay S et al (2007) Survival analysis of 130 patients with papillary renal cell carcinoma: prognostic utility of type 1 and type 2 subclassification. Urology 69:230–235

Poulakis V, Witsch U, de Vries R et al (2003) Quality of life after surgery for localized renal cell carcinoma: comparison between radical nephrectomy and nephron-sparing surgery. Urology 62:814–820

Przybycin CG, McKenney JK, Reynolds JP et al (2014) Rhabdoid differentiation is associated with aggressive behavior in renal cell carcinoma: a clinicopathologic analysis of 76 cases with clinical follow-up. Am J Surg Pathol 38(9):1260–1265
Ramon J, Rimon U, Garniek A et al (2009) Renal angiomyolipoma: long-term results following selective arterial embolization. Eur Urol 55(5):1155–1161
Rini BI, Campbell SC, Escudier B (2009) Renal cell carcinoma. Lancet 373:1119–1132
Rini BI, Escudier B, Tomczak P et al (2011) Comparative effectiveness of axitinib versus sorafenib in advanced renal cell carcinoma (AXIS): a randomised phase 3 trial. Lancet 378:1931–1939
Romis L, Cindolo L, Patard JJ et al (2004) Frequency, clinical presentation and evolution of renal oncocytomas: Multicentric experience from a European database. Eur Urol 45:53–57
Ross H, Martignoni G, Argani P (2012) Renal cell carcinoma with clear cell and papillary features. Arch Pathol Lab Med 136:391–399
Sheth S, Scatarige JC, Horton KM et al (2001) Current concepts in the diagnosis and management of renal cell carcinoma: role of multidetector ct and three-dimensional CT. Radiographics 21:S237–S254
Srigley JR, Delahunt B, Eble JN et al (2013) The International Society of Urological Pathology (ISUP) Vancouver Classification of Renal Neoplasia. Am J Surg Pathol 37:1469–1489
Sternberg CN, Davis ID, Mardiak J et al (2010) (2010) Pazopanib in locally advanced or metastatic renal cell carcinoma: results of a randomized phase III trial. J Clin Oncol 28:1061–1068
Störkel S, Eble JN, Adlakha K et al (1997) Classification of renal cell carcinoma: Workgroup No. 1. Union Internationale Contre le Cancer (UICC) and the American Joint Committee on Cancer (AJCC). Cancer 80(5):987–989
Sukov WR, Lohse CM, Leibovich BC et al (2012) Clinical and pathological features associated with prognosis in patients with papillary renal cell carcinoma. J Urol 187(1):54–59
Tannir NM, Jonasch E, Albiges L et al (2016) Everolimus versus sunitinib prospective evaluation in metastatic non-clear cell renal cell carcinoma (ESPN): a randomized multicenter phase 2 trial. Eur Urol 69:866–874
Toro JR, Glenn G, Duray P et al (1999) Birt-Hogg-Dubé syndrome: A novel marker of kidney neoplasia. Arch Dermatol 135:1195–1202
Truong LD, Shen SS (2011) Immunohistochemical diagnosis of renal neoplasms. Arch Pathol Lab Med 135:92–109
Urge T, Hes O, Ferda J et al (2010) Typical signs of oncocytic papillary renal cell carcinoma in everyday clinical praxis. World J Urol 28:513–517
Van Poppel H, Da Pozzo L, Albrecht W et al (2011) A prospective, randomised EORTC intergroup phase 3 study comparing the oncologic outcome of elective nephron-sparing surgery and radical nephrectomy for low-stage renal cell carcinoma. Eur Urol 59:543–552
Vera-Badillo FE, Conde E, Duran I (2012) Chromophobe renal cell carcinoma: a review of an uncommon entity. Int J Urol 19:894–900
Volpe A, Novara G, Antonelli A et al (2012) Chromophobe renal cell carcinoma (RCC): oncological outcomes and prognostic factors in a large multicentre series. BJU Int 110:76–83
Wang H-Y, Mills SE (2005) KIT and RCC are useful in distinguishing chromophobe renal cell carcinoma from the granular variant of clear cell renal cell carcinoma. Am J Surg Pathol 29(5):640–646
Zhou M, Magi-Galluzzi C (2007) Genitourinary pathology, foundations in diagnostic pathology. Churchill Livingstone, Philadelphia

Clinical Pathology of the Urinary Bladder

George Agrogiannis, Christos Alamanis,
Eleni A. Karatrasoglou, Georgios Kousournas,
Andreas C. Lazaris, Vasileios Spapis,
Georgia-Eleni Thomopoulou, and Dionysia N. Zouki

A. C. Lazaris (ed.), *Clinical Genitourinary Pathology*,
https://doi.org/10.1007/978-3-319-72194-1_2

A pathologic report for transurethral resection of bladder tumor (TURBT) specimens should include the following information: layers of bladder wall represented, adequacy of material for determining T category of pTNM stage, surface denuded or ulcerated, rough tumor size, tumor configuration (papillary, flat, solid/nodular, invasive, ulcerated, undetermined), histologic type [conventional, urothelial carcinoma with/without squamous differentiation, squamous cell carcinoma, adenocarcinoma (classical or variant), small cell carcinoma, undifferentiated, mixed cell type, undetermined], histologic grade (based on tumor type), microscopic extent of tumor/invasion/pathologic staging (noninvasive flat carcinoma in situ, invasive carcinoma involving lamina propria, muscularis propria; the latter present, absent, or indeterminate), lymphovascular invasion (present, not identified, indeterminate; should be assessed away from the main tumor and only if unequivocal; often is overdiagnosed), extension in prostatic chips sampled by TURBT [involvement of prostatic urethra, prostatic acini, and ducts (by carcinoma in situ) or prostatic stroma (by invasive carcinoma)], associated epithelial lesions [urothelial papilloma (classic or inverted type), papillary urothelial neoplasm of low malignant potential, other], and additional findings (carcinoma in situ, dysplasia, metaplasia, hyperplasia, inflammation, regenerative changes, treatment-related changes, or other). Some of these features may be difficult to identify on small biopsies. It is also recommended to include clinically relevant historical information.

With regard to cystectomy (total/partial), cystoprostatectomy, and pelvic exenteration specimens, in addition to the above data, the following should be included: specimen type/procedure; tumor site and multifocality; exact tumor size; pTNM stage; surgical margin status (specify margins involved by invasive carcinoma or in situ carcinoma; if uninvolved by invasive carcinoma, specify distance from invasive carcinoma to margin); presence of tumor at margins of the urethra, ureter, paravesicular soft tissue, or pelvic soft tissue; and involvement of adjacent structures, perivesical fat, ureter (specify laterality), urethra, vagina, uterus and adnexae, pelvic sidewall (specify laterality), prostate, seminal vesicle (specify laterality), rectum, or others.

2.1 Introduction to Bladder Neoplastic Clinical Pathology

Christos Alamanis, Eleni A. Karatrasoglou, Georgios Kousournas, Dionysia N. Zouki, and Andreas C. Lazaris

The urothelium (formerly known as "transitional epithelium") is the epithelium that lines much of the urinary tract (including the surface of the renal pelvis, the ureters, the urinary bladder, and proximal parts of the urethra). It is stratified and composed of three types of cells: basal precursor cells, intermediate cells, and large superficial umbrella cells. Normally, it consists of less than approximately seven layers of urothelial cells covered by a single umbrella cell layer. Umbrella cells are large and elliptical with abundant eosinophilic cytoplasm and often binucleation or prominent nucleoli. Intermediate urothelial cells are cuboidal to low columnar with well-defined borders and amphophilic cytoplasm, rich in glycogen. They present regularly arranged, ovoid nuclei, finely granular chromatin, and small nucleoli. Usually, there are no mitotic figures. Basal urothelial cells are more cylindrical, some with longitudinal nuclear grooves. They lie on the continuous basal lamina. In normal or reactive urothelium, p53 is generally expressed by only a few cells and with weak intensity, whereas cytokeratin 20 expression is limited to the umbrella cell layer.

Carcinoma of the urinary bladder is the fourth most common malignancy in men, and more than 90% of cases are urothelial carcinoma.

2.1.1 Principals in Bladder Neoplastic Pathology

2.1.1.1 Benign Urothelial Neoplasms

Urothelial Papilloma and Diffuse Papillomatosis

Urothelial papilloma is a benign exophytic urothelial neoplasm. The most common symptom it causes is hematuria. This tumor consists of a discrete papillary growth with a central fibrovascular core lined by cytologically and architecturally normal urothelium. The superficial cells are often prominent.

The designation "diffuse papillomatosis" is applicable when the mucosa is extensively occupied by multiple small delicate papillary processes. The malignant potential of this lesion is uncertain.

Inverted Papilloma

Inverted papilloma is a rare benign tumor. Hematuria and obstruction are the most common symptoms at presentation. Histologically, it shows an inverted growth pattern, usually composed of anastomosing islands and trabeculae of histologically and cytologically normal urothelial cells, invaginating from the surface urothelium into the subjacent lamina propria but not into the muscularis propria.

2.1.1.2 Flat Intraepithelial Lesions

Flat Urothelial Hyperplasia (Simple Hyperplasia)

Urothelial hyperplasia refers to a nonneoplastic epithelial abnormality. Generally, it is asymptomatic and by itself, it has no malignant potential. It may occur adjacent to low-grade papillary tumors or as an isolated lesion. It is characterized by markedly thickened mucosa with an increase in the number of cell layers, usually to ten or more. The cells show no significant cytologic atypia.

Urothelial Reactive Atypia

Reactive (inflammatory) atypia consists of mild nuclear abnormalities occurring in acutely or chronically inflamed urothelium. Nuclei are uniformly enlarged and vesicular, with central, visible nucleoli. Mitotic figures may be frequent but always occur in the lower epithelial layers of the urothelium. Inflammation is almost always present.

Urothelial Atypia of Unknown Significance

Urothelial atypia of unknown significance includes those instances where a lesion cannot be confidently placed in the reactive versus dysplastic categories. Inflammation is often present, and nuclear changes are similar to those seen in reactive atypia. However, the degree of cytologic atypia is greater, and dysplasia cannot be definitely ruled out.

Urothelial Dysplasia (Low-Grade Intraurothelial Neoplasia)

Urothelial dysplasia is defined as abnormal urothelium with cytologic and architectural changes that do not meet all the criteria for an unequivocal diagnosis of urothelial carcinoma in situ. However, it shares some abnormalities with carcinoma in situ and therefore likely represents a precursor lesion.

Urothelial Carcinoma In Situ (High-Grade Intraurothelial Neoplasia)

Urothelial carcinoma in situ is defined as a flat urothelial lesion comprised of cytologically high-grade malignant cells, which may involve either full or partial thickness of the urothelium.

2.1.1.3 Urothelial (Transitional Cell) Carcinoma

Urothelial carcinoma is the most common type of bladder cancer and cancer of the ureter and urethra. The majority of bladder cancer patients present with hematuria and a significant proportion of them also have irritative voiding symptoms.

The initial evaluation and management for patients with suspected bladder cancer involve cystoscopic evaluation of the bladder and prostatic urethra for mucosal lesions. Small lesions and flat lesions worrisome for carcinoma in situ can be sampled with cold cup biopsy forceps, and larger suspicious lesions are resected transurethrally as completely as possible. Transurethral resections and biopsies should include muscularis propria, if possible.

Urothelial carcinomas are often multifocal, with 30–40% of patients having more than one tumor at diagnosis. In fact, multiple coexisting tumors often arise before clinical symptoms are apparent. The separate tumors may or may not share a similar histology.

Diagnostic and prognostic information includes histologic type, histologic grading (using WHO grading scheme: WHO 1973, WHO 2016, or both, Hansel et al. 2013), and staging (using TNM staging system).

Histologic grading is one of the most important prognostic factors in bladder cancer (Hansel et al. 2013). The first grading system for papillary urothelial neoplasms – 1973 WHO classification – divided urothelial tumors into four categories: papilloma, grade (G) 1 (G1) carcinoma, grade 2 (G2), and grade 3 (G3), according to the degree of cellular anaplasia. The new system 2016 WHO/ISUP classification separates noninvasive papillary urothelial neoplasms into four categories, designated papilloma, papillary urothelial neoplasm of low malignant potential (PUNLMP), low-grade carcinoma, and high-grade carcinoma. Nevertheless, urothelial neoplasms frequently demonstrate features of more than one grade. The grading is typically based on the worse grade present. However, cancer heterogeneity could have a significant impact on patient outcome. Pathologic stage (Cheng et al. 2009) is most critical for assessing patient prognosis.

At gross examination, most tumors present as a single, solid, polypoid mass. Histologically, the neoplastic cells invade the bladder wall as nests, cords, trabeculae, small clusters, or single cells.

Urothelial carcinoma has a propensity for divergent differentiation. Histological variants of urothelial carcinoma include:

- Urothelial carcinoma with mixed differentiation
- Urothelial carcinoma, nested variant
- Urothelial carcinoma, inverted variant
- Urothelial carcinoma, micropapillary variant
- Urothelial carcinoma, microcystic variant
- Lymphoepithelioma-like urothelial carcinoma
- Lymphoma-like/plasmacytoma-like urothelial carcinoma

- Urothelial carcinoma, clear cell variant
- Urothelial carcinoma, lipoid cell variant
- Urothelial carcinoma with syncytiotrophoblastic giant cells
- Sarcomatoid urothelial carcinoma (see below)
- Small cell carcinoma
- Large cell undifferentiated carcinoma
- Urothelial carcinoma with rhabdoid features
- Urothelial carcinoma with prominent stromal reaction

Some of these variants have a different clinical outcome, and therefore their recognition is important.

2.1.1.4 Glandular Neoplasms

Villous Adenoma

Villous adenoma is an uncommon benign glandular epithelium neoplasm with exophytic growth. Patients often present with hematuria and/or irritative symptoms. Histologically, it is composed of columnar, mucin-filled, goblet cells lining delicate fibrovascular stalks.

Adenocarcinoma

Adenocarcinoma of the bladder is defined as a primary malignant neoplasm showing histologically *pure* glandular phenotype and mucin-producing cells. Adenocarcinoma of the bladder may show different histologic patterns, and it is not uncommon to find a mixture of them.

2.1.1.5 Squamous Cell Neoplasms

Squamous Cell Carcinoma

Squamous cell carcinoma of the bladder is defined as a malignant neoplasm derived from the urothelium that shows a *pure* squamous cell phenotype. Several morphologic variants of this carcinoma, including verrucous, basaloid, and clear cell pattern, have been recognized.

2.1.1.6 Neuroendocrine Tumors

Small Cell Carcinoma

Small cell carcinoma is a rare malignant neuroendocrine neoplasm of the urothelium which histologically mimics its pulmonary counterpart. Clinical presentations include hematuria, irritative symptoms, or localized pain. The majority of patients have advanced stage disease when first diagnosed. In most of the cases, this tumor appears as a single large, solid, polypoid mass. Histologically, it consists of sheets or nests of small cells with scant cytoplasm and irregular, hyperchromatic nuclei. Necrosis is common and vascular invasion invariably present.

Large Cell Neuroendocrine Carcinoma

Large cell neuroendocrine carcinoma is a poorly differentiated and high-grade neuroendocrine tumor, morphologically identical to its counterpart in the lung. It presents a combination of histologic (neuroendocrine morphology and necrosis), cytologic (large cell size, abundant cytoplasm, nucleoli, coarse chromatin, high mitotic rate), and immunohistochemical evidence of neuroendocrine origin.

Carcinoid

Carcinoid is a potentially malignant neuroendocrine neoplasm derived from the urothelium. Hematuria is common, but irritative voiding symptoms may be the first symptom. Histologically, tumor cells have abundant amphophilic cytoplasm and are arranged in insular, acinar, trabecular, or pseudoglandular pattern with a delicate vascular stroma.

2.1.1.7 Sarcomatoid Carcinoma

The term "sarcomatoid carcinoma" applies when a malignant neoplasm exhibits morphologic or immunohistochemical evidence of both epithelial and mesenchymal differentiation. The gross appearance is characteristically "sarcoma-like," with a dull gray fleshy cut surface and infiltrative margins. The tumors are often polypoid and tend to form large intraluminal masses. Microscopically, sarcomatoid carcinoma is composed of a urothelial, glandular, or small cell epithelial component showing variable degrees of differentiation and a mesenchymal component, usually with high-grade spindle cell morphology; high molecular weight cytokeratin and p63 immunohistochemical positivity is frequently detected in both components.

General Clinical Consideration

The urothelial/transitional cell carcinoma of the bladder (UC/TCC) in clinical practice and pathologic aspect can be easily divided into two major categories, depending on the infiltration or not of the detrusor muscle of the bladder:

1. The nonmuscle-invasive bladder cancer (NMIBC) or "superficial" bladder cancer (Ta, T1)
2. The muscle-invasive bladder cancer (MIBC) or invasive bladder cancer ($\geq$ T2)

Since the treatment and the follow-up, the prognosis is completely different among these two distinguished entities; a detailed histopathological examination is of great importance for the patient.

Symptoms

The main symptom is gross or microscopic hematuria. Many times these tumors remain asymptomatic and are identified in ultrasound scans of the abdomen performed for other reasons.

In many occasions, especially in cases of urothelial carcinoma in situ (CIS), the main symptom is irritative voiding, mainly dysuria, without gross hematuria.

Laboratory Investigation

1. Ultrasound: an exophytic hypoechoic lesion of the bladder wall is the most common finding. Non-exophytic, flat tumors such as CIS cannot be identified in ultrasound scans.

   The number of the lesions and their respective size must be also reported by the radiologist.

2. Intravenous urography or C/T urography
   In those two examinations, the tumor presents as a contrast media filling defect in the bladder.
   The pyelocalyceal system can also be assessed for filling defects or hydronephrosis (as a result of infiltration of the ureteric orifice by the tumor).
   Moreover, the C/T urography can provide information on the involvement of lymph nodes and the potential presence of visceral metastases.
3. Cytologic examination of the urine
   Urine cytology has a high positive predictive value, especially in cases of in situ or muscle-invasive TCC. In cases of low-grade tumors, cytology has low negative predictive value.

Treatment of NMIBC

The *treatment decision* depends on the *histological examination*:

Nonmuscle-invasive tumors are initially completely resected, and depending on the depth of infiltration, grade, size, and number, the resection may be followed by intravesical instillations of chemotherapeutic agents or BCG (Bacillus Calmette-Guerin), a live attenuated strain of *Mycobacterium bovis* (Babjuk et al. 2017a, b).

The prediction of disease recurrence and progression is very important. There are six predicting factors as follows:

1. Number of tumors (single, 2–7, ≥8)
2. Tumor diameter (<3 cm, ≥3 cm)
3. Prior recurrence rate (primary, ≤1 recurrence per year, >1 recurrence per year)
4. Category (Ta, T1)
5. Concurrent CIS
6. Tumor grade (low or high grade)

According to those, patients are stratified into three risk groups:

1. Low-risk tumors (primary, solitary, <3 cm, no CIS)
2. Intermediate risk (tumors not defined in the other two groups)
3. High-risk tumors [T1 or high grade (HG) or CIS or multiple and recurrent and large Ta G1/G2]

Treatment of Muscle-Invasive Bladder Cancer (MIBC)

The treatment of choice for localized MIBC is radical surgery and urinary diversion. It is recommended traditionally for patients with T2-T4a, N0-Nx, M0 tumors (Witjes et al. 2017a, b).

Other indications include high-risk and recurrent superficial tumors, BCG-resistant Tis, T1G3, and extensive papillary disease that cannot be controlled with resection and intravesical therapy alone.

Radical cystectomy in men includes removal of the bladder, prostate, seminal vesicles, distal ureters, and regional lymph nodes (LNs).

In women it includes removal of the bladder, entire urethra, adjacent vagina, uterus, distal ureters, and regional LNs.

Neoadjuvant, cisplatin-containing chemotherapy improves overall survival and especially in responders with a favorable pathologic staging. Currently, no tools are available to select patients who may benefit from neoadjuvant chemotherapy.

The options for urinary diversion following cystectomy depend on the age and the performance status of the patient. Therefore, orthotopic neo-bladder diversion is indicated for younger patients with a good performance status, in contrast to ileal conduits or cutaneous ureterostomies which are preferred for elderly patients or extended disease.

It is evident that the close cooperation between urologist and pathologist is essential for the diagnosis, the treatment, and the follow-up of the patients suffering from bladder cancer.

Treatment Options in Metastatic Bladder Cancer

Metastatic urothelial cancer (MUC) is associated with a poor prognosis and limited treatment options. It is a disease that has seen no major advances for more than 30 years outside of the United States. Urothelial cancer (UC) is the ninth most common cancer worldwide, with 430,000 new cases diagnosed in 2012, and it results in approximately 145,000 deaths globally each year. Men are three times more likely to suffer from UC, compared with women, and the disease is three times more common in developed countries than in less developed countries.

If metastasis is suspected, additional work-up to evaluate the extent of the disease is necessary. This includes a chest CT and a bone scan if enzyme levels (ALP-alkaline phosphatase) are abnormal or the patient shows signs or symptoms of skeletal involvement.

Patients who present with disseminated metastatic disease are generally treated with systemic chemotherapy. Management of persistent disseminated disease may involve chemotherapy, radiation, or a combination of these. Clinical oncologist decides for treatment options according to the performance status (PS), renal function, and comorbidities. Cisplatin-containing chemotherapy with GC (gemcitabine/cisplatin) or MVAC (methotrexate, vinblastine, adriamycin, and cisplatin) is standard in advanced surgically unresectable and metastatic patients fit enough to tolerate cisplatin. Median survival in these patients is about 14 months; long-term disease-free survival (DFS) has been reported in about 15% of patients; in 20.9% with lymph node-only disease compared with only 6.8% with visceral metastases (Loehrer et al. 1992; von der Maase et al. 2000, 2005). So far, no improvement in survival has been achieved with newer triplets, novel four-drug regimens, or dose-dense chemotherapy (Bellmunt et al. 2012; Galsky et al. 2007; Milowsky et al. 2009). GC is less toxic than MVAC (von der Maase et al. 2000). MVAC is better tolerated with the use of granulocyte colony-stimulating factor (G-CSF) (Bamias et al. 2004; Gabrilove et al. 1988). High dose intensity MVAC with G-CSF, delivered in half the time of traditional MVAC, is an option for fit patients with limited advanced disease, given its lower toxicity profile and superior response rate compared with standard MVAC (Sternberg et al. 2006).

About 50% of patients are unfit for cisplatin-containing chemotherapy due to poor performance status, impaired renal function, or comorbidity. Patients unfit for cisplatin-based chemotherapy may be palliated with a carboplatin-based regimen or single-agent taxane or gemcitabine. Methotrexate/carboplatin/vinblastine (M-CAVI) and carboplatin/gemcitabine (CarboGem) are active in patients unfit for cisplatin, but without a statistically significant difference in overall survival (OS) and progression-free survival (PFS). Severe acute toxicity was slightly higher on M-CAVI, which makes CarboGem the preferred and reference treatment in unfit patients (De Santis et al. 2012). Patients with PS 2 and impaired renal function have limited benefit from combination chemotherapy, and best supportive care is the best option for them (De Santis et al. 2012). For this group of patients, new strategies are needed, and therefore it could be very useful for them to enter into clinical trials.

Patients with disease progression below 12 months can either receive second-line chemotherapy or enter into a clinical trial. The only valid randomized phase III trial in patients progressing after first-line treatment with platinum-containing combination chemotherapy for metastatic disease tested vinflunine, a novel third-generation vinca alkaloid, plus best supportive care (BSC) versus BSC alone (Bellmunt et al. 2009). The results showed modest activity (overall response rate is 8.6%), a clinical benefit with a favorable safety profile and a survival benefit in favor of vinflunine, which was statistically significant in the eligible patient population. This trial reached the highest level of evidence ever reported for second-line treatment. In Europe, vinflunine is the only approved drug in this setting: however, it is unknown whether other agents used in this setting would have a similar benefit. Patients, whose disease has progressed during a period of up to 1 year after first-line treatment, can be managed with platinum-based chemotherapy.

Immunotherapy: A New Era in Treatment of Metastatic Bladder Cancer

Approximately half of patients with bladder cancer do not respond to their initial, or first-line, therapy, and only 10–15% of those patients respond to second-line chemotherapy. In May 2016 atezolizumab, which acts as a programmed cell death ligand-1 inhibitor, and in February 2017 nivolumab, which is a programmed cell death receptor-1 inhibitor, had received by the US Food and Drug Administration (FDA) an accelerated approval for the treatment of patients with locally advanced or metastatic urothelial carcinoma who have disease progression during or following platinum-containing chemotherapy (Hoffman-Censits et al. 2016; Sharma et al. 2017).

Atezolizumab is a monoclonal antibody designed to target and bind to a protein called PD-L1 (programmed death-ligand 1), which is expressed on tumor cells and tumor-infiltrating immune cells. PD-L1 interacts with PD-1, which is found on the surface of T cells, causing inhibition of T cells. By blocking this interaction, atezolizumab may enable the activation of T cells, restoring their ability to effectively detect and attack tumor cells. Further research in immunotherapy resulted in an accelerated approval by the FDA in April 2017 for atezolizumab as a frontline treatment for cisplatin-ineligible patients with locally advanced or metastatic urothelial carcinoma. The approval is based on the data that showed the objective response rate (ORR) with atezolizumab was 23.5%, including a complete response (CR) rate of 6.7% (Balar et al. 2017).

On the other hand, nivolumab is the second immune checkpoint inhibitor to be approved for the treatment of bladder cancer. The nivolumab approval is for patients with locally advanced or metastatic bladder cancer whose disease has gotten worse during or after first-line platinum-containing chemotherapy. By binding to a protein called PD-1 on the surface of T cells and preventing it from interacting with the PD-L1 protein on cancer cells, nivolumab releases the brakes on the immune system, allowing T cells to attack cancer cells. The approval was based on the results of a phase II clinical trial with objective response rate 19.6%, complete response rate 2.2%, and partial response rate 17.3% (Sharma et al. 2017).

Both nivolumab and atezolizumab received an accelerated approval on the basis of response rates; data on other outcomes, including survival, are awaited, and therefore there are a lot of ongoing clinical trials right now. These immunotherapy agents are for now approved only in the United States, and they offer clinicians new options in metastatic bladder cancer after more than 30 years without a new drug therapy.

2.2 Case 2.1: Reactive Changes of Bladder Mucosa

Case Study

Data Prior to Microscopy

A 70-year-old patient with a history of long-term indwelling bladder catheter removed 2 months ago, and radiotherapy after surgery for prostate cancer, presents with urinary frequency and urgency.

Cystoscopy reveals multiple areas of friable mucosal irregularity on the dome and posterior wall of the bladder and small submucosal cysts; transurethral biopsies are taken.

2.2.1 Microscopic Evaluation of Bladder Biopsy Specimens

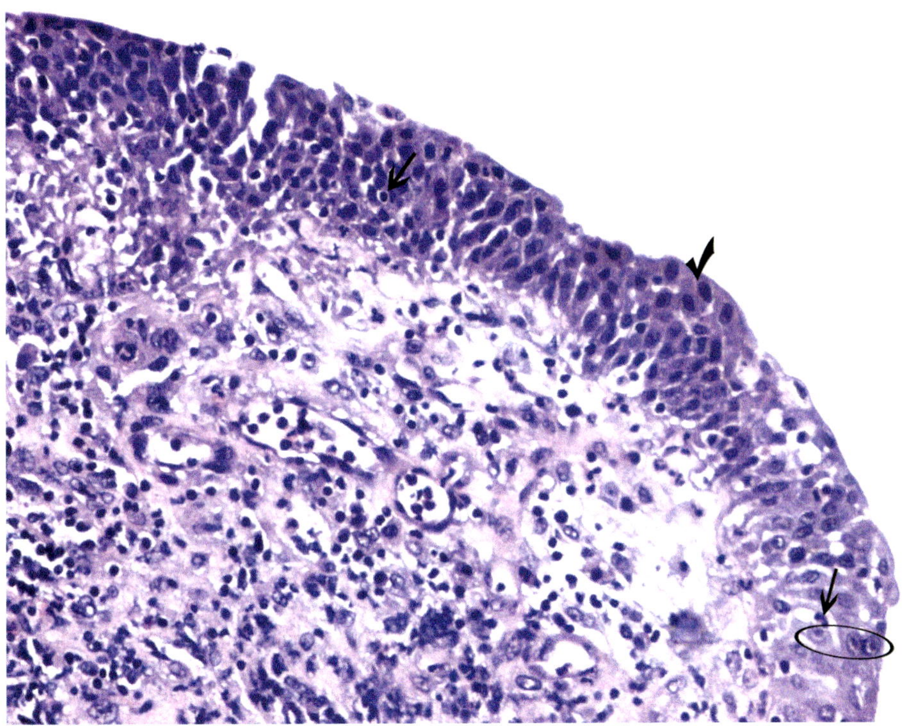

Fig. 2.1 (H-E, ×100) Inflammatory cells within urothelium (*arrows*) and in the lamina propria. The majority of cases of both acute and chronic cystitis show nonspecific histologic features of inflammation.

Reactive atypia of the urothelium. Urothelium is normal (*to slightly thickened*) and shows morphologic evidence of maturation, at least focally. Nucleomegaly is a prominent finding in reactive urothelial atypia; the nuclei often have conspicuous, usually centrally located, pinpoint nucleoli (*ellipse*). Nuclei are round and significant nuclear pleomorphism is lacking. The cells generally maintain their polarity perpendicular to the basement membrane. Reactive inflammatory atypia may have frequent mitotic figures involving the *lower* layers of urothelium. Typical umbrella cells (*tick*) are recognized but can be displaced so that they are not on surface.

We should have in mind that in thick sections, the urothelium may appear hyperchromatic and that the urothelium of the bladder neck is usually composed of cells with slightly larger nuclei and diminished cytoplasmic clearing; misinterpretation as dysplasia should be avoided

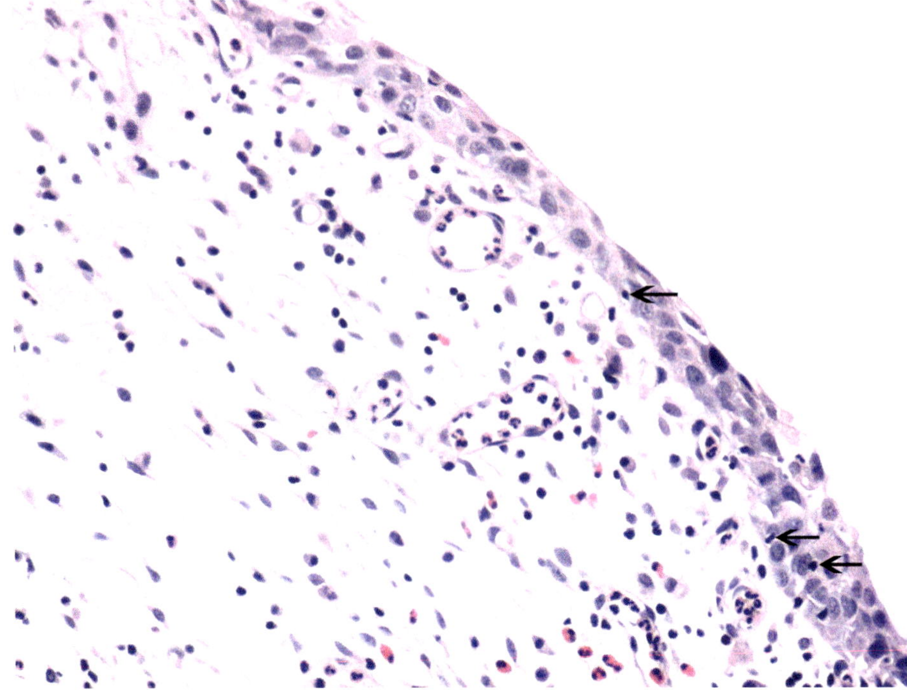

Fig. 2.2 (H-E, ×100) Variably sized and shaped nuclei in thinned bladder mucosa with some polarity loss. Sparse elements of inflammation in the lamina propria and within the urothelium (*arrows*).

The pathologist is uncertain whether these morphological alterations are reactive or neoplastic, and immunohistochemistry has not provided decisive help in this case. In order that the patient is followed up after inflammation subsides, the descriptive term "urothelial atypia of unknown significance" can be used in such a biopsy in which the severity of atypia in a flat urothelium appears to be out of proportion to the extent of inflammation, so dysplasia or carcinoma in situ (*CIS*) cannot be confidently excluded

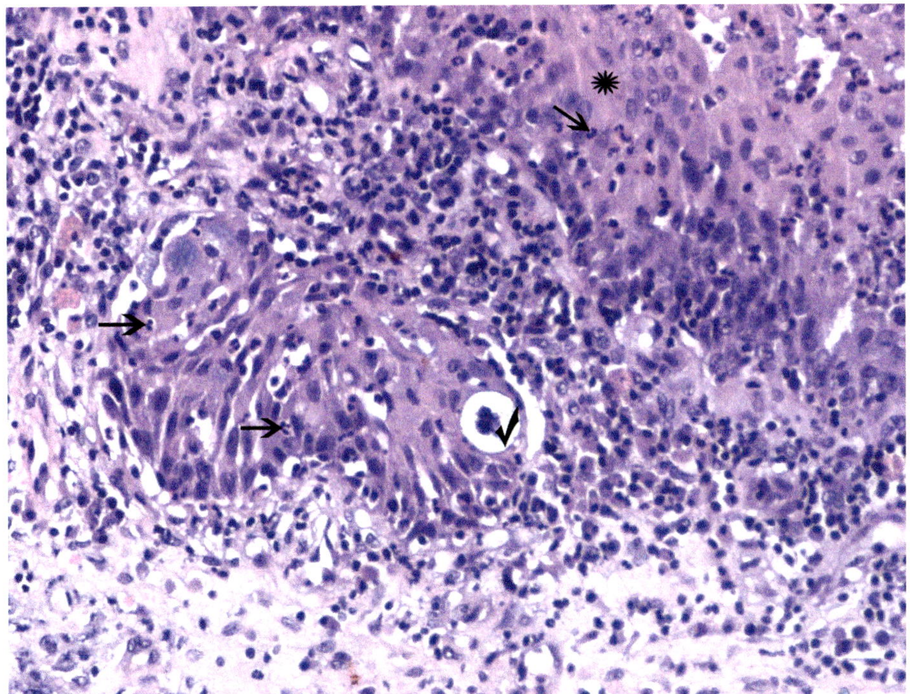

Fig. 2.3 (H-E, ×100) In cystitis, lamina propria is usually inflamed with inflammation extending to the mucosa. The presence of acute inflammatory cells in the inflammatory component (*arrows*) should be correlated with the results of bladder culture.

In reactive atypia, the cells are often larger than normal, with vesicular nuclei and more abundant cytoplasm (*asterisk*) than normal urothelial cells, occasionally acquiring a squamoid appearance. The most common reactive proliferative change within the urothelium is the formation of Brunn's nests, which represent invaginations of the surface epithelium into the underlying lamina propria. The Brunn's nest here shows cystic change (*cystitis cystica, tick*).

The presence of acute or significant chronic inflammation, particularly in an intraurothelial location, warrants caution in the interpretation of intraurothelial neoplasia (either low-grade, i.e., dysplasia, or high-grade, i.e., CIS), although inflammatory atypia may coexist with dysplasia or CIS. Inflammatory atypia and non-pleomorphic forms of CIS share in common the presence of enlarged nuclei with prominent nucleoli; attention to other nuclear characteristics is of fundamental importance in such a setting

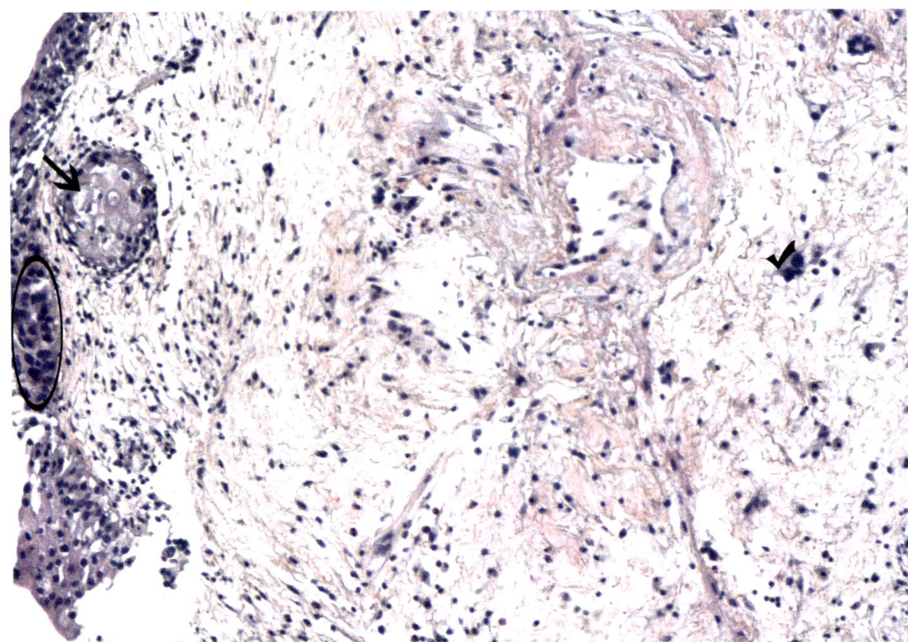

Fig. 2.4 (H-E, ×100) Postradiation changes. Lamina propria edema. Hyperchromatic nuclei of urothelial cells (*ellipse*). Mitotic activity in urothelium should be rare. The cytoplasm in radiation atypia is often prominent and may show degenerative changes with cytoplasmic and nuclear vacuolation (*arrow*) with normal nuclear/cytoplasmic ratio, as in the evenly spaced Brunn's nest above (*arrow*), which may resemble nonkeratinizing, glycogenated squamous metaplasia. There may be multinucleated cells with bizarre nuclei not typical of CIS. Reactive-appearing, multinucleated stromal mesenchymal cells (*tick*) with degenerative atypia and unremarkable mitotic activity are compatible both with radiation atypia and giant cell cystitis (the latter, not a clinical entity), while atypical fibroblasts and radiation vasculopathy may be identified in the bladder wall after radiation treatment

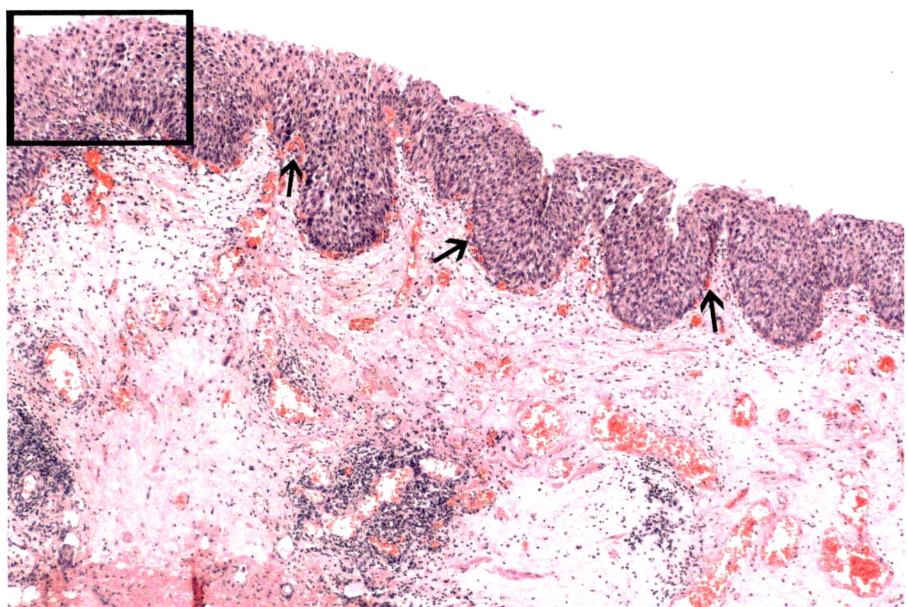

Fig. 2.5 (H-E, ×50) Urothelial hyperplasia is characterized by markedly thickened mucosa with an increase in the number of cell layers (usually to ten or more), in completely flat lesions. Marked thickening and/or increased cell density within urothelium (increased cells per unit area) is enough to diagnose hyperplasia. Adjacent, nonhyperplastic urothelium, when noticeable, can be used as a yardstick; counting cell layers is not recommended.

De novo "papillary" urothelial hyperplasia is a likely precursor lesion to low-grade papillary urothelial neoplasms. Undulating urothelium is arranged into mucosal narrow papillary folds of varying heights. We notice tenting folds *without* detached-appearing papillary fronds with fibrovascular cores, the latter being diagnostic of a papillary urothelial neoplasm. Lack of complex arborization. The tent-shaped folds lack the edema typical of polypoid cystitis (see Fig. 2.6). Increased vascularity may be noticed in the stroma at the base of the papillary folds (*arrows*). Adjacent flat mucosa is also thicker than normal (*flat hyperplasia, square frame*).

The cells in urothelial hyperplasia, either flat or papillary, should show no significant cytologic abnormalities. Loss of cell polarity and nuclear crowding and atypia should raise suspicion of concomitant dysplasia and warrant immunohistochemical investigation.

The term "urothelial proliferation of uncertain malignant potential" tends to replace "papillary and flat urothelial hyperplasia"

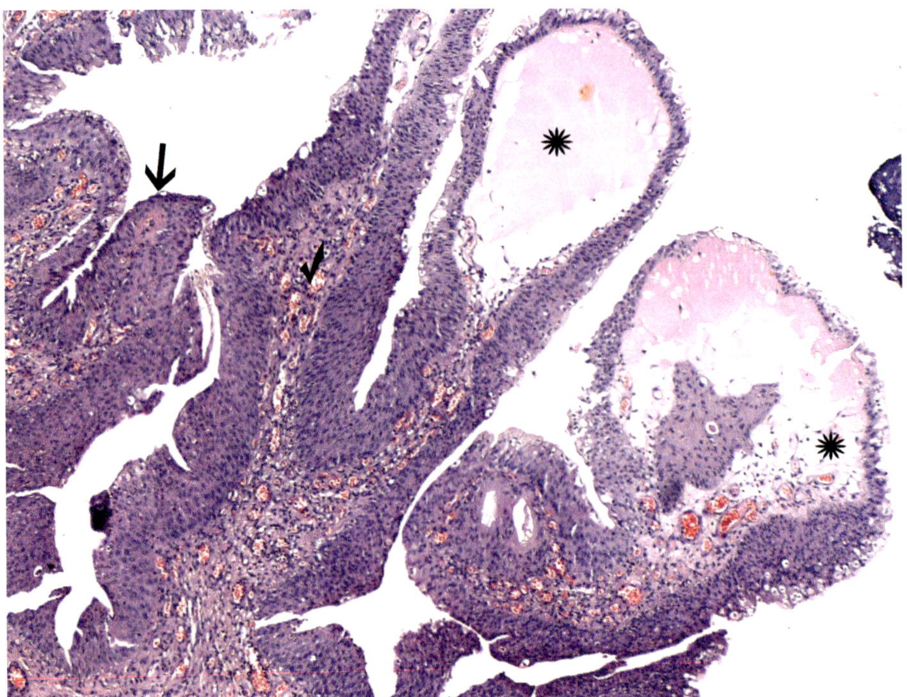

Fig. 2.6 (H-E, ×50) The term polypoid or papillary cystitis is ordinarily used to describe a nonneoplastic, noninfectious, exophytic, inflammatory lesion composed of normal or slightly reactive urothelium covering a focally edematous (*asterisks*) or fibrotic lamina propria. The exophytic projections are composed of inflammatory granulation tissue (*tick*) and are lined by hyperplastic/reactive urothelium or are denuded. The stromal cores often taper, pointing toward lumen. Slender papillary excrescences are occasionally seen (*arrow*) but always without complex secondary branching. Nevertheless, broad-based, nonbranching edematous fronds with bulbous tips typically predominate in polypoid cystitis, under *low magnification.*

Isolated papillary fronds within the otherwise classic polypoid cystitis may lack edema. With time, fronds of polypoid cystitis lesions become less edematous and are replaced by *dense* fibrosis, often associated with chronic inflammation; these lesions may be referred to as papillary cystitis. Papillary cystitis is the chronic phase of polypoid cystitis.

Chronic inflammation of the lamina propria and dilated blood vessels are prominent and diagnostically helpful features of both polypoid and papillary cystitis

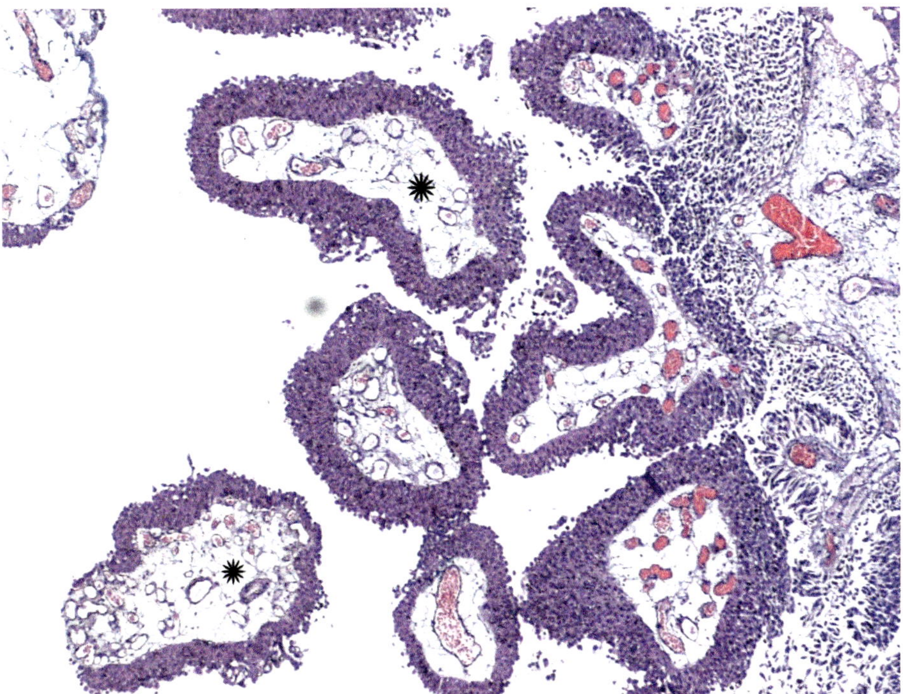

Fig. 2.7 (H-E, ×50) Broad, scattered, edematous fibrovascular cores (*asterisks*) with congested blood vessels of polypoid cystitis distinguish this entity from the narrow-necked, thin, and delicate fibrovascular cores of papillary urothelial neoplasms in which smaller papillae arise from larger papillae. The fronds in polypoid cystitis are simple and do not branch into smaller papillae. The urothelium lining the edematous stalks exhibits reactive atypia, at most.

When edema in the papillae is so extensive that width is greater than height, the term "bullous cystitis" is used.

Such configurations are often mistaken for neoplasms, cystoscopically. Any injurious agent, most often indwelling catheters, may give rise to polypoid cystitis; removal of the catheter typically results in resolution of cystitis.

The rare fibroepithelial polyps of the bladder are distinguished from polypoid cystitis by being solitary, with a more fibrous core and paucity of inflammatory cells

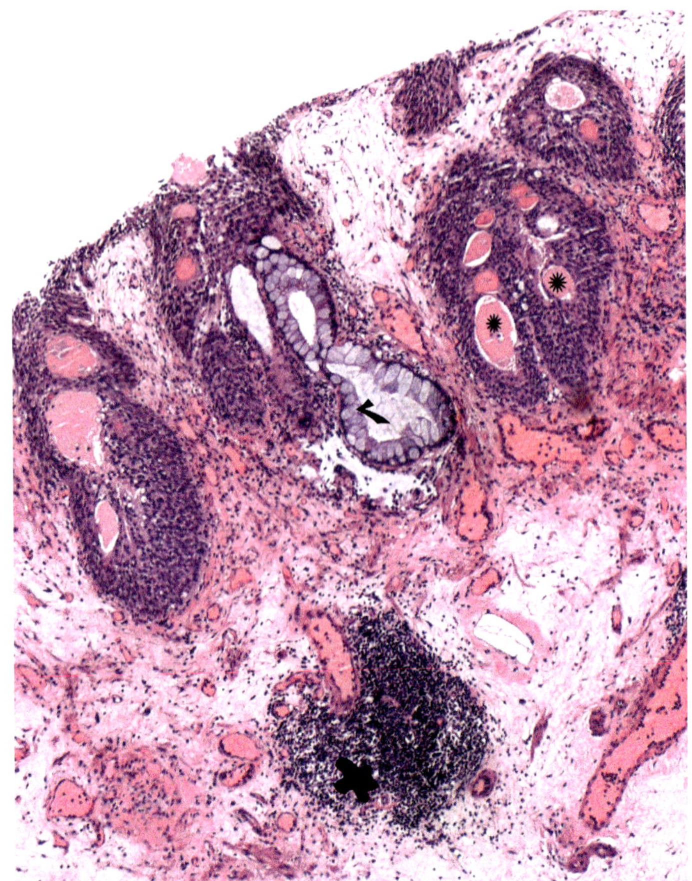

Fig. 2.8 (H-E, ×50) Cystitis cystica et glandularis (proliferative cystitis), most likely resulting from injury to the bladder mucosa and a local inflammatory insult, is a proliferation of Brunn's nests growing downward into the lamina propria, becoming cystically degenerated and either acquiring a luminal space lined by flattened urothelial lining and filled by pale, eosinophilic fluid (cystitis cystica, *asterisks*) or, in addition, acquiring a cuboidal/columnar glandular epithelium lining central lumens with luminally oriented cytoplasm (see Fig. 2.9) and indications of mucin secretion [cystitis glandularis (of nonintestinal, common type)].

In cystitis cystica, Brunn's nests grow into lamina propria and are transformed into urothelium lining slit-like or cystic spaces with pink fluid (*asterisks*). The cysts of cystitis cystica arise from obstruction of the pores of Brunn's nests and are usually 0.1–1 cm in diameter.

The two processes (cystitis cystica and cystitis glandularis) often coexist. The superficial location, the lobular growth pattern or the linear array, the regular spacing with a sharp linear border at the noninfiltrative base where no atypia or increased mitoses are observed, and the supposed accumulation of luminal "mucins" (this material is actually either negative or only weakly positive in mucin stains) rule out the nested type of urothelial carcinoma.

Intestinal metaplasia (*tick*) defines replacement of urothelium by colonic mucosa with obvious mucin production by at least scattered goblet cells which ordinarily lack cellular atypia and are confined to the area of the former urothelium; in such an instance, the term "cystitis glandularis with intestinal (colonic) metaplasia" is appropriate and is synonymous with the term "intestinal metaplasia." A benign behavior of colonic metaplasia has been supported; however, the presence of nuclear beta-catenin is suggestive of malignant potential, in contrast to cystitis glandularis of common type which expresses membranous beta-catenin.

A dense lymphocytic aggregate is noticed in the lamina propria (*blob*)

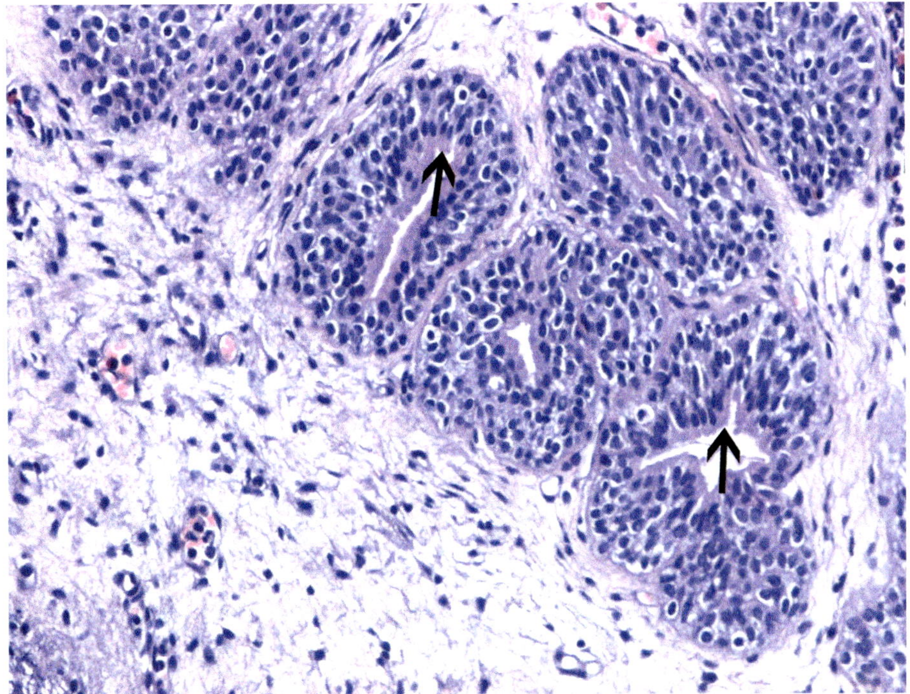

Fig. 2.9 (H-E, ×200) Cystitis glandularis (of common type): glands in lamina propria lined by columnar (*arrows*) or cuboidal epithelium (Pathology Outlines 2017). Apart from the luminal surface, the glands of cystitis glandularis (of common type) consist of layers of basal and intermediate urothelial cells. No intestinal metaplasia is noticed in this field. Cystitis glandularis of common type is more frequent than intestinal type, in most series

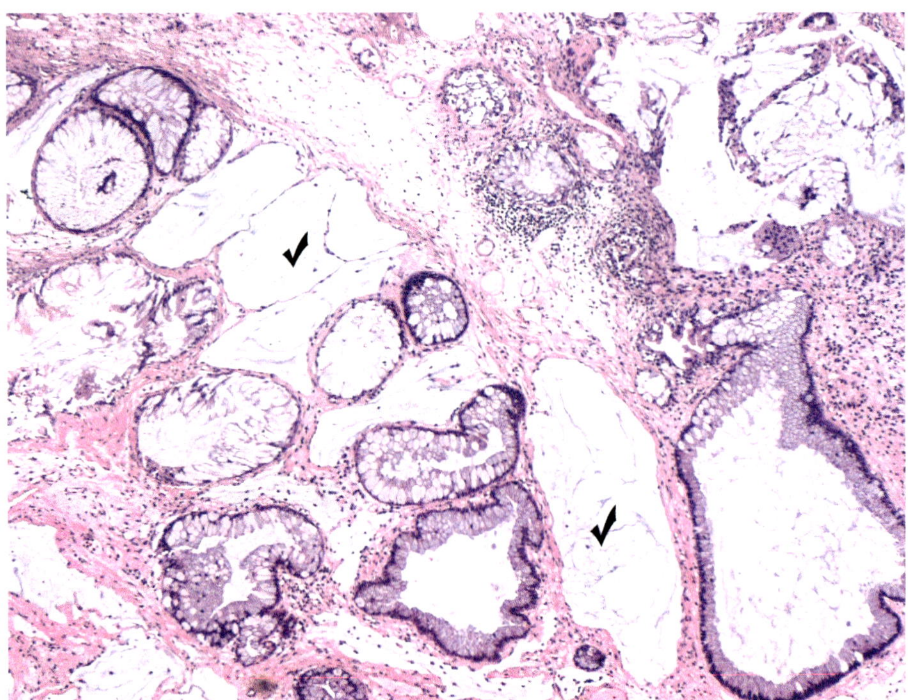

Fig. 2.10 (H-E, ×50) The cells of cystitis glandularis of intestinal type/intestinal metaplasia lack nuclear atypia, necrotic activity, and signet ring cells and involve the lamina propria and, rarely, the muscularis propria. *Focal* mucinous pools *lacking epithelial cells* (*ticks*) are not uncommon in cases of intestinal metaplasia, and their presence in a tissue sample is *not* diagnostic of adenocarcinoma. A suspicion of adenocarcinoma should be raised, however, when an irregular, haphazard arrangement of glands in the deeper lamina propria or muscularis propria combined with moderate to severe cytologic atypia are noticed, especially in small biopsies.

Metaplastic lesions of the urothelium are almost always associated with sources of chronic irritation and are of three basic types: squamous, intestinal, and nephrogenic

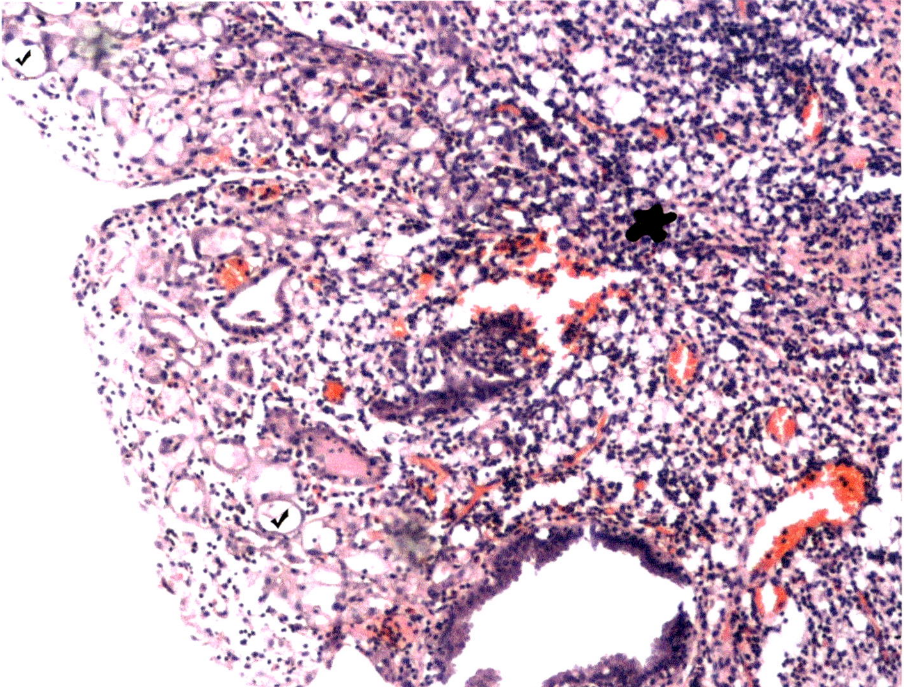

Fig. 2.11 (H-E, ×100) Nephrogenic metaplasia is a peculiar reactive process, usually of the posterior bladder wall, with a broad histologic spectrum, which often results in papillary and, most commonly, small round/cystically dilated tubular growths (*ticks*), reminiscent of immature structures, ordinarily involving the edematous lamina propria and sparing the muscularis propria. A *single layer of cytologically bland cuboidal cells* with scant, atrophic cytoplasm lines the tubules or stalks. Significant nuclear atypia is unusual in nephrogenic metaplasia and, when present, is focal. Mitotic figures are absent or rare. Hyalinized basal lamina and variable numbers of acute and chronic inflammatory cells of cystitis are commonplace in the background (*blob*). Immunohistochemically, nephrogenic metaplasia shows positive reaction for cytokeratins and PAX2 and lacks strong expression of prostatic antigens (PSA, PAP). The present lesion is composed solely of "vascular space"-like dilated tubules which, of course, are CD31-immunonegative.

Urothelial carcinoma with small tubules is a histological variant of urothelial carcinoma which can be distinguished from nephrogenic metaplasia by the former's diffusely infiltrative architecture, considerable variation of tubular shape with haphazard organization, and the frequent presence of muscle invasion. The neoplastic tubules are lined by urothelial cells

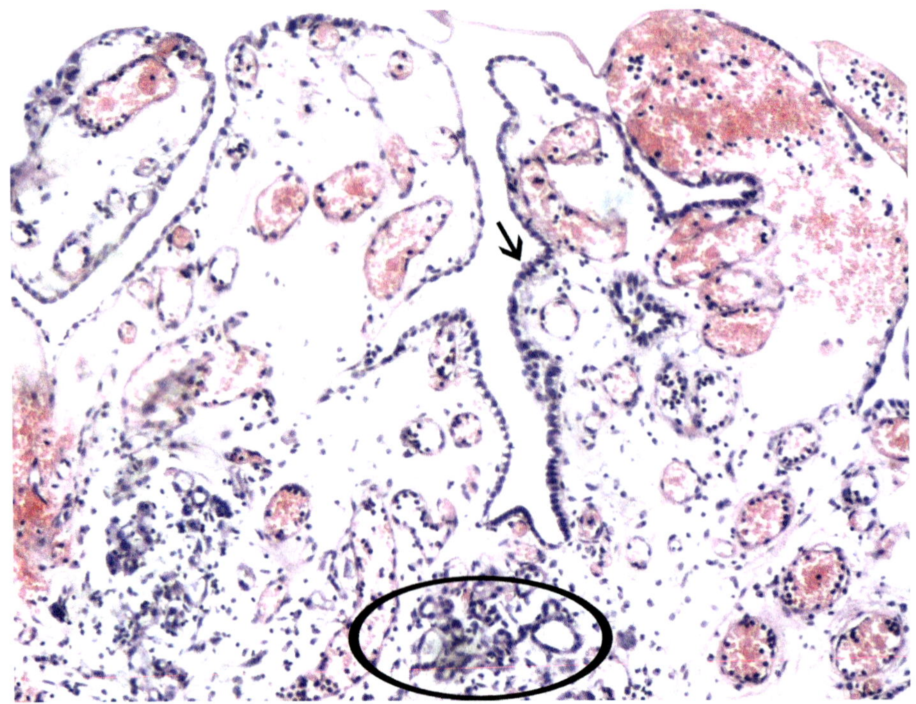

Fig. 2.12 (H-E, ×100) Papillary nephrogenic metaplasia lined by *single* (non-stratified) layer of cytologically bland cuboidal epithelium, which may have "hobnail" appearance (*arrow*). Recognition of admixed tubular/cystic pattern (*ellipse*) in the underlying lamina propria excludes papillary/polypoid cystitis.

The edematous and inflamed cores covered with a single layer of bland cuboidal or low columnar cells in nephrogenic metaplasia are in contrast to the delicate fibrovascular cores lined by stratified epithelium in papillary urothelial neoplasms.

In the next images, we are going to see some cases of bladder neoplasms with pure glandular differentiation

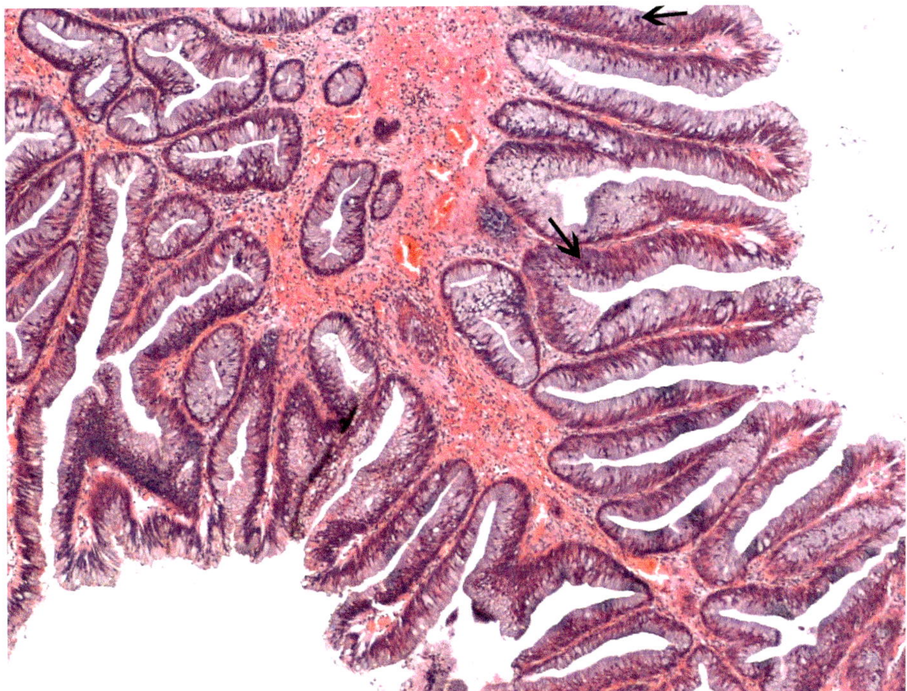

Fig. 2.13 (H-E, ×50) A well-circumscribed tumor arising at the bladder dome. Beyond diffuse cystitis glandularis of the intestinal type/intestinal metaplasia, the extensive presence of low-grade dysplasia (*arrows*) is compatible with tubulovillous adenomatous changes of the bladder mucosa on the background of cystitis glandularis, intestinal type

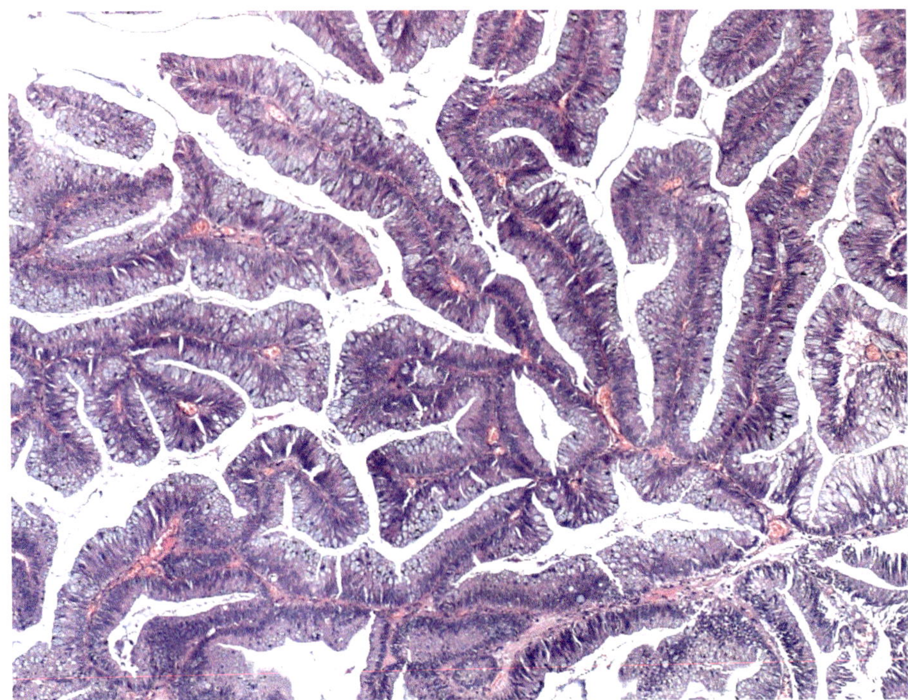

Fig. 2.14 (H-E, ×50) Villous adenoma of the urinary bladder with exophytic growth, histologically identical to its colonic counterpart and cystoscopically indistinguishable from a papillary urothelial neoplasm. Blunt, elongated villous structures with delicate, central fibrovascular stalks covered by a pseudostratified, dysplastic, intestinal-type epithelium with nuclear enlargement, crowding, and hyperchromasia and abundant, apically located cytoplasm, consistent with typical, adenomatous, low-grade dysplasia. The absence of destructive invasion in this field. This adenomatous epithelium is GATA3-immunonegative. Intestinal or squamous metaplasia and cystitis glandularis often occur in the adjacent urothelium.

Such adenomas should be examined in their entirety to exclude associated adenocarcinoma, in situ and invasive; complete excision is essential. On limited biopsy material, spread from an intestinal neoplasm should be clinically excluded

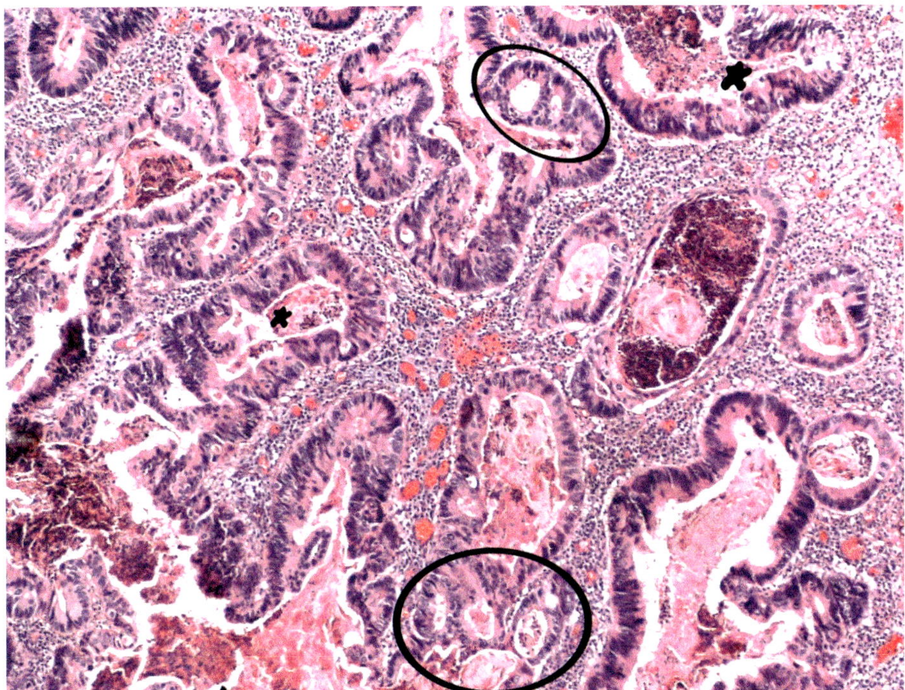

Fig. 2.15 (H-E, ×50) Primary nonurachal (pure) adenocarcinoma of the urinary bladder is a rare malignant neoplasm of ominous prognosis, derived from the urothelium, with a histologically *pure* glandular phenotype. In primary adenocarcinoma of the urinary bladder, admixed typical urothelial carcinoma (papillary, in situ, or invasive) should be absent. Two-thirds of adenocarcinomas are single discrete lesions, as opposed to urothelial carcinomas which tend to be multifocal.

Clearly, deeply infiltrating cancerous glands with *complex architecture* are evident at low power (*ellipses*), lined by pseudostratified, mucin-secreting, pleomorphic epithelium with central necrosis (*blobs*). This is the *enteric* type of bladder adenocarcinoma, identical to its gastrointestinal counterpart and thus easily distinguishable from urothelial neoplasms with glandular lumens; the latter are surrounded by cells with pseudostratified appearance and superficial cell differentiation of urothelium. We should point out that the presence of focal glandular formation in urothelial carcinomas is common and should not be regarded as adenocarcinoma. Urothelial carcinoma with glandular features/gland-like lumens doesn't differentiate toward colonic mucosa; there is usually minimal mucin and no goblet cells; "glands" are surrounded by urothelial-type cells (see Fig. 2.94).

Negative or even focal weak *nuclear* expression as well as strictly cytoplasmic expression of β-catenin favors primary origin of adenocarcinoma in the bladder against colonic origin, but clinical correlation and unremarkable colonoscopy is necessary for a definitive diagnosis of primary adenocarcinoma of the urinary bladder with enteric morphology. Identification of in situ adenocarcinoma after examining many sections of tumor-adjacent mucosa, when possible, confirms the primary location of the adenocarcinoma in the urinary bladder. Cystitis cystica and cystitis glandularis occur in approximately 50% of patients with adenocarcinoma located at the bladder base.

Urachal adenocarcinoma is primarily distinguished by its anatomic location in the bladder dome, within the anterior bladder wall, and the absence of surface intestinal metaplasia

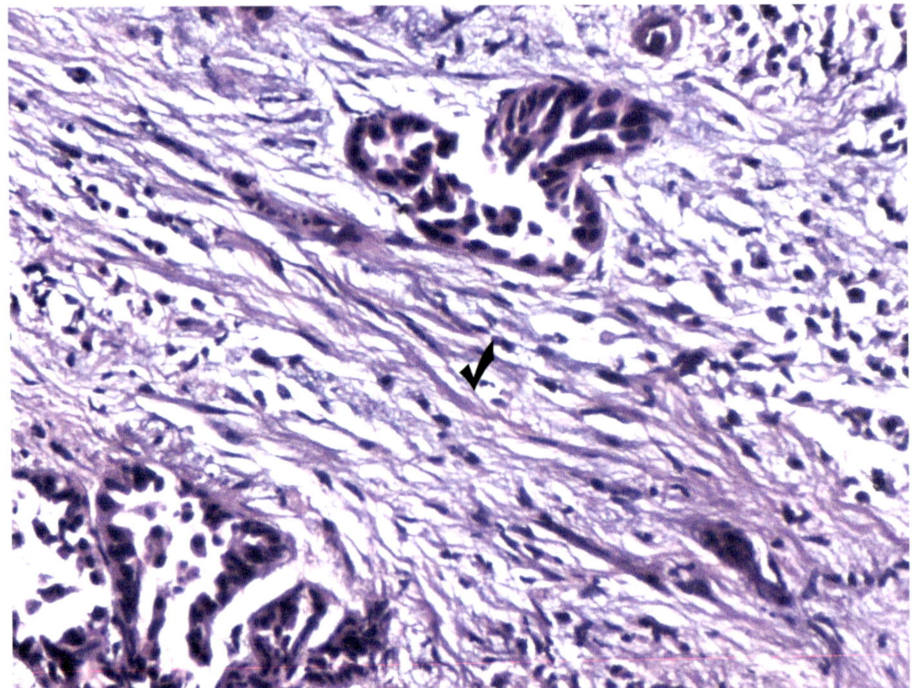

Fig. 2.16 (H-E, ×200) Bladder primary (pure) adenocarcinoma. Desmoplastic stromal response (*tick*) is absolutely compatible with destructive invasive growth of the evidently atypical glandular structures into lamina propria of the bladder

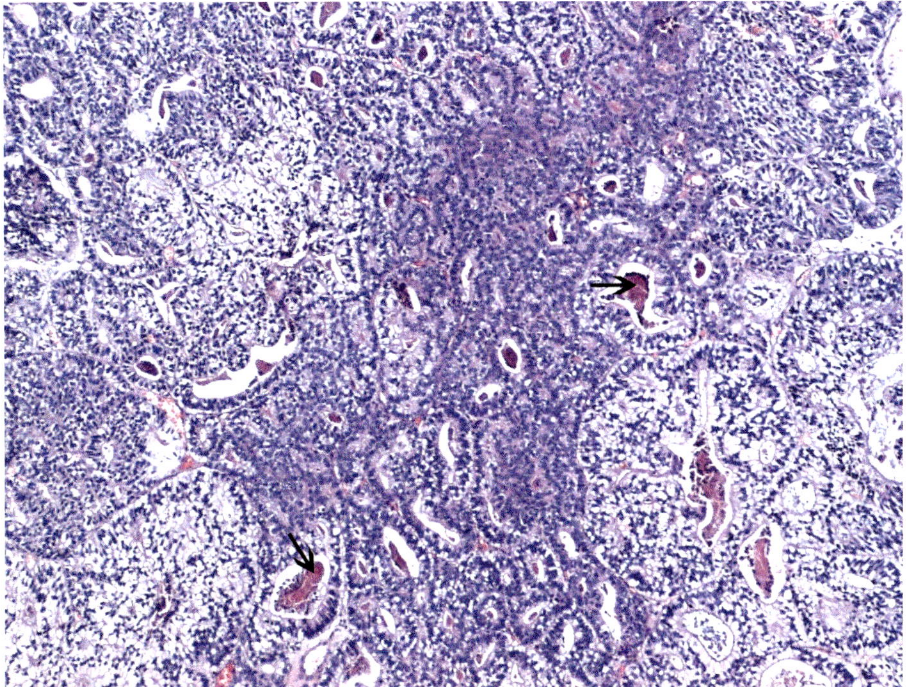

Fig. 2.17 (H-E, ×50) Clear cell carcinoma of the urinary bladder belongs to tumors of Mullerian type; it shows a tubulocystic pattern, which is this tumor's commonest pattern. The variably sized tubules contain secretions, here eosinophilic (*arrows*). Admixture of cells with clear or eosinophilic cytoplasm (image periphery and center, respectively)

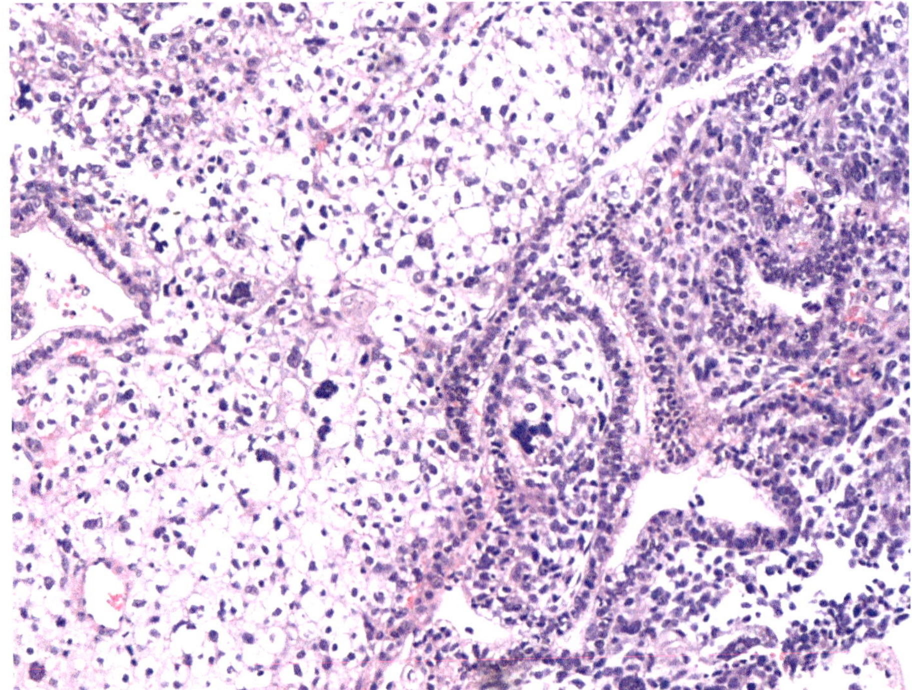

Fig. 2.18 (H-E, ×100) A mixture of architectural patterns is common in clear cell carcinoma. Diffuse, solid sheet of high-grade malignant cells with great variation in nuclear size, moderate to severe nuclear pleomorphism, and abundant clear cytoplasm, rich in glycogen, neighbor tubular structures often with a "hobnail" appearance. Clear cell carcinoma resembles urothelial carcinoma more than adenocarcinoma; however, typical urothelial carcinoma should be absent in order that clear cell carcinoma is diagnosed. Nuclear enlargement and hyperchromasia and abundant clear cytoplasm should be at least focally present in a clear cell carcinoma. Tumor cells are positive for CA-125, CEA, and Leu-M1. Extension or metastasis from gynecologic or other clear cell carcinoma (e.g., renal cell, urothelial) should be ruled out.

High-stage such tumors are typically associated with a poor outcome; low-stage clear cell carcinomas, particularly with exophytic growth, may have a favorable outcome, if treated aggressively

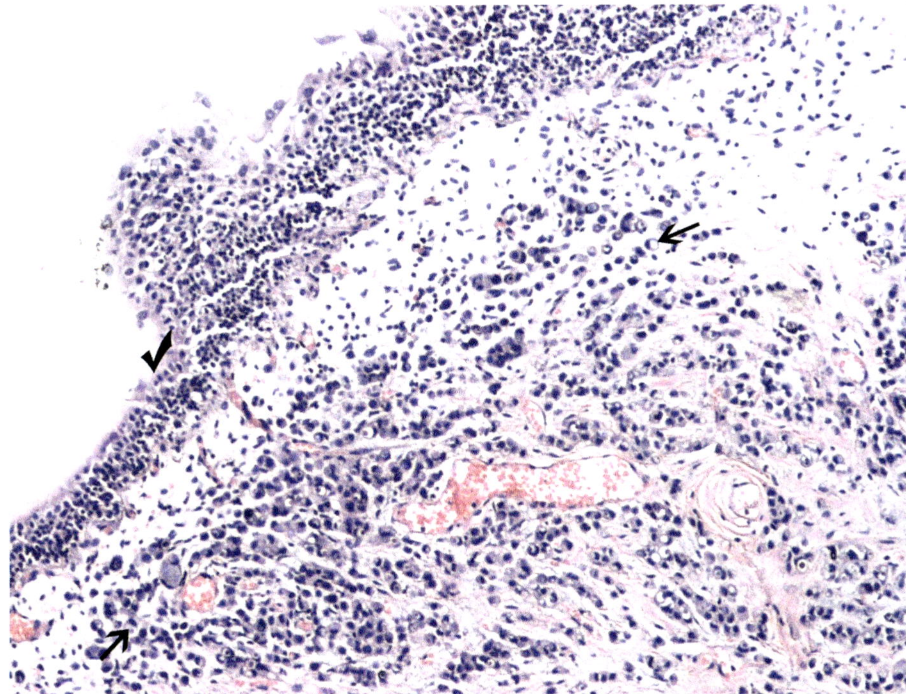

Fig. 2.19 (H-E, ×50) A strikingly dyscohesive, single cell, diffusely infiltrative growth pattern, similar to the "linitis plastica" seen in poorly differentiated stomach cancer, has been described in few cases of urothelial carcinoma. Furthermore, a few signet ring cells (*arrows*) are not uncommon in poorly differentiated bladder adenocarcinomas.

The submucosal location of the tumor and the benign appearing overlying urothelium with prominent umbrella cells (*tick*) necessitate exclusion of metastatic origin, since the urothelium is usually spared in metastatic disease. This is an exceptional case of a disseminating lobular breast carcinoma infiltrating the bladder wall. Attention to clinical history and immunohistochemical panel [positivity for ER, PR in particular, mammaglobin, and gross cystic disease fluid protein (GCDFP) combined with negativity for CK20] is mandatory.

Secondary involvement of the urinary bladder is more common than primary adenocarcinoma of the bladder. Extravesical tumors *usually* involve the urinary bladder by direct extension from adjacent pelvic organs

2.2.1.1 Clinical Commentary

Vasileios Spapis

This is a case of polypoid cystitis and other types of proliferative/inflammatory/reactive changes in the bladder mucosa and lamina propria of a patient with prolonged catheterization and radiation therapy.

Medical history of external beam radiation therapy (EBRT) is of great importance, since it is associated with increased risk of bladder cancer (BC). In a population-based cohort study, the standardized incidence ratio for bladder cancer developing after EBRT was 1.42 in comparison with the general US population (Nieder et al. 2008). Patients who have received radiotherapy (RT) for prostate cancer with modern modalities (such as intensity-modulated radiotherapy-IMRT) may have lower rates of bladder cancer (Zelefsky et al. 2012). However, since longer follow-up data are not available, all patients treated with radiation and with a long life expectancy are considered to be at a higher risk of suffering from BC.

Cystitis cystica and cystitis glandularis are common findings in urinary bladders, usually due to inflammation or chronic obstruction (Semins and Schoenberg 2007). They usually present with hematuria and irritative voiding symptoms. These benign conditions are typically associated with proliferation of von Brunn's nests. Even though they are not considered to be premalignant lesions, there have been some reports where they transformed into adenocarcinoma, and therefore, regular endoscopic evaluation of patients with these entities is recommended (Smith et al. 2008).

Polypoid or papillary cystitis is a nonspecific mucosal reaction secondary to chronically inflamed bladder. It is usually seen after repeated bladder catheterization and presents as a mass mimicking bladder carcinoma. For definitive diagnosis, biopsy is necessary. Treatment consists of removing the source of irritation and surgical excision of the suspicious mass (Ozaki et al. 2014).

Another lesion caused by chronic irritation of the urothelium is nephrogenic adenoma. This lesion may be vascular, which explains the presence of gross hematuria in most cases (Franke et al. 2011). In this case also, treatment consists of transurethral resection and elimination of the chronic irritation.

Hyperplasia is thought to be a precursor lesion for urothelial cancer. It is characterized by thicker mucosa with or without atypia. The urothelium is more than seven cells thick, and there is some disorganization of the cellular architecture (Epstein et al. 1998). Urothelial dysplasia has abnormal cytologic and nuclear changes that are preneoplastic but are not sufficient to be characterized as CIS (Sauter et al. 2004). However, dysplasia is a good marker of recurrence and progression in patients with known bladder cancer. Dysplasia progressing to CIS is believed to occur in about 20% of cases, but dysplasia with known history of urothelial cancer will progress to CIS in more than 60% of cases (Cheng et al. 1999).

Key Points

- Reactive proliferative changes of the urothelium such as Brunn's nests, cystitis cystica, and especially cystitis glandularis are not likely premalignant lesions. It is only the intestinal type of cystitis glandularis that, when persistent, extensive, or diffuse, may be associated with adenocarcinoma.
- Urothelial neoplasms should be diagnosed with caution in patients with indwelling catheters. The key to correctly diagnose polypoid/papillary cystitis is to recognize at low magnification the reactive nature of the process with an inflamed background that is edematous or densely fibrous, with predominantly simple, nonbranching, broad-based fronds of relatively normal thickness urothelium.
- All tissue of a villous adenoma should be submitted for histological evaluation so that invasive component is excluded.

2.3 Case 2.2: Recurring Bladder Carcinoma

Case Study

Data Prior to Microscopy

A 65-year-old male presents with painless intermittent microscopic hematuria. Urine cytology is negative. An elevated excrescence with a diameter of 1.8 cm is cystoscopically detected on the lateral wall of the bladder, close to the ureteral orifice, and is removed.

During the next programmed cystoscopy, a lesion of similar endoscopic appearance is detected and removed (first recurrence of disease).

Hematuria recurs after 6 months; this time, urine cytology is suspicious for cancer. Three either papillary or solid sessile lesions are cystoscopically detected and resected (second recurrence of disease).

2.3.1 Microscopic Evaluation of Transurethral Biopsy Specimens from the Three Cystoscopies

2.3.1.1 Material from the First Appearance of the Disease

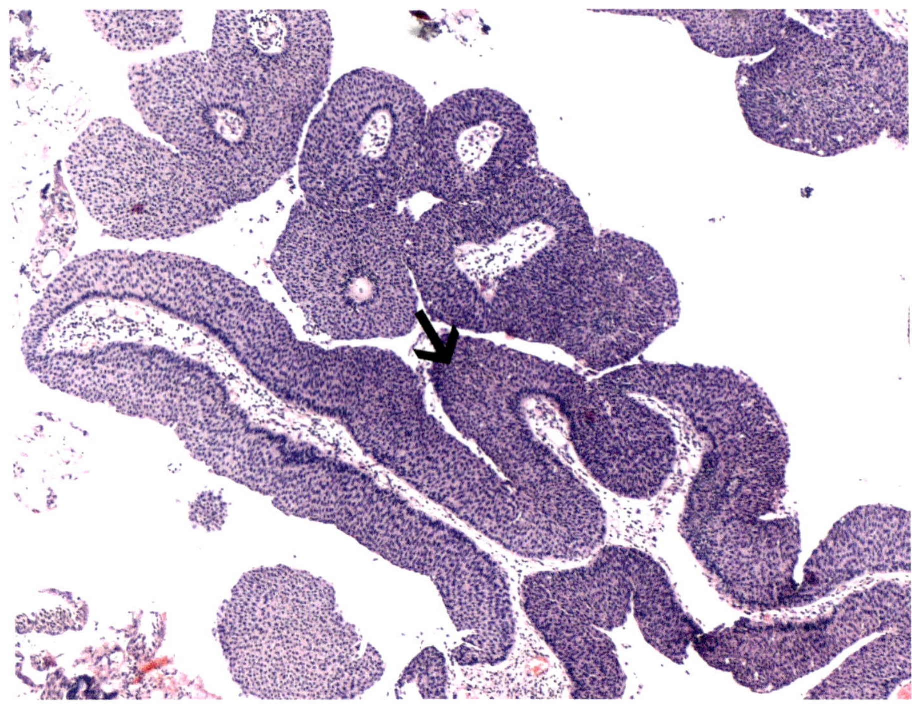

Fig. 2.20 (H-E, ×50) Papillary urothelial neoplasm of low malignant potential (PUNLMP). Discrete and slender papillary fronds lined by a *thickened* multilayered urothelium (*arrow*).

All such tumors would have been considered grade 1 urothelial carcinomas by the WHO 1973 three-tiered grading system; however, they apparently lack the capacity to invade or metastasize

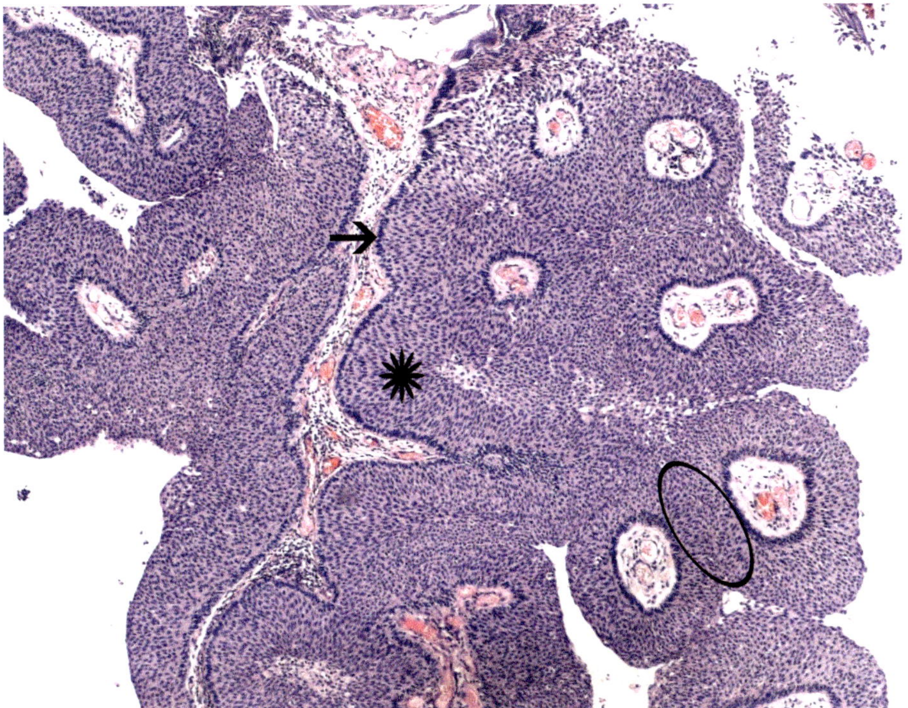

Fig. 2.21 (H-E, ×50) PUNLMP. Cell density and thickness appear to be *increased* compared with normal urothelium or that of papilloma (see Figs. 2.24, 2.25, and 2.26). Thickened urothelial lining that maintains normal perpendicular orientation to the basement membrane (i.e., order, *asterisk*) and minimal atypia are consistent with PUNLMP. The basal layers show palisading (*arrow*).

The thickness and cellularity of PUNLMP commonly exceeds that of normal urothelium. *Monotonous, bland*-appearing cells being virtually identical to each other, with no loss of order, are characteristic of PUNLMP. Fusion of adjacent papillae (*ellipse*) should not lead to overgrading because of its fake appearance of disorder

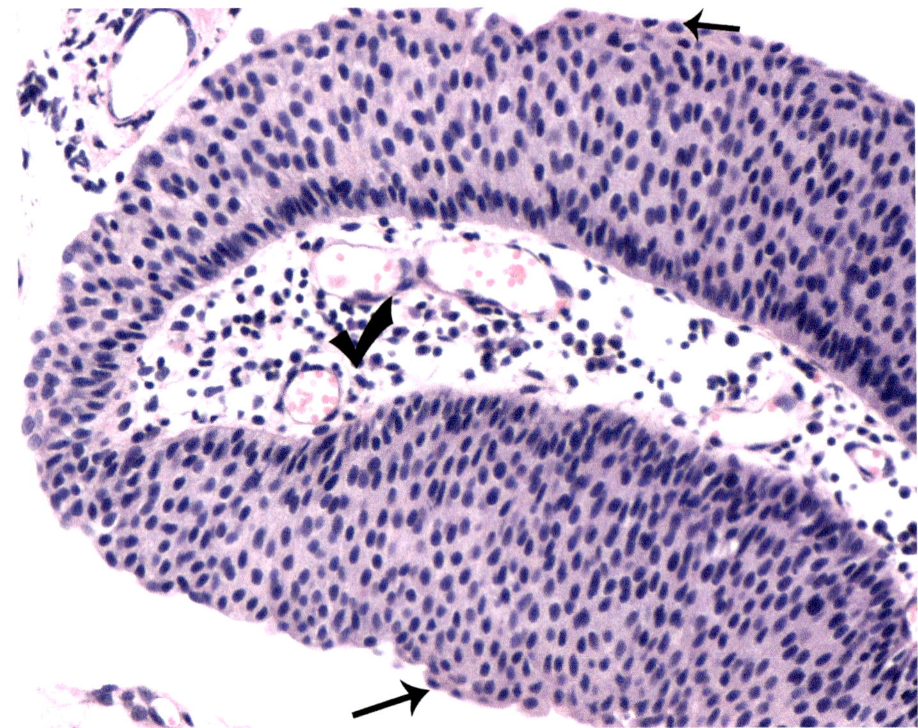

Fig. 2.22 (H-E, ×200) PUNLMP. The histologic architecture of the cells on the stalks is preserved, and the nuclear features are only slightly abnormal. The cells tend to be *evenly* distributed on the stalks; they have moderately distinct borders and homogeneous, amphophilic to acidophilic cytoplasm. Cytoplasmic clearing is almost always reduced when compared to normal cells from the same patient. Nuclei may be round or elongated, and they tend to maintain their normal perpendicular orientation to the surface and basal lamina. *Monotony* with regard to nuclear size and shape. Chromatin is evenly dispersed and finely granular. Minimal to absent cytologic atypia. The umbrella cell layer is often preserved (*arrows*), but it is less prominent than in urothelial papilloma. Mitoses should be rare and have a basal location.

When analyzing for the presence of order versus disorder, it is preferable to assess only those fibrovascular cores that have been cut perpendicular to the long axis of the papillary frond (*tick*). The stalks of PUNLMPs may have dilated blood vessels (*tick*), edema, or even foamy macrophages. Structures with broad stalks rich in connective tissue are not neoplasms.

PUNLMP shares many histologic features with papilloma (see Figs. 2.24, 2.25, and 2.26), the only differences being either thicker urothelium or diffuse nuclear enlargement in PUNLMP. At cystoscopy, PUNLMP tend to be larger than papillomas and may be indistinguishable from papillary carcinomas. In contrast to (noninvasive) low-grade papillary urothelial carcinoma, scattered cells with enlarged hyperchromatic nuclei are lacking in PUNLMP. Cytokeratin 20 (CK20) immunoreactivity should be confined to the umbrella cells of PUNLMP

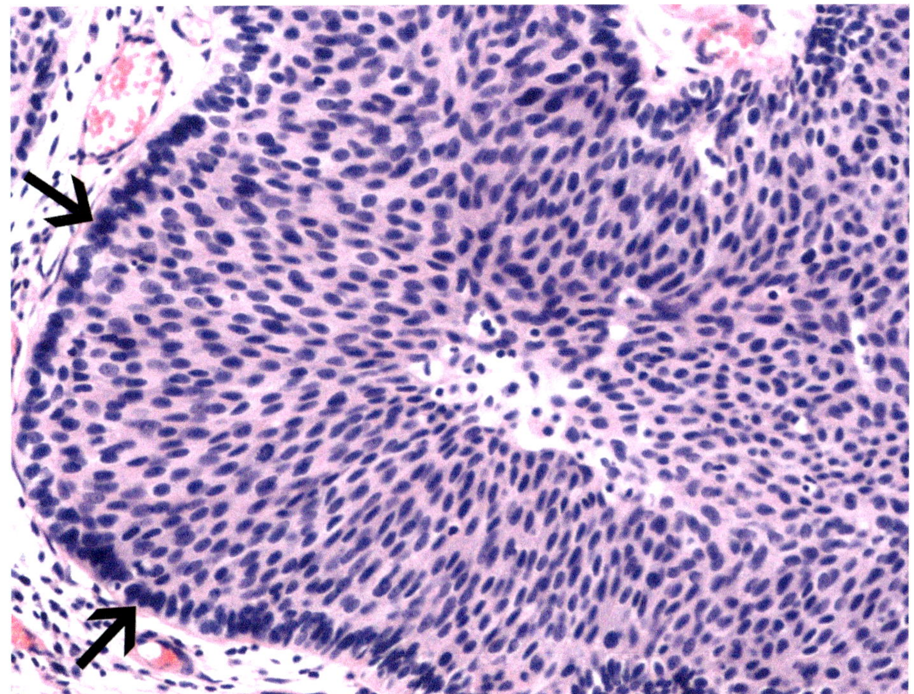

Fig. 2.23 (H-E, ×200) Signs of PUNLMP. Preservation of polarity of the multilayered urothelium, palisading of the basal layer (*arrows*). Neoplastic cells *streaming* upward from the basement membrane (i.e., normal polarity). Nuclear grooves may be seen in these tumors, but are not a common feature in higher-grade tumors. Mitoses should be exceedingly rare and with basal location, when the latter can be safely defined, of course. The mitotic activity observed in the lower left quartile of this image makes the diagnosis of PUNLMP controversial for this particular case. In low-grade papillary urothelial carcinoma, more than rare mitosis are counted, and scattered cells with enlarged hyperchromatic nuclei are observed. The simultaneous report of this tumor as a grade 1 urothelial carcinoma according to the WHO 1973 three-tired classification system appears, thus, quite informative.

Lesions which show no cytologic atypia and merely thickened urothelium with, at most, some degree of nuclear enlargement should be called PUNLMP according to the current WHO/ISUP two-tiered classification system; all these tumors would be classified as grade 1 tumors according to the WHO (1973) three-tiered classification system. However, other WHO (1973) grade 1 tumors with definite yet slight cytologic atypia should be diagnosed as low-grade urothelial carcinomas in the current system (see Fig. 2.30).

The following five images (Figs. 2.24, 2.25, 2.26, 2.27, and 2.28) derive from other patients, with totally benign urothelial neoplasms

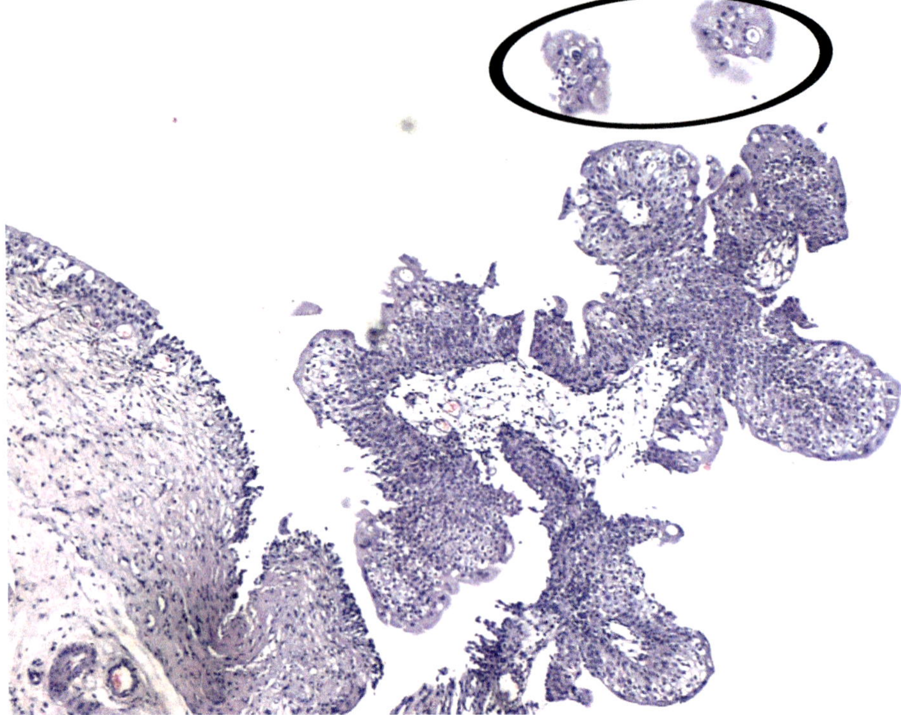

Fig. 2.24 (H-E, ×50) Exophytic urothelial papilloma is a very uncommon benign papillary urothelial tumor lined by normal-appearing urothelium. It may recur, but does not progress.

Most papillomas present as single lesions that are relatively small, delicate structures, superficially attached to the mucosa by a stalk. Exophytic pattern should predominate. Papillae appear to float above urothelial surface (*ellipse*) due to sectioning of branching papillae. Papillae are usually small with scant stroma and slender fibrovascular cores. Minimal epithelial confluence can be noticed between papillae

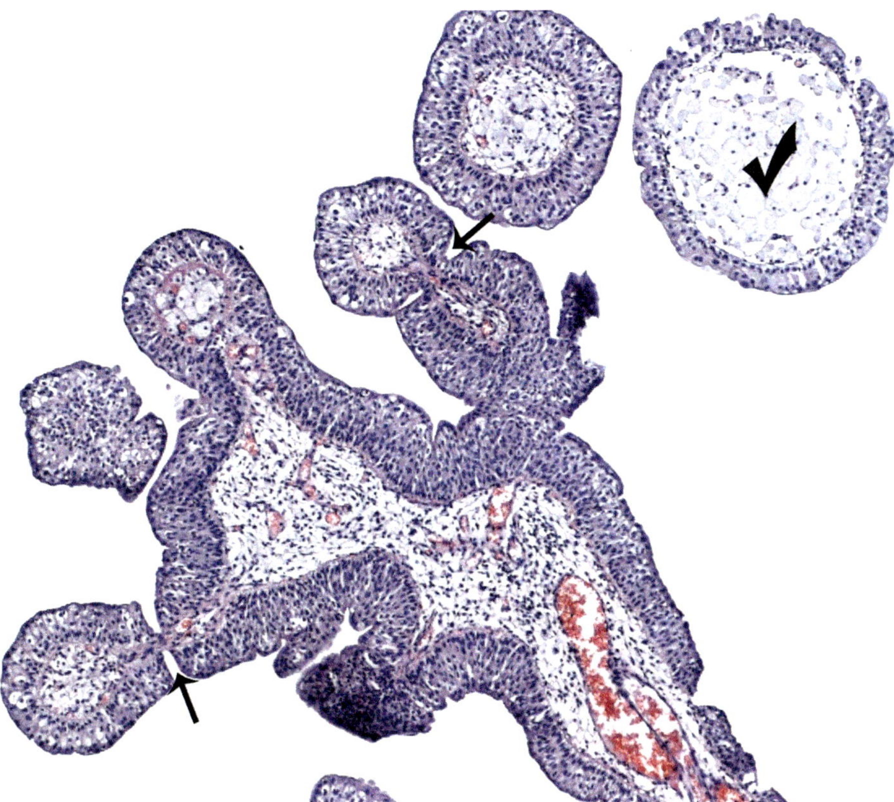

Fig. 2.25 (H-E, ×50) Urothelial papilloma. Simple, minimally branching arrangement, slender fibrovascular stalks lined by cytologically and architecturally normal-appearing urothelium with no more than seven layers of cells, in urothelial papilloma. The stroma shows inflammatory cells. Occasionally, foamy histiocytes accumulate within the fibrovascular stalks (*tick*).

Secondary budding of small fronds from larger simple primary papillary fronds (*arrows*) is commonly observed.

Arborization and the presence of *detached*-appearing papillary fronds exclude papillary hyperplasia.

In contrast to PUNLMP, lining urothelium in urothelial papilloma is of *normal* thickness

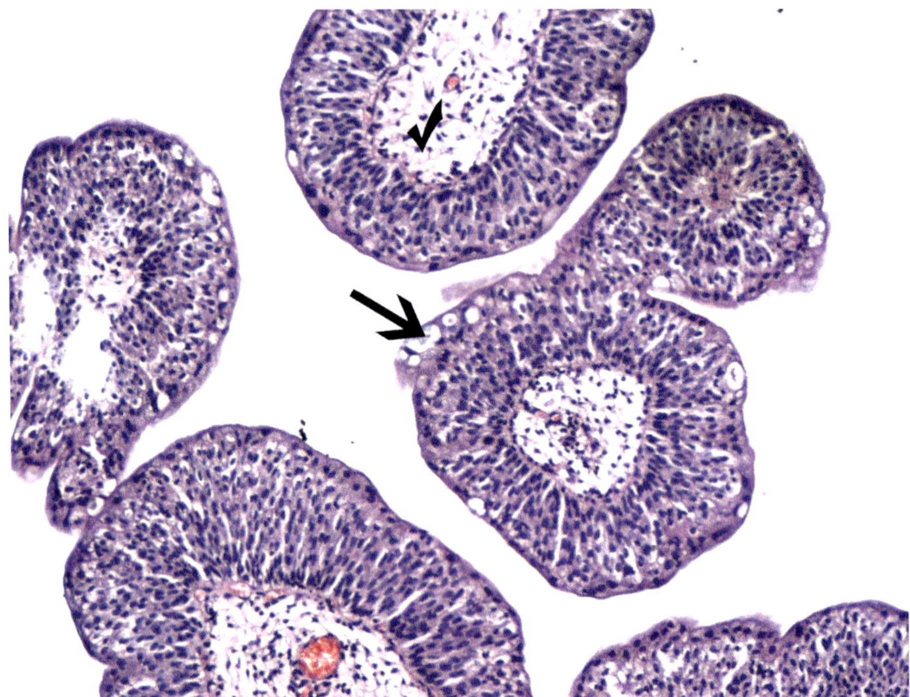

Fig. 2.26 (H-E, ×100) Superficial umbrella cells, with abundant eosinophilic cytoplasm and cytoplasmic vacuolization (*arrow*), can often be prominent in urothelial papilloma. Urothelial atypia, other than that which can be seen in umbrella cells, excludes the diagnosis of papilloma. Linear orientation of urothelial cells is perpendicular to the basement membrane. Mitoses should be rare or absent in urothelial papilloma and, when present, are located in the basal cell layer. The stroma shows edema (*tick*).

There is a decrease in nuclear size and hyperchromasia compared to PUNLMP.

Similarly to normal urothelium, in urothelial papilloma, cytokeratin 20 (CK20) is confined to umbrella cells, and accumulation of p53 is not seen or is very limited

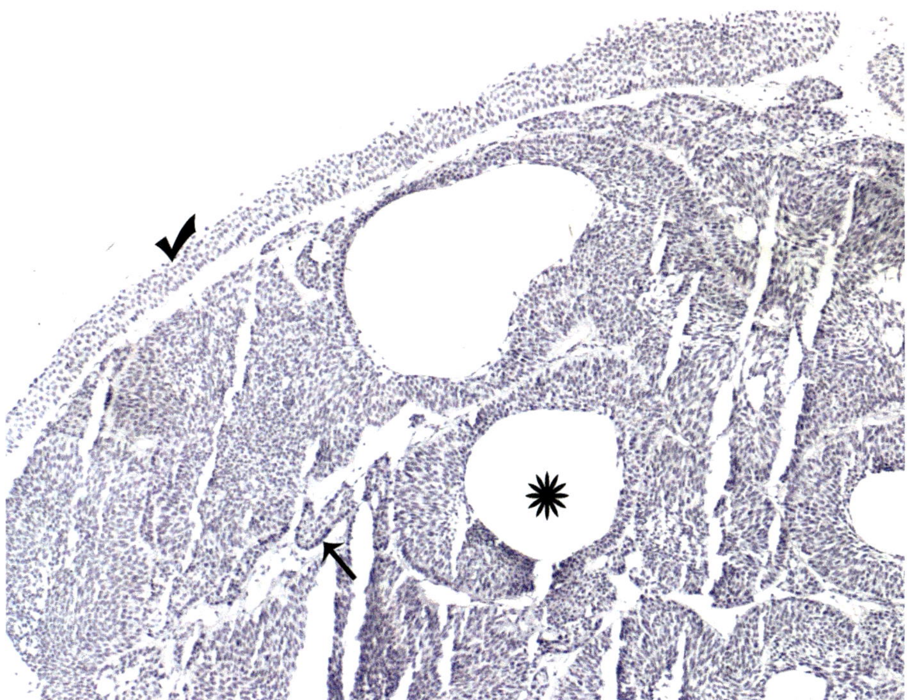

Fig. 2.27 (H-E, ×50) Inverted urothelial papilloma is a rare benign urothelial tumor involving the bladder trigone and neck or the prostatic urethra and typically appears as a solitary flat or slightly raised polypoid mass, frequently under 3 cm in greatest dimension, with smooth or nodular contours.

Microscopically, the surface urothelium may be compressed but otherwise unremarkable (*tick*). True papillae should be absent in inverted urothelial papillomas; when one or two small, apparently true fronds are present, they probably represent a tangential section off a polypoid growth, especially in cases of inverted papilloma fragmented during transurethral resection. Any exophytic component in a papillary urothelial neoplasm essentially excludes inverted papilloma.

Undermining overlying benign urothelium (*tick*), regular, *anastomosing* islands of histologically normal urothelium occupy the lamina propria (inverted pattern) but do *not* extend into the muscularis propria. This invagination should *not* be confused with invasion. Inverted papillomas are discrete lesions and do *not* exhibit an infiltrative border. Their base has a smooth interface with the subjacent stroma.

The neoplastic cells within the cords and nests of urothelium often have a spindled appearance. Focal minor cytologic atypia of degenerative nature may be seen in some cases. The periphery demonstrates palisading basaloid cells, at least focally (*arrow*). In the central portions of the invaginating growths, urothelial cells' streaming in parallel to the invaginating growths (i.e., normal maturation) is noticed in inverted papilloma. Small cystic spaces may be seen (*asterisk*). Minimal stromal component lacks inflammation and usually any other response (it can be fibrotic, though) and is relatively uniform between the inverted structures.

Round, non-anastomosing Brunn's nests, the florid proliferation of which should be distinguished from especially the glandular variant of inverted papilloma, are absent.

Compared with inverted papilloma, a urothelial carcinoma invading into Brunn's nests exhibits more atypia and mitotic activity and often demonstrates a papillary component

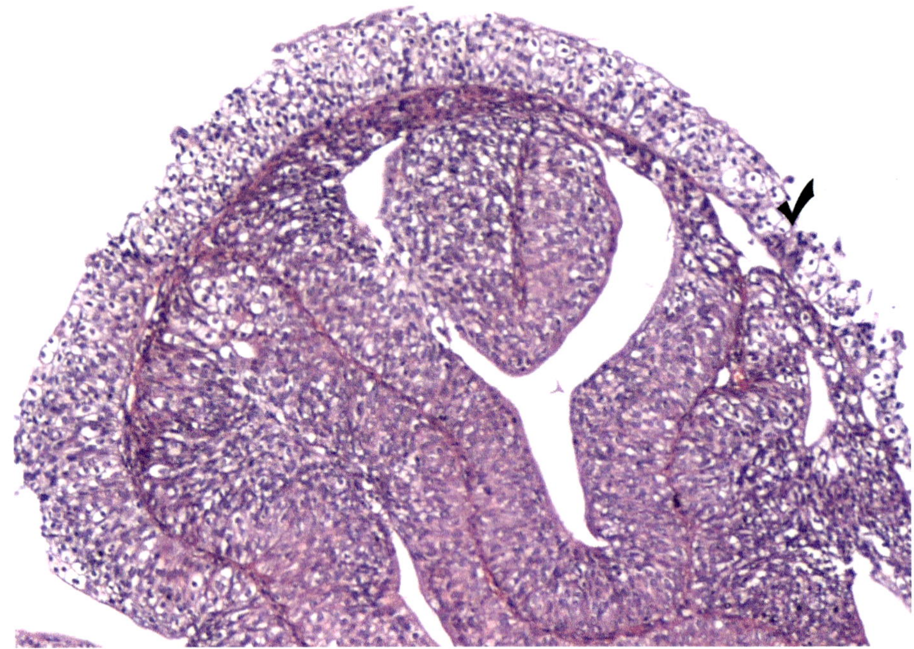

Fig. 2.28 (H-E, ×100) Inverted urothelial papilloma. Inter-anastomosing structures of cytologically bland urothelium extending down into the lamina propria, as if a papillary lesion had invaginated into the lamina propria.

The smooth, dome-shaped surface of an inverted papilloma consists of usually intact, cytologically unremarkable urothelium (*tick*). The tumor invaginates down from a smooth surface into the lamina propria as regular anastomosing trabeculae and cords of oval or spindle-shaped urothelium, usually with orderly maturation. The muscularis propria of the bladder wall should of course be uninvolved. These endophytic proliferations represent inversion of papillae.

The branching trabeculae are orderly, of relatively uniform width, in contrast to the thick and irregular tumor columns of a urothelial carcinoma with inverted growth pattern, in which transition to more solid areas is frequently observed. In inverted papilloma, cell layers vary from five to ten; thicker or more nodular or solid areas without cytologic atypia denote inverted PUNLMP or urothelial carcinoma with an inverted pattern of growth; some degree of nuclear atypia is necessary for the diagnosis of the latter, though. Minimal to absent cytologic atypia and absent or rare mitotic activity characterize inverted papilloma.

Three features are key to the recognition of inverted papilloma (and the exclusion of inverted pattern of urothelial carcinoma which may be difficult, especially in limited biopsy specimens with crush artifacts):

1. A relatively smooth surface with minimal to absent exophytic component
2. Lesional circumscription with a smooth base without obvious infiltration
3. Minimal to absent cytologic atypia
4. There is no evidence that inverted papilloma predisposes to the development of carcinoma, but the occasional coexistence of the two lesions suggests a pathogenetic relationship

2.3.1.2 Material from the Patient's First Recurrence

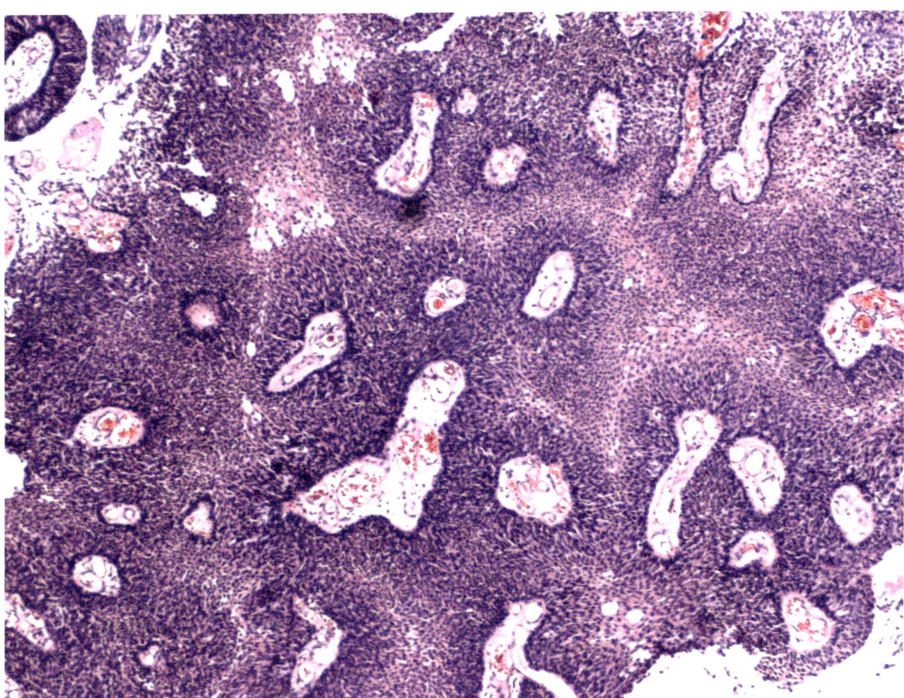

Fig. 2.29 (H-E, ×50) Noninvasive low-grade papillary urothelial carcinoma. Minimal variability in architecture and cytologic features is easily recognizable at scanning magnification; however, tangential sections near the base of the fronds may be misleading. Complex anastomosing epithelial growth entraps cores of adjacent papillae; final grading, however, should be based on cytoarchitectural features of the neoplastic epithelium as evaluated at medium power. At low magnification, there is a relatively orderly appearance, but at medium magnification, some loss of polarity as well as mild nuclear irregularity and pleomorphism is evident (see Fig. 2.30).

The absence of monotony is incompatible with PUNLMP

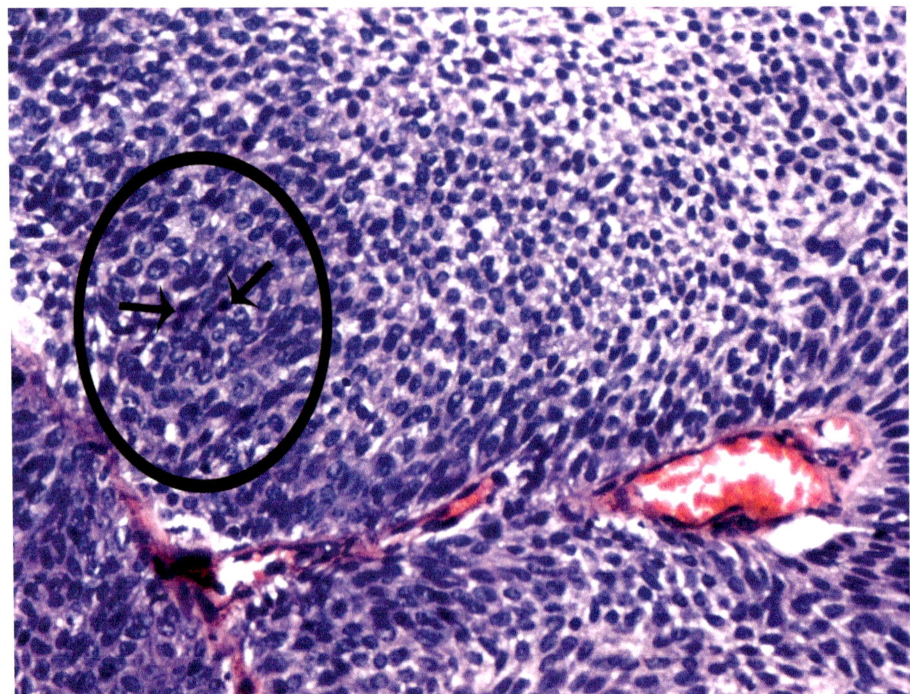

Fig. 2.30 (H-E, ×200) Noninvasive low-grade papillary urothelial carcinoma. Appearance looked orderly at low magnification, but mild variations in architectural and cytologic features (polarity, nuclear size, shape, contour, and chromatin texture) are easily recognizable at medium magnification; so the diagnosis of PUNLMP is not appropriate here.

In particular, loss of orientation to the basement membrane (*ellipse*) precludes a diagnosis of PUNLMP. Randomly distributed nuclei are located in varying directions. Subtle variation in nuclear size and shape. Nuclei are often rounded with occasional irregularities of nuclear contour. Nuclei tend to round up, thus creating a slight distortion of the cellular architecture. Relatively fine to slightly abnormal chromatin distribution. Many nuclei are uniformly enlarged with vesicular chromatin and present but inconspicuous nucleoli; nuclear grooves are usually present. Mitoses are still infrequent but can be noticed at any level, although they are usually limited to the lower half. Indistinct cell borders.

There is minimal but definite evidence of nuclear atypia consisting of scattered hyperchromatic nuclei (*arrows*), infrequent mitotic figures predominantly toward the base, and mild variation in nuclear size and shape. The finding of scattered hyperchromatic nuclei and scattered "typical" mitotic figures best distinguishes low-grade papillary urothelial carcinoma from PUNLMP. This particular tumor, which is classified as a noninvasive low-grade papillary urothelial carcinoma according to the current two-tiered WHO/ISUP classification, might still arguably fit in the grade 1 category of the three-tiered WHO 1973 classification system. The majority of low-grade papillary urothelial carcinoma cases, however, would have been considered as grade 2 in the WHO (1973) three-tiered classification

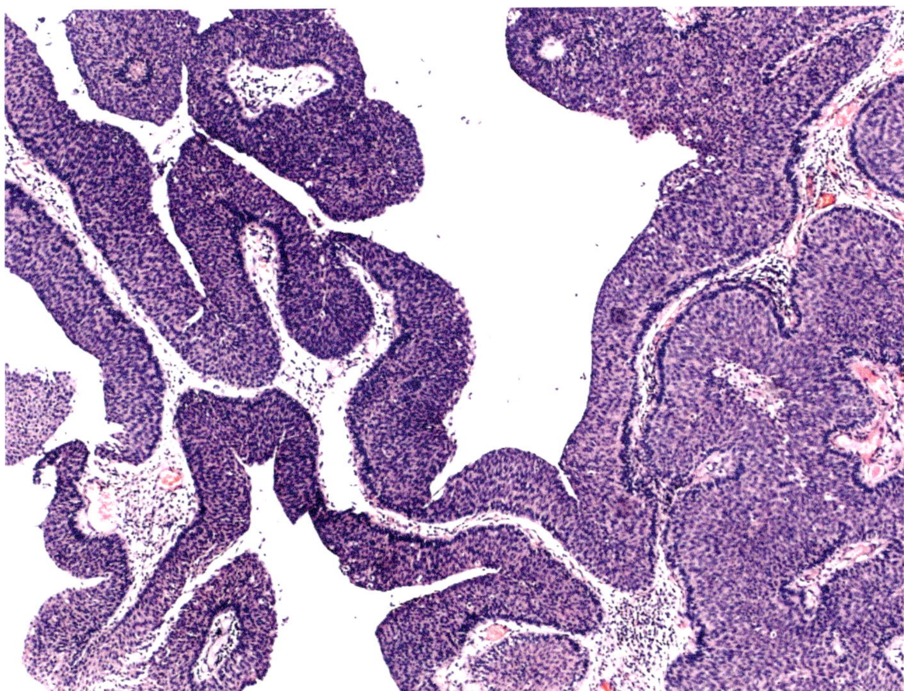

Fig. 2.31 (H-E, ×50) Noninvasive low-grade papillary urothelial carcinoma. Well-oriented longitudinal sections of papillae should be chosen for evaluation to avoid artifactual crowding from tangential sectioning. Slender papillary fronds are now showing frequent, extensive branching (left half of the image); fusion is minimal or totally absent (severe architectural distortion is still lacking).

At low magnification, the cells are uniform in size, predominantly cohesive, and evenly spaced (i.e., maintain polarity) but densely packed. At low and intermediate magnification in histologic sections, the cells of low-grade urothelial carcinoma are smaller and more densely arranged on the fibrovascular stalks than the cells of PUNLMP.

Thin papillary fronds with frequent branching and minimal fusion are characteristic of noninvasive low-grade papillary urothelial carcinoma. Tumor configuration is an important prognostic variable. Papillary tumors tend to be of lower-grade, earlier stage, and less aggressive behavior than nonpapillary tumors.

Papillary tumors may also exhibit an endophytic/inverted pattern (right one third of the image). Urothelial neoplasms exhibit two patterns of endophytic/inverted growth: (a) broad front verrucous carcinoma-like growth and (b) inverted papilloma-like growth (see Figs. 2.27 and 2.28).The two patterns may coexist, and either pattern may or may not be associated with frank stromal invasion (see Figs. 2.40, 2.41, 2.42, and 2.43).

In contrast to inverted papilloma, inverted urothelial carcinomas usually have a variable proportion of exophytic component.

If the endophytic/inverted component has markedly thickened but cytologically and architecturally unremarkable neoplastic formations and the exophytic component is similar, the designation of inverted PUNLMP seems appropriate.

Nearly all low-grade urothelial carcinomas are papillary, and invasive components are documented in less than 20% of cases

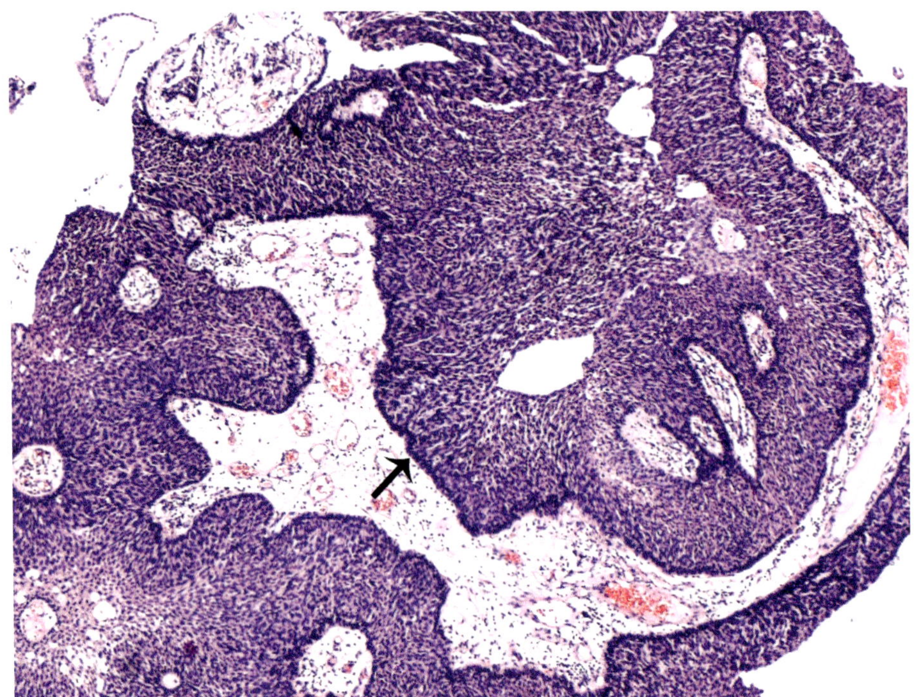

Fig. 2.32 (H-E, ×50) Noninvasive low-grade (papillary) urothelial carcinoma with an inverted growth. More expansile, thick structures of endophytic low-grade urothelial carcinoma, by comparison to inverted papilloma. Cellular disorder, but no pleomorphism.

In tumors with inverted papilloma-like growth, the basic configuration is like inverted papilloma, that is, endophytic, expansile growth with (or without) peripheral palisading of basaloid cells (*arrow*). Central streaming, seen in inverted papilloma, is lacking here, and the trabeculae are thick. By comparison with inverted papillomas, within inverted carcinomas, the ramifying structures are less uniform, sometimes solid without polarity, and typically consist of large, well-circumscribed rounded nests as opposed to anastomosing islands/trabeculae/cords of inverted papillomas. Nuclear pleomorphism, architectural abnormality, and increased mitotic activity are noticed in the inverted growth of urothelial carcinoma, and the surface of the neoplasm shows a typical exophytic papillary carcinoma (see Fig. 2.31). Whereas inverted papillomas usually do not demonstrate immunoreactivity for ki-67, p53, or CK20, urothelial carcinomas with inverted growth pattern frequently overexpress one or more of these biomarkers

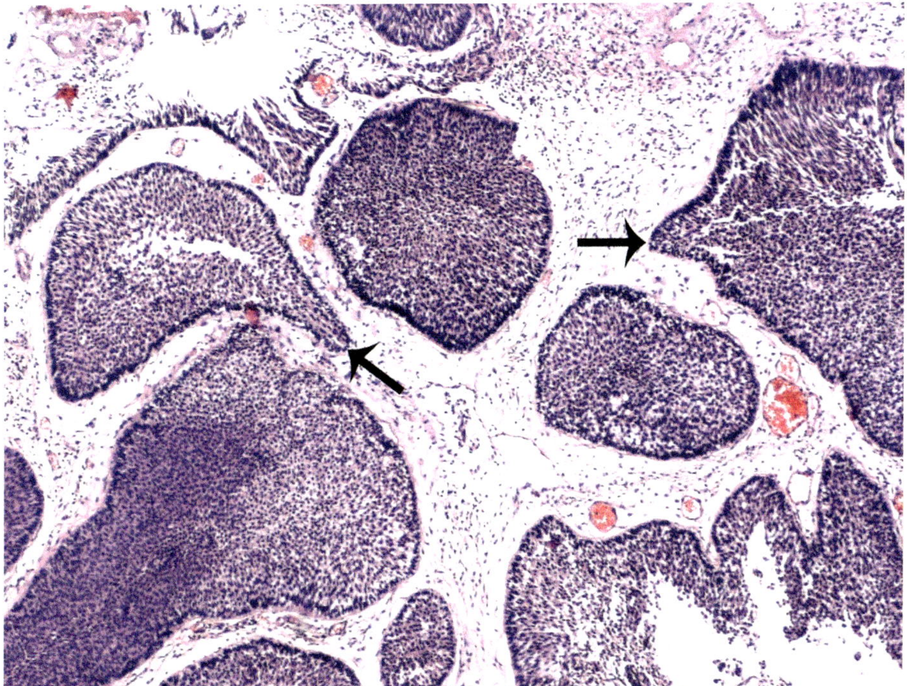

Fig. 2.33 (H-E, ×50) Broad-front inverted growth in the same tumor with often *large*, mostly *rounded* but focally irregularly shaped nests (*arrows*). Bulbous tongues of neoplastic urothelium extend deep into the lamina propria and sometimes may reach up to the muscularis propria but should *not* be encountered *within* the muscularis propria. Despite the deep penetration in the lamina propria, invasion is not present if the basement membrane is smooth, and the likelihood of metastasis is minimal. However, in case the inverted/endophytic growth of smooth-outlined neoplastic formations/nodules is not related to a diverticulum, and it clearly involves the muscularis propria, the perivesical tissue and possibly the stroma of the prostate gland, then invasion is documented; the carcinoma is staged accordingly (pT2-T4).

This tumor exhibits cytologic atypia elsewhere (see Fig. 2.30); so it should be designated as a low-grade urothelial carcinoma with both a papillary and an endophytic/inverted (i.e., not invasive) component (stage pTa).

Endophytic neoplasia of the urinary bladder includes inverted papilloma, endophytic urothelial neoplasm of low malignant potential, and endophytic urothelial carcinoma, low grade and high grade

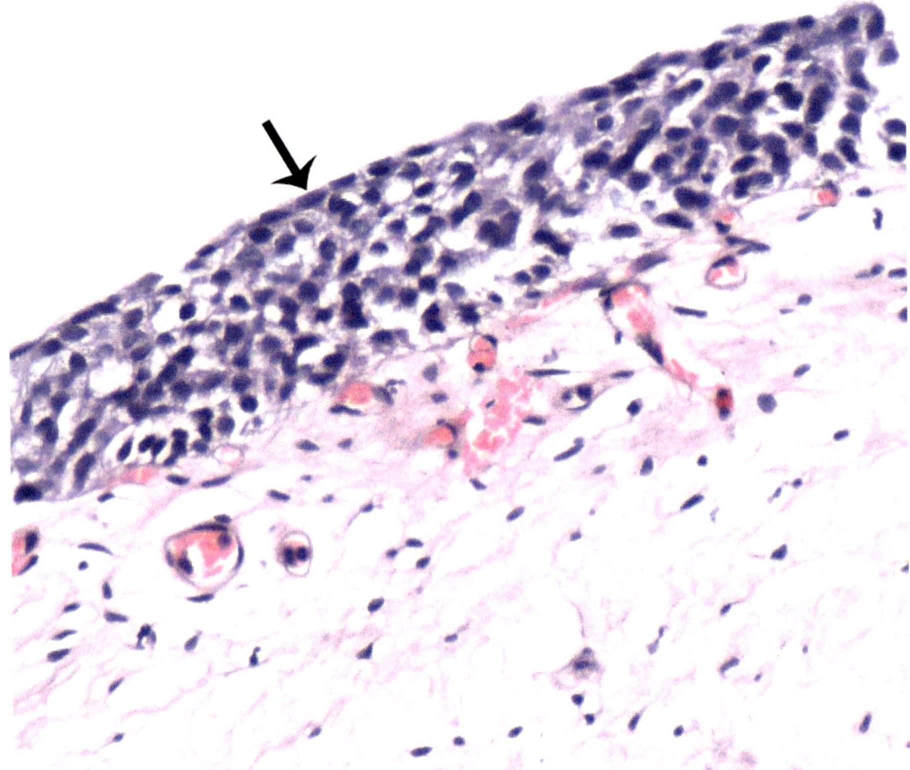

Fig. 2.34 (H-E, ×200) Urothelial dysplasia in random biopsies from mucosa adjoining the previous noninvasive low-grade papillary carcinoma. Distinct, appreciable nuclear abnormalities in the urothelium that occur in the absence of inflammation or that appear disproportionate to the amount of inflammation (if present) but are not severe [i.e., falling below the threshold of carcinoma in situ (CIS)] may be designated as urothelial dysplasia (low-grade intraurothelial neoplasia), characterized by cellular crowding, lack of orderly maturation, and cellular polarity in basal and intermediate cell layers (not full thickness). Grading of urothelial dysplasia is *not* recommended since urothelial dysplasia is synonymous with low-grade intraurothelial neoplasia (LG IUN). The term urothelial dysplasia describes lesions of flat, noninvasive urothelium with appreciable cytologic and architectural changes indicative of neoplasia but less than CIS; dysplasia represents an early morphologic manifestation of progressive alterations between normal urothelium and CIS.

The urothelium shows loss of cell polarity and crowding of slightly enlarged nuclei (increase in N/C ratio). Notching of cell borders. Nucleomegaly and loss of polarity can be better assessed when more normal-appearing urothelium is present in the same or other biopsy specimens of the same patient. Normal urothelial thickness (may be increased or decreased) and superficial umbrella cells (*arrow*) are intact.

Loss of the perpendicular arrangement of the dysplastic urothelial cells with a minimal degree of nuclear enlargement or irregularity is similar to that or low-grade papillary urothelial carcinoma; the latter entities are by definition papillary and/or inverted, in contrast to dysplasia which is flat by definition

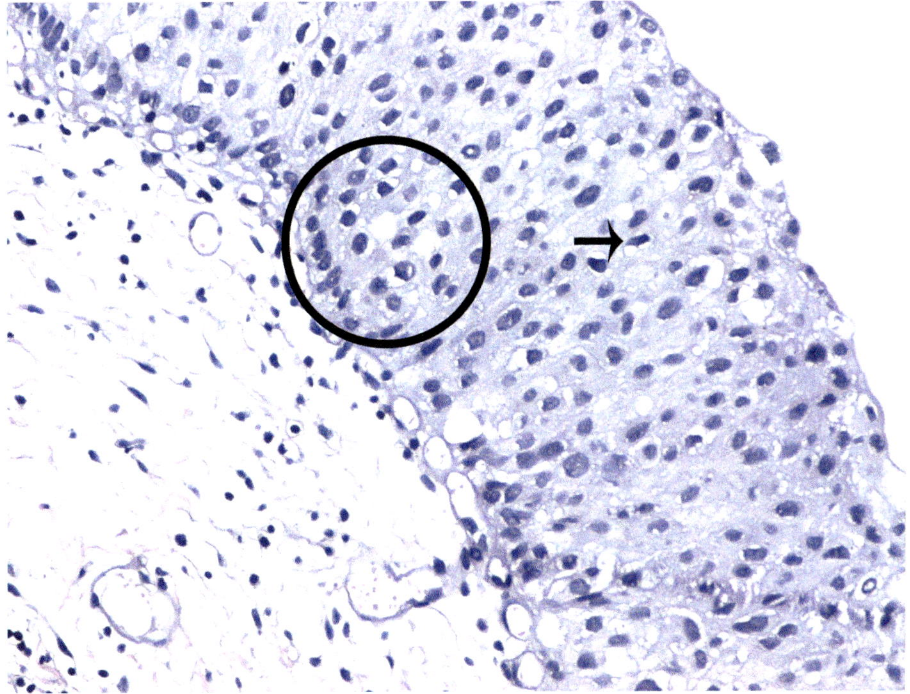

Fig. 2.35 (H-E, ×200) Urothelial dysplasia. Small yet hyperchromatic nuclei and scattered, enlarged nuclei. Mildly altered chromatin distribution, inconspicuous nucleoli in dysplastic urothelium. Irregularity of nuclear contours (*arrow*). Cytologic atypia is *not* severe enough to merit a diagnosis of CIS.

There is some loss of cytoplasmic clearing; increased cytoplasmic eosinophilia is observed along with nuclear enlargement, nuclear membrane irregularities, nuclear hyperchromasia, and at least loss of nuclear polarity (*circle*).

Lamina propria is normal in urothelial dysplasia; no evidence of acute or chronic inflammation rules out two other flat lesions, namely, reactive atypia and atypia of unknown significance

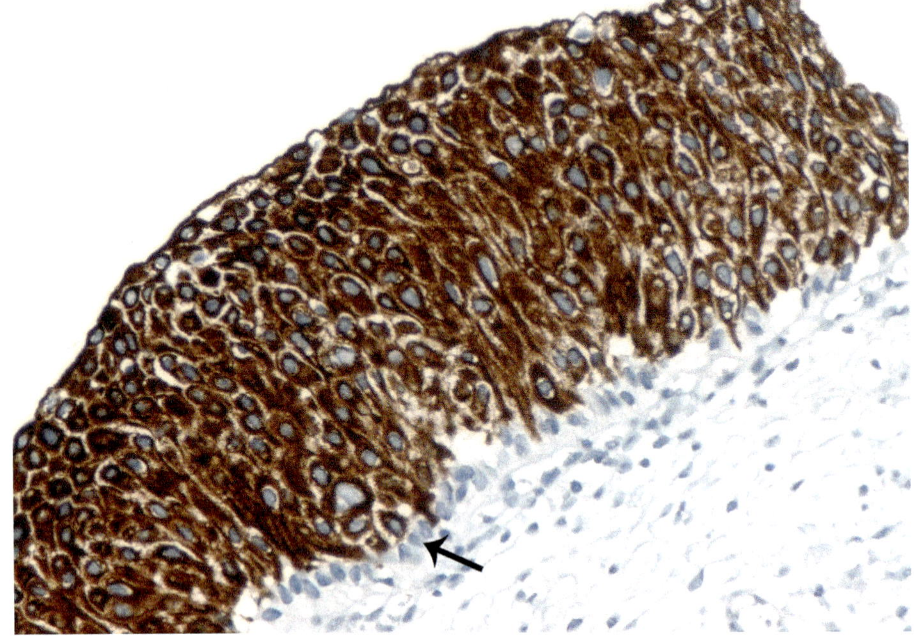

Fig. 2.36 [Cytokeratin20 (CK20) immunohistochemistry, ×200] Urothelial dysplasia. Low interobserver agreement on morphologic diagnosis of urothelial dysplasia, even among experts, is a fact; immunohistochemistry is therefore helpful. Aberrant CK20 expression confirms the diagnosis of urothelial dysplasia. CK20 is limited to the superficial cell layers in normal urothelium; in contrast, CK20 immunostaining is usually present in the superficial and *at least* in the intermediate layers of dysplastic epithelium; here it occupies almost its whole thickness; only basal cells remain unstained (*arrow*).

Overexpression of p53 and ki-67 also provides diagnostic aid as they are indicators of dysplastic change in urothelial in urothelial mucosa in conjunction with morphology; the latter immunomarker being reliable in the absence of severe inflammation. The ki-67 proliferation index in urothelial dysplasia is typically >50%, versus <10% in nonneoplastic urothelium. Positive CD44 immunostaining is observed only in the basal and parabasal cells in normal urothelium and is either absent entirely or present only in scattered cells in urothelial dysplasia, whereas full thickness positive membranous CD44 staining is typical of reactive urothelium

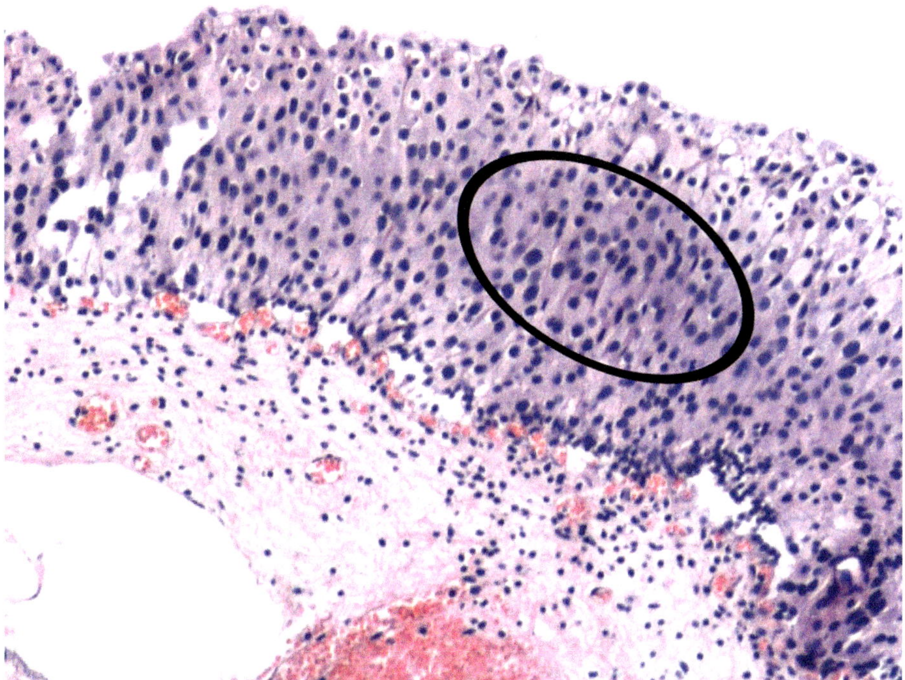

Fig. 2.37 (H-E, ×200) Urothelial dysplasia. Loss of polarity, evidenced by crowding of nuclei (*ellipse*), in flat urothelium. More rounded to polygonal cells with nuclei still parallel to the long axis. Increased cytoplasmic eosinophilia (*ellipse*). Atypical cytologic changes are restricted to intermediate and basal cells.

Mitotic figures, when present, should generally be basally located, while in CIS, mitoses can be observed in the upper epithelium.

A way to conceptualize the difference between dysplasia and CIS, which are both *flat* urothelial lesions, is that the cytological findings seen in dysplasia are analogous to those seen in noninvasive low-grade papillary urothelial carcinoma, whereas CIS is analogous in its histology to high-grade papillary urothelial carcinoma

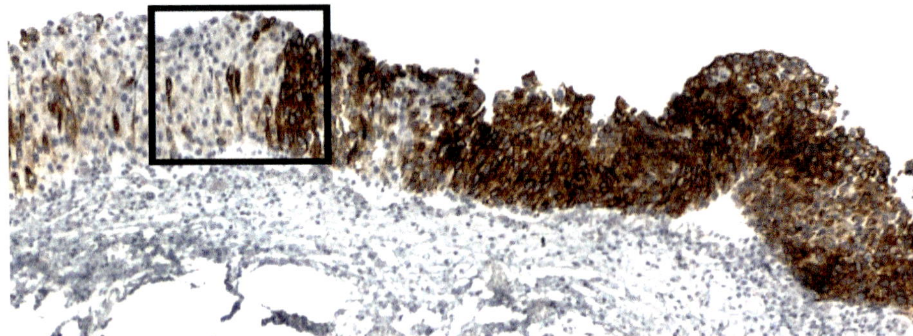

Fig. 2.38 (CK20 immunohistochemistry, ×100) As previously stated, urothelial dysplasia is the most difficult category to define, due to significant interobserver variability. So, increasing thickness of CK20 immunostaining in dysplastic urothelium is crucial for the diagnosis of dysplasia.

The transition from normal to abnormal is subtle (*square frame*); non-dysplastic unstained urothelial cells are often dispersed among the dysplastic immunostained cells

2.3.1.3 Material from the Patient's Second Recurrence

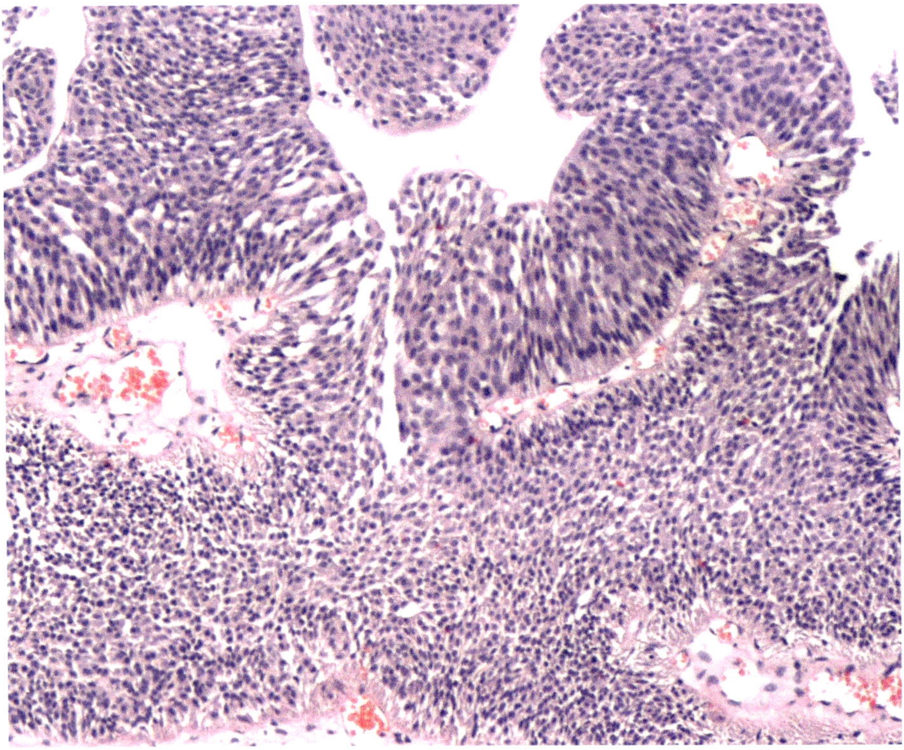

Fig. 2.39 (H-E, ×100) Noninvasive low-grade papillary urothelial carcinoma (pTa in this field).

Remember that only papillary fronds cut perpendicular to long axis of papillary frond (i.e., longitudinal sections) should be assessed

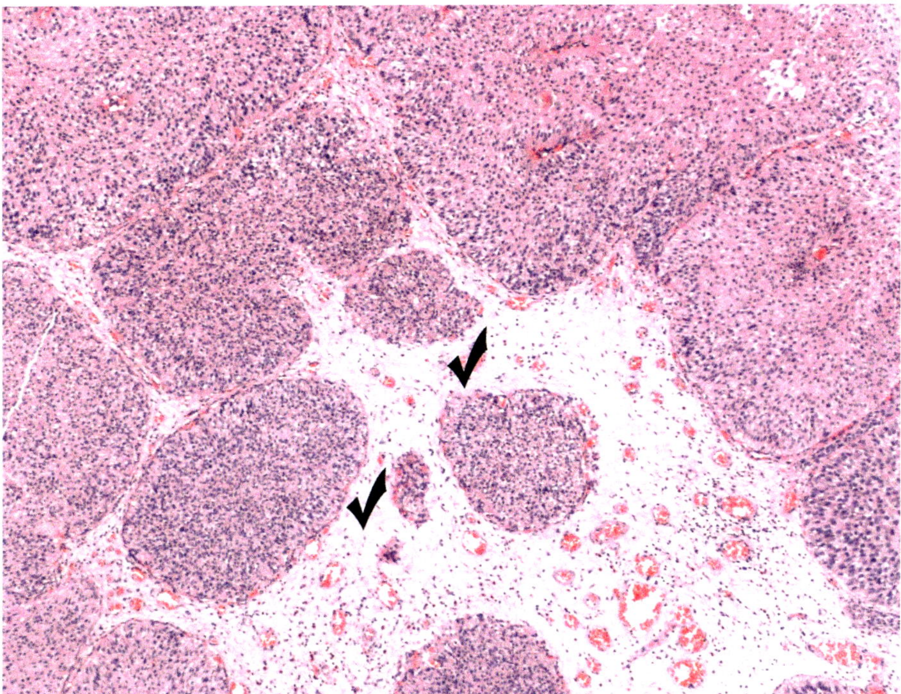

Fig. 2.40 (H-E, ×50) Noninvasive low-grade papillary urothelial carcinoma (pTa in this field). The present tumor, in addition to its exophytic papillary component, is associated, as usually happens, with an inverted element (*ticks*), shown in this image.

Tangentially sectioned, densely packed, noninvasive papillary tumors with an inverted component exhibit a stromal-epithelial interface that is smooth and regular (stage pTa, as in this field). The endophytic growth appears to extend into the lamina propria with a pushing border in which the basement membrane is not truly breached. Unless this pattern is accompanied by true destructive stromal invasion or extension into the muscularis propria, the likelihood of metastasis is minimal.

In the inverted pattern of this case, due to cancer heterogeneity, a very minor high-grade component of the tumor was detected and is shown in the remaining four images, highlighting this particular tumor area which, however, represents <5% of the whole tumor mass. More than 95% of the tumor mass corresponds to low-grade urothelial carcinoma as shown in Figs. 2.39 and 2.40

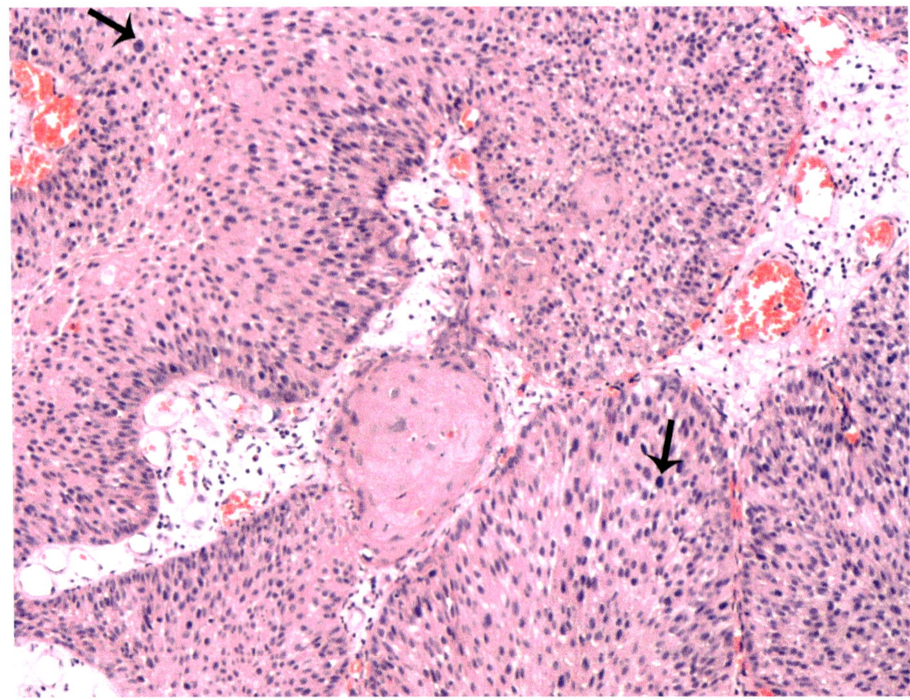

Fig. 2.41 (H-E, ×100) The minor high-grade tumor component with microinvasion of the lamina propria.

The WHO classification system requires the evaluation of the level of cytological and architectural disorder at low and medium magnification.

These cytologic abnormalities are recognizable even at low magnification (a feature which, by the way, is certainly incompatible with PUNLMP, as previously stressed). Low-grade papillary urothelial carcinoma features include loss of cellular polarity, random distribution of cells in urothelium, and loss of linear perpendicular orientation to basement membrane. Invasion both within the papillary cores and at the base of such a lesion should be meticulously investigated.

Cellular disorder and *scattered* pleomorphic/hyperchromatic cells (*arrows*) are sufficient for a high-grade carcinoma diagnosis in this field. Under the recent WHO/ISUP system, diffuse nuclear anaplasia is *not* necessary for a high-grade diagnosis

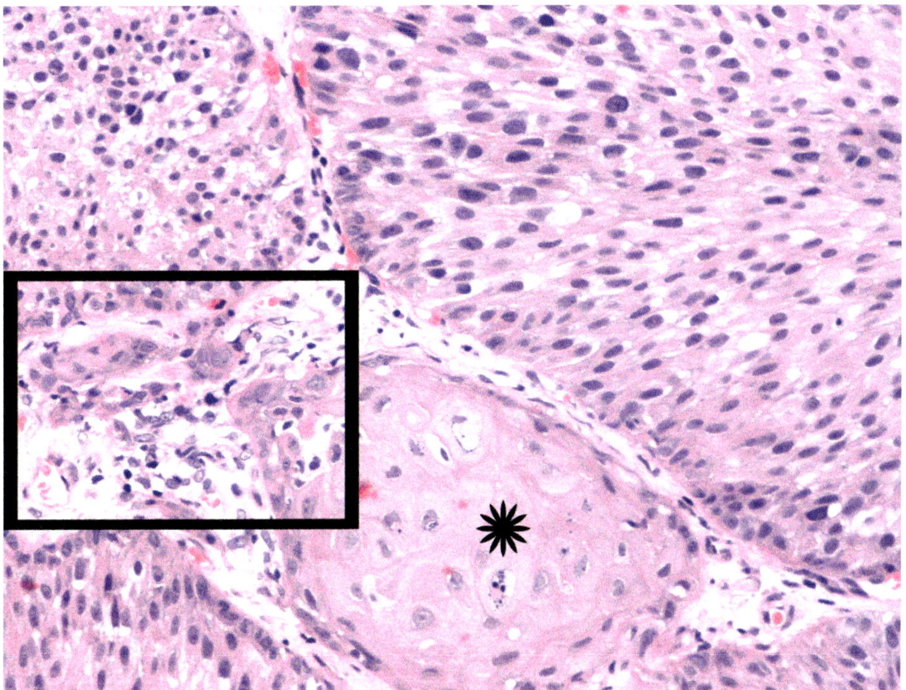

Fig. 2.42 (H-E, ×200) The minor high-grade component with microinvasion of the lamina propria.

Architecturally, the neoplastic cells are irregularly oriented and disorganized. Cellular pleomorphism is moderate; coarsely textured nuclei are obvious. In such tumors with variable histology, the tumor should be graded according to the *highest* grade, although current practice is to note minor components (<5%) of high grade yet grade the tumor still as low grade.

The features in this particular minor tumor area are incompatible with low-grade urothelial carcinoma. Disorderly appearance upgrades this tumor area to the high-grade (papillary) carcinoma category according to the current WHO/ISUP classification, although it might still be assigned grade 2 in the WHO (1973) three-tiered classification. We should have in mind that all tumors classified as grade 3 in the 1973 WHO three-tiered scheme, as well as *some* assigned grade 2 in that classification, would be considered high-grade carcinoma in the current, two-tiered WHO/ISUP classification. Urologists should be aware that "grade 2" does not equal low grade in all cases.

A focus of lamina propria microinvasion is noticed in the form of an irregularly shaped nest and individual tumor cells insinuating within the stroma (*square frame*). Particularly in microinvasive disease, the invasive tumor cells may acquire abundant eosinophilic cytoplasm; either paradoxical differentiation or squamous differentiation is implied (*asterisk*).

Invasive cells, in general, show moderate to abundant amphophilic or eosinophilic cytoplasm; their nuclei have irregular contours with angular profiles.

Although invasion beyond the basement membrane into the lamina propria (but not the muscularis propria) (stage pT1) is not necessarily an unexpected finding in low-grade carcinomas, it is much more commonly encountered in high-grade carcinomas

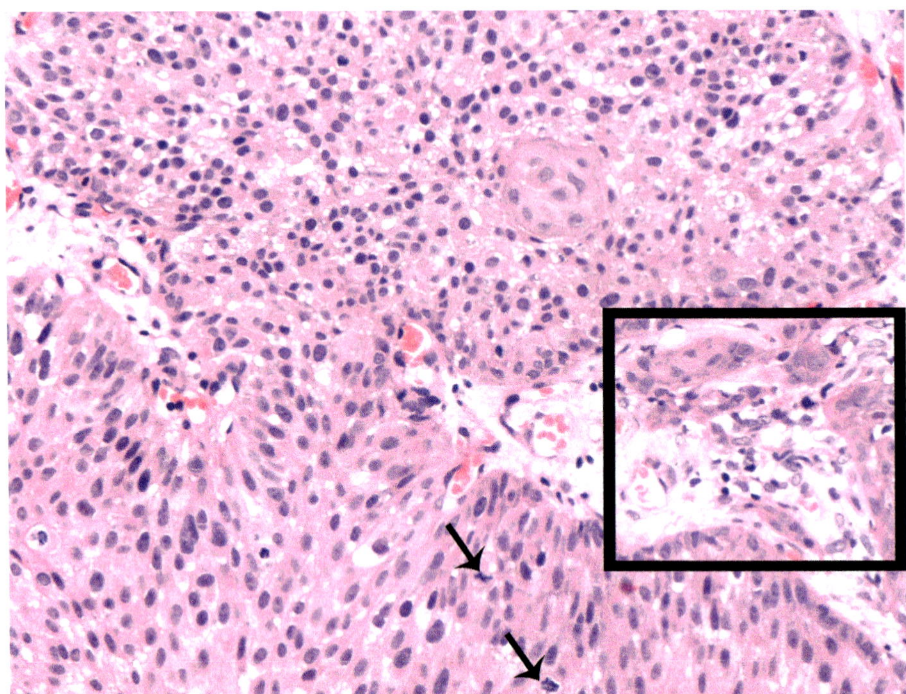

Fig. 2.43 (H-E, ×200) The minor high-grade component with microinvasion of the lamina propria.
Marked variation in nuclear polarity, size, shape, and chromatin pattern. This obviously disordered arrangement with cytologic atypia upgrades this minor tumor area to the current WHO/ISUP "high-grade" category. The neoplastic epithelium is still clearly of urothelial origin. Mitotic figures are frequently encountered (*arrows*). Foci of invasion are generally characterized by irregular urothelial nests, clusters, or single urothelial cells at the base of the lesion within the lamina propria (*square frame*) or within the papillary cores of the exophytic pattern (both staged as pT1)

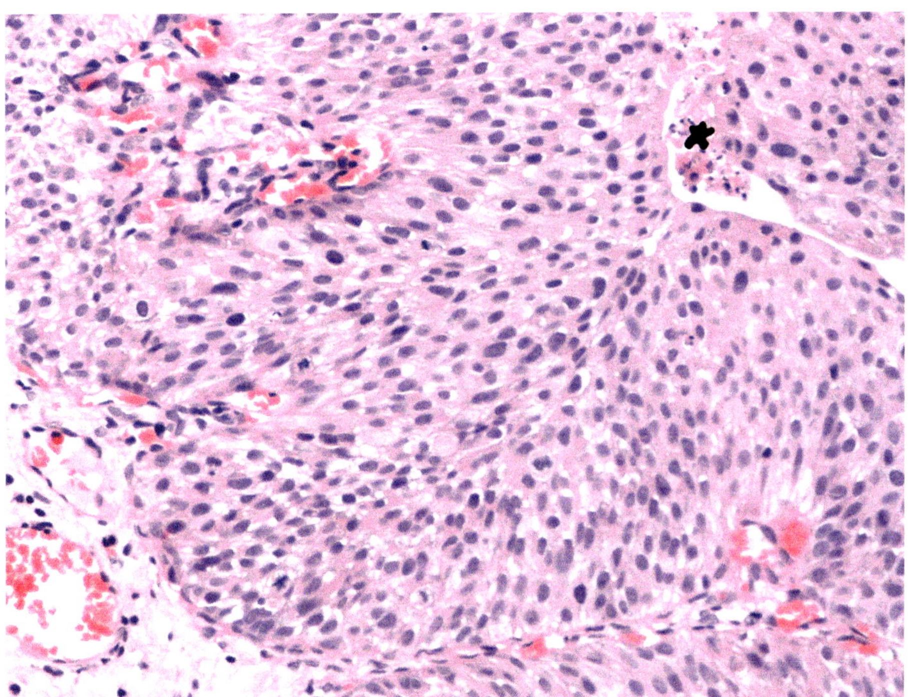

Fig. 2.44 (H-E, ×200) Area of high-grade urothelial carcinoma as a very minor component in the present tumor. Focal necrotic activity is suggested in this field (*blob*), another indicator of high grade.

Urothelial tumors may show heterogeneity of grade. Tumors are graded based on the higher grade exhibited. If the tumor is predominantly low grade and there is a high-grade component occupying more than 5% of the tumor, it should be classified as high-grade papillary carcinoma. For the uncommon case like this one, with a very minor (<5%) high-grade component, the lesion is diagnosed as low grade with a comment as to the presence of focal higher-grade tumor.

In conclusion, in this case, the diagnosis of high-grade papillary urothelial carcinoma component is based on scattered pleomorphic/hyperchromatic cells and easily identified mitotic figures. Such a lesion would possibly have been classified as grade 2 in the WHO 1973 system but should be classified as high grade according to the current WHO/ISUP classification

2.3.1.4 Clinical Commentary

Vasileios Spapis

The initial pathology report for the present patient was that of a PUNLMP. The next one was of a noninvasive low-grade papillary urothelial carcinoma (stage pTa) with dysplasia in the neighboring urothelium. The most recent pathology report speaks of low-grade papillary urothelial carcinoma with a very minor high-grade component within the tumor's inverted pattern where focal lamina propria microinvasion is detected (stage pT1).

Painless hematuria is the most common symptom in bladder tumors, and all patients with painless hematuria suffer from urothelial cancer unless proven otherwise. CT urography is used to detect papillary tumors mostly in the upper urinary tract. US is helpful for detection of renal masses and hydronephrosis, but cannot exclude the presence of bladder neoplasms (Babjuk et al. 2017a, b). Urine cytology has high sensitivity in grade 3 (G3) and high-grade tumors (84%) but low sensitivity in G1 and low-grade tumors (16%) (Yafi et al. 2015). Cystoscopy remains the most useful tool for diagnosis of papillary bladder masses. The suspected mass is then resected and histologically evaluated.

Papillary urothelial neoplasms of low malignant potential (PUNLMP) are essentially benign papillary tumors with minimal architectural abnormalities and minimal nuclear atypia (Jones 2016). In older grading systems, these tumors were classified as papillomas or grade 1 "transitional cell" carcinomas (TCCs). Now they are considered benign because they are unlikely to progress. However, patients with these tumors are at risk of developing new bladder tumors, usually of similar histology. Sometimes though, progress has been reported, so follow-up of the patient is warranted (Jones 2016).

In this case, recurrence and progression did eventually happen, and a lesion was visible during the first programmed cystoscopy (usually at 3 months). Low-grade, Ta carcinomas are characterized as low-risk tumors, and, after transurethral resection, six weekly bladder instillations (followed by six monthly instillations) with epirubicin is the treatment of choice. Follow-up of these patients should be continuous including cystoscopy every 3 months initially and yearly after 12 months (Babjuk et al. 2017a, b; Konety and Carol 2013; Solsona et al. 2000).

A second recurrence and further tumor progression are now observed. The tumor now is considered to be high risk and even early radical cystectomy could be offered. However, the most appropriate choice is the patient to be offered treatment with BCG instillations and closer follow-up (cystoscopy and urine cytology every 3 months for 2 years and then every 6 months). BCG failure (recurrence or tumor progression) even for nonmuscle-invasive bladder cancer (NMIBC) should lead to radical cystectomy (Babjuk et al. 2017a, b).

Key Points

- PUNLMP is a papillary urothelial tumor which resembles the exophytic urothelial papilloma but with increased cellular proliferation exceeding the thickness of normal urothelium. Recurrence of PUNLMP is at a lower frequency than with low-grade papillary urothelial carcinoma.
- The diagnosis of urothelial dysplasia can be made in cases in which the urothelium demonstrates significant cytologic atypia that cannot be attributed to inflammation or a reparative process and yet lacks the full complement of cytologic abnormalities that characterize carcinoma in situ (CIS).
- Dysplasia in patients with a history of or concomitant presence of noninvasive papillary neoplasms indicates urothelial instability and is a marker for progression or recurrence.
- A diagnosis of primary dysplasia (i.e., no prior history or concomitant urothelial neoplasia) should be made with great caution.
- Heterogeneity in grade is a characteristic of papillary carcinoma. Distinguishing low-grade papillary urothelial carcinoma from high grade is important, because therapy is different (intravesical therapy for high grade). It may be prudent to state the proportion of high-grade disease.

2.4 Case 2.3: High-Grade Bladder Carcinoma

Cytological Assessment by Dr. med. Georgia-Eleni Thomopoulou

Case Study

Data Prior to Microscopy

A 68-year-old woman presents with dysuria following a period of painless gross hematuria. Initial treatment for a presumed urinary tract infection had been ineffective. Urine cytology is positive and subsequent cystoscopy reveals a single, solid, sessile, polypoid mass at the bladder neck which is transurethrally resected. Sampling of the underlying muscularis propria (detrusor muscle) is performed, but no random biopsies from bladder mucosa are taken.

Based on the histological findings, cystoscopy is programmed 6 weeks after the initial resection. This time the patient complains about frequency, dysuria, and suprapubic fullness. Microscopic hematuria is found. Urine cytology is again positive for high-grade urothelial malignancy. Multiple granular areas are cystoscopically detected, and multiple biopsies are taken.

2.4.1 Microscopic Evaluation of the Initial Cytology Smears and Transurethral Resection of Bladder Tumor (TURBT) Specimen

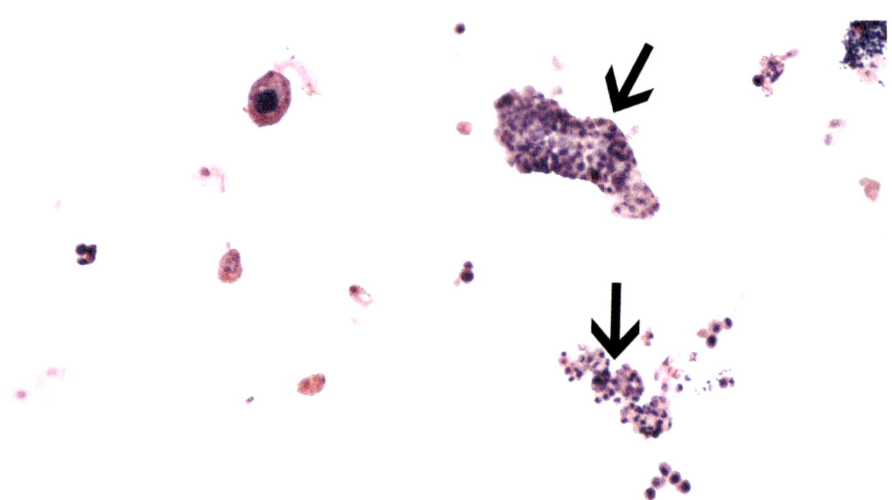

Fig. 2.45 (Papanicolaou stain, ×100) High-grade papillary urothelial carcinoma. Two recognizable papillae (*arrows*).

Exfoliative cytology is important for the *initial* diagnosis of bladder tumors but is of little practical value in the evaluation of *most* bladder tumors, which can be readily performed by urologists, since the majority of bladder urothelial tumors have an exophytic component or are exclusively exophytic/papillary. The major deficiency with cytologic examination is the under-recognition of low-grade papillary neoplasms (see Case 2.2.); in the latter neoplasms, the principle cytological clue is abundance of cells. In high-grade neoplasia, however, the diagnostic value of voided urine cytology is of vital importance

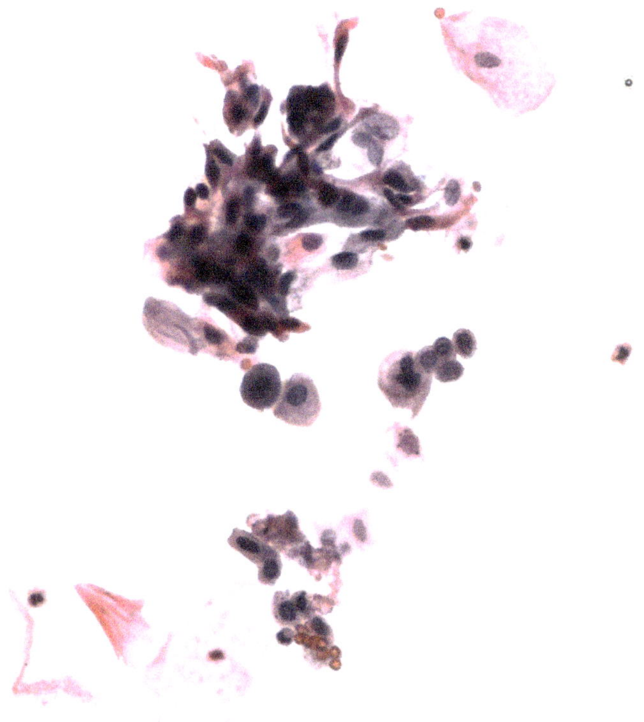

Fig. 2.46 (Papanicolaou stain, ×200) High-grade papillary urothelial carcinoma. Unlike benign urothelial cells, the majority of the above cells have substantial nuclear and cytoplasmic abnormalities. Clusters and single, markedly atypical cells with high nuclear/cytoplasmic ratio, pleomorphic nuclei, coarse, irregularly distributed chromatin. The nuclear contours are irregular.
The major cytological diagnostic criteria for high-grade urothelial neoplasia include:

- Spindle, pyramidal, and racquet shapes
- Increased numbers of irregular, three-dimensional cell groups
- Intracytoplasmic vacuoles
- Marked pleomorphism with enlarged hyperchromatic nuclei, coarse chromatin, increased N/C ratio, and prominent nucleoli

The presence of necrosis, lysed blood, and degenerated red blood cells is most suggestive of invasion, but invasion cannot be conclusively diagnosed on cytology specimens

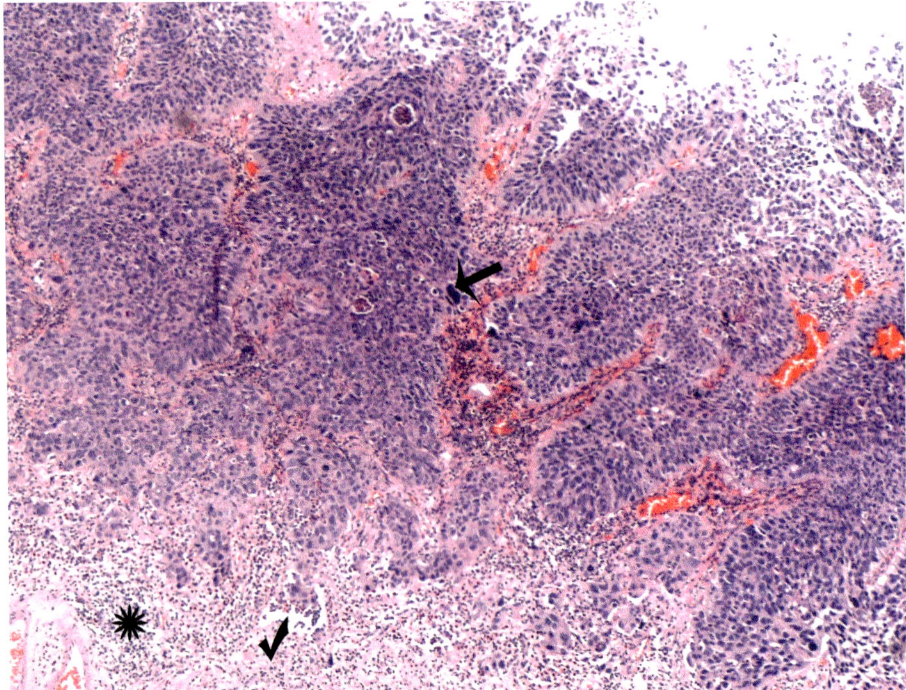

Fig. 2.47 (H-E, ×100) High-grade papillary urothelial carcinoma. Nuclei tend to cluster; among them separate, markedly pleomorphic nuclei are easily observed (*arrow*) under low magnification.

Invasive front of the carcinoma: irregularly shaped nests of tumor within the evidently inflamed stroma (*asterisk*); the interface between epithelium and stroma may be obscured.

There is a well-established invasion into underlying lamina propria in this field (stage pT1). The neoplastic cells in typical or conventional patterns of invasive urothelial carcinoma are usually of moderate size and have modest amounts of pale to densely eosinophilic cytoplasm and infiltrate the bladder wall as nests, cords, trabeculae, small clusters, or single cells. Invasive foci are often associated with retraction artifacts, mimicking vascular invasion (*tick*). The *extent of spread at the time of initial diagnosis* is the most important factor in determining the outlook for a patient

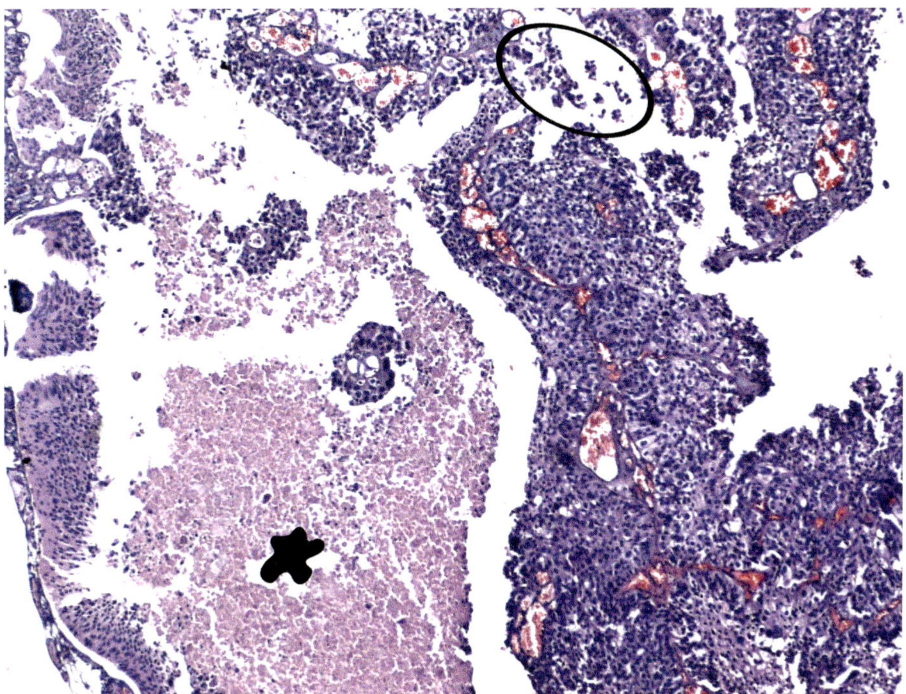

Fig. 2.48 (H-E, ×100) High-grade papillary urothelial carcinoma. In general, high-grade urothelial carcinomas have a relatively nondescript morphology, similar to that of poorly differentiated carcinomas of other types. Urothelium thickness may vary considerably. Necrotic activity (*blob*) can be considerable.

Obvious urothelial disordered arrangement and loss of polarity are observed at scanning magnification. Increased cellularity, nuclear crowding, and random cellular polarity. Vacuolization may be common. The superficial cell layer is partially or completely absent, often accompanied by prominent cellular dyscohesion (*ellipse*)

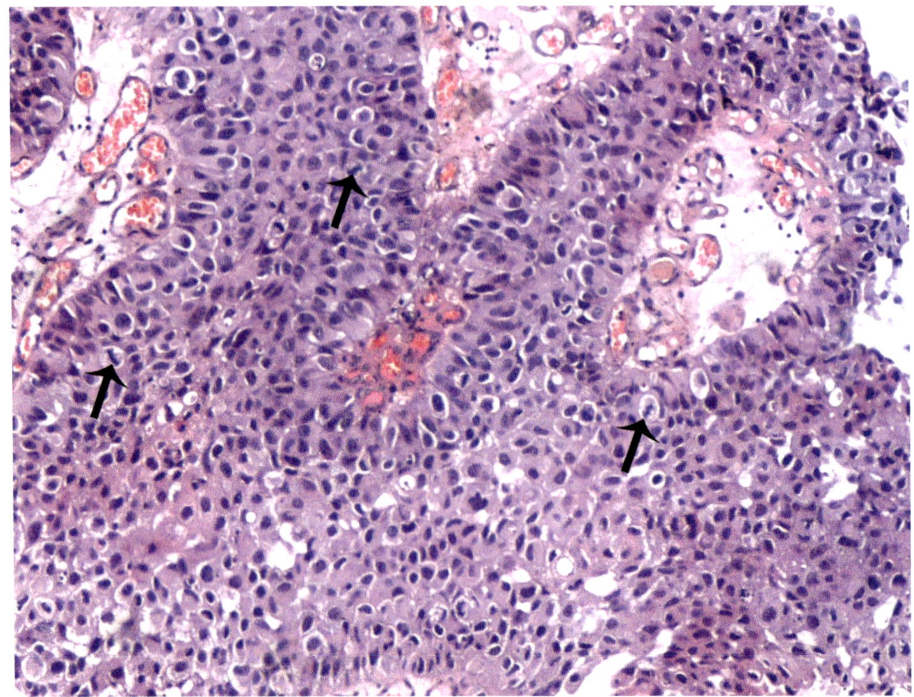

Fig. 2.49 (H-E, ×200) High-grade papillary urothelial carcinoma, here noninvasive. Papillary cores or lamina propria invasion should be carefully sought, especially in high-grade papillary carcinomas. If the tumor is high grade and noninvasive, complete submission is necessary to rule out invasion both within the papillary cores and at the base of the lesion.

Urothelium lining the fused and branching papillary fronds is characterized by a disorderly appearance resulting from marked architectural and cytologic abnormalities, recognizable even at lower magnifications. Nuclei vary considerably in shape, although sometimes not so much in size. Mitotic figures are frequently seen (*arrows*) at all levels of the urothelium.

All such tumors, classified as grade 3 in the three-tiered 1973 WHO scheme, are considered high grade in the current WHO/ISUP 2016 classification. High-grade morphology in this case corresponds to much more than 5% of the whole tumor – even though less than 50%; the tumor is thus classified as high grade, despite the predominance of low-grade areas

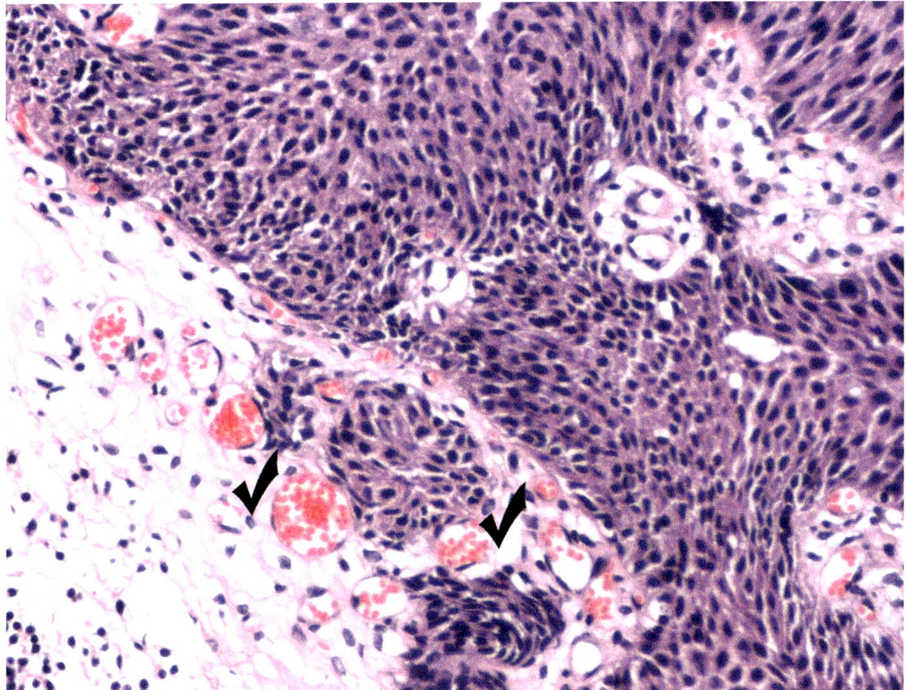

Fig. 2.50 (H-E, ×200) A low-grade area within the high-grade papillary urothelial carcinoma of the previous images. High-grade urothelial carcinomas are distinguished from low-grade carcinomas by their nuclear clustering, pleomorphism, and chromatin pattern; based on the latter criteria, this area can be comparatively classified as low grade.

Tangentially sectioned, densely packed, noninvasive papillary tumors exhibit a stromal-epithelial interface that is smooth and regular (*ticks*). No retraction artifact is against invasion. There is a parallel array of thin-walled vessels that evenly line the basement membrane of noninvasive nests (*ticks*); these are absent in invasive tumors

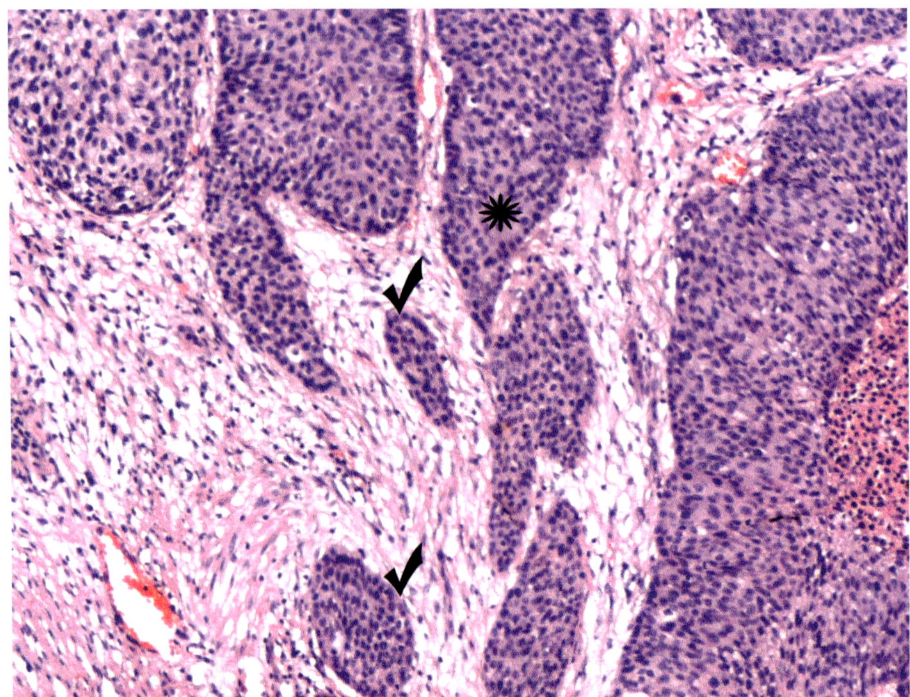

Fig. 2.51 (H-E, ×200) The smoothness of the epithelial-stromal/lamina propria interface.

Smooth, round, and predominantly regular contours (*ticks*) favor tangential sectioning, whereas irregular, jagged nests with a haphazard arrangement favor stromal invasion. Also, if the nests in question have the same cytology as the adjacent noninvasive component (*asterisk*), as opposed to the more abundant cytoplasm (i.e., paradoxical differentiation; see Fig. 2.42), one must consider the possibility of tangential sectioning.

Although invasion is not necessarily an unexpected finding in low-grade tumors, it is much more commonly encountered in high-grade lesions

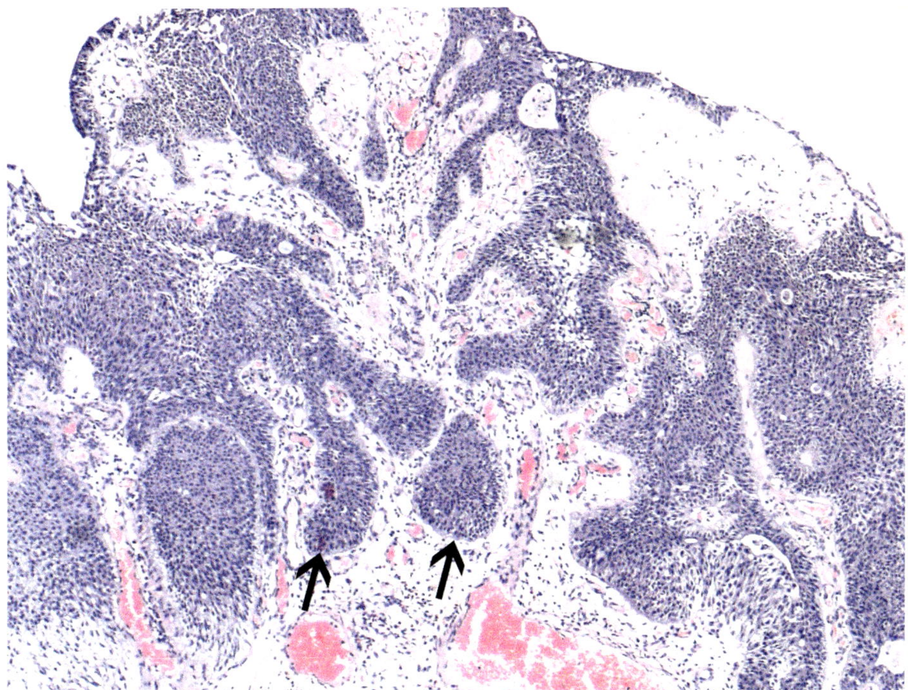

Fig. 2.52 (H-E, ×50) A low-grade area of urothelial carcinoma with a predominantly inverted/endophytic or broad-front growth pattern (*arrows*) which is difficult to be defined as invasive when this growth pattern is restricted in the lamina propria. Of course, when this growth pattern is observed in the muscularis propria or beyond, invasiveness is clearly defined.

When the specimen includes tangential sections through noninvasive tumor, the basement membrane preserves a regular, smooth contour (*arrows*), whereas in areas of frank invasion, it is frequently absent or disrupted

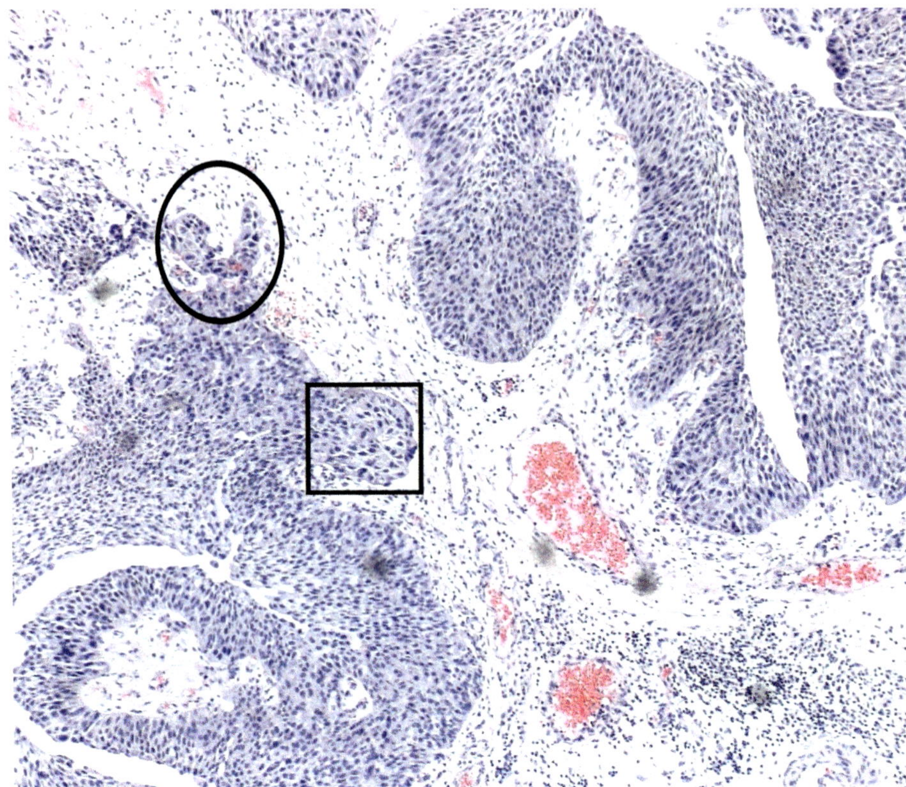

Fig. 2.53 (H-E, ×100) Expansile appearance predominates in this field. Classically, noninvasive tumors are devoid of a stromal reaction, retain delicate vascular architecture at the stromal-epithelial interface, and do *not* involve the muscularis propria. Characteristic features of stromal invasion are absent in this field; however, stromal response in areas of microinvasion is often absent. Some irregularity at the tumor border is focally noticed (*ellipse*); invasion seems imminent. At scanning magnification, nuclear atypia is detected at the above area (*ellipse*) and elsewhere (*square frame*). Several foci of high-grade cells in a predominantly low-grade carcinoma should alter the interpretation to high-grade carcinoma. There is some evidence, however, that purely high-grade papillary carcinomas are more aggressive than are mixed low- and high-grade lesions

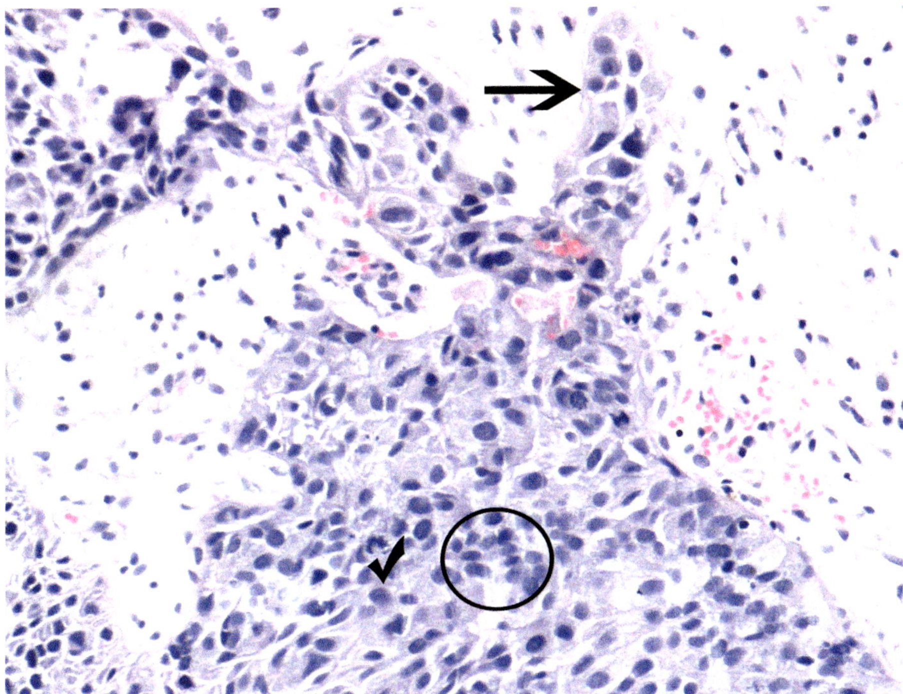

Fig. 2.54 (H-E, ×200) Imminent invasion of the high-grade tumor area with irregular contour, under higher magnification. As previously stated, the stromal response in areas of microinvasion is often absent.

Finger-like extension (*arrow*) starts arising from the base of the papillary tumor. Architecturally, there is disarray with loss of polarity.

Nearly all invasive urothelial carcinomas are high grade, at least in the foci of invasion. The nuclei of high-grade carcinoma cells tend to cluster in tissue sections (*ellipse*) like those of low-grade carcinomas. They exhibit marked variation in shape, not necessarily in size, and have coarsely clumped, unevenly distributed chromatin. Mitoses (*tick*) are readily apparent

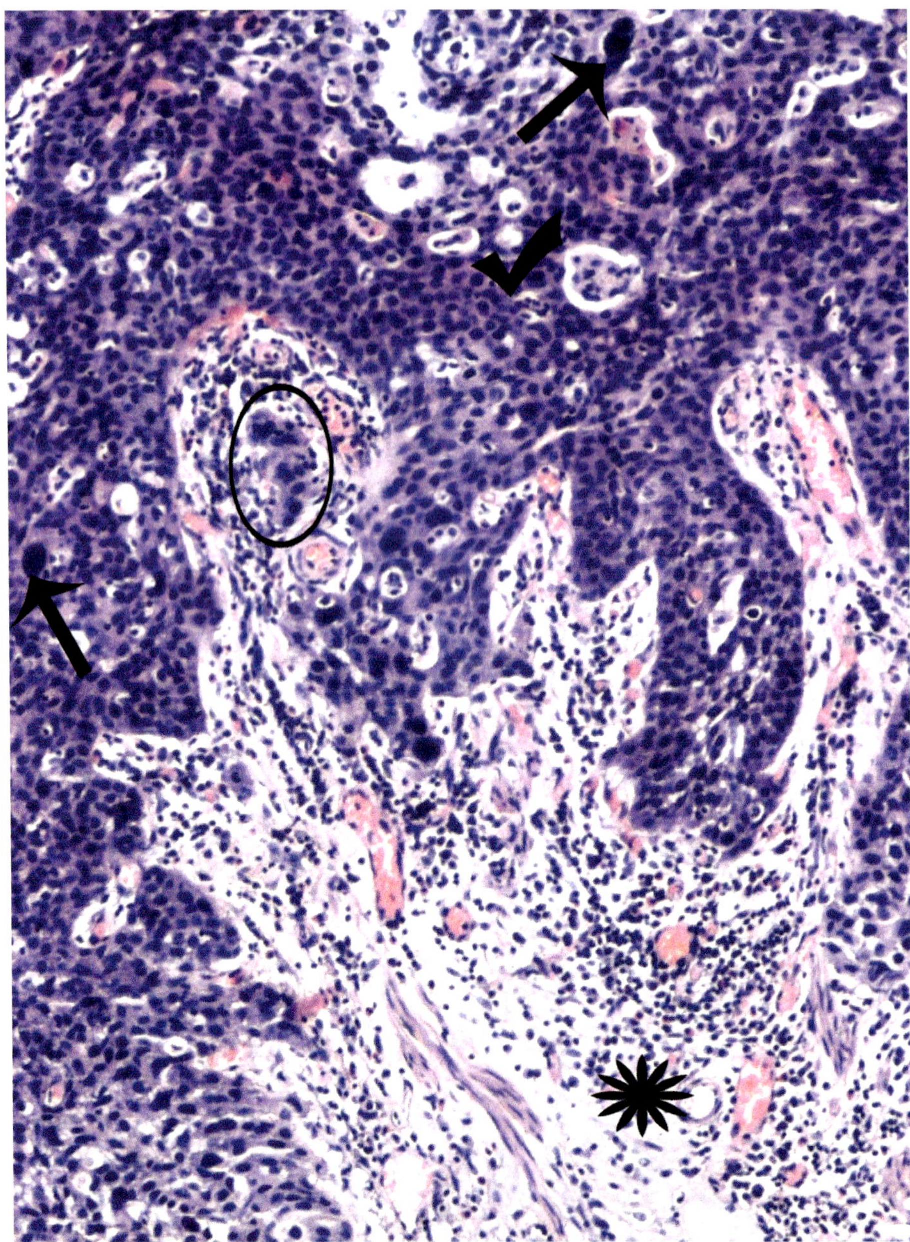

Fig. 2.55 (H-E, ×200) A clearly invasive border of the high-grade carcinoma. A focus of substantial nuclear pleomorphism with giant cell formation (*arrows*) and architectural abnormalities. Frank anaplasia is evident here. The cells of high-grade urothelial carcinomas tend to have indistinct borders. The cytoplasm is usually homogeneous. Gland-like lumina (*tick*) may be formed in urothelial carcinomas and should not be regarded as adenocarcinoma. Invasive tumors are mostly high grade. Small clusters (*ellipse*) invade the lamina propria (stage pT1). The inflammation (*asterisk*) may appear to be an integral component of the neoplasm

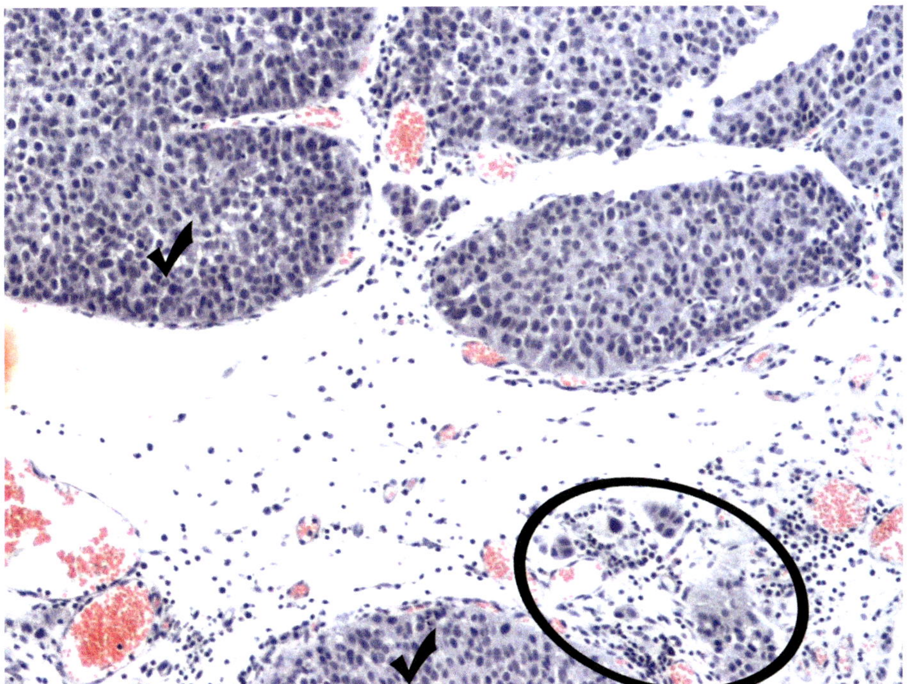

Fig. 2.56 (H-E, ×200) Tumor cells involving Brunn's nests (*ticks*) may mimic lamina propria invasion. However, apart from Brunn's nests, true microinvasion is easily detected in this field (*ellipse*).

Single cell invasion or small clusters of invasion (*ellipse*) may sometimes be camouflaged by intense background inflammation; in such instances, immunohistochemical studies with anti-cytokeratin antibodies are justified. As mentioned before, a stromal response may be absent, particularly in areas of microinvasion

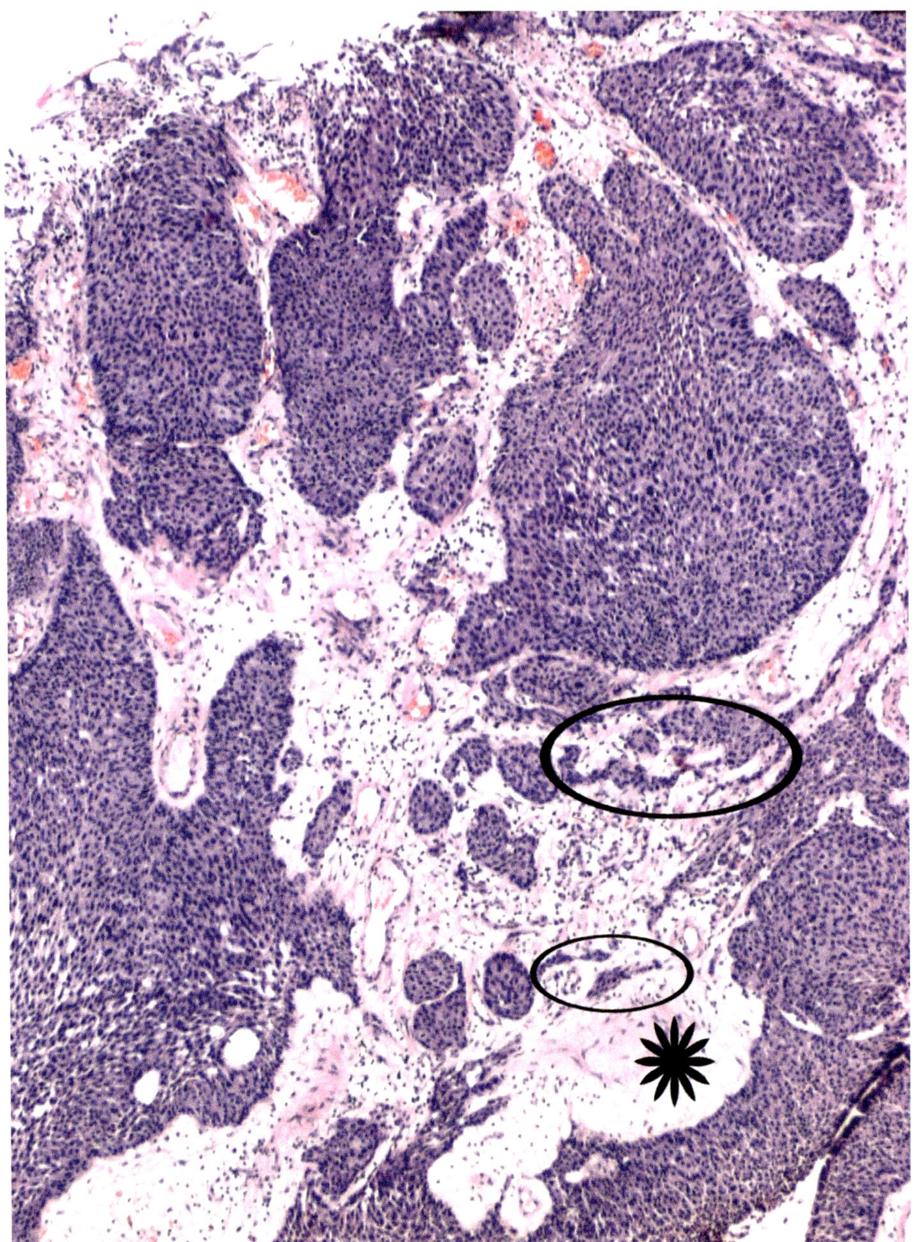

Fig. 2.57 (H-E, ×50) Inverted growth pattern in the lamina propria, raising the question of invasion. Small nests and tentacular extensions of invasive urothelial carcinoma (*ellipses*) within edematous/myxoid stroma (*asterisk*). Irregular contour of invading fronts. In instances of true invasion, variably sized and irregularly shaped nests or individual tumor cells are observed.

When there is pronounced irregularity of the basement membrane of the bulbous endophytic tongues of broad-front growth, and when there is retraction artifact, desmoplasia, or other features suggestive of destructive invasion, the tumor must be designated as invasive (stage pT1)

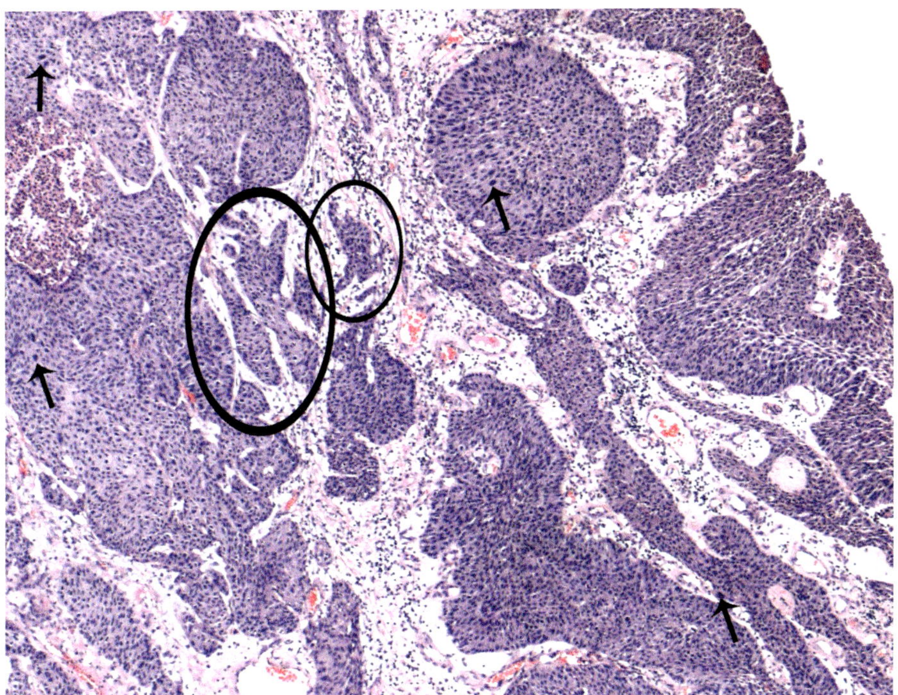

Fig. 2.58 (H-E, ×50) Architectural complexity of the tumor base in the form of tentacular or finger-like extensions, not conforming to the usual regularity of papillary neoplasms. Irregularly shaped, jagged nests (*ellipses*) with haphazard arrangement favor lamina propria invasion (stage pT1).

Nuclear atypia is focally detected (*arrows*) even under low magnification, as occurs in high-grade areas. In invasive bladder carcinomas, however, prognosis is dependent on *depth of invasion* rather than grade

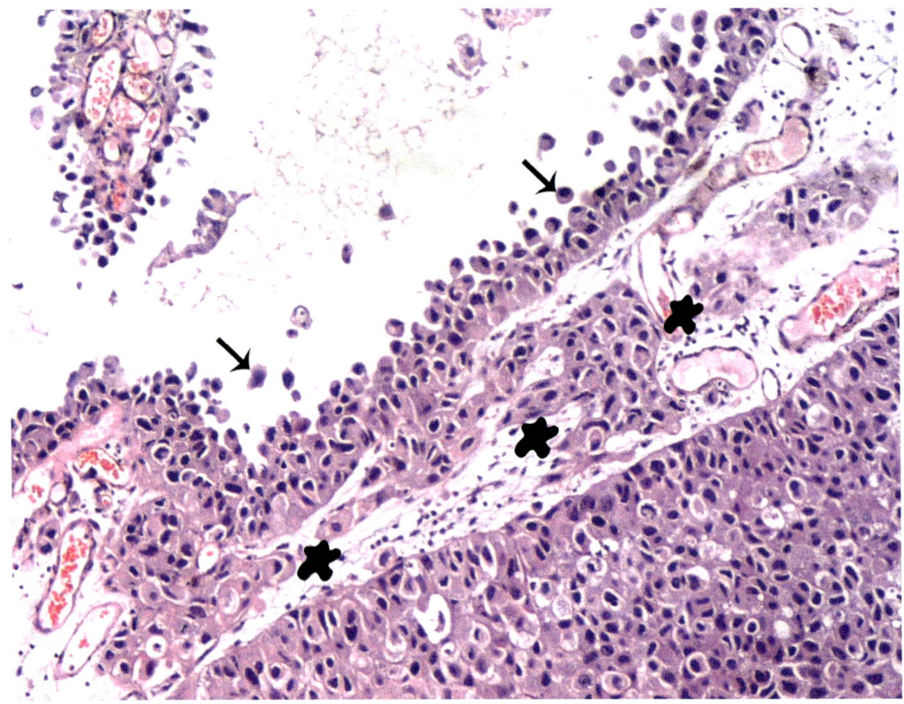

Fig. 2.59 (H-E, ×200) High-grade papillary urothelial carcinoma with microinvasion (2 mm or less) into stalk (stage pT1). Dyscohesive cells with large, hyperchromatic nuclei (*arrows*).

Irregular nests of infiltrating urothelial carcinoma in a fibrovascular stalk (*blobs*); appreciation of stalk invasion requires optimal orientation of the entire or large parts of the papillary tumor.

The cytoplasm of invasive cells here is abundant and eosinophilic. The sufficient amount of eosinophilic cytoplasm may give a distinctly squamoid appearance which should be distinguished from true squamous differentiation; the latter is defined by the presence of intercellular bridges and/or keratinization. Glycogen can also accumulate in the cytoplasm, resulting in a clear cell appearance. The presence of scattered mucin-containing cells or cytoplasmic mucin detected on histochemical stains is not considered to indicate glandular differentiation

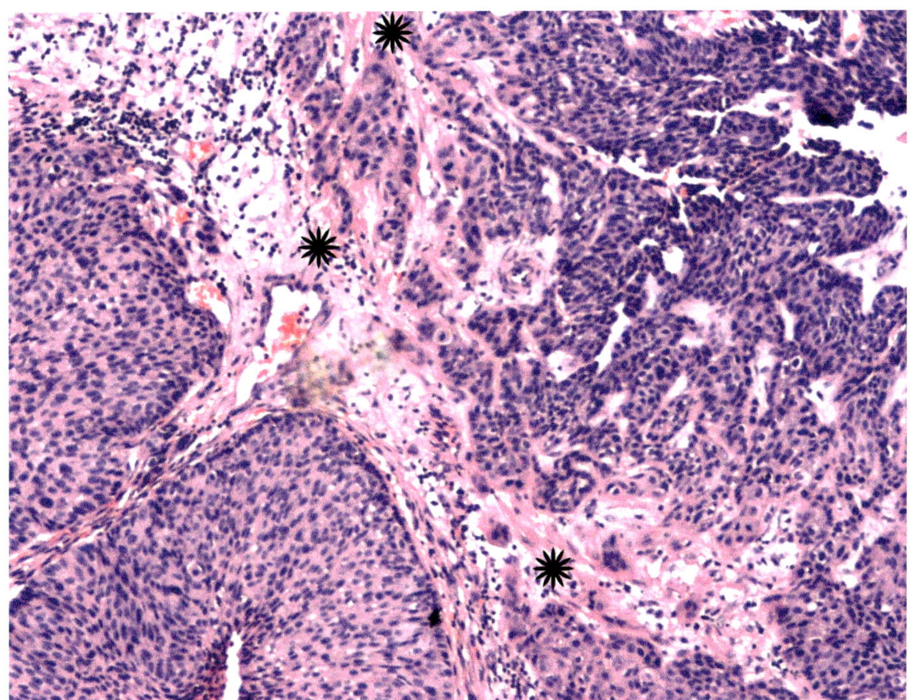

Fig. 2.60 (H-E, ×100) The neoplastic cells clearly invade lamina propria as cords, trabeculae, and clusters, separated by desmoplastic/collagenized stroma (*asterisks*). Irregular tongues of epithelium are in continuity with overlying component

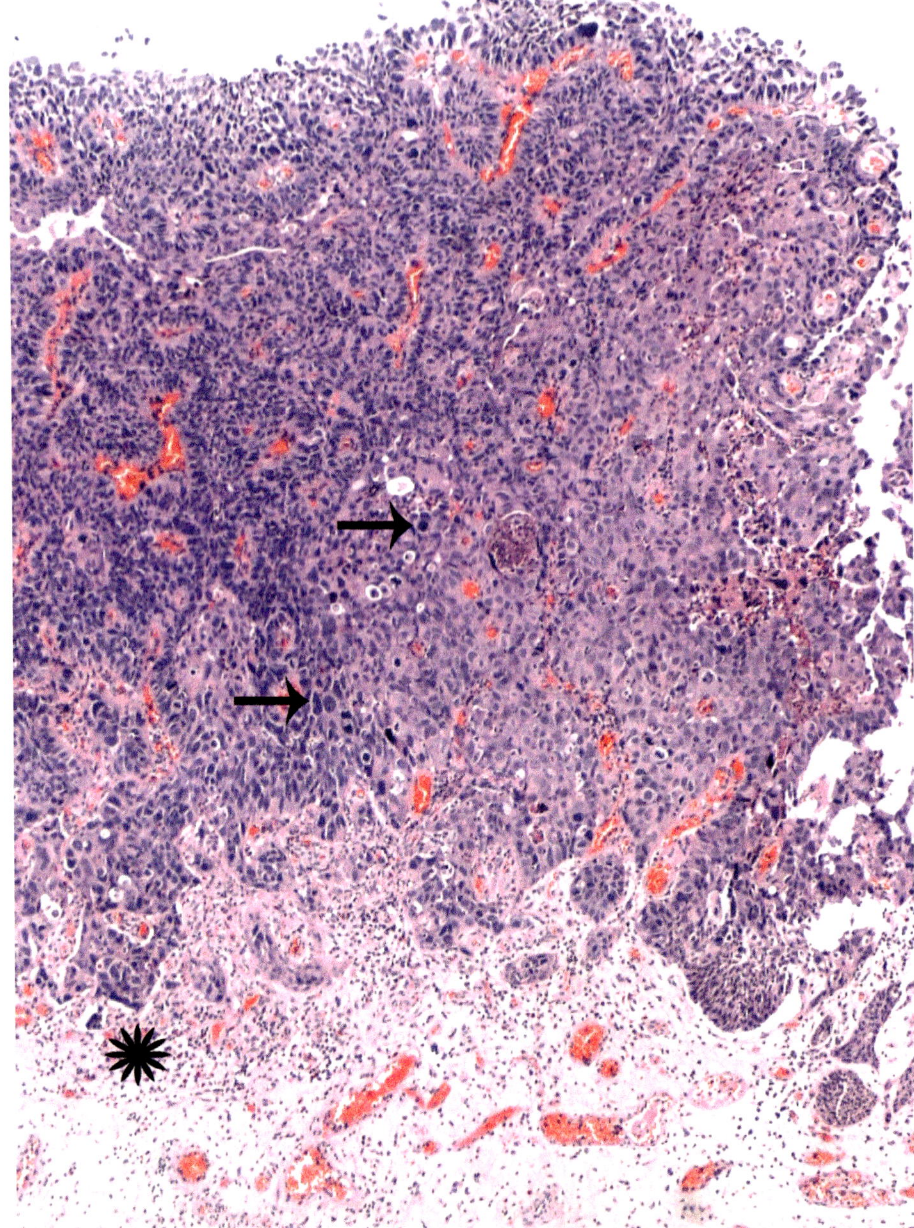

Fig. 2.61 (H-E, ×50) High-grade papillary urothelial carcinoma invading lamina propria (stage pT1). Complex, papillary architecture with anastomosis and excessive confluence of papillae. In high-grade lesions, the papillae may be fused, giving them a more solid exophytic appearance.

The presence of nuclear pleomorphism visible at low-power magnification (*arrows*) warrants a diagnosis of high-grade urothelial carcinoma.

Inflammatory stromal reaction in the lamina propria and retraction artifacts are associated with invasive tumor (*asterisk*). Although invasion into the lamina propria worsens the prognosis, the major decrease in survival is associated with tumor invading the muscularis propria (detrusor muscle)

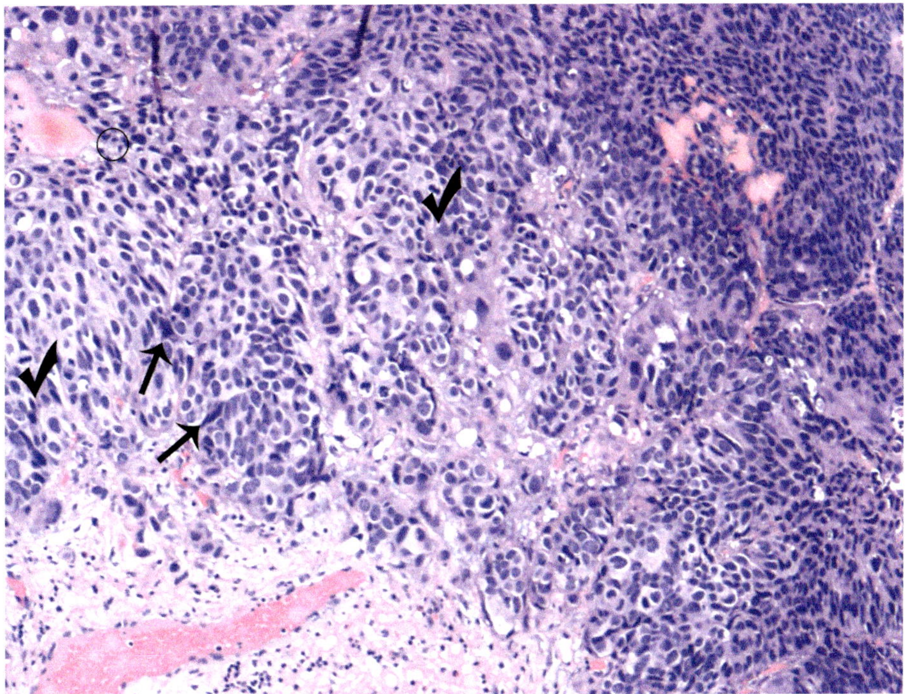

Fig. 2.62 (H-E, ×200) High-grade urothelial carcinoma invading lamina propria (stage pT1).

Crowded invasive nests with typically pleomorphic nuclei with angular profiles (*arrows*) or often rounded nuclear contours, mitotic activity (*ticks*), and apoptotic debris (*circle*). No papillary configuration in this field.

Cases with *extensive* invasion of fibrous tissue (lamina propria) require complete tissue submission in search of muscularis propria invasion

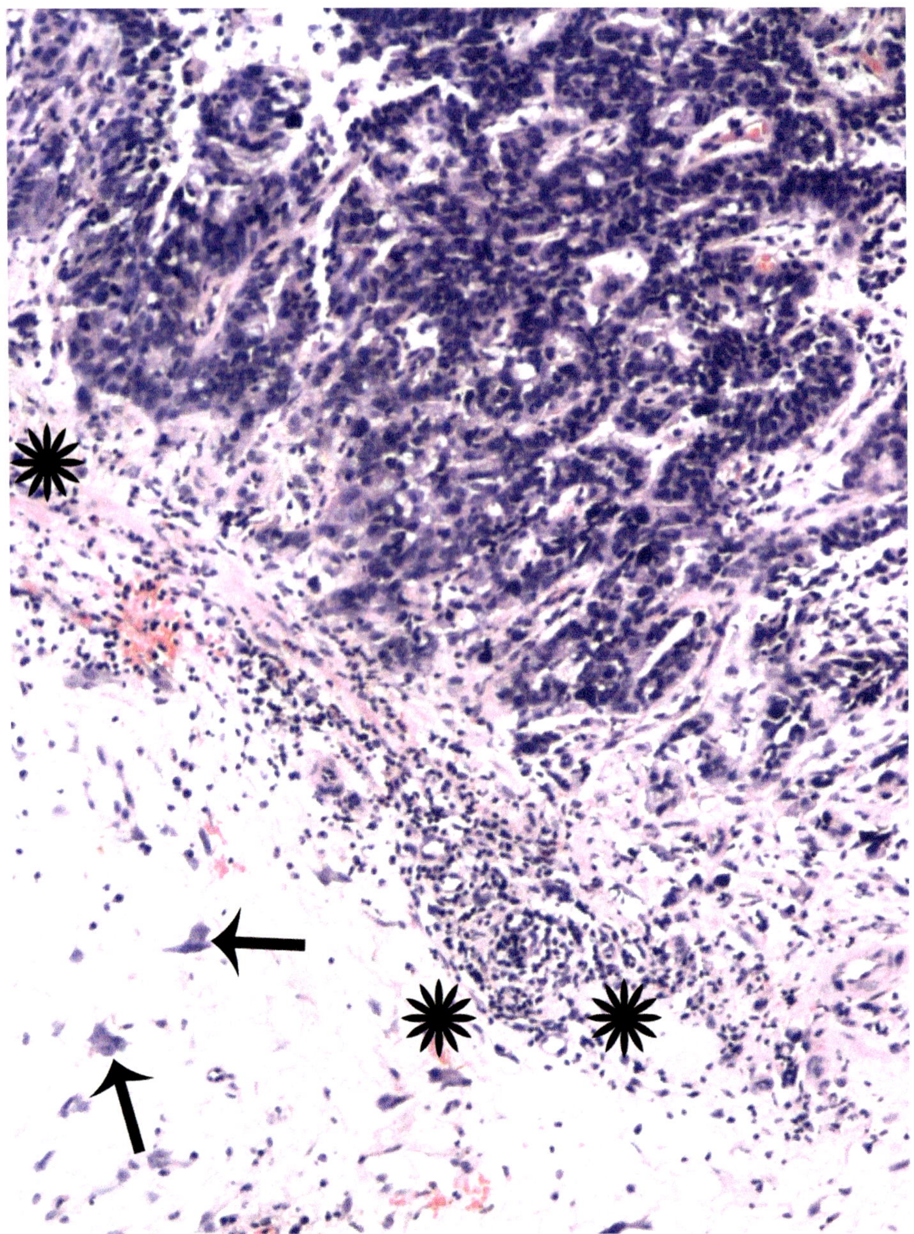

Fig. 2.63 (H-E, ×200) High-grade urothelial carcinoma invading lamina propria (stage pT1). There is a need to express some assessment of the *degree or extent of invasion* in the pathology report.

Assessment of differences in stromal pattern provides an important diagnostic clue for invasion. Invasive cords within *myxoid*, *desmoplastic*, and *inflamed stroma* (*asterisks*) with multilobated elements (*arrows*) with dark smudgy chromatin, a normal variation in stromal cells which should not be confused with a malignant spindle cell neoplasm and does not indicate prior radiation

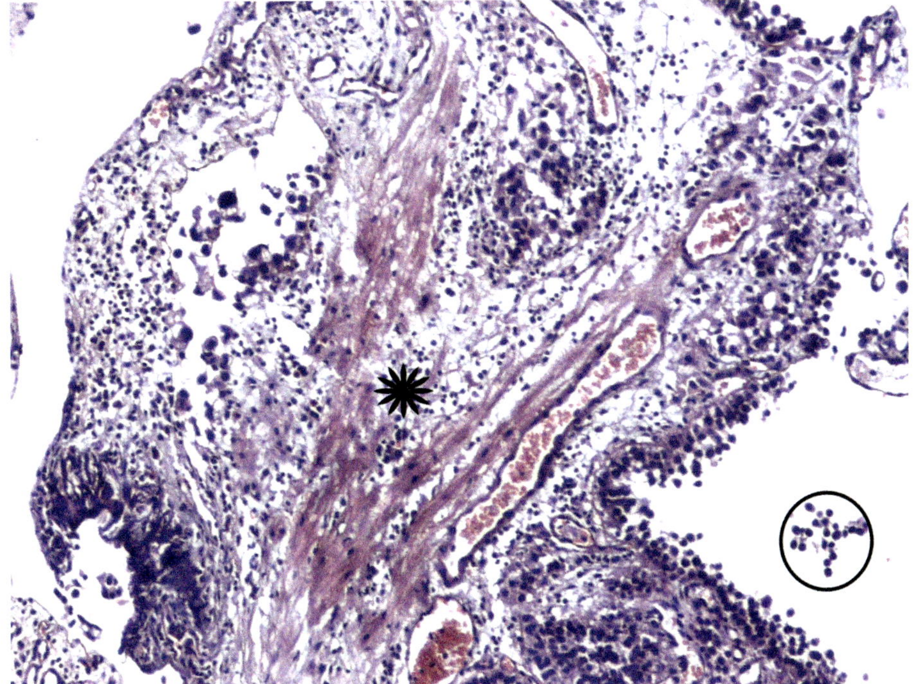

Fig. 2.64 (H-E, ×100) High-grade urothelial carcinoma invading muscularis mucosae elements (*asterisk*) of the lamina propria (stage pT1).

Cellular dyscohesion (*circle*) and denudation are common in high-grade tumors.

Orientation is to some degree maintained in this specimen. When possible, pathologists should provide an assessment of the depth of lamina propria invasion or the extent of disease.

A well-developed muscularis mucosae is not uniformly present as a continuous layer in the lamina propria of human urinary bladders. An anatomic layer identical to the muscularis mucosae of the gut does *not* exist in the human urinary bladder.

Small, discontinuous, slender layers of smooth muscle fibers of the muscularis mucosae (*asterisk*) adjacent to a linear vascular plexus of large, thin-walled blood vessels, surrounded by loose fibro-connective tissue, are observed in the lamina propria and should not be confused with the thick and compact smooth muscle bundles of muscularis propria. The distinction of hypertrophic smooth muscle fibers of the muscularis mucosa is made possible by their location in the lamina propria and their being distinct from recognizable deeper muscularis propria muscle. Muscularis mucosae invasion (pT1) should *not* be mistaken for muscularis propria invasion (pT2) which is currently regarded as the crossroad between conservative management and definitive therapy. In the present case, all muscularis propria segments were tumor-free

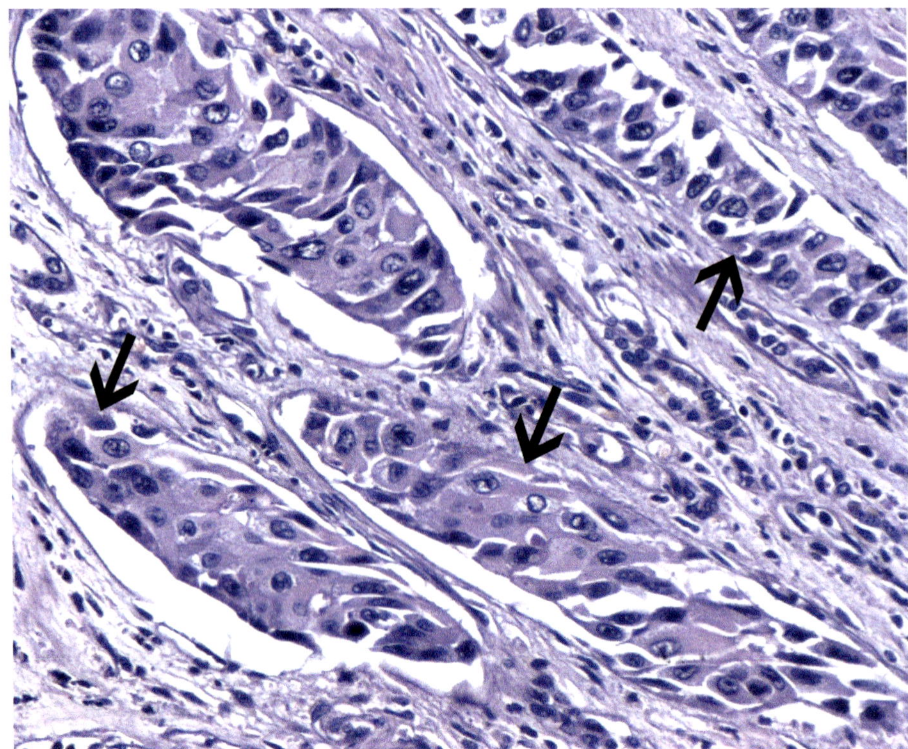

Fig. 2.65 (H-E, ×200) A subset of infiltrating urothelial carcinomas may exhibit peritumoral vascular invasion. Small vessel infiltration affects prognosis. Tumor thrombi are attached to the walls of lumens (*arrows*) and conform to the shape of the vessels.

Retraction artifact (see Figs. 2.47 and 2.61), observed particularly in those carcinomas with limited or early invasion as well as in micropapillary tumors, mimics vascular-lymphatic invasion. Caution is hence warranted, and strict criteria should be used, possibly augmented with immunohistochemistry for vascular/lymphatic markers

2.4.2 Microscopic Evaluation of the Second Cytology Smears

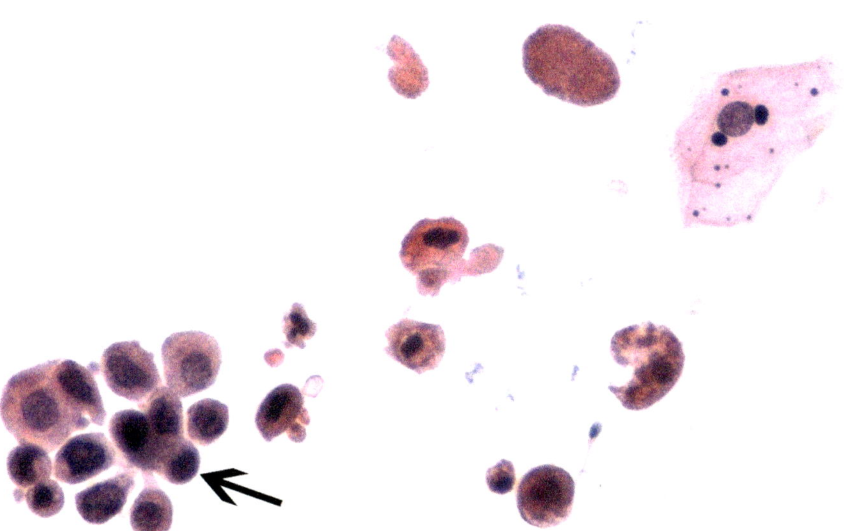

Fig. 2.66 (Papanicolaou stain, ×400) High-grade cancer cells. Cytology is 95% sensitive for carcinoma in situ (CIS). In case subsequent biopsy is negative, bladder washing cytology is mandatory because tissue sampling might have not been representative.
Urine cytology is performed:
1. In patients with painless hematuria or hematuria of unknown origin
2. For screening of urothelial carcinoma in high-risk population
3. *Follow-up procedures* of the patients previously diagnosed with bladder cancer in order to early detect recurrence or new primary

CIS can be cytologically diagnosed 6 months earlier than by cystoscopy. The voided specimen from this case with CIS contains a population of markedly atypical cells (*arrow*) of uniform size with scanty to moderate amount of cytoplasm, which are present mostly as single cells. Hyperchromatic angulated nuclei, *coarse chromatin pattern*, irregular nuclear contours, and occasional prominent nucleoli may be seen. If the chromatin pattern cannot be evaluated, a diagnosis of malignancy should not be given. Nuclear pyknosis is frequently present.
The cytological diagnosis of CIS is based on the following features:
- Nuclear changes of carcinoma with evident pleomorphism, possibly, single bizarre cells.
- Numerous, isolated, high-grade neoplastic cells.
- Absence of papillae.
- Relatively clean background. In contrast to invasive urothelial carcinoma, generally no necrosis and scanty erythrocytes or leukocytes (i.e., a generally clean background) are found in the background of samples containing cells of urothelial CIS (Strojan Flezar 2010).

The absence of characteristic nuclear inclusions rules out polyoma virus infection

2.4.3 Microscopic Evaluation of the Bladder Re-biopsy Specimen

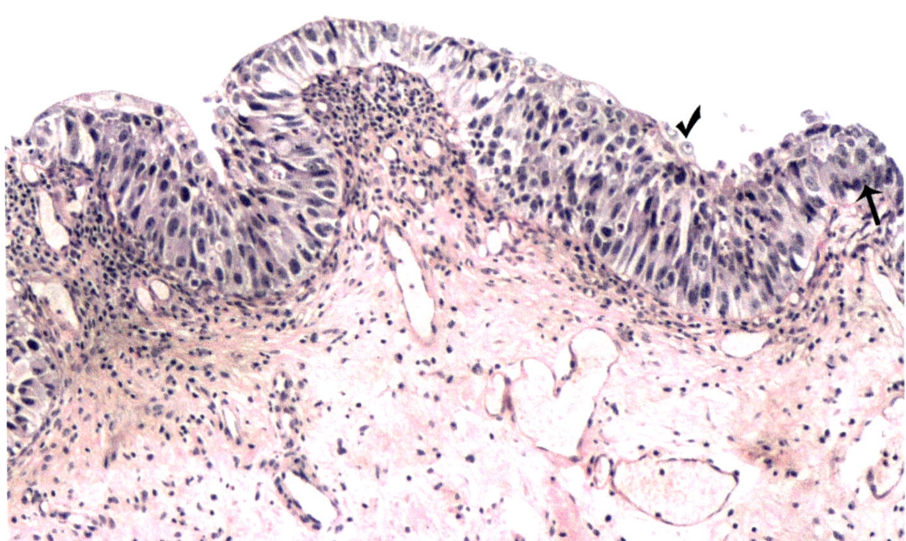

Fig. 2.67 (H-E, ×100) Urothelial CIS (also known as high-grade intraurothelial neoplasia). By definition, no invasion into lamina propria.

De novo CIS constitutes less than 3% of all urothelial neoplasms but occurs in 45% with concurrent invasive bladder carcinoma.

Nonpapillary, flat, by definition *high-grade* lesion of variable thickness, composed of malignant cells in mid to upper epithelium with high cytologic grade (anaplasia). Atypia may not be full thickness; CIS may show the presence of maturation on the surface. The neoplastic cells of CIS need not occupy the entire thickness of the urothelium.

Unequivocal severe cytologic atypia (i.e., changes thought to represent clear-cut neoplasia at the light microscopic level) is necessary for the diagnosis of CIS. Disorganization of cells is characteristic. Alteration of polarity, some degree of nuclear anaplasia, not so excessive on this focus of CIS; large nucleoli are noticed in some of the cells (*arrow*). Moderate to abundant cytoplasm. Umbrella cells are usually absent but can rarely be present (*tick*).

In some CIS, neoplastic cells may be monomorphic and uniform with conspicuous eosinophilic cytoplasm mimicking reactive urothelial atypia (large cell non-pleomorphic CIS) (see Figs. 2.1, 2.2, and 2.3) *or* with scant cytoplasm, a high nucleus to cytoplasmic ratio, without pleomorphism (small cell CIS). Markedly enlarged nuclei with high-grade cytologic features (either consistent, prominent nucleoli or unequivocal irregular nuclear chromatin distribution and irregular cell borders) favor CIS. Immunohistochemistry provides diagnostic help as an adjunct to morphology, particularly in such cases: CIS frequently shows diffuse, strong, *full thickness* cytoplasmic reactivity for CK20 and for p53, while CD44 reactivity is often absent in CIS cells and is limited to residual basal cells, if present. The typical immunophenotype for CIS cells is CK20+, p53+, Ki-67+, and CD44-.

There is no evidence that immunohistochemistry can differentiate CIS from urothelial dysplasia. Both urothelial CIS and dysplasia are *flat* lesions. The presence of pleomorphism comparable to that seen with high-grade papillary carcinoma, dyscohesion, or mitoses (particularly atypical ones) in the upper urothelium favors the diagnosis of CIS over dysplasia; in the latter, cellular pleomorphism is comparable to that seen with low-grade papillary carcinoma.

With regard to the distinction of reactive atypia, in the latter, intraepithelial inflammation is usually prominent. Although there is nuclear enlargement in reactive atypia, it is usually uniform and usually <3× size of a normal lymphocyte nucleus

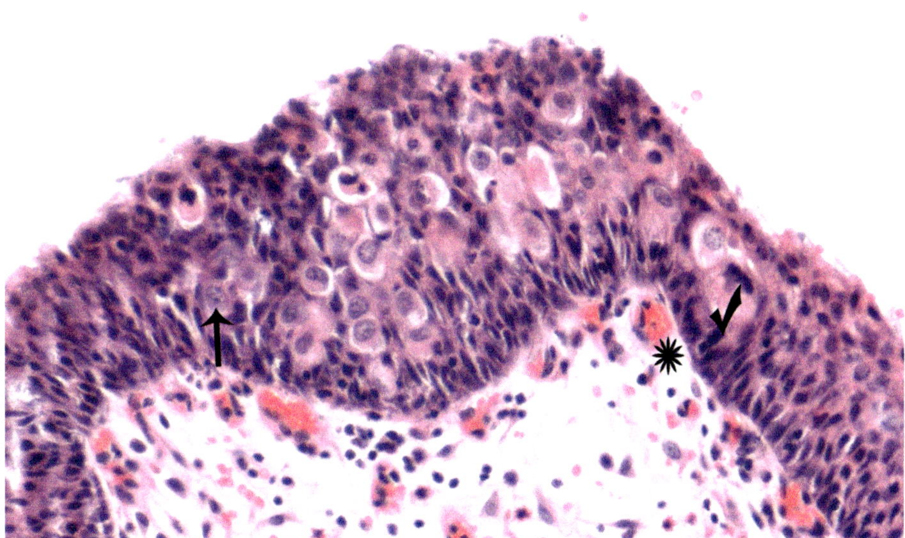

Fig. 2.68 (H-E, ×200) Multifocality of CIS is common. Pagetoid cancerization of normal urothelium by large single cells with enlarged nuclei (*arrow*) or small clusters of cells within otherwise normal urothelium. Chromatin tends to be coarse and clumped in CIS cells. Definite nucleomegaly with nuclear hyperchromasia and irregular chromatin is required for the diagnosis of CIS. Elevated mitotic rates (*tick*) are not sufficient as they may be seen in reactive lesions.

Proliferation of small capillaries in the lamina propria (*asterisk*).

Pagetoid CIS is rarely, if ever, the primary lesion and usually comprises only small foci in a CIS of the usual pattern (see Fig. 2.67). Extramammary Paget's disease can be ruled out by cytokeratin 20 and thrombomodulin immunopositivity of urothelial cancerous cells

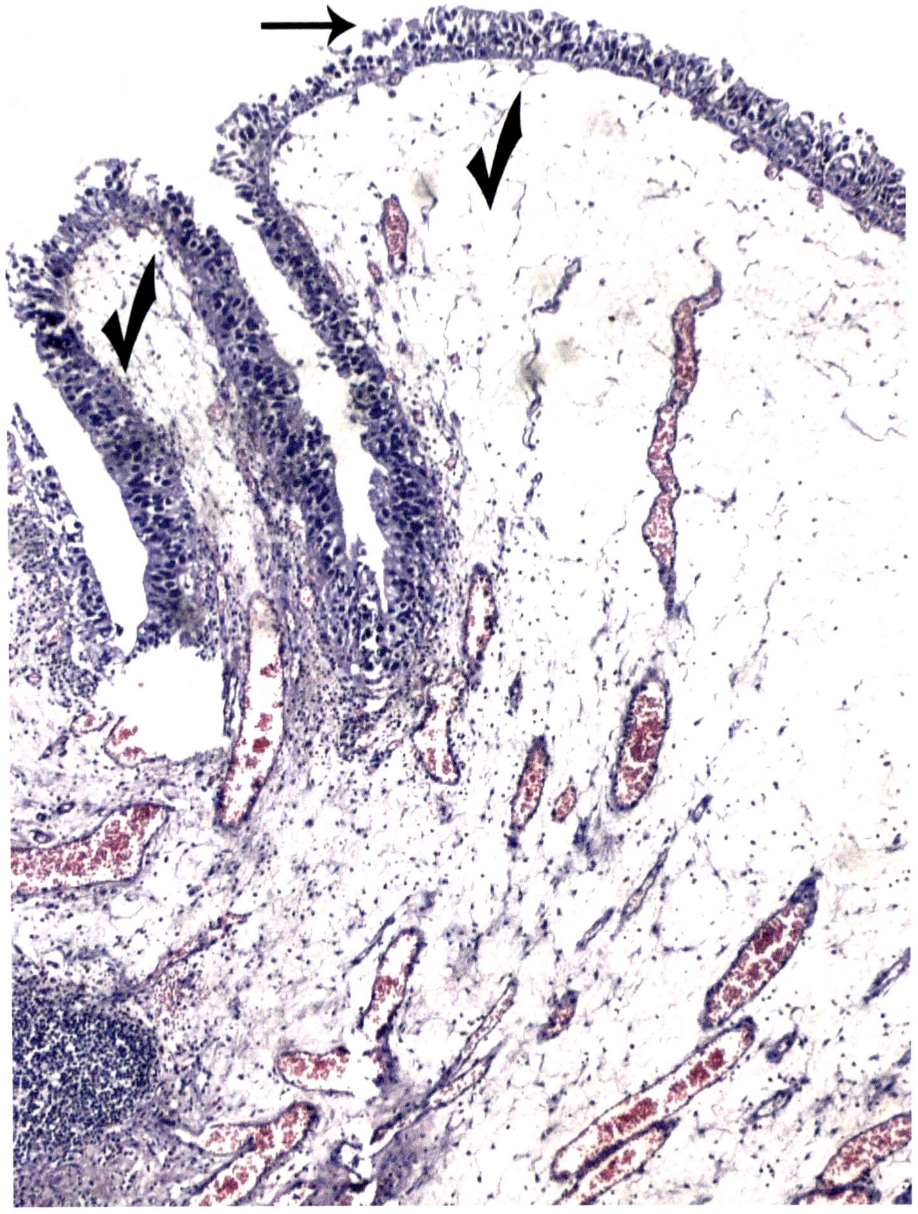

Fig. 2.69 (H-E, ×50) CIS. Edematous papillary – polypoid structures of cystitis (*ticks*) (without branching architecture) lined by CIS urothelium. The lack of intercellular cohesion toward the surface of CIS (*arrow*). CIS on the background of polypoid cystitis should not be confused with noninvasive (pTa) high-grade papillary urothelial carcinoma

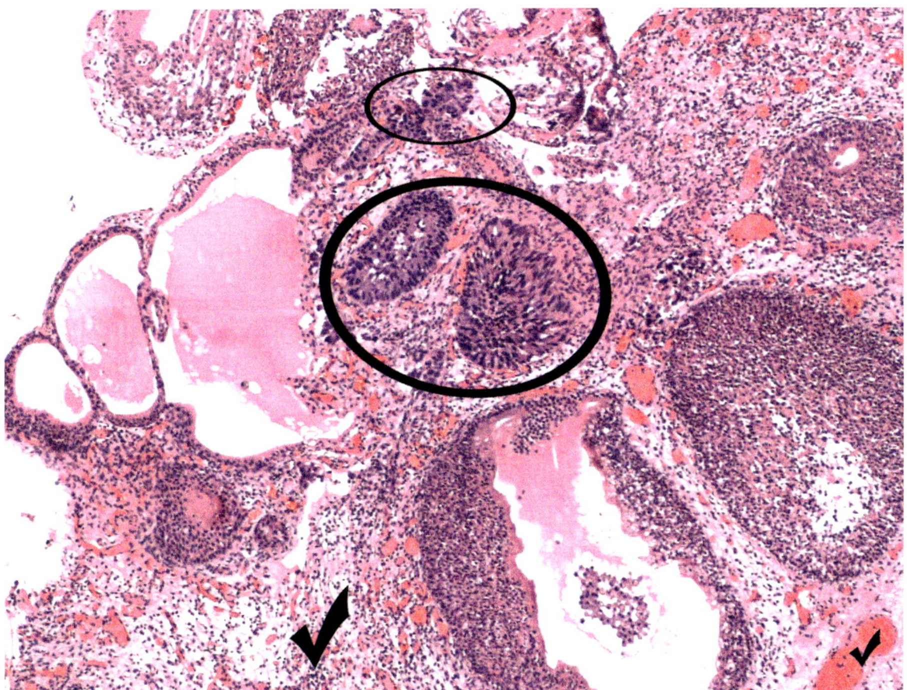

Fig. 2.70 (H-E, ×50) The level of cytological disorder in CIS (*ellipses*) is such that it is visible at low to medium magnification. Brunn's nests and cystitis cystica et glandularis may be completely or partially replaced by the cytologically malignant cells, easily recognizable at scanning magnification. The demarcation between CIS and the adjacent mucosa is nearly always *sharp*. The lamina propria usually shows an inflammatory infiltrate, some degree of edema, and vascular congestion/ectasia (*ticks*).

Adenocarcinoma in situ should be excluded in the absence of concurrent invasive adenocarcinoma

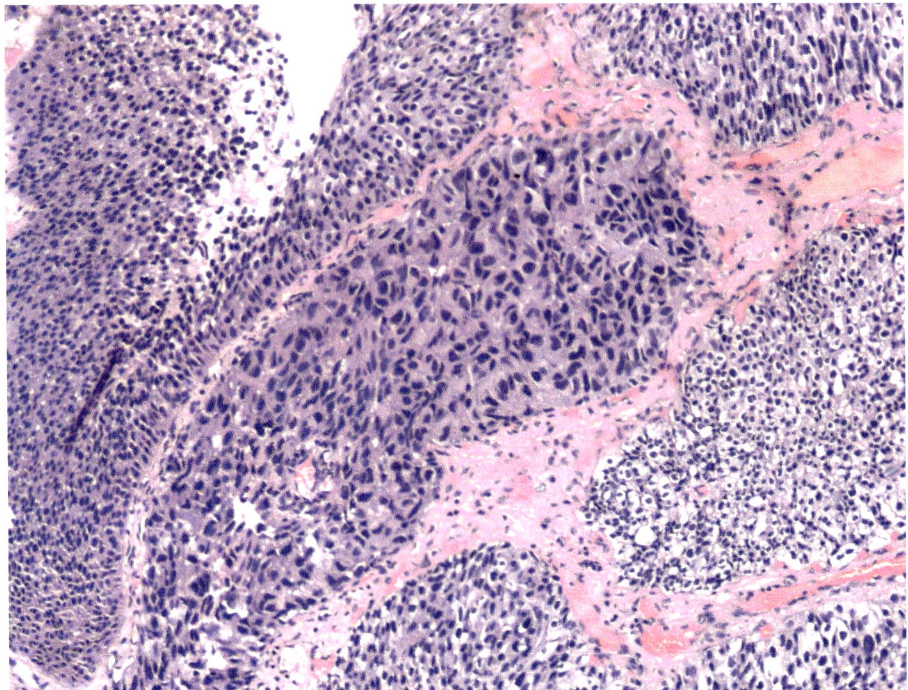

Fig. 2.71 (H-E, ×200) CIS involving a hyperplastic Brunn's nest (image center). Nuclear pleomorphism and crowding, loss of polarity of high-grade cells in a prominent nest within the lamina propria. Microinvasion should be investigated. The most atypical CIS nuclei are approximately five times the size of adjacent stromal lymphocytes, a useful gauge of nucleomegaly, compared with normal urothelium (right and left part of the image) in which they are only two times the size of stromal lymphocytes. In CIS, the cytoplasm is often eosinophilic or amphophilic and cellular borders are indistinct

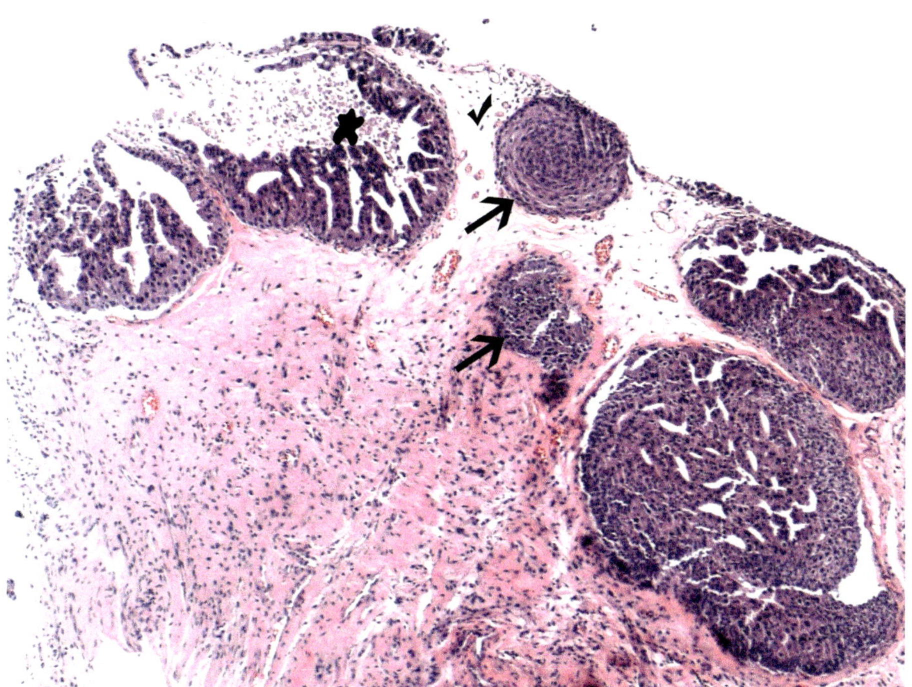

Fig. 2.72 (H-E, ×50) CIS can involve Brunn's nests within the superficial lamina propria. Despite a focal retraction artifact (bottom right) and a collagenized stroma, the round contours (*arrows*) prevent an overdiagnosis of invasion. Tissue edema in superficial lamina propria (*tick*).

CIS with micropapillary features is an unusual form of CIS (upper left part of the figure, combined with necrotic activity, *blob*). CIS pattern need not be included in surgical pathology report

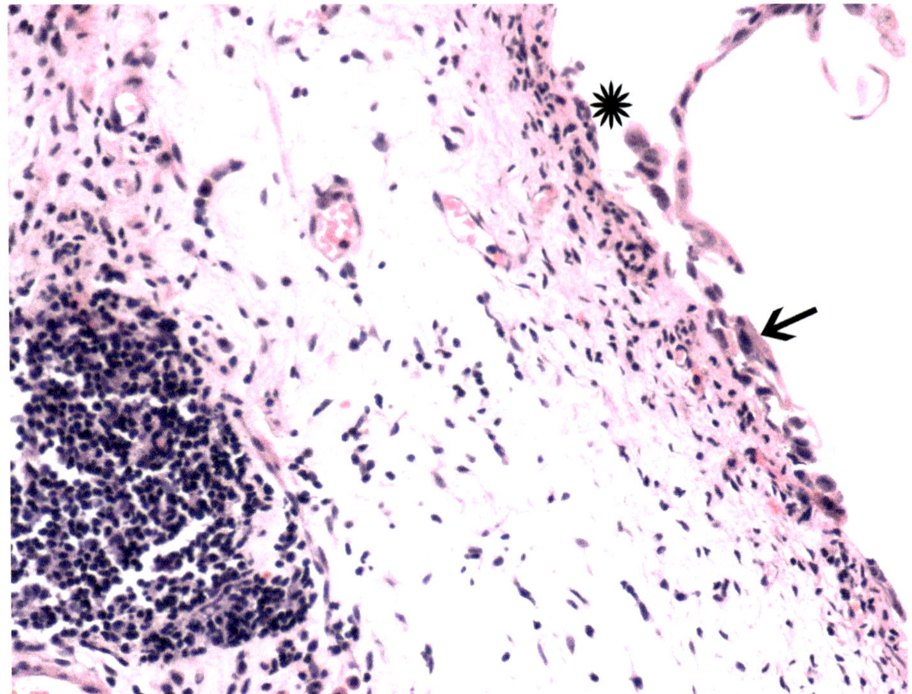

Fig. 2.73 (H-E, ×200) Clinging CIS. A common CIS feature shared with high-grade papillary urothelial carcinoma is the lack of cohesiveness, which leads to the shedding of malignant cells into the urine.

In this focus of CIS, the urothelium lifts off (*asterisk*), and the basement membrane is denuded, either reflecting the dyscohesive nature of the cells or, artifactually, when the biopsy is performed with a hot wire loop. Some single-layered cells retain eosinophilic cytoplasm (*arrow*) and meet the morphologic criteria for CIS.

The main conditions associated with urothelium denudation are trauma due to instrumentation, prior therapy, and CIS. CIS cells are not cohesive, leading to shedding into urine; in contrast, cells are still cohesive in radiation effect

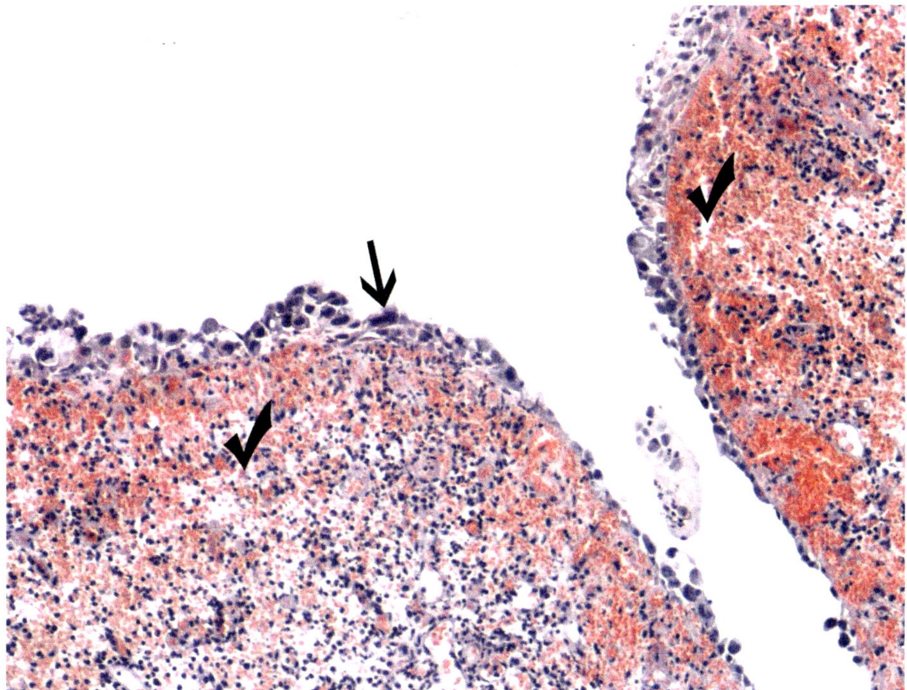

Fig. 2.74 (H-E, ×100) CIS. Hypervascular/hemorrhagic and inflamed lamina propria (*ticks*) is a clue that the overlying epithelium is abnormal. Unequivocal severe cytologic atypia (*arrow*) is necessary for the diagnosis of CIS. CIS shows nuclear anaplasia identical to high-grade papillary urothelial carcinoma. The presence of nuclear pleomorphism, nuclear size >5–6 lymphocytes, and brisk mitotic activity favors CIS over dysplasia.

In case the overlying epithelium is absent, deeper sections may help identify it; correlation with prior to cystoscopy, urine cytology findings should be suggested

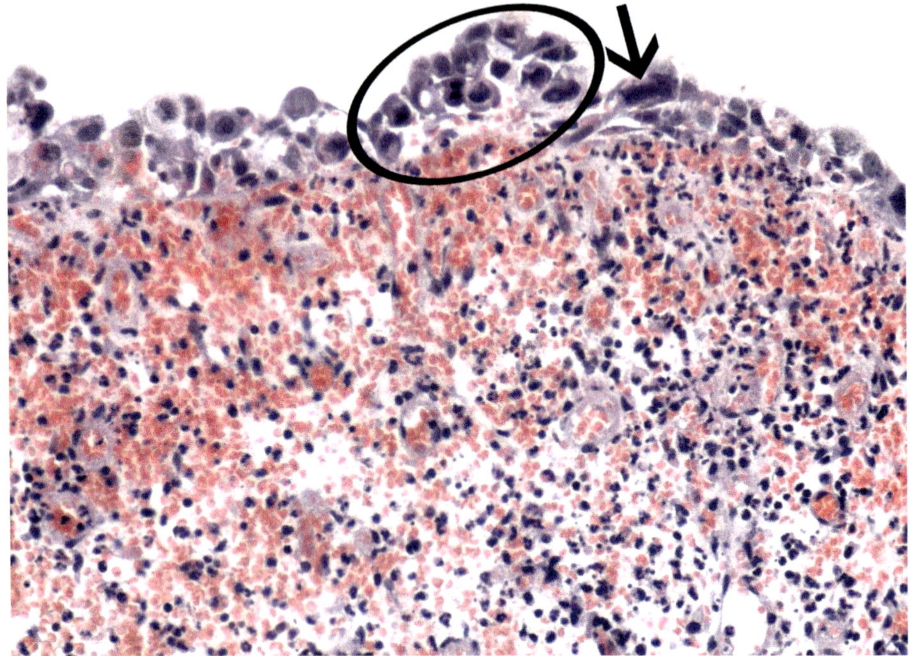

Fig. 2.75 (H-E, ×200) Large cell CIS with pleomorphism. Complete loss of polarity and nucleomegaly with hyperchromasia (*ellipse*) and marked variation in nuclear shape and size (*arrow*). Coarse or condensed chromatin. In CIS, nuclear size is five times that of lymphocytes vs. two times lymphocytes for normal urothelium. Nuclear anaplasia is identical to high-grade papillary urothelial carcinoma

2.4.3.1 Clinical Commentary

Vasileios Spapis

This is a case of a high-grade, pT1 urothelial carcinoma with papillary and inverted growth pattern, with tumor emboli in small vessels of the lamina propria. On re-biopsy, multifocal CIS is detected.

Painless hematuria is usually the first sign of bladder cancer. Gross hematuria though is associated with higher-stage disease at first presentation, compared to microscopic hematuria (Ramirez et al. 2016). In patients with lower urinary tract symptoms (LUTS) and especially irritative voiding, the presence of in situ carcinoma might be suspected (Babjuk et al. 2017a, b).

Urinary cytology is a useful tool especially for detecting high-grade tumors. In these cases, its sensitivity is about 84% but falls below 16% for low-grade tumors (Yafi et al. 2015). Sensitivity in CIS detection varies from 28% to 100% (Tetu 2009). It should be noted though that urinary cytology is most useful complementary to cystoscopy, as a positive outcome can indicate a urothelial tumor *anywhere* in the urinary tract but negative cytology cannot exclude the presence of a tumor. CT urography and US imaging will be used to detect papillary masses mostly in the upper urinary tract. Cystoscopy itself cannot be replaced by any other examination.

In this patient, the tumor was characterized as T1, high grade. This means that the patient should be treated with BCG because T1 tumors have a 20% chance of disease progression, if left untreated (Cambier et al. 2016). Also, all patients with T1 tumors should undergo a second transurethral resection (TUR) of all suspicious lesions 2–6 weeks after the initial TUR because of the danger of understaging (Babjuk et al. 2017a, b). Suspicious lesions include possible residual mass and velvety red patches; even random biopsies from otherwise normal-appearing mucosa could be performed.

CIS is a flat, noninvasive tumor that is high grade by definition and is regarded as a precursor to the development of invasive cancer. If left untreated, approximately 54% of the patients will progress to muscle-invasive disease (Jones 2016; Lamm 1992). Response to intravesical treatment with BCG is an important prognostic factor for subsequent disease progression (Fernandez-Gomez et al. 2009; Takenaka et al. 2008). Detection of concurrent bladder CIS, associated with T1 G3/HG tumors, means that the patient is at the highest risk of progression, and early cystectomy should be discussed (Babjuk et al. 2017a, b).

Key Points

- Urine cytology represents a major tool in the diagnosis of high-grade urothelial carcinomas and CIS in particular, since cystoscopy has a lower sensitivity of CIS detection due to denudation of the urothelium. The greatest value of urinary bladder cytology is in the follow-up of patients who have received some treatment for bladder carcinoma.
- Invasive bladder carcinomas (especially high-grade tumors) are often associated with adjacent or subsequent zones of carcinoma in situ remote from the main tumor mass.
- High-grade noninvasive papillary lesions are not designated as carcinoma in situ to avoid lumping together two conditions with markedly different architectural features, natural history, and probably molecular pathways.
- The most important factors for progression-free survival of patients with urothelial carcinoma are the presence of lamina propria invasion, grade, and associated CIS.

2.5 Case 2.4: Muscle-invasive Bladder Carcinoma

Case Study

Data Prior to Microscopy

A 66-year-old male is being investigated for painless, gross hematuria. After bimanual examination, cystoscopy is programmed. In the meantime, urinary cytopathology reveals malignant tumor cells consistent with a high-grade neoplasm. Cystoscopic examination identifies a single, sessile, solid, ulcerated mass with a maximum diameter of 8 cm, at the left ureteral orifice extending into the bladder neck. There is evidence of hydronephrosis of the left kidney on ultrasound. Multiple biopsies are taken, and the pathology report renders cystectomy under consideration.

After a month, radical cystectomy and pelvic lymph node dissection including the common iliac lymph nodes were performed. Adjacent organs are uninvolved. Perivesical infiltration is not macroscopically evident. Nodal dissection specimens were submitted in separate packets; all resected lymph nodes were tumor-free.

2.5.1 Microscopic Evaluation of the Initial Transurethral Resection of Bladder Tumor (TURBT) Specimen

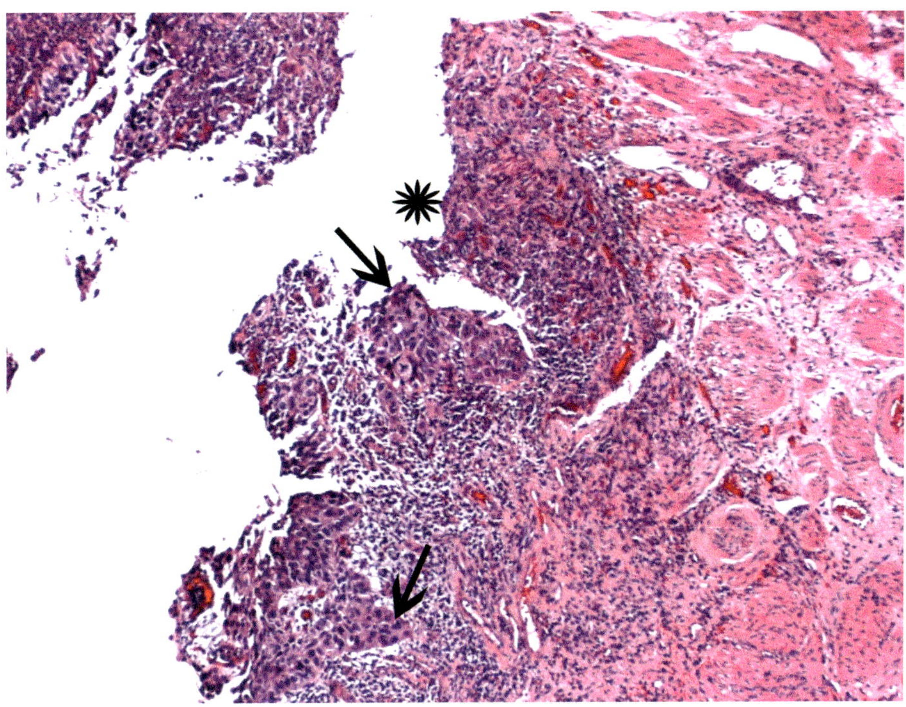

Fig. 2.76 (H-E, ×50) The epithelial surface is focally denuded (*asterisk*). Denudation is common in high-grade urothelial carcinomas and uncommon in low-grade urothelial carcinomas unless cautery is utilized. The malignancy of the remaining urothelium is clearly high grade at scanning magnification (*arrows*). Hyperplastic smooth muscle bundles of the muscularis mucosae are noticed in the lamina propria (right side of the figure, also see Fig. 2.85)

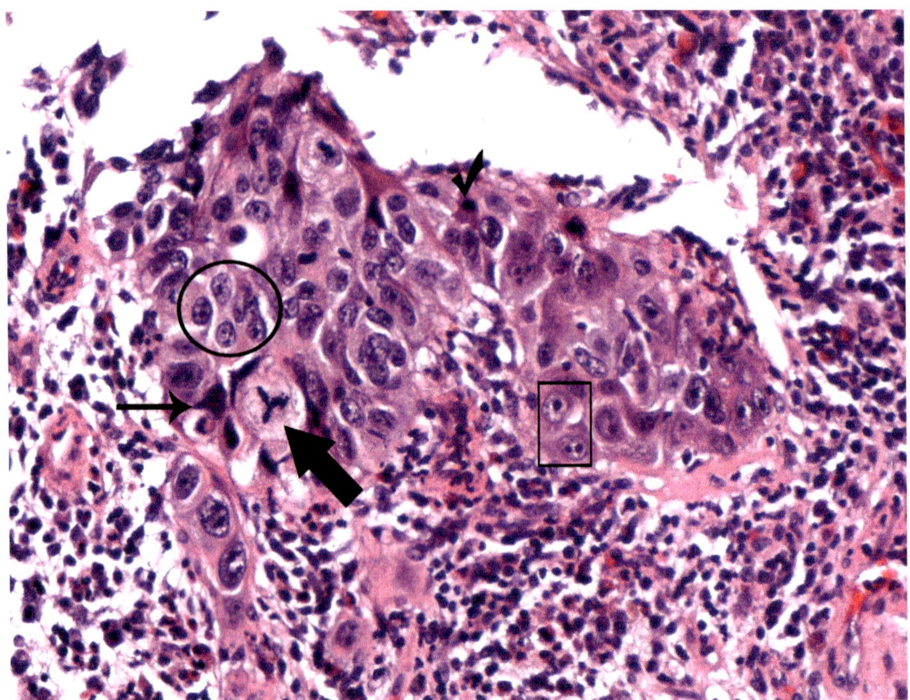

Fig. 2.77 (H-E, ×200) High-grade urothelial carcinoma commonly has rounded nuclear contours, obvious pleomorphism, often large, hyperchromatic nuclei (*thin arrow*), coarse, unevenly dispersed, clumped chromatin (*ellipse*), brisk mitotic activity including abnormal mitoses (*thick arrow*), and apoptotic cells (*tick*). Large nucleoli (*square frame*) may be observed in some cells. Architecturally, there is disarray with loss of polarity, i.e., loss of normal perpendicular alignment to the basement membrane.

High-grade urothelial carcinomas are distinguished from low-grade carcinomas by their nuclear clustering, pleomorphism, and chromatin pattern. In most analyses, less than 10% of low-grade cancers invade, but as many as 80% of high-grade papillary urothelial cell carcinomas are invasive (Epstein 2005)

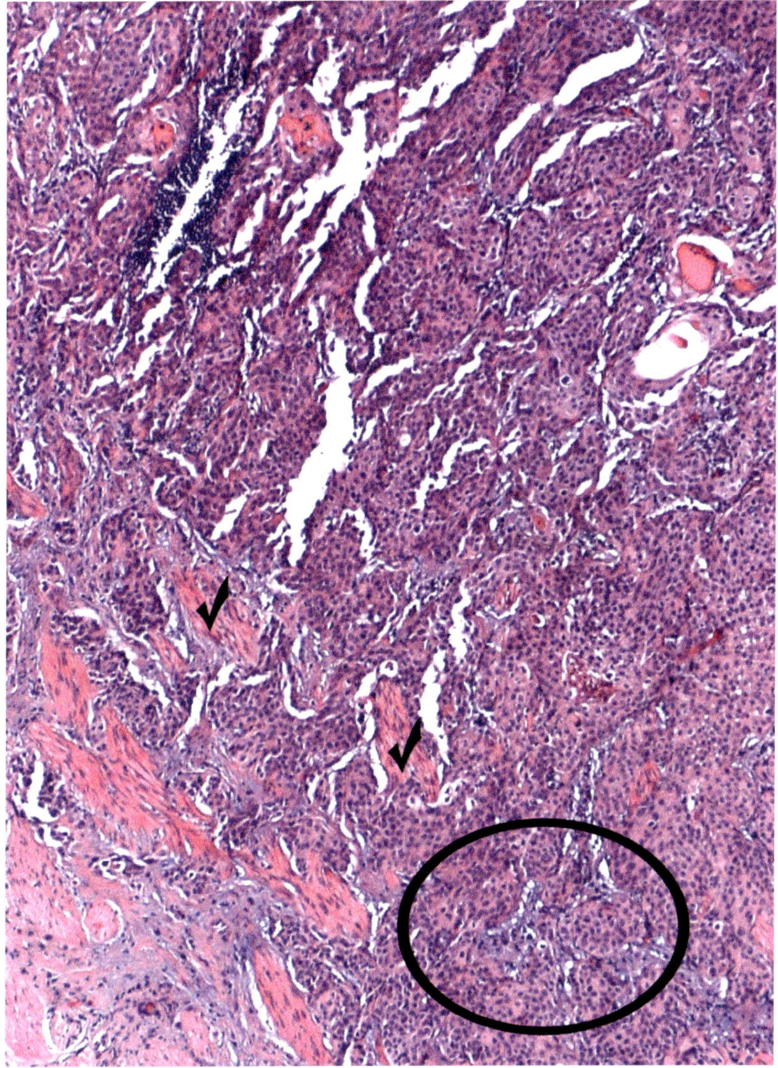

Fig. 2.78 (H-E, ×50) Invasive urothelial carcinoma among muscularis mucosae (*ticks*). The tumor infiltrates in a diffuse pattern but focal nests and clusters are present (*ellipse*). The cells show moderate eosinophilic cytoplasm.

In few urothelial carcinomas, tumor urothelial cells may resemble plasma cells and/or monocytes (plasmacytoid urothelial carcinoma) as urothelial cancer cells may have eosinophilic cytoplasm and central or eccentrically placed, enlarged hyperchromatic nuclei (see also Fig. 2.87).

The presence of tumor among small, separate, individual smooth muscle bundles (*ticks*) which do not extend throughout the biopsy specimen [and are adjacent to a linear vascular plexus (see Fig. 2.64)] is consistent with muscularis mucosae invasion (stage pT1). This case of so far pT1 disease is unequivocal and extensive, and this should be noted in the pathology report. Deep lamina propria invasion, as here observed, identifies a subset of patients with T1 disease with a more adverse prognosis; therefore, the need to express some assessment of the degree or extent of invasion in the pathology report of TURBT specimens is encouraged.

On the other hand, we should have in mind that numerous muscle bundles that are too extensive for muscularis mucosae, no matter how thin they are, may represent muscularis propria, partly destroyed by invasive carcinoma

2

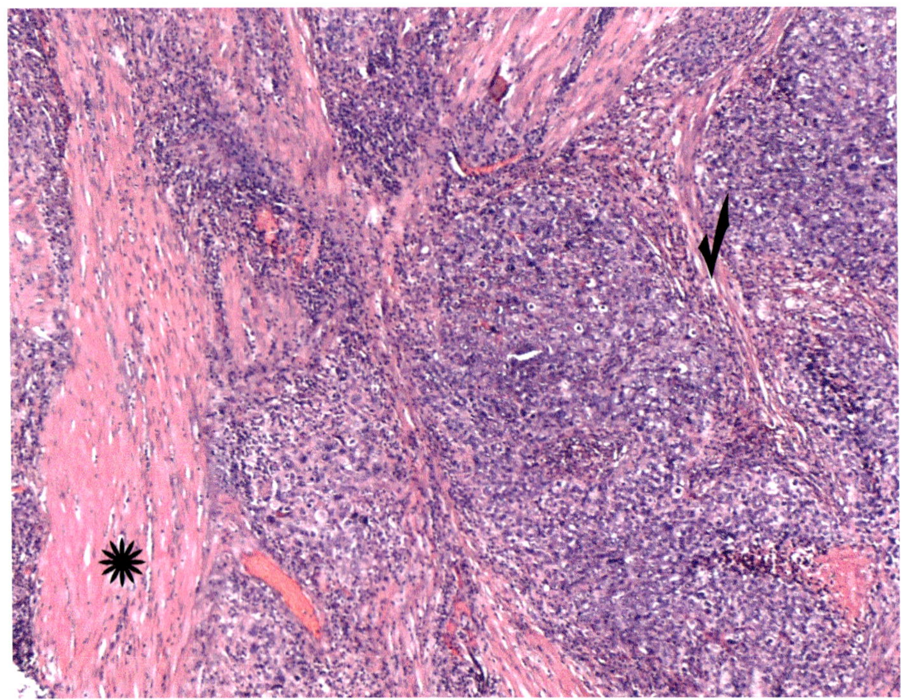

Fig. 2.79 (H-E, ×50) Stage pT2.
In evaluating biopsy specimens, the pathologist should always state what components of the bladder wall are represented (i.e., mucosa, lamina propria, muscularis propria).

Usually, nonpapillary tumors are those which infiltrate the underlying muscularis propria (stage pT2). Muscularis propria invasion implies tumor-infiltrating *thick* smooth muscle bundles (*asterisk*). When there is extensively destructive invasion, the residual muscularis propria bundles may appear thin (*tick*), mimicking the bundles of muscularis mucosae. Muscle-invasive tumors often seem to carve out the muscle bundles, thus conforming to their contours and preserving a rim of residual muscle tissue. The presence of one relatively large muscle bundle (*asterisk*) *and* several smaller bundles of smooth muscle is diagnostic of muscularis propria invasion. The presence of smooth muscle aggregates *throughout* an entire tissue fragment is strongly suggestive of muscularis propria, even if the smooth muscle aggregates are thin.

As a rule, muscularis propria consists of thick aggregated muscle bundles of detrusor muscle which, as previously stated, must be distinguished from muscularis mucosa. Assessment of muscularis propria invasion is very important (pTa/pT1 vs. pT2). The pathologist should mention whether muscularis propria is present in biopsies, and if invasion is present, he/she should not confuse occasionally prominent fascicles of muscularis mucosa that is part of lamina propria (hypertrophic muscularis mucosa, being more common in women) with muscularis propria invasion. Smoothelin antibody may be useful to distinguish muscularis propria from muscularis mucosa. Smoothelin is a smooth muscle-specific contractile protein expressed only by fully differentiated smooth muscle cells, and not by proliferative or noncontractile smooth muscle cells and myofibroblasts. Smoothelin immunostaining may be useful when tumor obliterates muscularis propria and only scant residual muscle is seen; weak, patchy smoothelin immunoreactivity is observed in muscularis mucosae, whereas *strong*, *diffuse* reactivity is observed in *muscularis propria*; nevertheless, an internal control of definite muscularis mucosae should be present so that the stain is useful.

In cases of detrusor muscle invasion, the pathologist cannot substage pT2 as pT2a or pT2b unless he/she has full thickness and well-oriented biopsy of bladder; so, he/she can assess the presence but not depth of muscularis propria invasion in TURBT specimen. pT2 tumors can be reliably substaged in cystectomy specimens

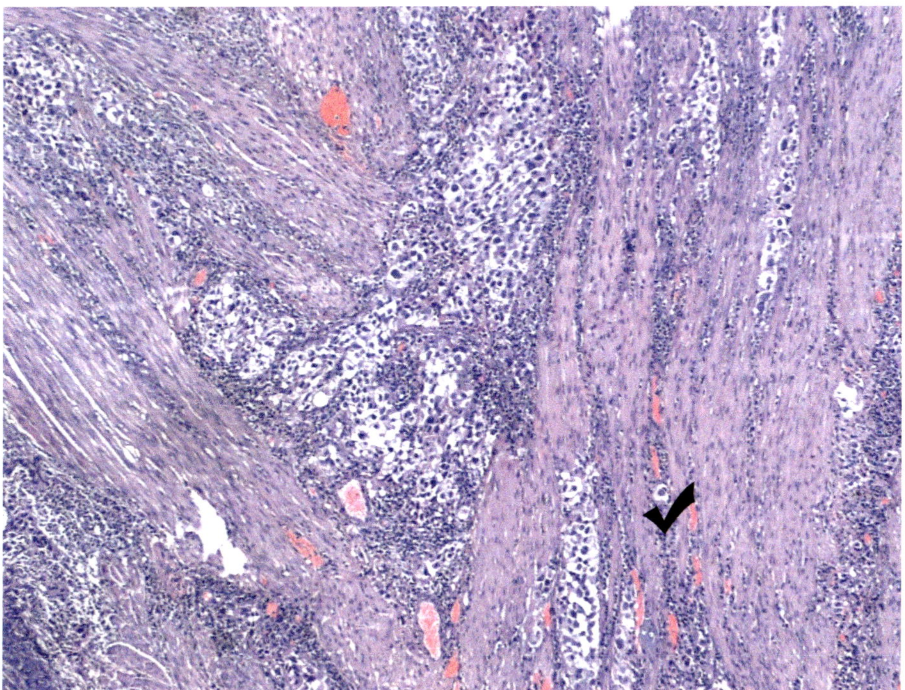

Fig. 2.80 (H-E, ×50) Invasive high-grade urothelial carcinoma dissects between confluent thick bundles of smooth muscle, a finding diagnostic of muscularis propria invasion. This feature classifies the tumor as at least pathologic stage pT2 in transurethral resections.

Subtle foci of carcinoma, within muscularis propria (*tick*) or in cases of severe biopsy crush artifact, can be identified by pancytokeratin stains; however, they should not be confused with cytokeratin-positive myofibroblasts; morphologic correlation is mandatory

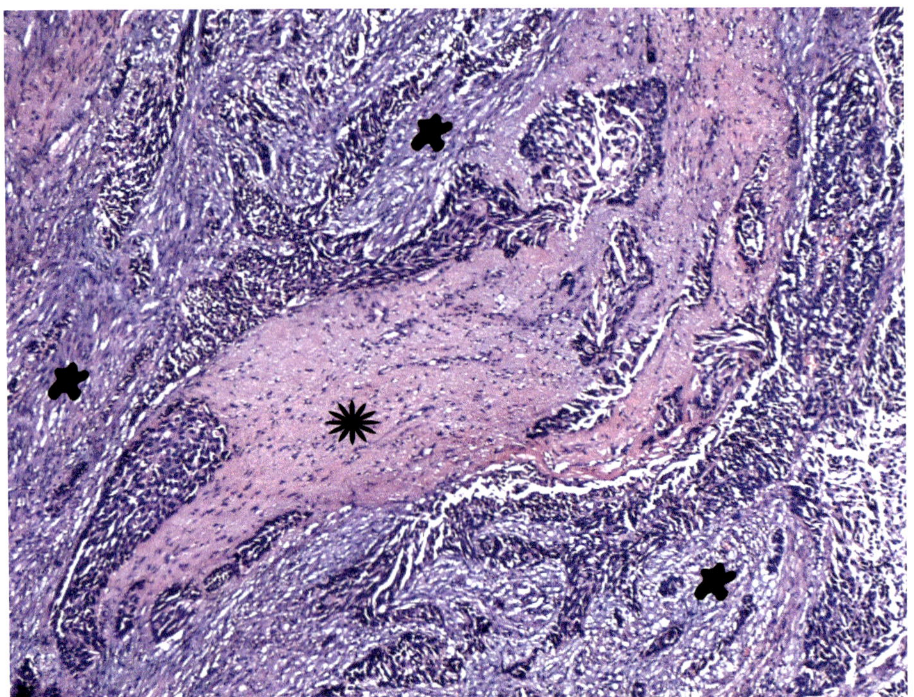

Fig. 2.81 (H-E, ×50) Stage pT2. Irregular, jagged nests of urothelium invade a thick bundle of muscularis propria (*asterisk*). Tumor cells should "carve out" the muscle bundles of detrusor muscle. In pT2 tumors, a clearly infiltrative pattern of growth arguably predicts worse prognosis than a nodular or trabecular pattern of muscle-invasive growth. The large size of this smooth muscle bundle (*asterisk*), which is arranged in a fascicular pattern, is diagnostic of muscularis propria. Because TURBT specimens lack orientation with respect to bladder anatomy, substaging of T2 disease should be performed in cystectomy specimens alone.

Muscle-invasive carcinoma may or may not elicit a desmoplastic stromal response (*blobs*) which sometimes should be discriminated from muscle tissue by special stains. The pathologist can use trichrome stain to highlight all smooth muscle tissue, discriminate it from any desmoplastic response, and determine if muscularis mucosa or muscularis propria is invaded. A desmoplastic reaction (*blobs*) is not diagnostic of detrusor muscle invasion but should raise the suspicion of muscle wall invasion. The desmoplastic reaction may be so extensive as to replace large areas of the detrusor muscle; specimens composed of large, high-grade urothelial carcinomas interspersed with desmoplastic tissue are especially likely to be invasive

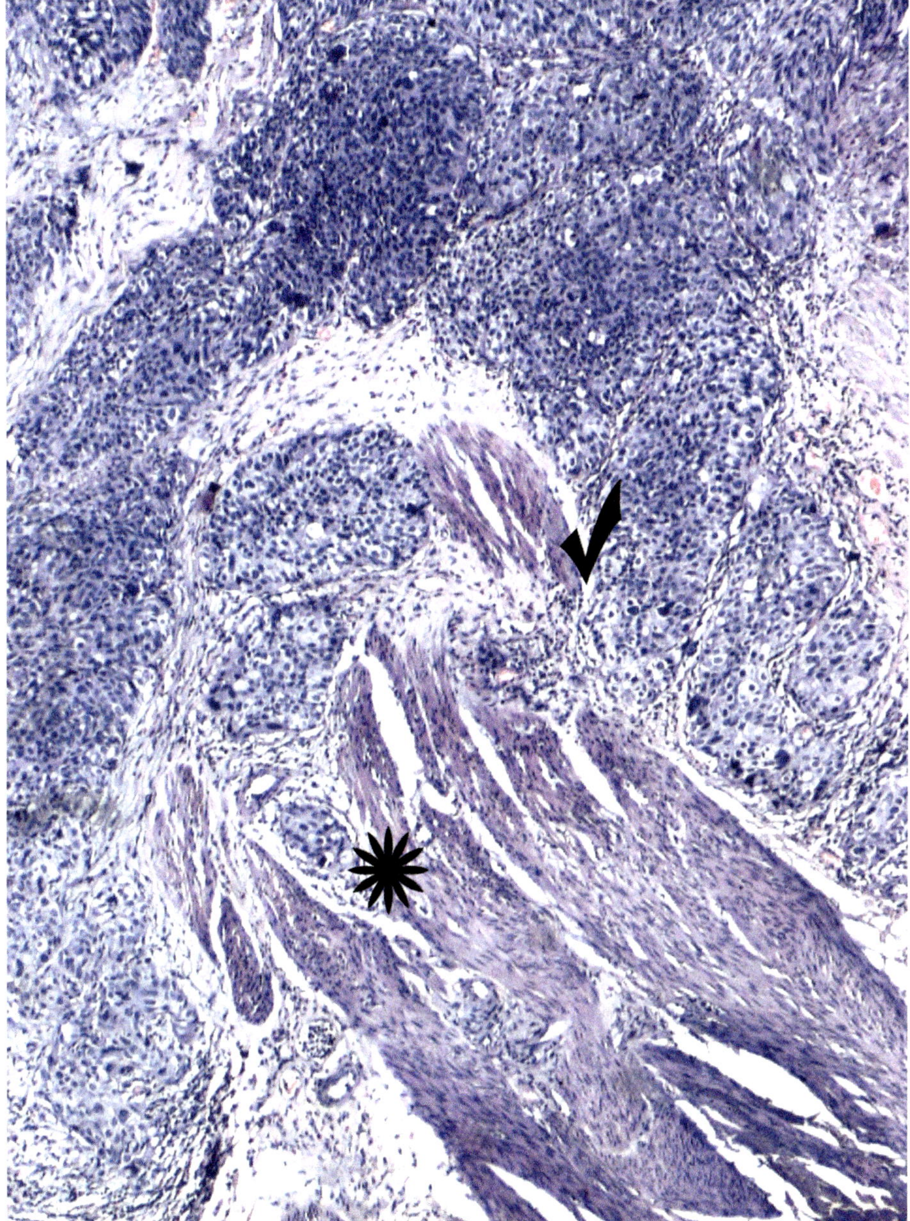

Fig. 2.82 (H-E, ×50) Stage pT2. Adequate transurethral resection of bladder tumor includes resection of all visible tumors *and* sampling of the underlying muscularis propria to assess whether muscle invasion has occurred. To be certain the tumor is infiltrating muscularis propria, one must see tumor cells osculating (*tick*) or extending (*asterisk*) among broad bundles of smooth muscle

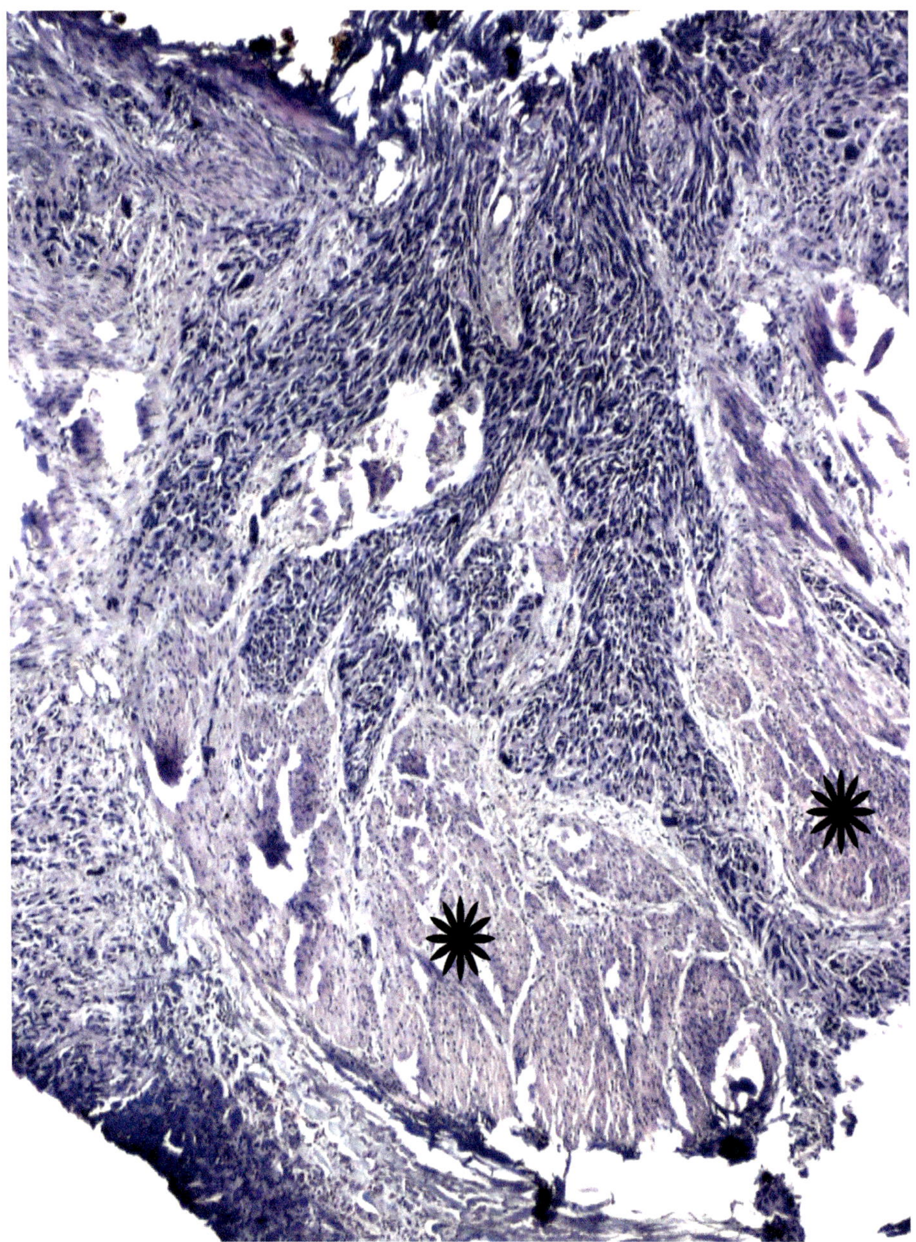

Fig. 2.83 (H-E, ×50) High-grade invasive urothelial carcinoma, stage pT2.

With rare exceptions (i.e., nested or tubular variants), invasive urothelial carcinoma is morphologically high grade. We should have in mind, however, that a poorly differentiated bladder cancer in a male patient should raise the possibility of prostate carcinoma, particularly if the specimen is obtained from the trigone or bladder neck.

Large aggregates of confluent dense smooth muscle, which in some regions may be very superficially located, do correspond to muscularis propria (detrusor muscle). The presence of muscle infiltration should be reported only when it is certain that the tumor has penetrated into the muscularis propria. The confluent mass of tightly aggregated smooth muscle (*asterisks*) is characteristic of muscularis propria

2.5.2 Microscopic Evaluation of the Subsequent Cystectomy Specimen

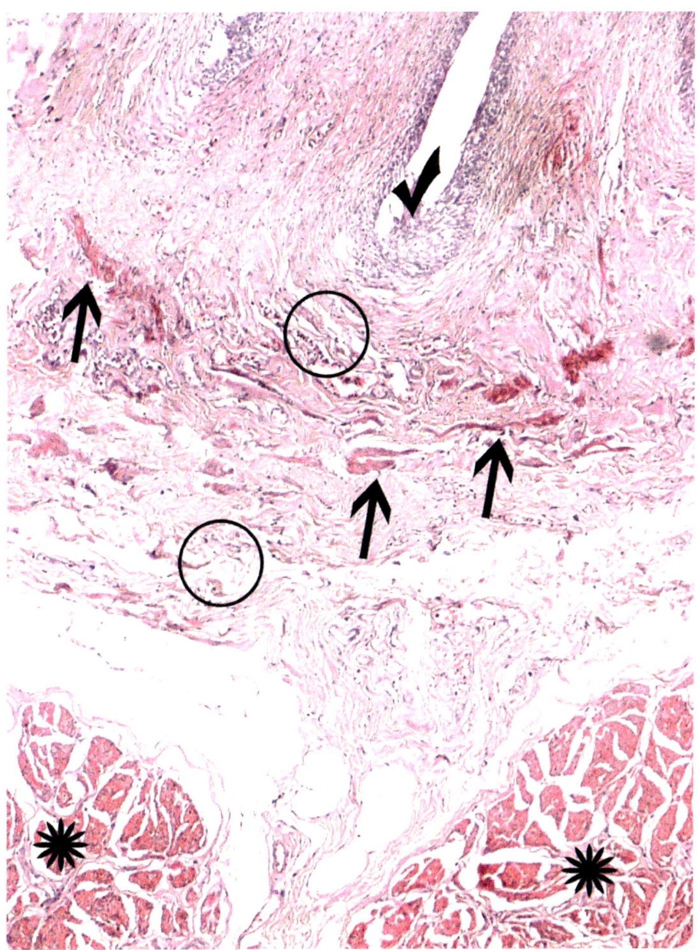

Fig. 2.84 (H-E, ×50) The normal urinary bladder wall. Urothelium (*tick*), here projected within lamina propria (*circles*) and muscularis propria/detrusor muscle (*asterisks*). Vestigial remnants of muscularis mucosae (*arrows*) do not form a plane sufficiently distinctive for substaging the lamina propria.

The few wisps or small separate individual rounded bundles of smooth muscle (*arrows*) that are commonly seen within the lamina propria must not be mistaken for fascicles of the muscularis propria (*asterisks*) in coming to a decision about the depth of invasion. Their configuration is different from the muscle bundles of the detrusor.

Patients with noninvasive tumors with exophytic and/or inverted growth (stage pTa) and tumors confined to lamina propria (pT1) are treated by transurethral resection and possibly intravesical chemotherapy, while patients with "muscle-infiltrating tumors" (at least T2 lesions) are offered radical cystectomy. For this reason, the pathologist must be very careful in assessing depth of invasion on a biopsy specimen. With regard to epithelial tumors arising in an acquired bladder diverticulum, no pT2 stage can be assigned because in this case the detrusor muscle layer cannot be assessed

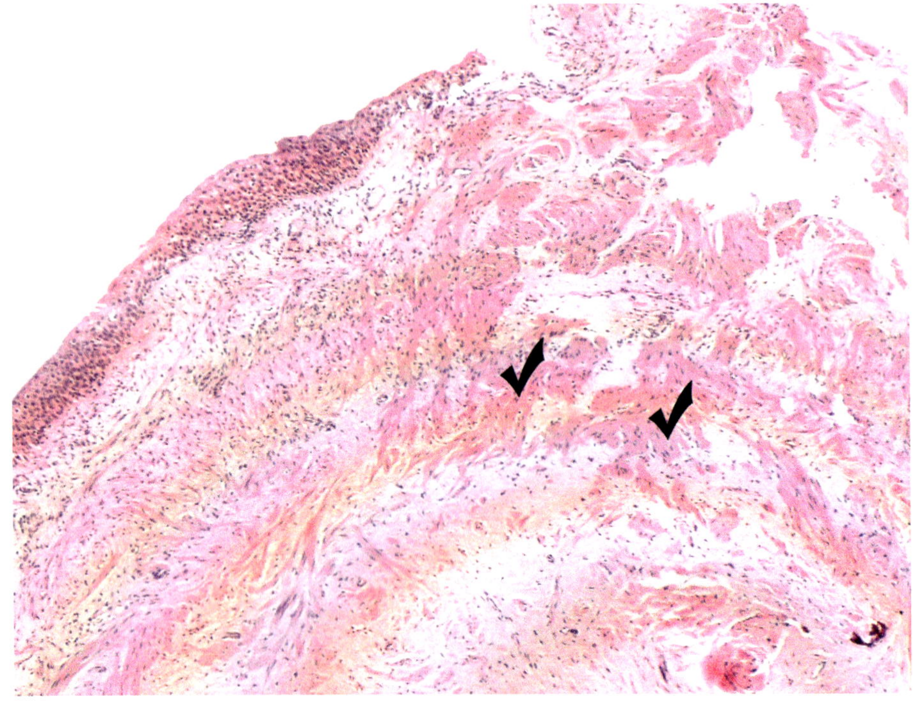

Fig. 2.85 (H-E, ×50) Hyperplastic fascicles of muscularis mucosae (*ticks*) may become thicker and disorganized with dispersion in multiple directions

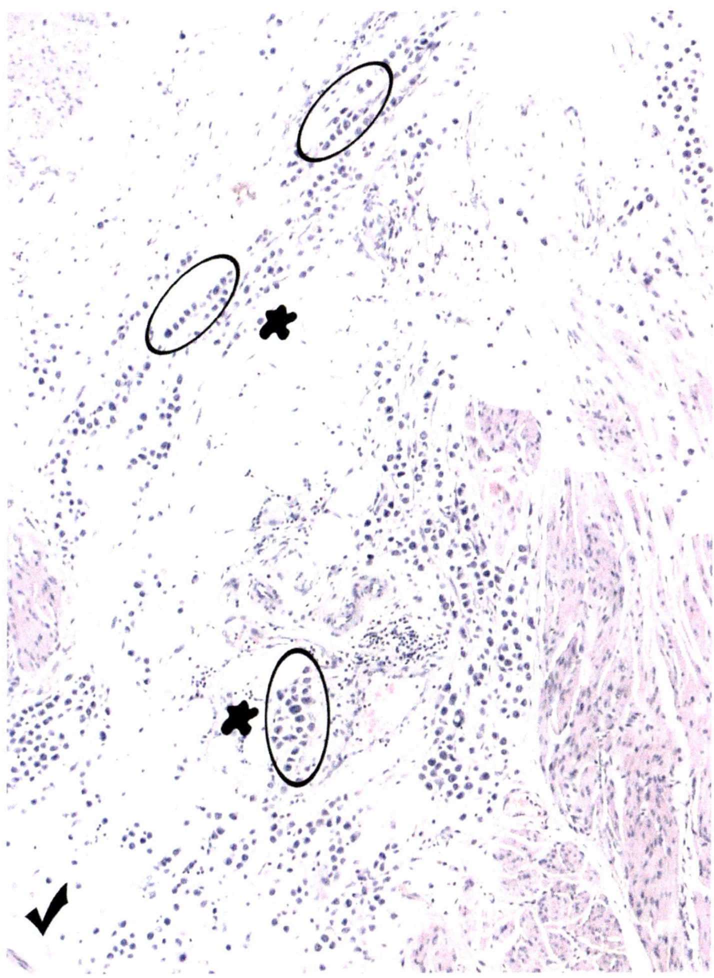

Fig. 2.86 (H-E, ×100) Invasion of lamina propria adipose tissue (*blobs*) by urothelial carcinoma cells. In addition to perivesical tissue, adipose tissue is present throughout the entire bladder wall, including lamina propria and muscularis propria; therefore, tumor infiltration of adipose tissue is *not* a reliable criterion to assess the depth of invasion. Invasion into fat, on its own, does not indicate extravesical spread.

With regard to the morphology of these cancer cells, they may be confused with mononuclear inflammatory cells at this magnification, and they infiltrate in a pattern similar to signet ring adenocarcinoma.

Plasmacytoid urothelial carcinoma is a distinct variant of urothelial carcinoma, characterized by the presence of single, dyscohesive, monotonous malignant cells (*ellipses*), resembling lobular breast carcinoma or diffuse type of gastric cancer, in a loose or myxoid, edematous stroma (*tick*). Retraction spaces around tumor cells (*ellipses*) can be noticed. Cytologic atypia can be minimal. Classic urothelial carcinoma is usually also present elsewhere. A lymphoma-like urothelial carcinoma has also been described; its epithelial nature is confirmed by immunohistochemistry. Positive stains include cytokeratin (strong immunoreactivity for CK7, CK20), uroplakin III, and, possibly, CD138, a finding further mimicking a plasma cell infiltrate. Nevertheless, plasma cell and lymphocyte markers, gamma globulin, and light chains are consistently negative (unlike primary plasmacytomas or lymphomas of the bladder). Membranous E-cadherin is usually absent, a feature related to the poor cohesion of malignant cells of this variant

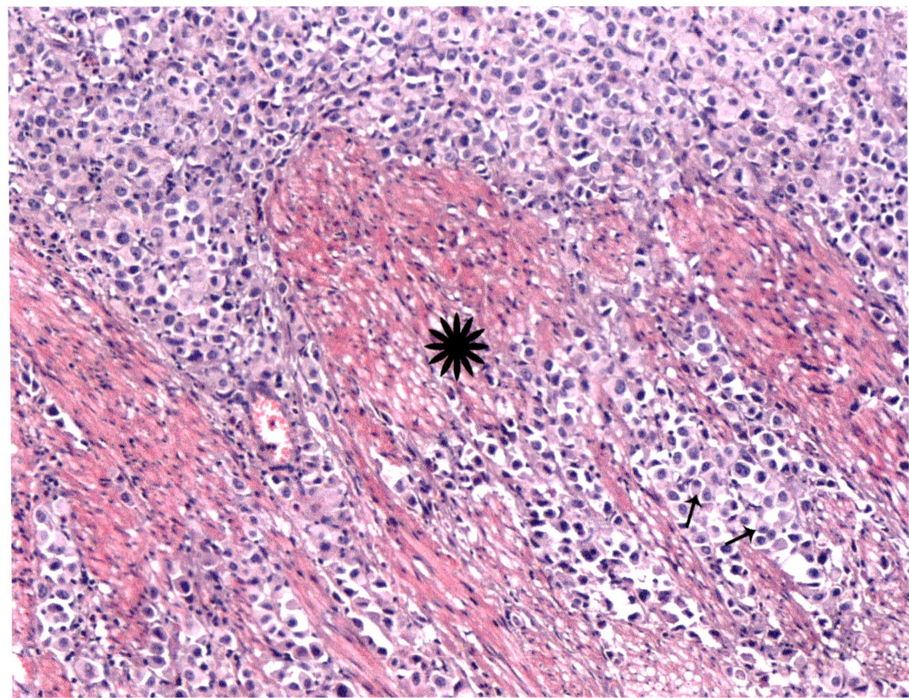

Fig. 2.87 (H-E, ×100) Large cell, high-grade tumor area with muscularis propria invasion (*asterisk*) and some tumor cells reminiscent of plasmacytic origin (*arrows*). In so called plasmacytoid urothelial carcinoma, tumor cells have features of plasma cells, due to abundant, glassy, eosinophilic cytoplasm, round, eccentrically placed, enlarged, hyperchromatic nuclei with indistinct nucleoli. The tumor cells themselves, rather than a surrounding infiltrate (see Figs. 2.103 and 2.104), have lymphoma-like features

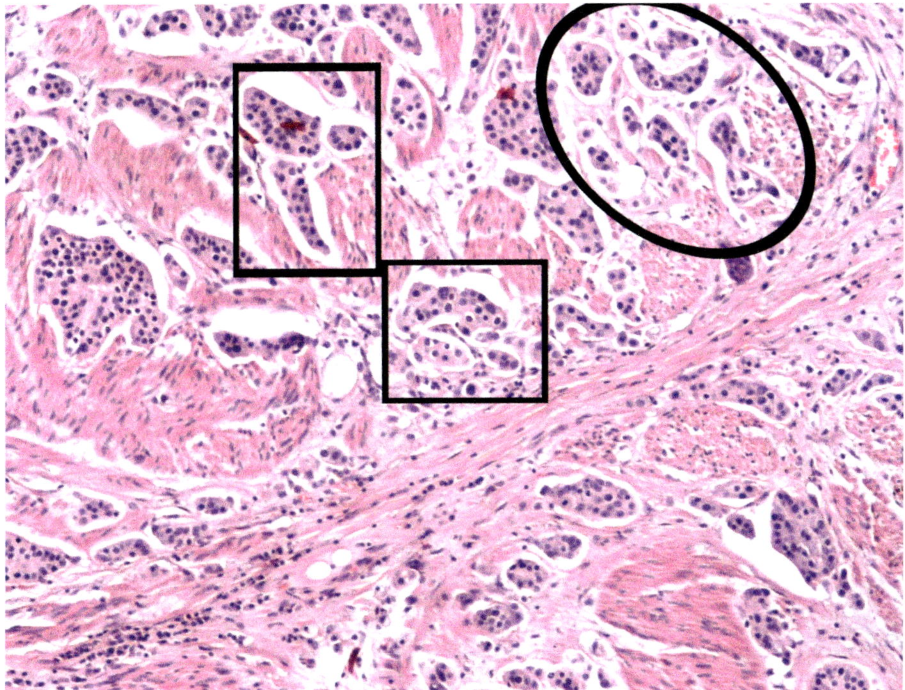

Fig. 2.88 (H-E, ×100) Stage pT2. Deep invasion of detrusor muscle by a micropapillary tumor component (*ellipse*).

There is a high association of the micropapillary variant of urothelial carcinoma with muscle-invasive disease. Surrounding retraction artifact (*ellipse*) is prominent in this site of detrusor muscle invasion by small nests and micropapillae of malignant urothelial cells and should not be overinterpreted as vascular invasion; of course, stromal retraction is immunohistochemically negative for CD31, CD34, and D2–40. In contrast to micropapillary carcinoma, typical invasive urothelial carcinoma with stromal retraction exhibits larger nests and no micropapillae and does not show multiple small nests in the same retraction space (*square frames*)

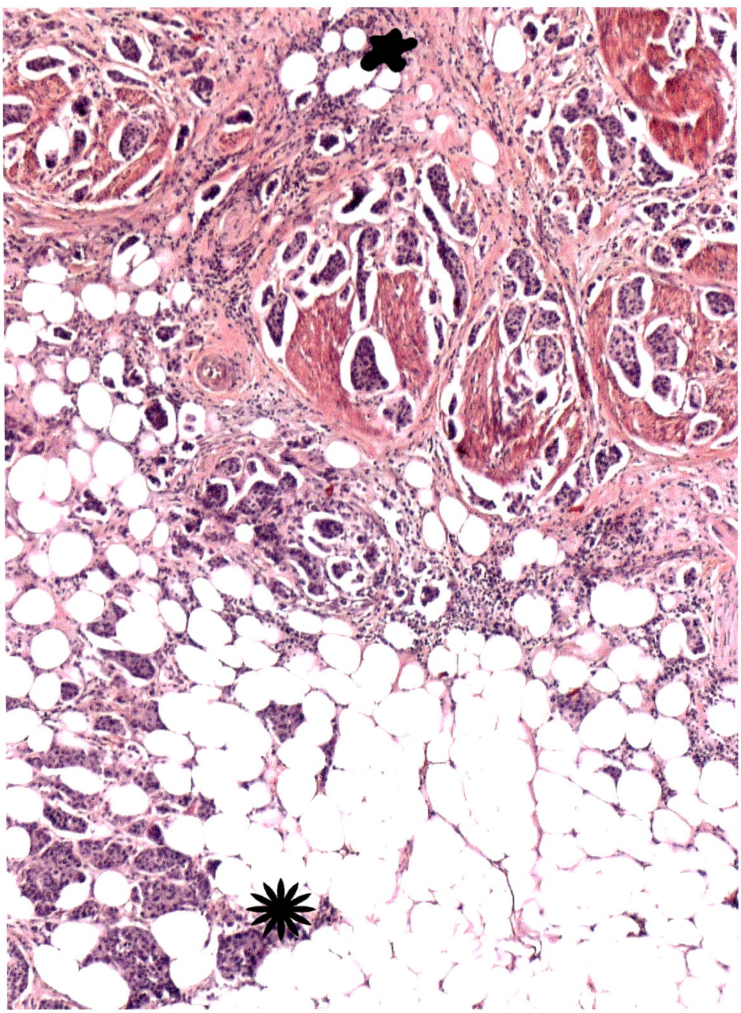

Fig. 2.89 (H-E, ×50) Stage pT3a. *Micro*scopically detected perivesical fat invasion (*asterisk*). Perivesical adipose tissue is deep to muscularis propria but is also present within deep lamina propria, usually as small localized aggregates and within all muscularis propria (superficial and deep). As previously stressed, we should beware of inappropriate staging as pT3 due to tumor infiltration of adipose tissue, particularly in TURBT specimens. At cystectomy, histological distinction between muscularis propria outer half invasion (pT2b) and microscopic perivesical fat invasion (pT3a, as here) can be difficult, because the boundary between the outer muscularis propria and perivesical fat is not well defined. Adipose tissue is often present between detrusor muscle bundles (*blob*). The junction between the muscularis propria layer and perivesical fat is not well demarcated; so, while determining the status of a tumor as T2 or T3, an imaginary line may be drawn at low power to demarcate the boundary between the bladder wall in a cystectomy specimen and perivesical tissue.

The present patient was node-negative. For node-positive radical cystectomy patients with meticulous lymph node dissection and thorough histologic examination, lymph node extracapsular extension has prognostic value, but N1 vs. N2 does not. Metastases to lymph nodes are detected in 25% of invasive tumors; also, metastatic dissemination may affect the lung, liver, bone, and CNS.

In cystectomy specimens, dysplasia or carcinoma in situ is often found elsewhere in the bladder including the bladder neck but also in the ureters, urethra, prostatic ducts, and seminal vesicles. The 10-year survival is only 40% for high-grade tumors (Pathology Outlines 2017)

2.5.3 Microscopic Images of Urothelial Carcinoma Variants in Other Cases

The variant histology should be documented in the pathology reports because metastatic tumors usually continue to exhibit the distinctive histologic pattern, and knowledge of the variant histology facilitates association of the metastasis with the primary tumor.

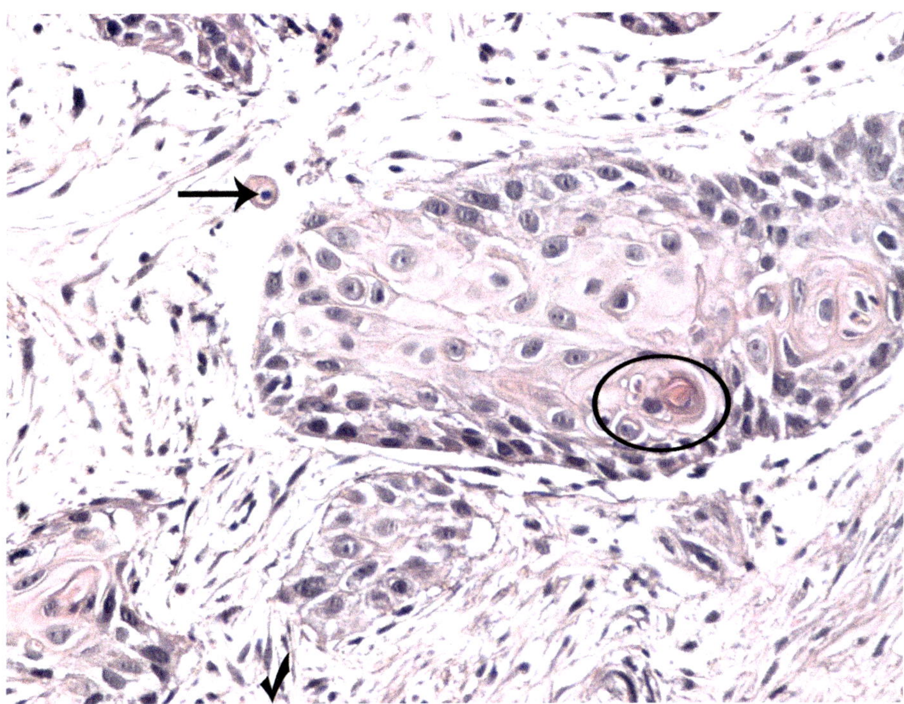

Fig. 2.90 (H-E, ×200) Invasive urothelial carcinoma with squamous differentiation. Invasive nests and islands of malignant squamous epithelium are observed, and, by definition, an identifiable malignant urothelial component (which may be only carcinoma in situ) should be encountered elsewhere. This is the most common type of divergent differentiation of high-grade urothelial carcinoma and is defined by the presence of intercellular bridges and/or evidence of keratinization either individual cell keratinization (dyskeratosis) or formation of keratin pearls (*ellipse*). The squamous component has nests of malignant squamous epithelium characterized by polygonal malignant cells with irregularly distributed chromatin and evident or prominent nucleoli (*arrow*). The cytoplasm is more eosinophilic than typical urothelial carcinoma. Interestingly, the squamous component may have basaloid or clear cell features. Associated florid stromal myofibroblastic proliferation (*tick*) and/or eosinophils are frequent. Immunohistochemically, the squamous component is positive for CK14 and Mac387 (L1 antigen) and negative for uroplakins (the latter are positive in urothelial component) and also negative for CK20

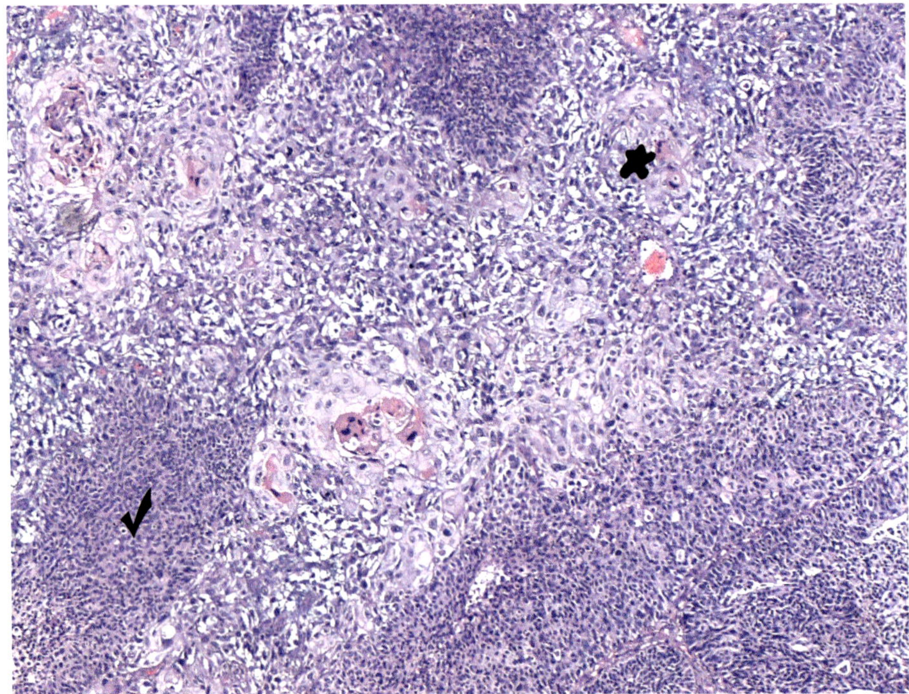

Fig. 2.91 (H-E, ×50) This mixed variant with malignant urothelial (*tick*) and squamous (*blob*) components is most often encountered.

Either component may be in situ only (see Fig. 2.92).

It is recommended to report the percentage of the squamous component.

Because focal squamous cell changes are common in high-grade urothelial tumors, as above, the term "squamous cell carcinoma" should be reserved for those tumors that are squamous throughout, lacking a urothelial component [the same applies to (*true*) glandular differentiation and the term "adenocarcinoma"]. So, in squamous cell carcinoma, there is no associated urothelial component (i.e., pure squamous cell tumor parenchyma). True squamous carcinomas of the bladder certainly do occur, usually as solid invasive lesions; they are rare in areas where schistosomiasis is not endemic, although they may occur in chronically irritated and inflamed bladders, possibly through a process of metaplasia of the urothelium. The presence of squamous metaplasia, however, is not an obligate phase in the pathogenesis of (pure) squamous cell carcinomas

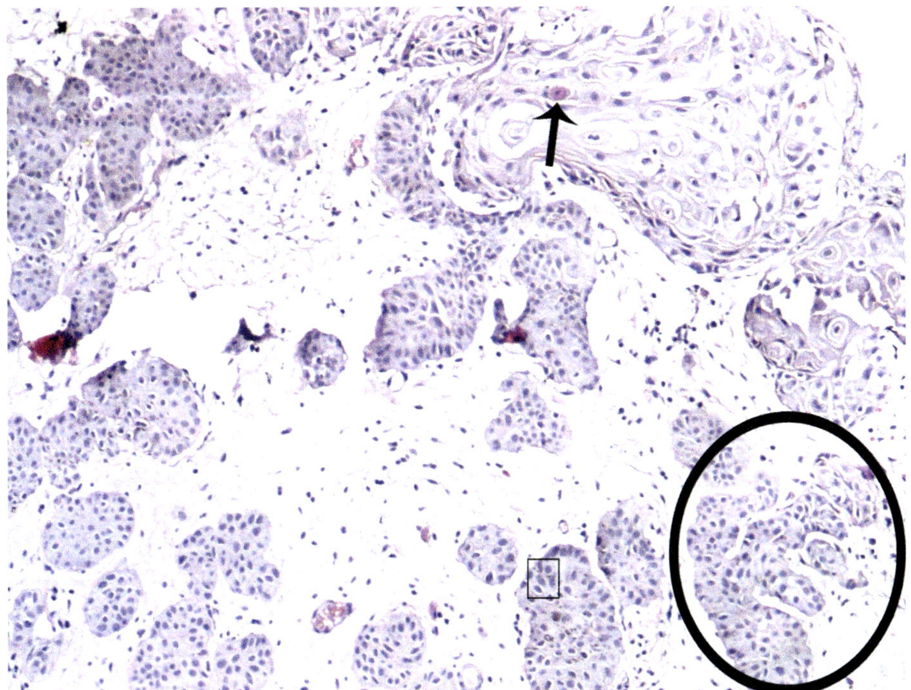

Fig. 2.92 (H-E, ×100) Urothelial carcinoma with in situ squamous (upper right part) and invasive nested-type components.

Individual cell keratinization/dyskeratosis (*arrow*) in the former component. Well-defined cellular borders.

The nested type is a rare bladder tumor in which neoplastic urothelial cells are arranged in irregular and confluent small nests (*ellipse*) and abortive tubules composed of urothelial cells infiltrating the lamina propria or muscularis propria, usually without surface involvement. Tumor nests often have some degree of complex anastomosis, at least focally (*ellipse*). Most of the neoplastic cells are only slightly atypical but *scattered anaplastic elements* are found in every case (*square frame*). There is often more atypia and focal anaplasia with increasing depth of invasion.

These structures, when noticed within the lamina propria, may resemble proliferations of Brunn's nests. The seemingly benign architecture and cytology belie the potentially aggressive behavior of the nested variant of urothelial carcinoma. Nested (and tubular) variants of urothelial carcinoma generally lack significant cellular atypia; however, grading of invasive component does not affect prognosis as all invasive urothelial carcinomas have recurring and metastatic potential. Nested urothelial carcinomas differ from proliferations of Brunn's nests by their invasive growth pattern and focal nuclear anaplasia; often, increasing levels of atypia are noticed toward deeper portions of tumor. Urothelial carcinoma, nested type, grows by *invasion* of the bladder wall. Muscularis propria is commonly involved by nested urothelial carcinoma.

When deceptively bland patterns of urothelial carcinoma (e.g., nested and microcystic patterns) are limited to the lamina propria, they may make the recognition of T1 disease extremely difficult. Attention should be paid to general features useful in assessing invasion, such as cytologic atypia, infiltrative architecture, desmoplasia, and architectural complexity, especially because these features may appear subtle in superficial biopsies

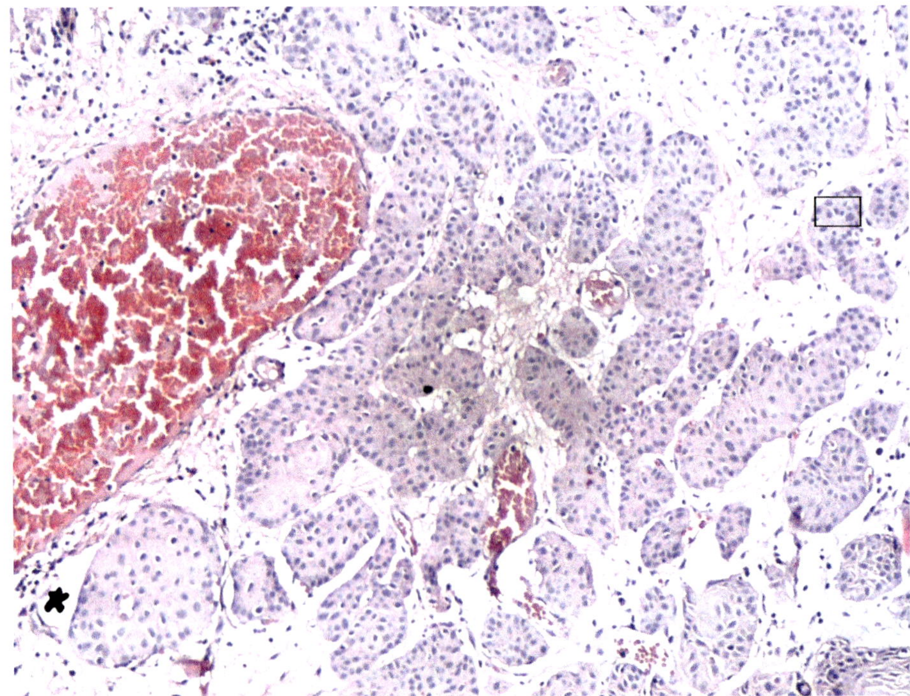

Fig. 2.93 (H-E, ×100) Nested variant urothelial carcinoma infiltrating the lamina propria. There is a disorderly proliferation of discrete to confluent crowded small nests (image center) beneath the urothelium. There is little or no intervening stroma. *Haphazard* distribution of nests. The nests are too small and crowded to represent Brunn's nests. Architectural complexity, confluence, and anastomosis between the nests. Abortive tubules may be observed. Retraction artifact may be seen (*blob*). Typical urothelial carcinoma is often present elsewhere.

By definition, these tumors cannot be high grade or have overlying surface urothelial CIS. Tumor cells have only mild atypia (mild pleomorphism, slightly increased N/C ratios, occasional prominent nucleoli, rare mitotic figures) and resemble cystitis glandularis et cystica; however, at least some nests should have more pleomorphic nuclei, coarse nuclear chromatin, and large nucleoli (foci of unequivocal cancer). Some cytologic atypia should be seen (*square frame*), particularly at the lesion's base.

Irregular infiltrating border with lamina propria is characteristic. Deep tumor-stroma interface is jagged and *infiltrative* in contrast to benign conditions which extend to a uniform level within the lamina propria creating a sharp, linear border at their base; the latter also occurs in Brunn's nests of the ureter and renal pelvis which, noteworthily, tend to be smaller and more crowded than in the bladder and so more easily confused with the nested variant of urothelial carcinoma. In small superficial bladder biopsy specimens, a definitive diagnosis may sometimes be impossible. In nested urothelial carcinoma, epithelial nests are present *deeper in the lamina propria*; we also notice areas with *more complex architecture* than seen in benign mimics such as florid Brunn's nests. Significantly greater MIB-1 and p53 expression, compared to florid Brunn's nests, is reported in the nested variant of urothelial carcinoma.

Several nonurothelial tumors (e.g., paraganglioma, carcinoid tumor, melanoma, alveolar soft part sarcoma) involving the urinary bladder may have a nested pattern; in such cases an appropriately constructed immunohistochemical panel will permit their distinction

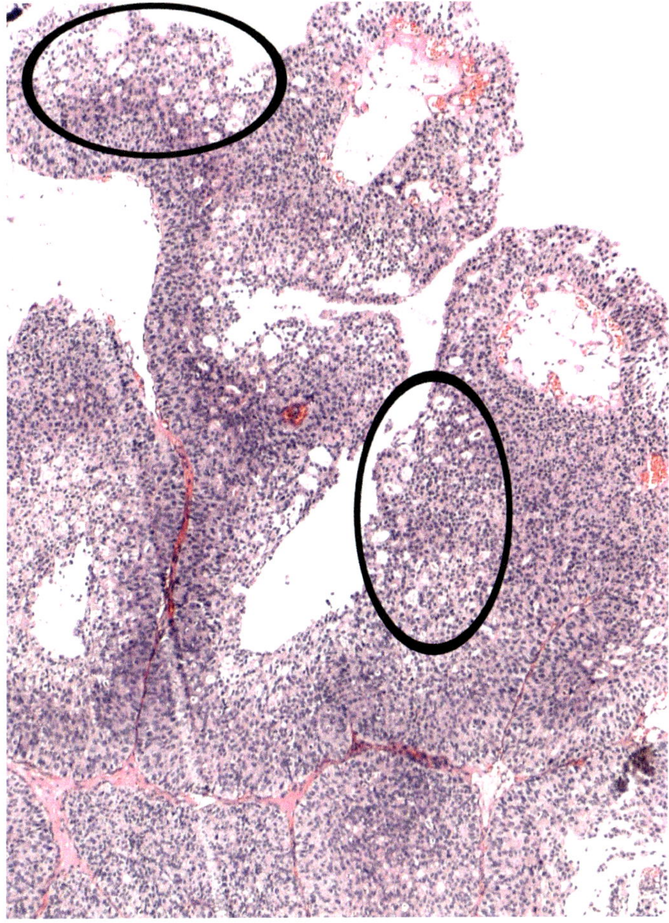

Fig. 2.94 (H-E, ×50) Urothelial carcinoma with gland-like lumens (*ellipses*), which represent microcystic change *within* urothelial carcinoma. The cells surrounding these lumens have an architectural pattern reminiscent of urothelium rather than colon. There is the absence of true glandular spaces within the urothelial component. Predominant features of urothelial carcinoma but with prominent inter- or intracellular lumens surrounded by neoplastic urothelial (or squamous cells) and no true glands. Lumens are usually empty but may contain granular eosinophilic debris, necrotic cells, or mucin. Intracytoplasmic mucin, on its own, is not considered to represent glandular differentiation in a urothelial carcinoma. Urothelial carcinoma with gland-like lumens often contains mucin yet lacks the apical cytoplasm and basally situated nuclei of true glandular differentiation. Urothelial carcinoma with prominent *inter*cellular or *intra*cellular gland-like lumens (for the latter see Fig. 2.95) is close to the microcystic variant of urothelial carcinoma [which should be distinguished from (pure primary) adenocarcinoma of the bladder]. Lumens are usually small but may reach cystic proportions. Most appear empty in usual histologic preparations. Cysts vary in size, are round/oval, are up to 2 mm, and are lined by urothelium, flattened cells, or low columnar cells, but *not* colonic epithelium or goblet cells. Cysts should be infiltrative and may invade the muscularis propria

Fig. 2.94 (continued)

A urothelial carcinoma variant with small tubules has been described; it's an invasive carcinoma with small gland-like spaces lined by urothelial cells without intracellular mucin or columnar lining. Some consider this part of the nested variant.

1. Urothelial carcinoma with gland-like lumens should be distinguished from:
2. Urothelial carcinoma with (*true*) glandular differentiation

   (Pure, primary) Adenocarcinoma of the bladder

   1. Urothelial carcinoma with glandular differentiation is *primarily* a urothelial tumor [in contrast to (pure) adenocarcinoma], but, in contrast to urothelial carcinoma with gland-like lumens, urothelial carcinoma with glandular differentiation has *true* glands lined by goblet cells or colonic epithelium.
   2. Adenocarcinoma is *diffusely* lined by goblet cells or intestinal cells, not flattened urothelial-like cells; it is usually deeply invasive and high grade (see Figs. 2.15 and 2.16)

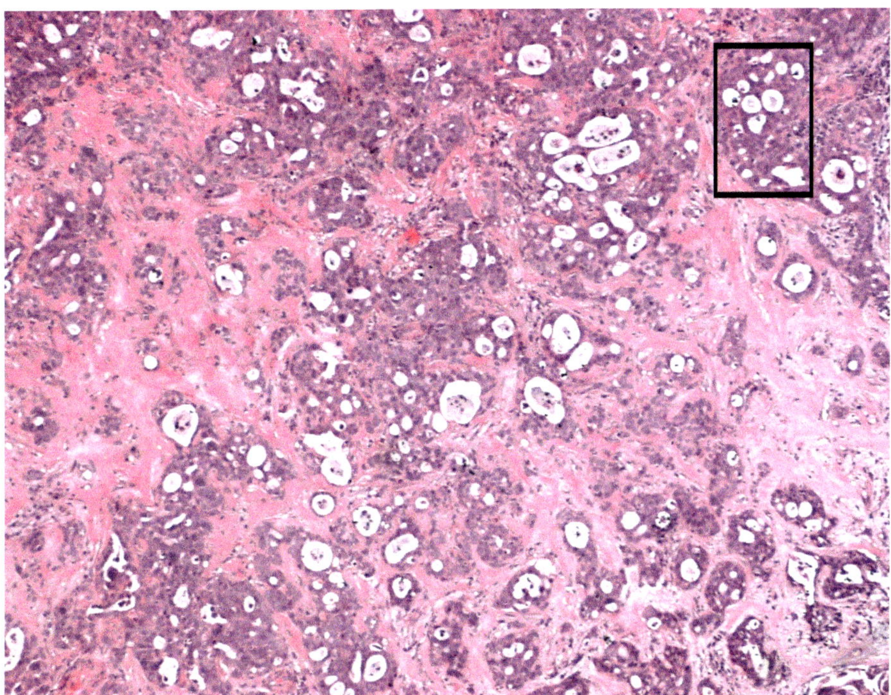

Fig. 2.95 (H-E, ×50) (High-grade) urothelial carcinoma with glandular differentiation is a *urothelial* carcinoma with *focal true glands* with goblet cells *or* columnar intestinal epithelium and mucin. This glandular component should *resemble adenocarcinoma* (*square frame*). Conventional urothelial carcinoma (in situ, noninvasive papillary or invasive) should be present elsewhere. Tubular *or* enteric glands with mucin secretions may be present in about 6% of urothelial carcinoma of the bladder. Small amounts of predominantly acid mucins can be revealed by appropriate histochemical reactions. Goblet cells were not identified in this case. Immunohistochemically, areas of glandular differentiation within urothelial carcinomas are positive for CK7, CK20, and MUC5AC-apomucin. Glandular differentiation must be distinguished from the gland-like lumens (pseudoglandular spaces) that can occur in usual urothelial carcinoma (see Fig. 2.94). Immunohistochemistry shows the acquisition of an enteric expression pattern (CDX2 *and* CK20 reactivity) in areas of glandular differentiation; villin is negative, however.

The distinction of urothelial carcinomas with gland-like lumens from urothelial tumors with glandular differentiation is somewhat arbitrary, and it's important only when the urothelial neoplasm is of low cytologic grade. The histologic architecture of the variant of urothelial carcinoma with gland-like lumens is distinctly urothelial throughout. Extracellular lumens are lined by flattened cells rather than goblet cells, and the pattern may be reminiscent of cystitis glandularis et cystica. Nevertheless, distinction between true glandular differentiation with glandular lumens (with colonic epithelium or goblet cells) and gland-like lumens (lacking these cells) appears to have no clinical significance, since the overlying pattern is clearly *urothelial*.

In addition, a urothelial carcinoma with villoglandular differentiation has been described. These cases are defined as having villoglandular features if they contain superficial finger-like processes lined by epithelium having true glandular lumina (Lim et al. 2009).

The important differential diagnosis is that of (pure primary) adenocarcinoma of the bladder; in the latter, there is *no* urothelial component. Adenocarcinoma of the bladder is a tumor consisting *exclusively of pure glandular components* with glands lined by goblet cells or intestinal cells (not flattened urothelial-like cells); adenocarcinoma is usually deeply invasive and high grade

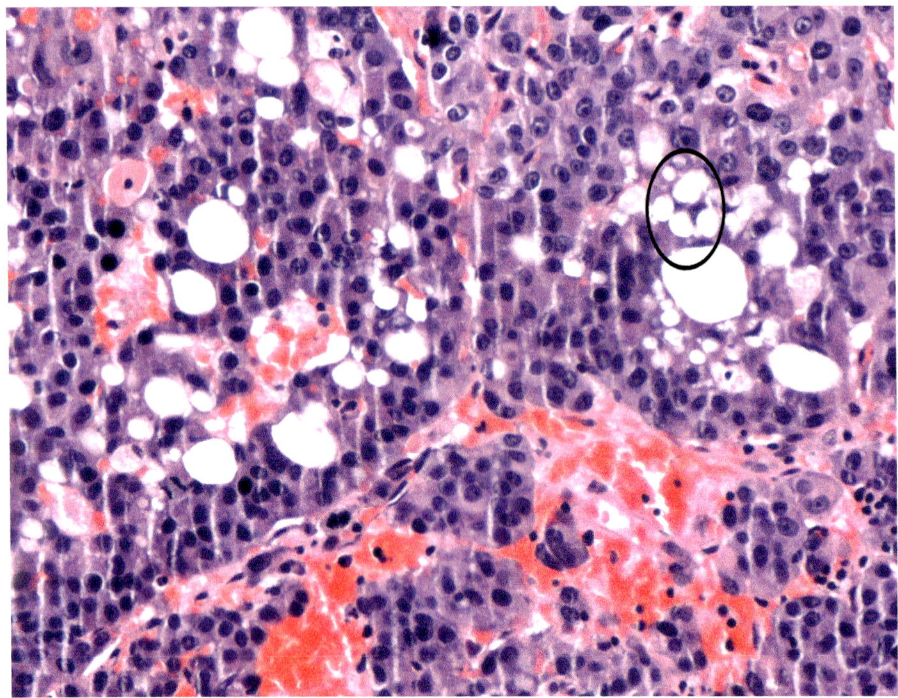

Fig. 2.96 (H-E, ×100) Lipid-rich urothelial carcinoma is characterized by the presence of large signet ring/lipoblast-like cells with intracellular lipid-forming one or more clear cytoplasmic vacuoles that indent the nucleus (*ellipse*). In contrast to liposarcoma, these lipid-rich cells maintain cytokeratin AE1/AE3 immunoreactivity and are S100-negative. The background urothelial carcinoma is invariably high grade and invasive.

Large carcinoma cells with optically clear, empty, multivacuolated cytoplasm resemble lipoblasts. When lipid-rich cellular areas are prominent, the possibility of a signet ring component (glandular differentiation) or liposarcomatous elements of a sarcomatoid carcinoma should be investigated.

Foci of glandular metaplasia are common usually in the form of *intra*cytoplasmic mucin-containing vacuoles. Exceptionally, a microcystic pattern develops as the result of enlargement of the mucin-filled cavities, which can reach a diameter of 1 mm or more. Microcystic urothelial carcinoma is characterized by predominantly round to oval microcysts (1–2 mm in size) lined by a bland or denuded-looking epithelium. The irregular and haphazard nature of the proliferation, the overt size variation, and the widespread involvement of lamina propria aid in recognition as carcinoma (and distinction of cystitis glandularis; see Figs. 2.8, 2.9, and 2.10). The microcystic pattern often coexists with the nested variant of urothelial carcinoma.

A clear distinction between *urothelial* carcinomas with focal mucin production and/or some true glandular differentiation and the (pure, primary) *adenocarcinomas* of the bladder should be made (Rosai and Ackerman 2007)

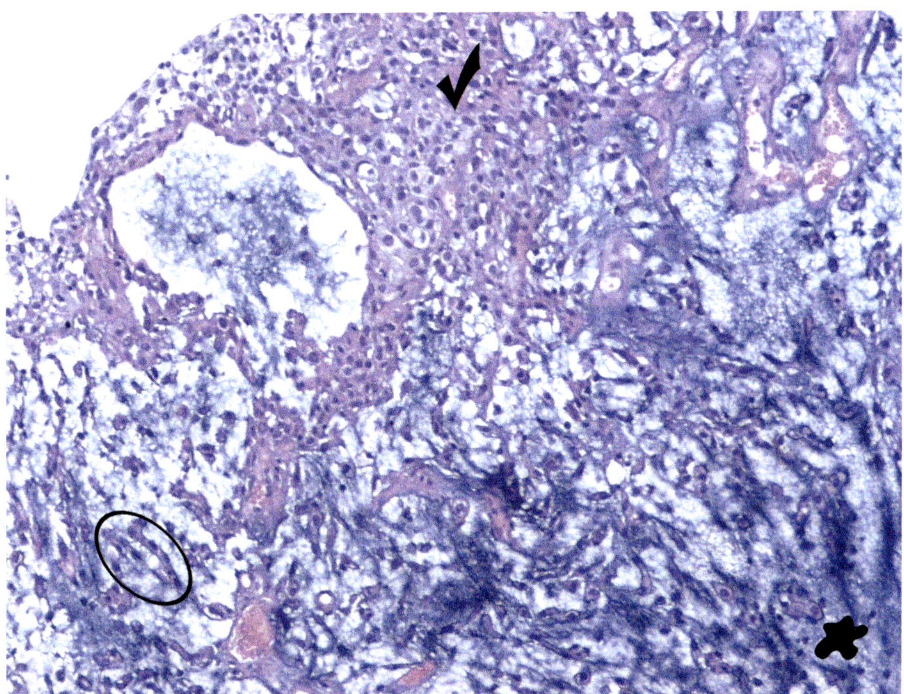

Fig. 2.97 (H-E, ×100) A urothelial carcinoma with prominent myxoid stroma. Small neoplastic cells with eosinophilic cytoplasm may "float" in myxoid matrix (*blob*) in aggregates or chains (*ellipse*) and maintain epithelial immunophenotype. This morphologic pattern can cause confusion with myofibroblastic lesions; the degree of nuclear chromatin changes of the former is more than that seen in myofibroblastic lesions. Typical urothelial carcinoma is almost always present (*tick*).

The cord-like growth (*ellipse*) and the absence of *intra*cytoplasmic mucin exclude a mucinous adenocarcinoma

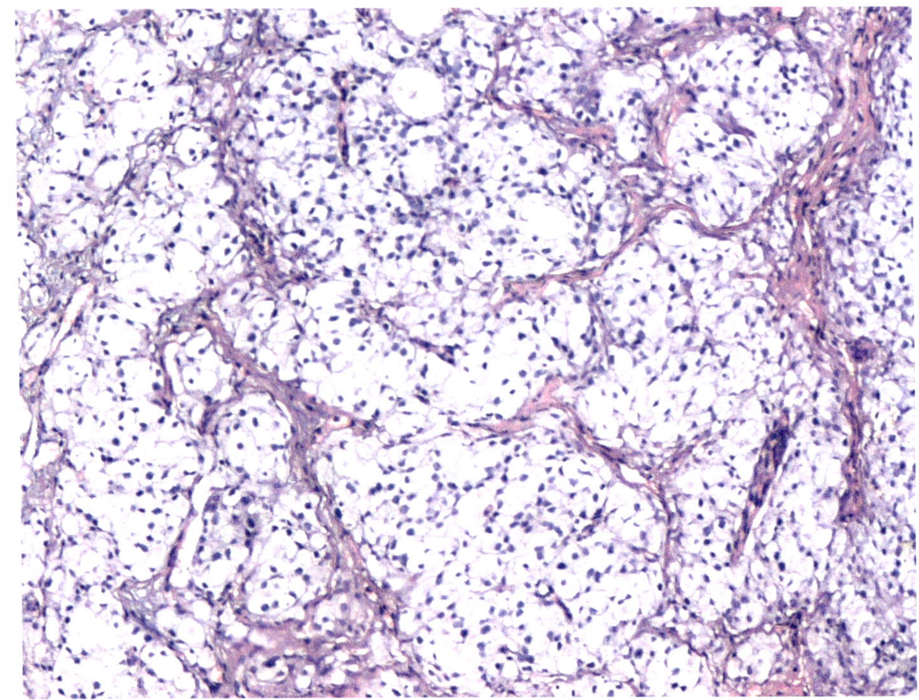

Fig. 2.98 (H-E, ×100) Clear cell (glycogen-rich) *urothelial* carcinoma. Abundant clear cytoplasm secondary to glycogen accumulation.

This variant is reminiscent of clear cell renal cell carcinoma. The clear cells of clear cell (glycogen-rich) urothelial carcinoma show the usual immunohistochemical profile of urothelial carcinoma (e.g., CK7 positivity), however.

This variant of urothelial carcinoma is also different from the rare instance that a urothelial carcinoma demonstrates Mullerian differentiation, manifesting as a clear cell (adeno)carcinoma (see Figs. 2.17 and 2.18).

Finally, cytoplasmic clearing as a result of thermal artifact in transurethral resections should not be mistaken for this variant of bladder cancer

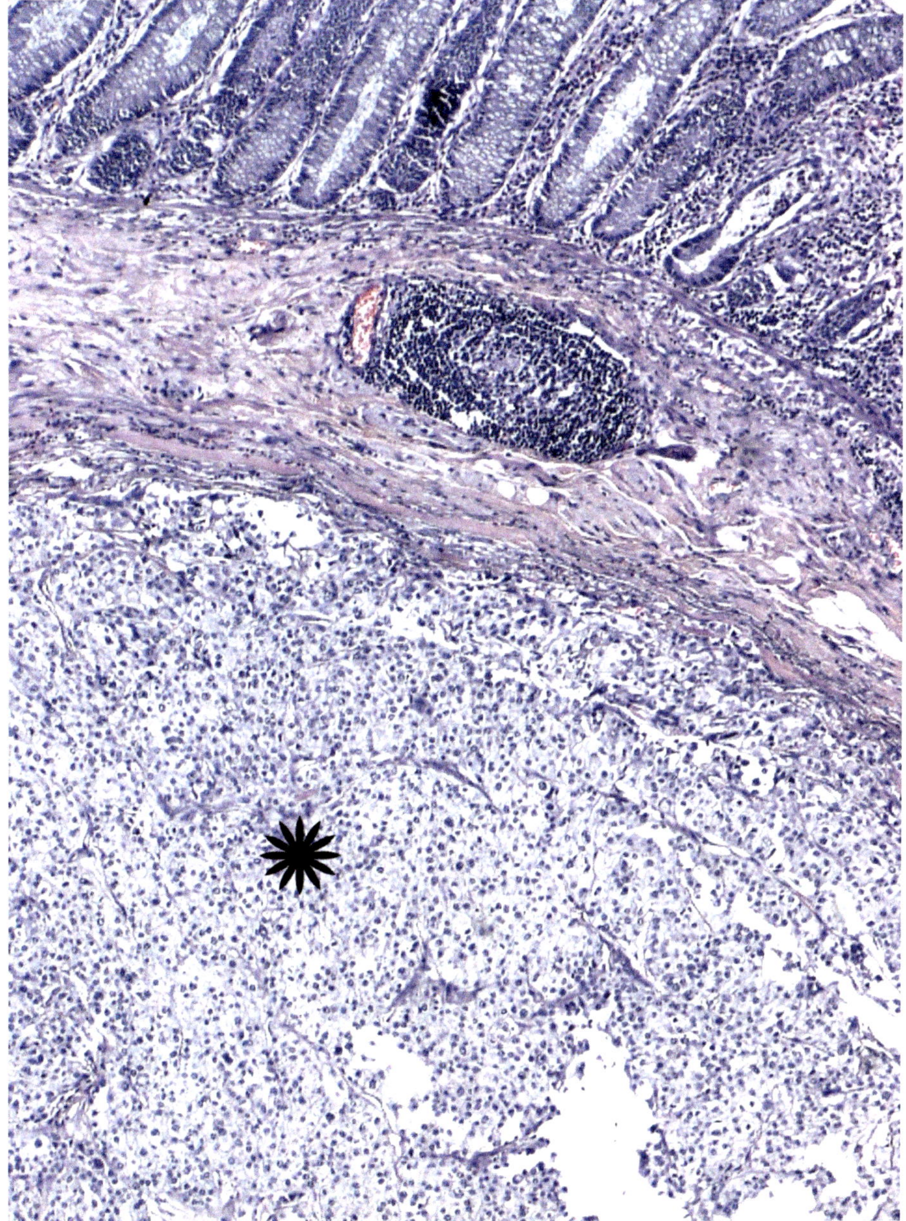

Fig. 2.99 (H-E, ×50) Clear cell (glycogen-rich) *urothelial* carcinoma invading colon wall (extension to adjacent organ, stage pT4).

Clear cell urothelial carcinomas are typically high grade, so the differential diagnosis includes in addition to clear cell (adeno)carcinoma and high-grade renal cell carcinoma and high-grade prostatic carcinoma as well.

Poorly differentiated urothelial carcinomas with clear cell features have a more sheet-like growth pattern (*asterisk*) and often have more *characteristic* appearing *areas*, at least focally, of *urothelial* carcinoma with conventional morphology (Epstein et al. 2010)

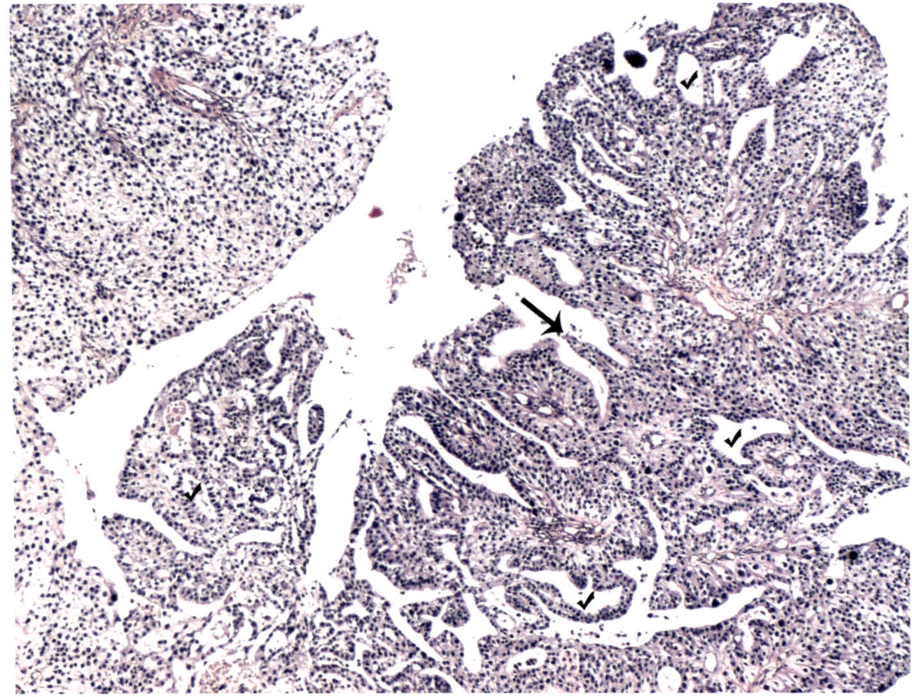

Fig. 2.100 (H-E, ×50) A clear cell urothelial carcinoma component (on the upper left side) neighboring another superficial component with villiform processes (*arrow*) and glandular formations (*ticks*)

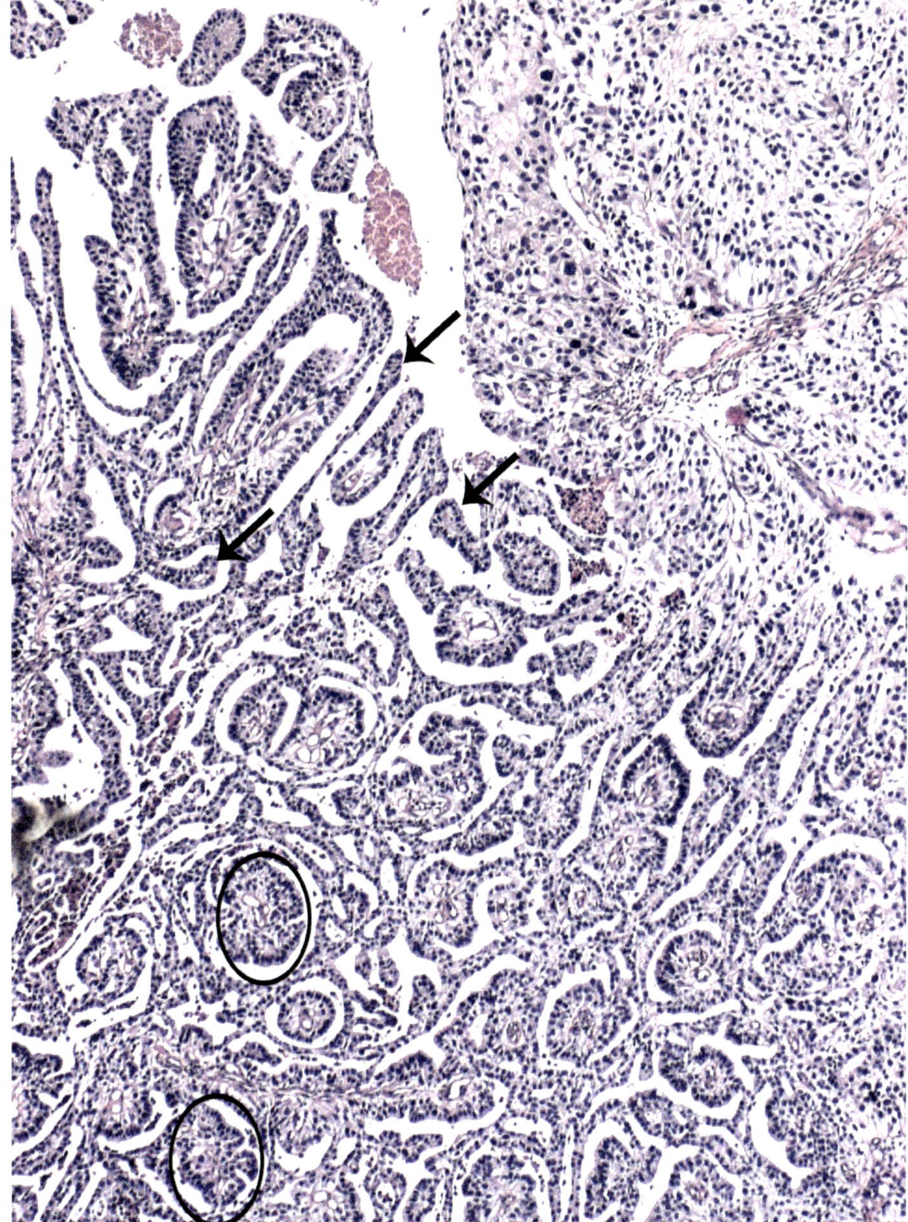

Fig. 2.101 (H-E, ×50) Slender, delicate filiform processes (*arrows*), rarely with a fibrovascular core. When cut in cross sections, these micropapillae appear as glomeruloid bodies (*ellipses*).
A high-grade tumor component is identified in the upper right part of the image

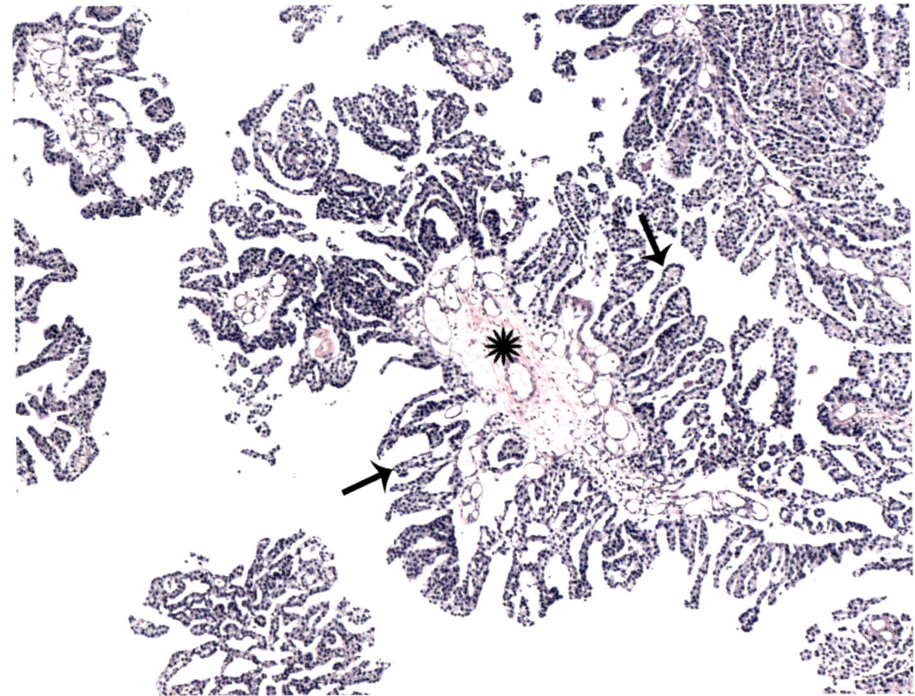

Fig. 2.102 (H-E, ×50) When micropapillary processes are *only* present in the superficial, noninvasive component, the tumor should *not* be classified micropapillary carcinoma.

This example of noninvasive carcinoma has extensive micropapillary architecture characterized by elongated filiform papillae (*arrows*) arising from the main papillary core (*asterisk*).

If surface micropapillary carcinoma is present in biopsy without muscularis propria, deeper biopsy to determine muscular invasion is recommended since muscle invasion by the micropapillary component is a significant concern (see Figs. 2.88 and 2.89). Most micropapillary urothelial carcinomas tumors are muscle invasive (Pathology Outlines 2017)

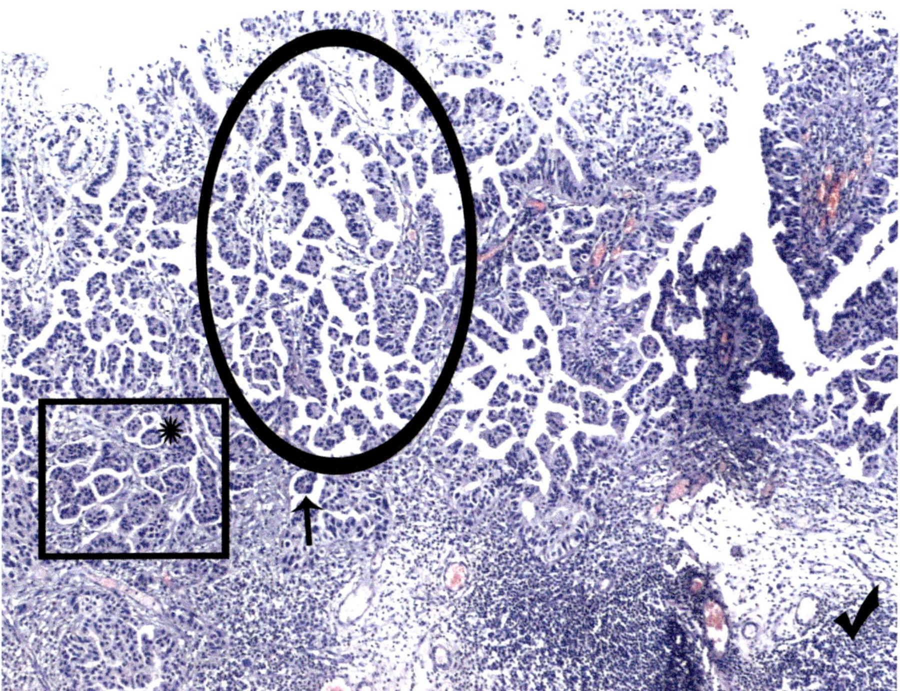

Fig. 2.103 (H-E, ×50) Micropapillary variant of bladder urothelial carcinoma. Delicate papillae, one to four cell layers thick, sometimes with thin stromal cores and numerous secondary micropapillae (hierarchical branching). Confluent retraction spaces (*square frame*) are characteristic and simulate lymphovascular invasion. In the invasive component and in all metastatic sites, the tumor cells are arranged in small tight nests or balls, aggregated in lacunae, which mimic vascular invasion. Edematous stroma with chronic inflammatory infiltrate (*tick*).

In the invasive portion, minute nests and fine papillae often lacking true fibrovascular cores, with surrounding lacunae (*ellipse*)/retraction spaces (*arrow*), are observed, resembling ovarian serous borderline tumor. Back-to-back lacunar spaces. Multiple small nests, without vascular cores, in the *same* single lacunar space (*ellipse*), are characteristic. Numerous mitoses. Nuclear grade is typically high in deeper portions but may have lower grade appearance at surface. Rather bland cytology at surface and possible peripheral orientation of the nuclei can be encountered. Clusters of cells with peripherally oriented nuclei may create a rosette-like pattern (*asterisk*). Psammoma bodies, a feature of ovarian papillary serous neoplasia, are exquisitely rare in micropapillary carcinoma of the urinary bladder. Mucins tend to be absent. Many of the spaces surrounding the clusters are artifacts – no lining endothelial cells are demonstrable by immunohistochemistry – but true lymphovascular invasion is common. Most micropapillary carcinomas are muscle invasive with vascular invasion. CD31, CD34, and podoplanin may help to distinguish true lymphatic invasion from retraction artifact.

Micropapillary urothelial carcinoma is often mixed with urothelial carcinoma in primary, but metastases usually have only micropapillary pattern.

Immunohistochemically, MUC 1 is limited to basal surface of cells, compared to apical, intracytoplasmic, or intracellular staining in conventional urothelial papillary carcinomas.

The micropapillary variant grows by invasion and dissemination. Any amount of micropapillary carcinoma, even <10%, is significant and should be reported since it represents a more aggressive clone of neoplastic cells.

In a bladder tumor, pure micropapillary histology (without a conventional urothelial carcinoma component) may raise concern for a primary or metastatic adenocarcinoma, the latter probably deriving from the ovary, lung, or breast, and for a mesothelioma. Immunohistochemistry provides substantial diagnostic aid in such cases

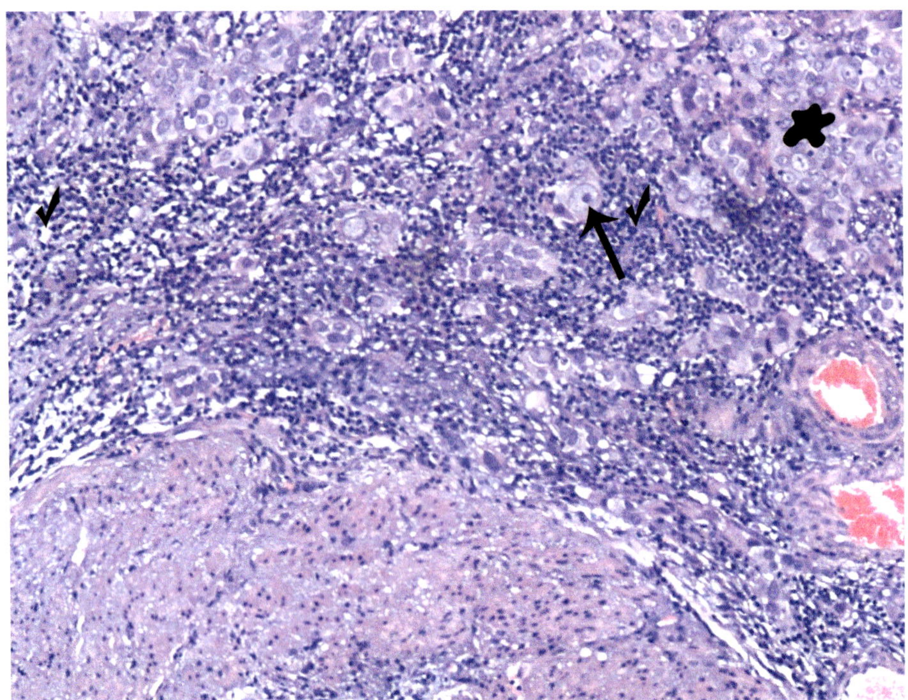

Fig. 2.104 (H-E, ×100) Lymphoepithelioma-like carcinoma. Undifferentiated tumor cells with indistinct, poorly defined cytoplasmic borders, in syncytial sheets (*blob*), nests, or cords, often with minimal cytoplasm, large pleomorphic nuclei with prominent nucleoli (*arrow*), numerous mitoses, and the background consisting of a prominent lymphoid infiltrate (*ticks*). This rare bladder tumor is usually muscle invasive; it may have a markedly pleomorphic epithelial component and resembles undifferentiated nasopharyngeal carcinoma (lymphoepithelioma) but is EBV-negative.

When lymphoepithelioma-like carcinomas occur in a *pure* form, they are more responsive to systemic chemotherapy than typical urothelial carcinoma, providing the potential to salvage bladder function. The lymphoepithelioma-like component should be >50% for the diagnosis of lymphoepithelioma-like carcinoma; however, the often coexisting urothelial carcinoma and urothelial carcinoma in situ make the outcome similar to that of conventional urothelial carcinoma. The percentage of lymphoepithelioma-like areas is important for treatment and should thus be accurately estimated and reported.

With regard to the differential diagnosis of lymphoepithelioma-like carcinoma, large cell undifferentiated carcinoma is distinguished by its distinct cell borders and *no* prominent lymphocytic component. Large cell undifferentiated carcinoma exhibits sheets of large polygonal or round cells with moderate to abundant cytoplasm and distinct cell borders; usually, >90% of the tumor is composed of the large cell component. The tumor is either infiltrative or has solid expansile nests with variable dyscohesive growth.

The syncytial arrangement and typical cytology are essential for the discrimination of a lymphoepithelioma-like carcinoma from a high-grade urothelial or squamous cell carcinoma with a brisk inflammatory infiltrate.

As far as the discrimination of melanoma is concerned, epithelioid neoplastic cells with prominent nucleoli are again observed, but spindle cells may also be encountered, and there is positivity for melanocytic immunohistochemical markers

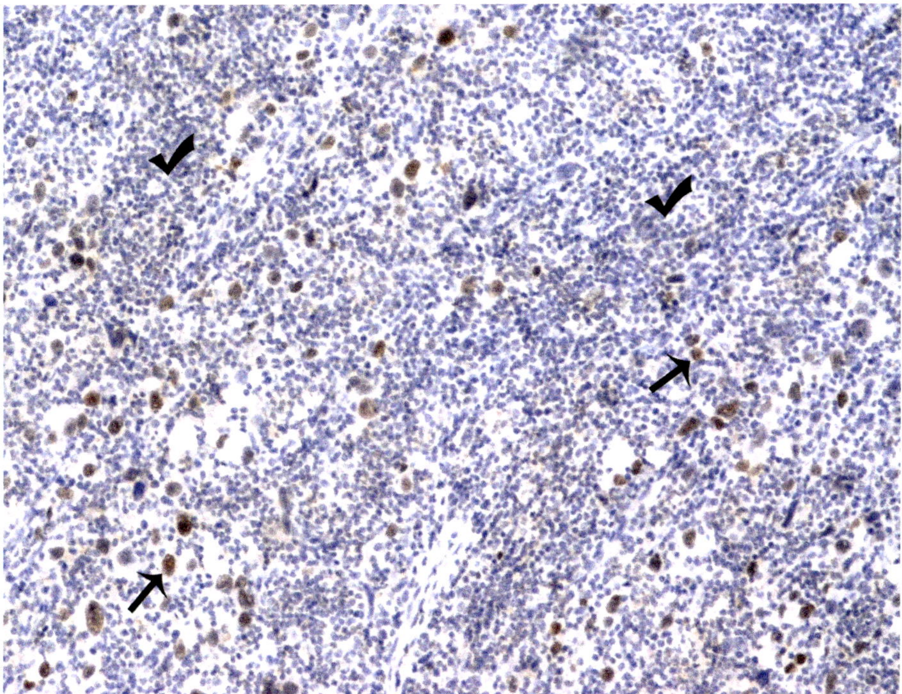

Fig. 2.105 (p63 immunohistochemistry, ×50) Lymphoepithelioma-like carcinoma. The sine qua non for the diagnosis of this histologic pattern of urothelial carcinoma is the presence of a prominent lymphoid infiltrate (*ticks*). Chronic inflammation may frequently obscure tumor cells. Nonneoplastic cells are a mixture of polyclonal B and T lymphocytes, histiocytes, eosinophils, and plasma cells. The differential diagnosis of lymphoepithelioma-like carcinoma includes lymphoma and, in limited and crushed biopsies, marked chronic cystitis. p63 highlights the urothelial tumor cells (*arrows*); GATA3 is an alternative immunomarker

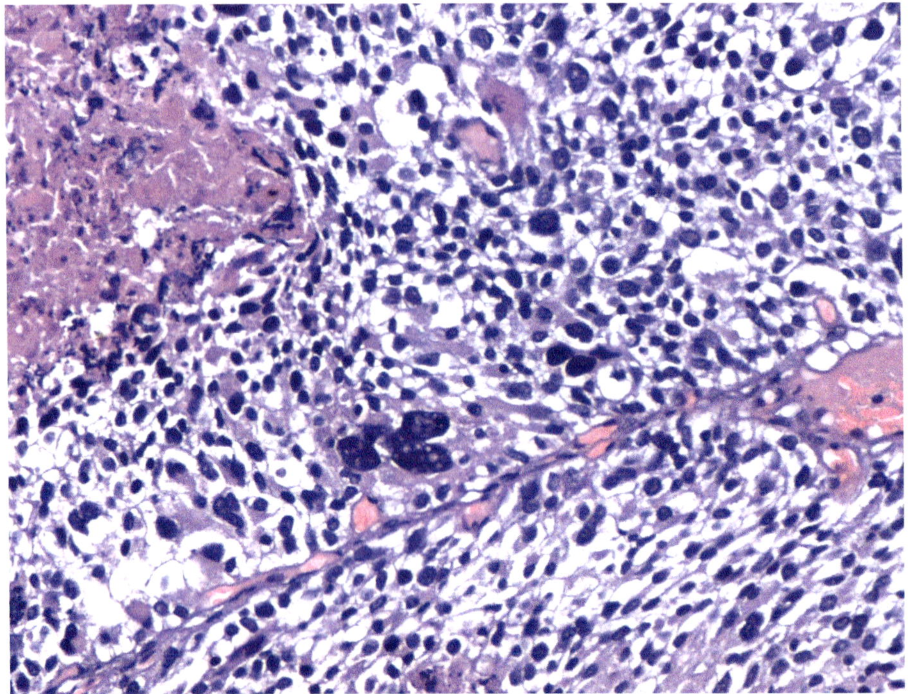

Fig. 2.106 (H-E, ×200) In a small percentage of high-grade invasive urothelial carcinomas, there are prominent markedly pleomorphic, highly bizarre giant tumor cells scattered throughout (image center), sometimes resembling cells of giant cell carcinoma of other sites (e.g., large cell undifferentiated carcinoma of the lung). Anaplasia is not graded separately but may be noted in the report. These giant cells should be distinguished from those that exhibit trophoblastic differentiation or those with osteoclast-like features (see Figs. 2.106 and 2.107).

Cells with bizarre nuclei are relatively common in high-grade urothelial carcinomas. Only a few cells react with antibodies to human chorionic gonadotropin (HCG); the positive reaction may be seen in giant cells as well as smaller mononucleated cells. When in an invasive urothelial carcinoma, giant cells, and occasionally other cells are HCG+, trophoblastic differentiation is documented. Morphologic context is critical to rule out choriocarcinomatous differentiation. The group of urothelial carcinomas with trophoblastic differentiation is divided into three categories (the first two being similar to testicular germ cell tumors): (a) urothelial carcinoma with scattered syncytiotrophoblasts, (b) urothelial carcinoma with choriocarcinomatous differentiation or pure choriocarcinoma, and (c) urothelial carcinoma with immunohistochemical expression of HCG, but no recognizable trophoblasts, probably a metaplastic phenomenon

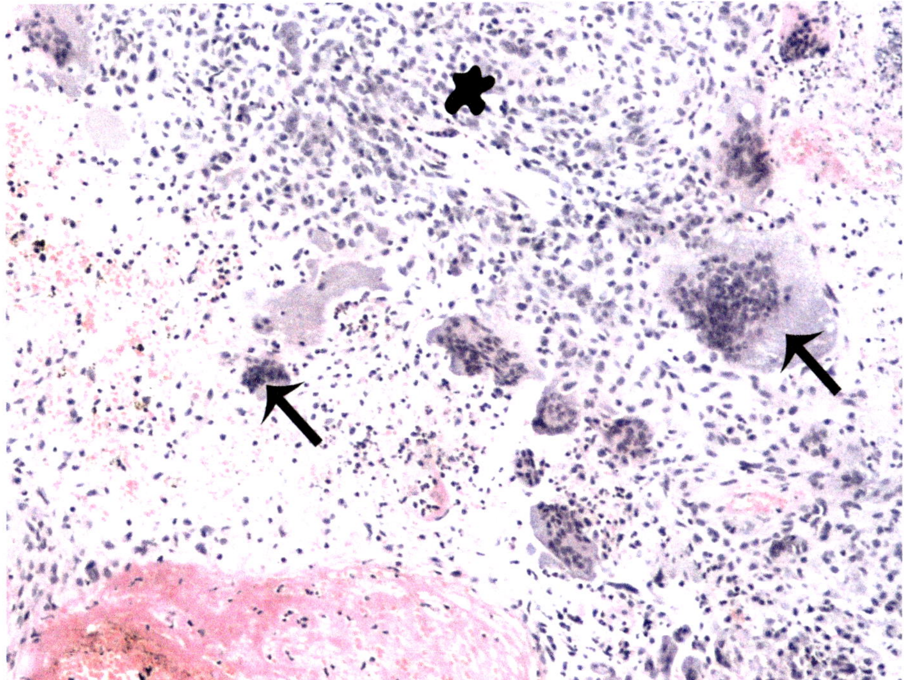

Fig. 2.107 (H-E, ×100) Undifferentiated urothelial carcinoma with many osteoclast-like giant cells in its stroma (osteoclast-rich undifferentiated carcinoma of the bladder).

Giant cells resembling osteoclasts are occasionally present in the stroma of conventional high-grade bladder carcinoma as well as in the stroma of the osteoclast-rich undifferentiated carcinoma variant. These giant cells (*arrows*) are histiocytic in origin (CD68-, CD51-, and CD54-positive) and have no prognostic significance; in the above rare variant, background spindled and *mononuclear* cells (*blob*) are pancytokeratin, EMA, CAM 5.2, and CK7-positive, confirming an epithelial lineage of the latter. Simultaneous, usual urothelial neoplasia may be recognized in varying proportions with matched p53 positivity in *mononuclear* cells and conventional urothelial tumor cells

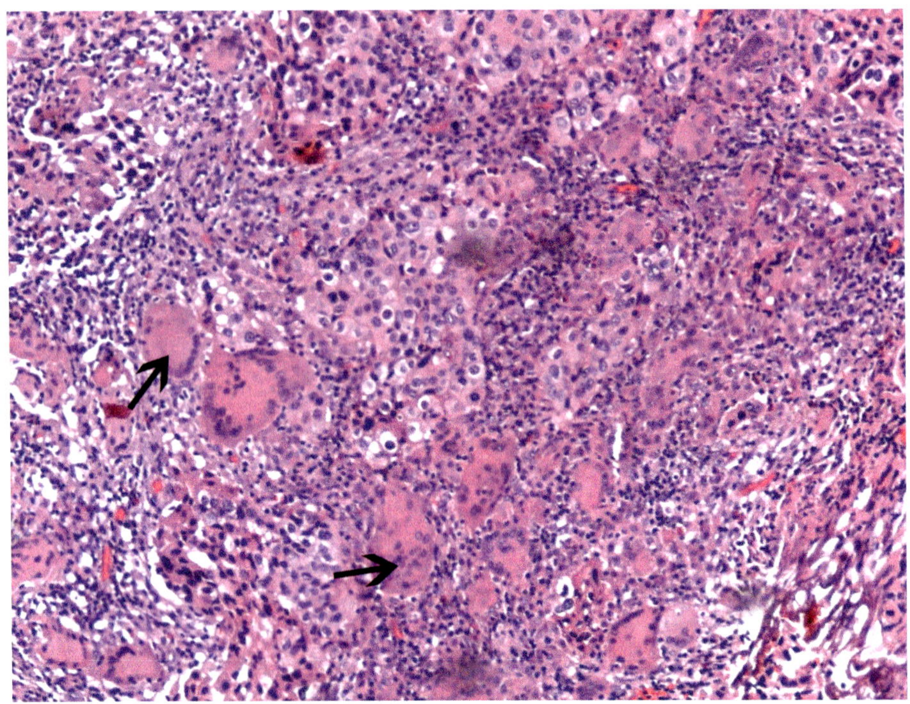

Fig. 2.108 (H-E, ×100) Osteoclast-like giant cells (*arrows*) can be detected in the stroma of a conventional invasive high-grade urothelial carcinoma.

In contrast, undifferentiated urothelial carcinoma with many osteoclast-like giant cells in its stroma (osteoclast-rich undifferentiated carcinoma) is an extremely rare variant of high-grade urothelial carcinoma with an aggressive behavior and poor outcome. It is composed of a mixture of undifferentiated *mononuclear* carcinoma cells and osteoclast-like reactive giant cells. Mononuclear cells have abundant cytoplasm, round to oval vesicular nuclei, possibly mild atypia, and variable mitotic activity (see Fig. 2.107). The giant cells are morphologically and immunohistochemically identical to osteoclasts and are regarded as being of histiocytic origin; they are cytologically bland and may exhibit phagocytic activity but no mitotic activity; they are generally evenly distributed among mononuclear cells but may condense around hemorrhagic foci.

These tumors should be differentiated (a) from giant and spindle cell carcinoma in which there is mitotic activity in both the large, multinucleated, obvious malignant bizarre giant cells as well as in the smaller spindle cells, and the whole tumor population contains epithelial markers, (b) from the non-epithelial giant cell tumor of mesenchymal derivation, and (c) from a foreign-body type giant cell reaction which is characterized by an inflammatory infiltrate, no atypia, and no invasion

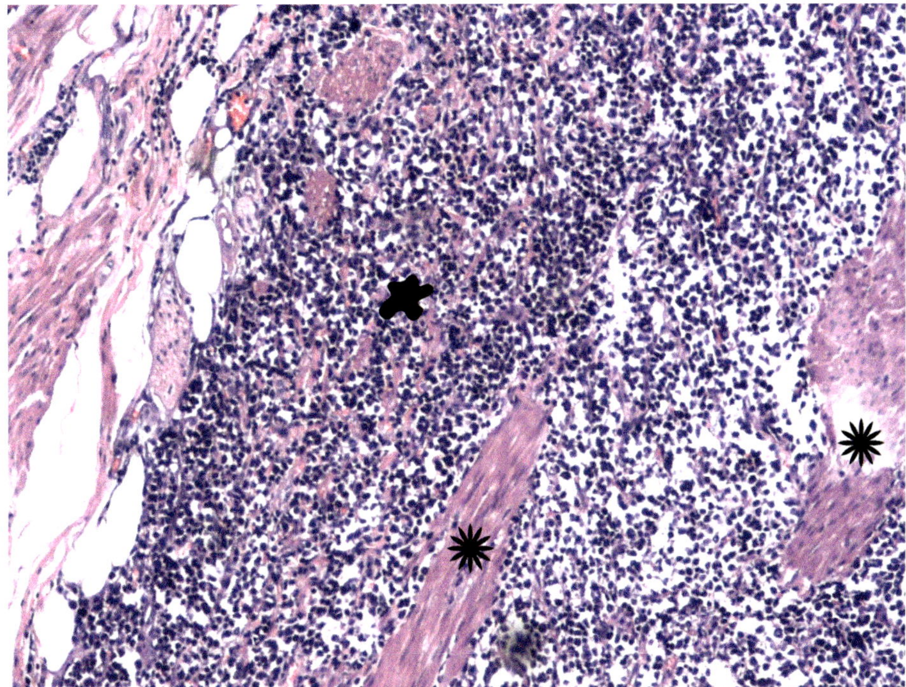

Fig. 2.109 (H-E, ×100) The best characterized poorly differentiated carcinoma of the urinary bladder is histologically similar to small cell carcinoma of the lung and may be mistaken for lymphoma, poorly differentiated urothelial carcinoma with scant cytoplasm (see Fig. 2.86) and even inflammation in a crushed, cauterized, superficial, or scant specimen.

This highly aggressive, small cell carcinoma is a malignant neuroendocrine neoplasm derived from the urothelium that mimics its pulmonary counterpart; it is of interest that TTF-1 may be positive in almost 40% of the small cell carcinomas of the bladder. Immunohistochemically, many of these tumors have neuroendocrine features. All small cell neuroendocrine carcinomas are invasive (*asterisks*) at presentation. In almost half of small cell carcinomas, an admixed coexisting epithelial component of urothelial carcinoma including CIS is found, supporting a bladder primary. Even a focal small cell component within a conventional urothelial carcinoma should be reported, and tumors with any appreciable small cell component could be classified as small cell carcinoma.

Loosely cohesive sheets of small- to intermediate-sized cells with scant cytoplasm (*blob*), inconspicuous nucleoli, and evenly dispersed, finely stippled chromatin. Hyperchromatic nuclei. Sheets of small cells are separated by scant stroma (*blob*). Well-formed epithelial structures are absent. A "patternless" pattern of diffuse growth predominates; focal nesting may be present. Nuclear molding (but perhaps no nuclear overlapping) and punctate or geographical necrosis are common. Mitotic figures and vascular invasion are readily evident.

Simultaneous synaptophysin, CD56 and CK7 and CAM5.2 positivity, the latter frequently with a cytoplasmic dot-like positivity, is of help; however, neuroendocrine stains are considered of questionable value by many since this is a diagnosis which can be made on morphologic grounds alone. On the other hand, it is also accepted that many such poorly differentiated carcinomas do not react with cytokeratin cocktails.

An important reason for the accurate recognition of a small cell carcinoma component is that it is recognized as a systemic disease and apparently has response to newer chemotherapy protocols. The recognition of an undifferentiated carcinoma as small cell carcinoma is important because it requires a *different* chemotherapeutic regimen.

The differential diagnosis includes metastasis of a small cell carcinoma from another site (very uncommon), malignant lymphoma, and poorly differentiated urothelial carcinoma.

The range of neuroendocrine tumors in the bladder also includes carcinoid tumor, large cell neuroendocrine carcinoma (with a more discernable architecture and prominent nucleoli), and mixed patterns

2.5.3.1 Clinical Commentary

Vasileios Spapis

This is a case of a high-grade, detrusor muscle-invasive urothelial carcinoma (stage pT2 on transurethral resection specimen). Cystectomy with lymph node dissection was performed, and the carcinoma was finally staged as pT3aN0. Areas of very poorly differentiated cancer cells of plasmacytoid, often dyscohesive appearance, as well as others of micropapillary morphology, particularly in areas of detrusor muscle invasion, were noticed.

Apart from this case, some other specific variants of aggressive invasive urothelial carcinoma, which often coexist as components of a conventional invasive urothelial carcinoma, are highlighted.

About 75% of patients with bladder cancer (BC) present with a disease confined to the mucosa or submucosa (stages Ta-T1-CIS). In younger patients (< 40 years), this percentage is even higher (Hansel et al. 2013). Patients at early stages have a significantly lower risk of cancer-specific mortality compared to patients with T2–4 tumors (Burger et al. 2013). Tobacco smoking, occupational exposure to chemicals (aromatic amines), radiotherapy, and chronic urinary tract infection are the most common etiologic factors for BC. Another interesting fact is that although men are more likely to develop BC, women present with more advanced disease and have worse survival rates, possibly because women experience longer delays in diagnosis than men, as the differential diagnosis in women includes diseases more prevalent than BC (Hansel et al. 2013).

After initial TURBT (transurethral resection of bladder tumor) where muscle infiltration is detected, careful staging must be performed, providing information regarding extent of local tumor invasion, tumor spread to lymph nodes (LNs), and tumor spread to the upper urinary tract (UUT) and other distant organs (e.g., liver, lungs, bones, peritoneum, pleura, and adrenal glands). The TNM classification is recommended (Brierley et al. 2017). Blood vessel, lymphatic vessel invasion (LVI), and lymph node (LN) infiltration have an independent prognostic significance (Hansel et al. 2013). Both CT and MRI can be used in clinical practice for assessment of local invasion, but they are not able to safely detect microscopic invasion of perivesical fat (T2 vs. T3a) (Hansel et al. 2013). The purpose of using CT and MRI is therefore to detect T3b disease or higher. LN metastasis cannot be assessed by either MRI or CT scan for normal-sized lymph nodes. Bone and brain metastases are rare at the time of presentation of invasive BC, and therefore, additional imaging (bone scanning, brain CT) is not routinely recommended. However, abdominal and chest CT should be performed (Witjes et al. 2017a, b).

Radical cystectomy (RC) is currently the gold standard for localized MIBC (muscle-invasive bladder cancer) (Hansel et al. 2013) and should be performed within 3 months from initial diagnosis. Patient's performance status (PS), age, and quality of life (QoL) may influence that decision, though. Bladder-preserving treatment especially for the elderly could be offered. However, most patients with MIBC T2-T4a, N0-Nx, and M0 disease will undergo RC (Hansel et al. 2013). Lymphadenectomy is an integral part of RC, and removal of at least ten LNs is recommended as sufficient for evaluation of LN status, as well as being beneficial for overall survival (Wright et al. 2008). The type of urinary diversion is an important topic that should be discussed with the patient taking into consideration his comorbidities, life expectancy, tumor stage, and location. Adjuvant chemotherapy after RC for patients with pT3/4 and/or LN positive (N+) disease without clinically detectable metastases (M0) is still under debate and is still infrequently used (Hansel et al. 2013).

Key Points

- In invasive urothelial carcinoma, it is important to state depth of invasion by clearly reporting invasion of lamina propria or muscularis propria. In contrast to superficially invasive tumors (pT1/lamina propria), deeply invasive tumors (pT2 or greater/muscularis propria and beyond) have poor prognosis. Invasion of muscularis propria often constitutes the crossroads between conservative and aggressive management.
- Pathologic staging in TURBT specimens is limited to whether the tumor is Ta, T1, or T2. The distinction between T2a (inner half/superficial detrusor muscle invasion), T2b (outer half/deep detrusor muscle invasion), and pT3 (perivesical tissue invasion) cancer is, hence, performed only in cystectomy specimens.
- Invasion of the muscular wall (detrusor, muscularis propria) is best appreciated when nests of tumor cells insinuate between thick distinct rounded muscle fascicles. Care should be exercised not to misinterpret the inconsistent but sometimes prominent fascicles of muscularis mucosae (particularly common in women) as belonging to the muscularis propria.
- The mature adipose tissue commonly present in the lamina propria or muscularis propria should not be misinterpreted as perivesical soft tissue in order that a tumor adjacent to fat in a biopsy specimen is not badly overstaged.
- Urothelial neoplasia has a pronounced ability for divergent differentiation. Variants of invasive urothelial carcinoma have poor prognosis and, as a rule, occur as part of a high-grade, high-stage carcinoma. Variant histology must be documented, including percentage, if not pure in histology.
- Urothelial tumors with foci of malignant squamous or glandular differentiation are essentially always high-grade lesions whose clinical course, stage for stage, is not different from that of a high-grade urothelial carcinoma.

2.6 Case 2.5: Spindle Cell Neoplasm of the Bladder

Advisory Opinion from Dr. med. George Agrogiannis

Case Study

Data Prior to Microscopy

Male smoker, 72 years old, with a history of prostate acinar adenocarcinoma treated by radiation, presents with recurrent urinary tract infections and bladder outlet obstruction.

Cystoscopically, a large intraluminal mass of 11 cm in diameter, with a polypoid surface, cavitation, and a well-recognizable base with infiltrating margins, was detected. There is nodal metastatic disease at the initial presentation.

2.6.1 Microscopic Evaluation of the TURBT Specimens

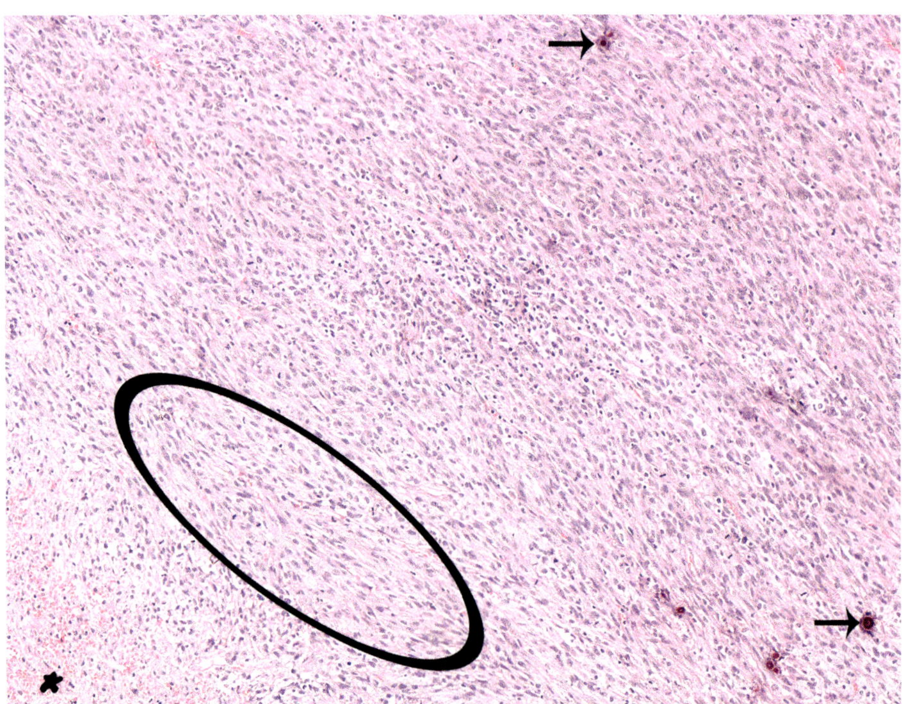

Fig. 2.110 (H-E, ×40) In most areas, the tumor shows sarcomatoid morphology, being composed by predominantly spindle or ovoid cells, arranged in long fascicles (*ellipse*). Extravasated erythrocytes (*blob*) and isolated calcifications are present (*arrows*)

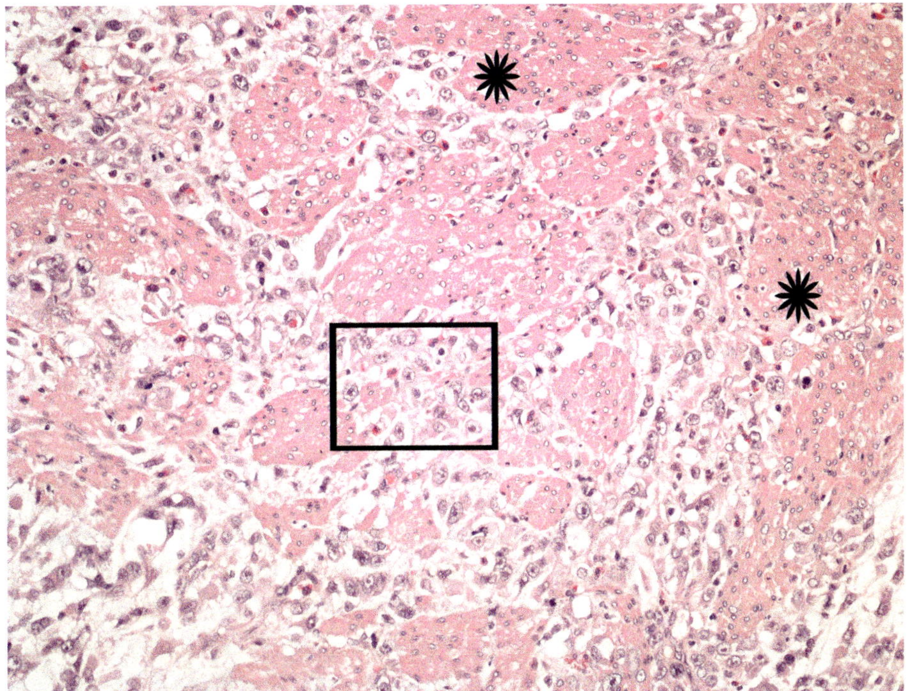

Fig. 2.111 (H-E, ×200) Foci with a more epithelioid morphology of tumor cells (*square frame*) are detected and thus prompt careful consideration of a carcinoma, on morphological grounds. This epithelioid component may indeed represent a high-grade carcinoma which diffusely infiltrates the muscularis propria (*asterisk*, stage at least pT2 in the TURBT specimen), but the urothelial nature of these cells is morphologically uncertain.

In any case, such a lesion warrants appropriate immunohistochemical evaluation of both cell types [i.e., spindle (sarcomatoid) and epithelioid].

Sarcomatoid carcinoma is a tumor showing both a malignant spindle cell component *and* a malignant epithelial component, although the latter may only be identifiable immunohistochemically

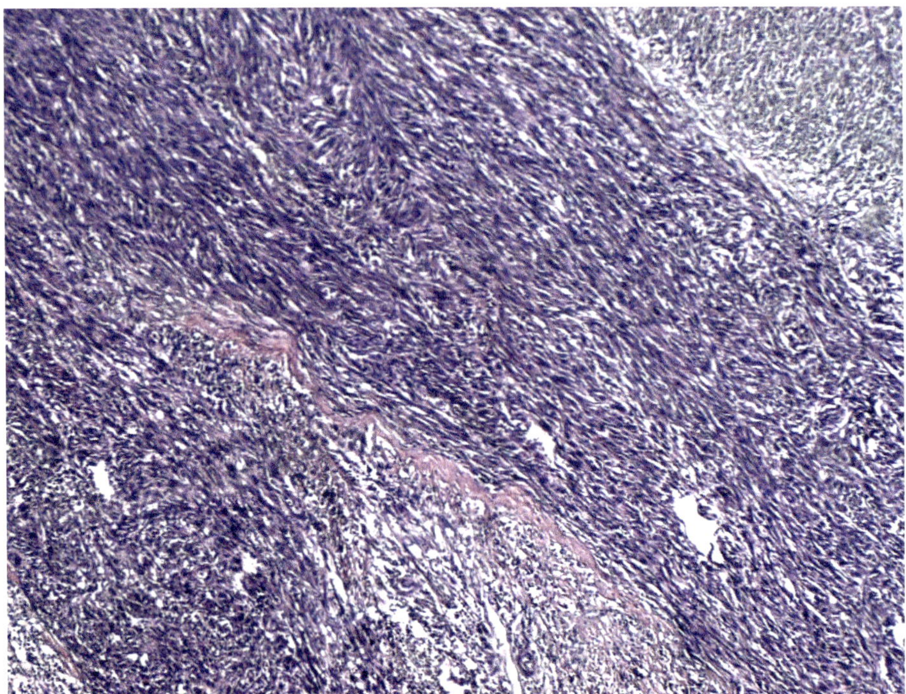

Fig. 2.112 (H-E, ×100). Sarcomatoid carcinoma of the bladder. The sarcomatoid component of a sarcomatoid urothelial carcinoma usually exhibits features of an undifferentiated high-grade spindle cell sarcoma. This area of sarcoma-like appearance necessitates differential diagnosis between sarcomatoid carcinoma and leiomyosarcoma of the bladder.

Intersecting fascicular growth and increased cellularity, as seen above, are indeed features of leiomyosarcoma. True sarcomas are distinctly uncommon in the bladder. The most common sarcoma in the bladder in adults is leiomyosarcoma which is a highly cellular tumor with common necrosis and possible pseudoepitheliomatous hyperplasia. Interestingly, up to 23% of primary leiomyosarcomas of the urinary bladder are reported to express p63; *focal* aberrant weak cytokeratin (CK) of low molecular weight (LMW), pancytokeratin AE1/AE3, and EMA staining can also be observed. Strong *h-caldesmon* positivity confirms the diagnosis of *leiomyosarcoma*. Of course, in all primary sarcomas of the bladder, there is no carcinomatous component (see Fig. 2.115) or recent history of urothelial carcinoma.

The mesenchymal component of sarcomatoid urothelial carcinomas usually has high-grade sarcoma-like, spindle cell morphology. When a carcinomatous component is not present, immunohistochemical reactions for cytokeratins may be essential in arriving at the appropriate diagnosis of sarcomatoid carcinoma of the bladder. Evidence of the epithelial nature of these proliferations is provided by the immunoreactivity for keratin, which can often, but not always, be detected in the sarcoma-like component. Immunohistochemical expression of pancytokeratin, high molecular weight (HMW) CK (34βE12, CK5/6) and p63 is often detected in both the epithelial and spindled component of the sarcomatoid variant of urothelial carcinoma. Smooth muscle actin may be only variably positive, at best

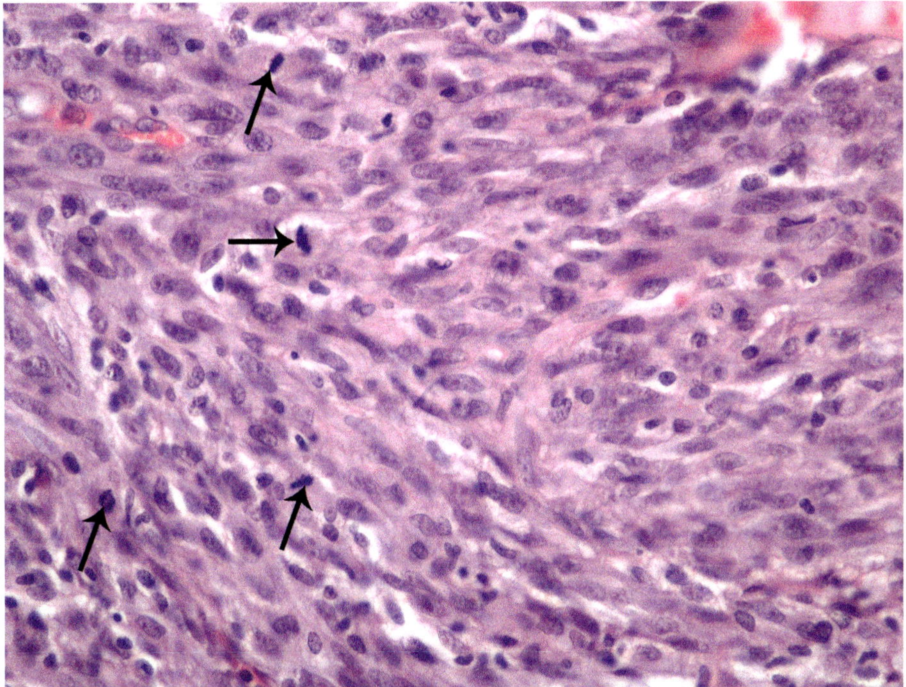

Fig. 2.113 (H-E, ×200) Sarcomatoid carcinoma of the bladder. Mitotic rate is high (*arrows*).

The sarcomatoid component may occasionally have a relatively bland cytology. These cells show myofibroblastic morphology, being ovoid or spindle shaped, with occasional nucleoli. The degree of nuclear chromatin irregularity can be diagnostic of epithelial malignancy; cytology can be the most useful feature in the distinction of a myofibroblastic proliferation from a sarcomatoid carcinoma. The definite cytologic atypia at least focally present in epithelial malignant lesions and the concurrent presence of neoplastic epithelial elements elsewhere (see Fig. 2.115) should exclude nonneoplastic lesions such as inflammatory myofibroblastic tumor/pseudosarcomatous myofibroblastic proliferations. Nevertheless, pure spindled sarcomatoid carcinomas may be deceptively bland with only subtle nuclear chromatin changes; evaluation of the *entire* tumor should, however, reveal areas with more pronounced atypia, beyond that seen in myofibroblastic lesions. Anaplastic lymphoma kinase-1 (Alk-1), a marker expressed in a varying proportion of inflammatory myofibroblastic tumors, is negative in sarcomatoid urothelial carcinoma

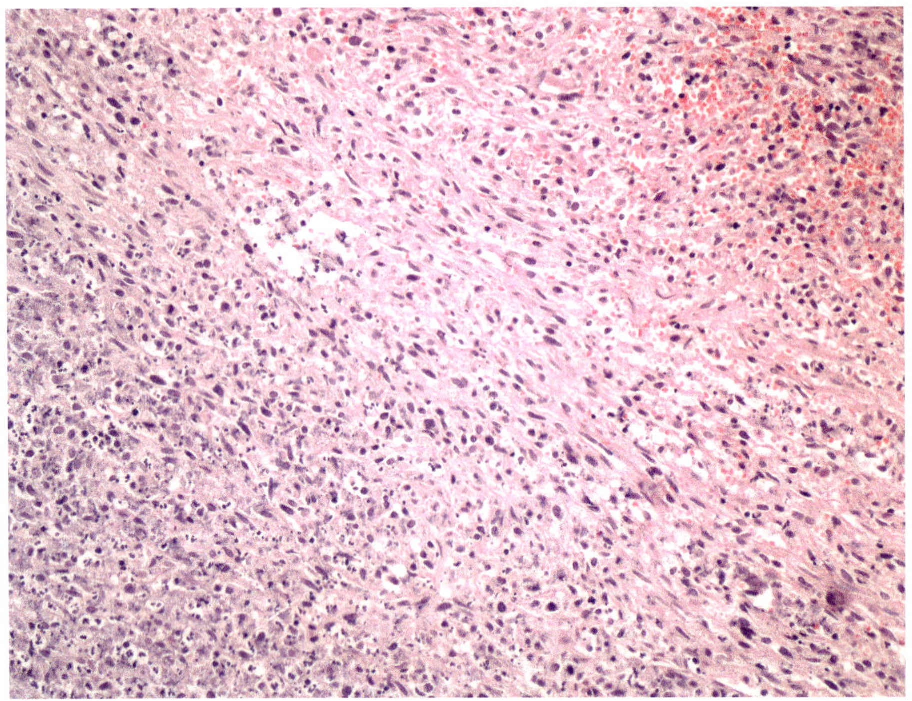

Fig. 2.114 (H-E, ×200) Sarcomatoid carcinoma of the bladder.

Extensive intratumoral necrotic areas are present (lower left side), an additional finding necessitating the exclusion of a high-grade sarcoma. A large hemorrhagic focus is also seen at the upper right side.

In the absence of an obvious invasive urothelial carcinoma or other epithelial (i.e., homologous) differentiation, the history of prior urothelial carcinoma, the coexistence of urothelial CIS, or *strong* cytokeratin immunoreactivity is helpful in making the diagnosis of sarcomatoid carcinoma over a primary sarcoma. The epithelial elements of a sarcomatoid urothelial carcinoma are consistently positive for cytokeratin, but we should have in mind that the reactivity in the malignant spindle cell component of the sarcomatoid urothelial carcinoma varies. The spindle cell component is consistently positive only for vimentin

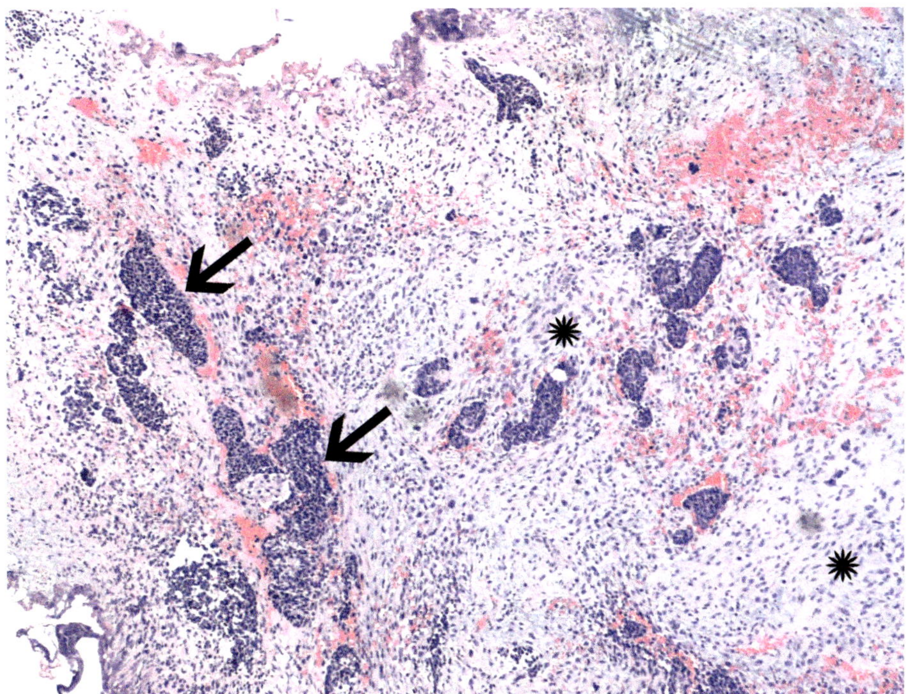

Fig. 2.115 (H-E, ×50) Sarcomatoid carcinoma of the bladder. The presence of a malignant epithelial component (homologous) differentiation, here easily identifiable as urothelial carcinoma (*arrows*), rules out the diagnosis of a primary sarcoma. Multiple tissue sections may be necessary to uncover the islands of epithelial differentiation or foci of CIS that are diagnostic of sarcomatoid carcinoma of the bladder, since sarcomatoid areas usually predominate.

Spindle cells (*asterisks*) surround isolated islands and nests of malignant epithelial cells; the latter allow the distinction from sarcoma. The homologous type of the sarcomatoid variant is best recognized by the identification of malignant epithelial islands within the spindle cells, as above, or CIS in the overlying mucosa. A previous history of urothelial carcinoma may also be helpful. In addition, immunohistochemistry *may* identify cytokeratins diffusely expressed among the spindle cells and thus provide significant diagnostic aid. The islands of epithelial differentiation expectedly react for pancytokeratin, whereas the predominant spindle cell elements may not. On the other hand, as mentioned before, *focal* positivity for cytokeratins, especially low molecular weight ones, can occur in true sarcomas.

Apart from sarcomas, sarcomatoid carcinoma should be distinguished from urothelial carcinoma associated with an unusual, degenerative yet atypical appearing, stromal reaction. Urothelial carcinomas may have a pseudosarcomatous stromal response with mesenchymal cells of degenerative atypia in primary or metastatic sites. This stromal response rarely displays sufficient cellularity and cytologic atypia in the spindle cell proliferation or a myxoid appearance to raise serious concern about sarcomatoid carcinoma; this unusual stroma lacks mitotic activity or an expansile growth, and there is a lack of morphologic transition between the spindle cells and the carcinoma cells. This reactive stroma is negative or only focally positive for epithelial markers (e.g., cytokeratin), in contrast to sarcomatoid carcinoma of the bladder which commonly (but not always) expresses cytokeratins diffusely.

Invasive urothelial carcinomas may also be associated with a myofibroblastic proliferation in their stroma; generally bland morphology of myofibroblasts rules out sarcomatoid carcinoma

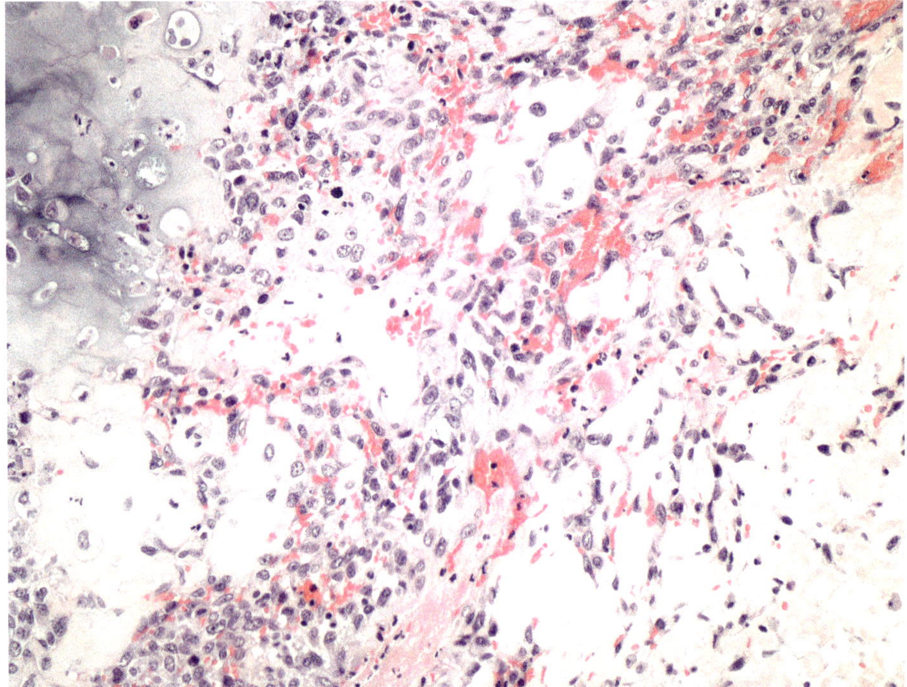

Fig. 2.116 (H-E, ×200) The mesenchymal-like component of a sarcomatoid urothelial carcinoma may sometimes show completely heterologous differentiation. In this field, there is deposition of amorphous eosinophilic and amphophilic material with features of osteoid and cartilaginous differentiation, respectively, at the left side. This is an example of osteosarcomatous differentiation. Notably, the osteoblasts are atypical, and some mitotic figures are also present, a key fact that excludes cartilaginous and osseous metaplasia (see Fig. 2.117). Osteosarcomas and chondrosarcomas are rare in the bladder and, when present, should prompt search for a carcinomatous component so that the diagnosis of sarcomatoid urothelial carcinoma is established. In exceptional cases, more than one type of sarcoma can be present (Lopez-Beltran et al. 1998); these are foci of malignant mesenchymal elements.

To sum up, this is a sarcomatoid urothelial carcinoma of the bladder. This high-grade biphasic tumor is composed of sarcomatoid (predominantly high-grade spindle cells), osteosarcomatous, and carcinomatous components. The presence of heterologous elements (i.e., osteosarcoma) should be mentioned in the diagnosis. Immunohistochemically, spindle cells *and* carcinomatous elements of this case expressed pancytokeratin, high molecular weight cytokeratin, EMA, *and* vimentin, while the osteosarcomatous component was expectedly immunonegative for all epithelial markers.

Sarcomatoid carcinoma is a high-grade neoplasm of the bladder in which a malignant epithelial component, clearly identifiable as such of urothelial, glandular, squamous, or undifferentiated type, coexists with areas having a sarcoma-like/sarcomatoid or truly sarcomatous appearance. The sarcoma-like/sarcomatoid component usually has a nonspecific, spindle cell or pleomorphic look, but a truly sarcomatous component exhibiting specific features of heterologous-specific mesenchymal differentiation, such as rhabdomyosarcoma, chondrosarcoma, osteosarcoma (see Fig. 2.116), liposarcoma, or malignant fibrous histiocytoma, can coexist and should be reported. Whether areas of specific mesenchymal differentiation occur or not, transitions may be seen between the two major components (epithelial and sarcomatoid), suggesting that the sarcomatoid areas are also epithelial in nature. The nonspecific sarcomatoid component of sarcomatoid urothelial carcinomas can be cytokeratin-negative but usually retains, at least focally, some cytokeratin expression. Similarly, the epithelial component can be vimentin-negative (20% of cases). Smooth muscle markers are typically negative except for areas with heterologous differentiation. Immunohistochemical results should be interpreted with caution and always in relation to morphologic characteristics

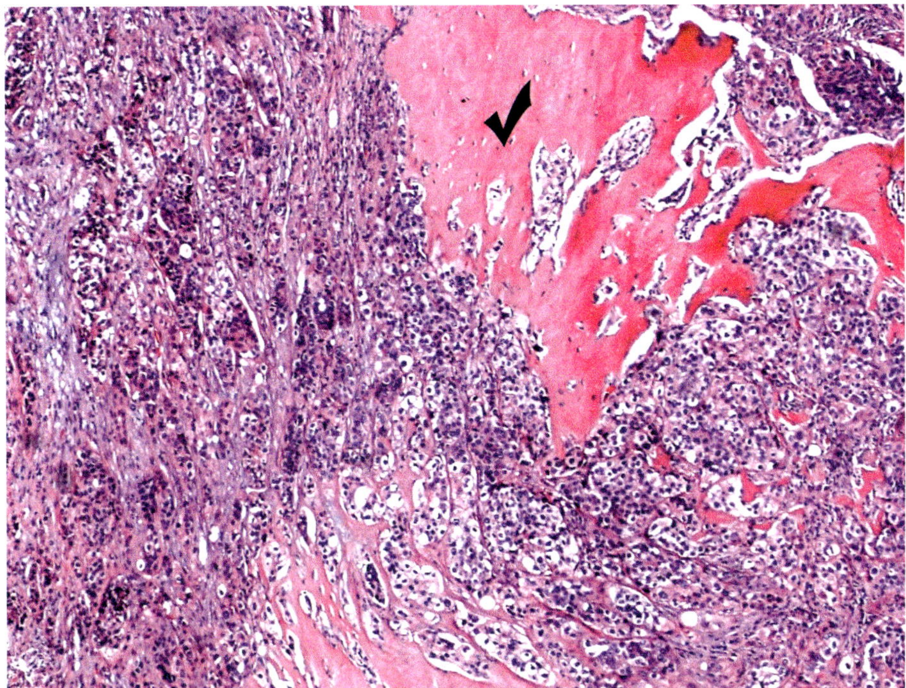

Fig. 2.117 (H-E, ×100) Not all heterologous elements are malignant. This image derives from another case; it is an invasive high-grade urothelial carcinoma with benign-appearing osseous metaplasia of its stroma (*tick*). The stroma of urothelial carcinomas or their metastases may rarely undergo osseous (or cartilaginous) metaplasia. This feature should not be mistaken for heterologous differentiation in a sarcomatoid carcinoma (see Fig. 2.116). Tumor-associated osseous (or chondroid) metaplasia is a stromal reaction in which metaplastic tissue is histologically benign.

It is a fact that urothelial carcinomas of high grade may manifest heterogeneous elements of *both* epithelial (e.g., squamous, glandular) and stromal origin. Such variations should be recognized by the pathologist to avoid interpretive errors, but they have no other known implications for patient care, and there is no compelling reason to include stroma subtype designations such as osseous metaplasia, in the final diagnosis, where their presence might confuse the unsophisticated.

The following images (Figs. 2.118, 2.119, 2.120, 2.121, and 2.122) come from another case with features of a myofibroblastic lesion partially compatible with an inflammatory myofibroblastic tumor. Potential malignancy of this case warrants close follow-up of the patient, analogous to that for patients with low-grade myofibroblastic sarcomas. The patient was a middle-aged woman who presented with gross hematuria and irritative symptoms

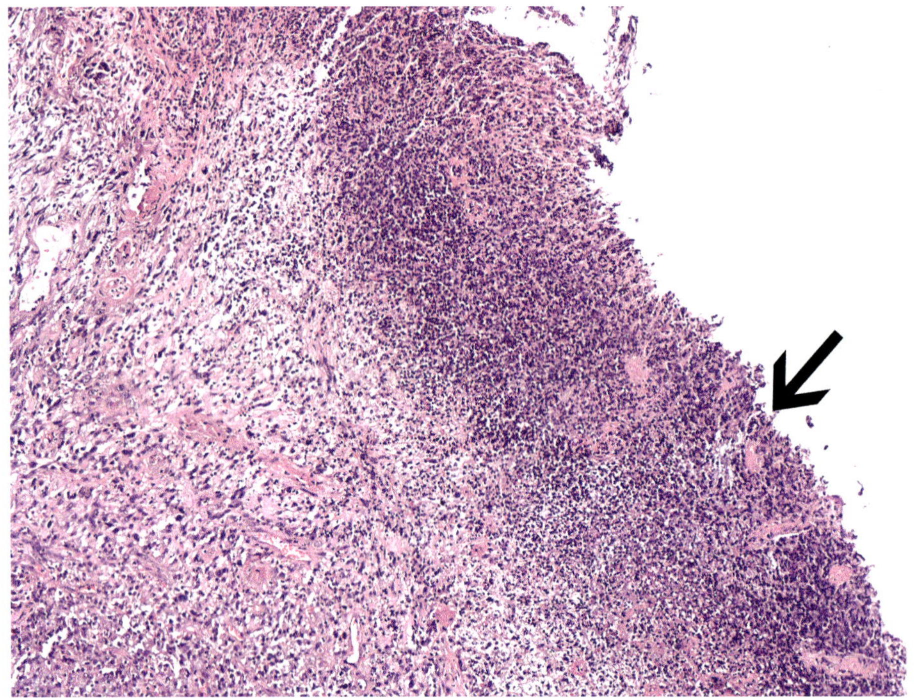

Fig. 2.118 (H-E, ×100) The tumor is infiltrating and is associated with surface ulceration. The tumor extensively ulcerates the surface bladder epithelium (*arrow*) which is almost totally replaced by a superficial acute inflammatory infiltrate and dense granular tissue.

Myofibroblastic proliferations often exhibit superficial hypocellularity with higher cellularity at deeper sites. Some degree of cytologic atypia is compatible with inflammatory myofibroblastic tumor. Inflammatory myofibroblastic tumor may be cellular and infiltrative with mucosal ulceration and *necrosis at the site of surface ulceration*. Myofibroblastic proliferations are generally characterized by distinct fascicular architecture, often loose. Involvement of muscularis propria does *not* denote malignancy. As a rule, the tumor-muscle interface is sharply demarcated, and any necrotic areas should be *superficial* in inflammatory myofibroblastic tumors. *Intra*tumoral necrosis may only rarely be seen in inflammatory myofibroblastic tumors. Deep necrosis, as may be seen in a sarcoma, is not encountered in inflammatory myofibroblastic tumors

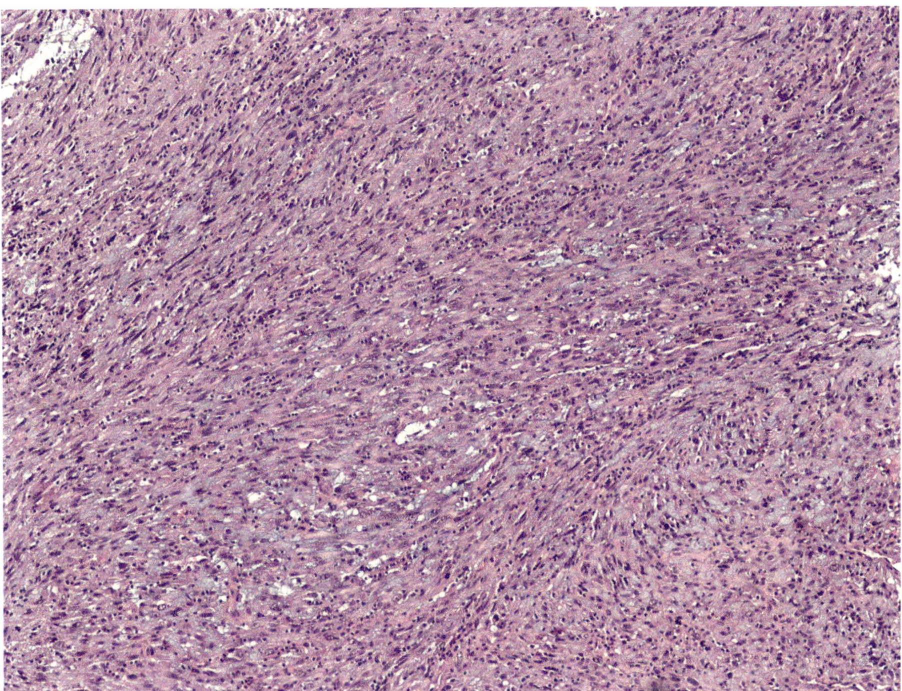

Fig. 2.119 (H-E, ×40) At low magnification, the tumor shows increased cellularity, with spindle cells arranged in a compact fascicular or storiform pattern (fibrous histiocytoma-like pattern). There is also accompanying interspersed inflammatory cell infiltrate.

This neoplasm is composed of spindle cells which are rather cohesive and show a moderate to *severe* degree of atypia in this field, a rather worrisome feature.

An area with more rounded cells of epithelioid appearance is observed elsewhere (see Fig. 2.121)

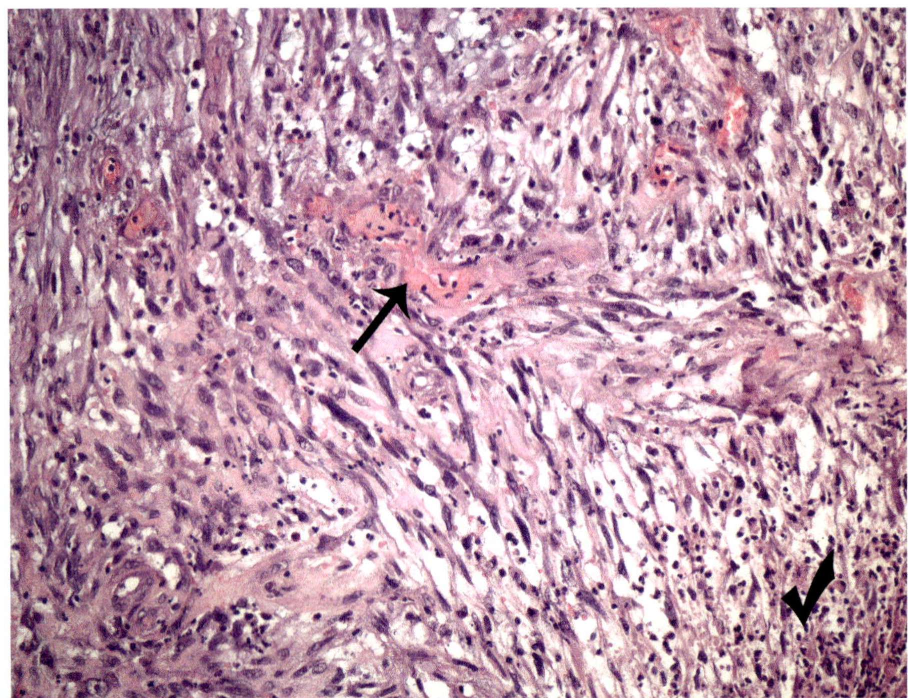

Fig. 2.120 (H-E, ×200) Myofibroblastic cells resemble tissue culture fibroblasts arranged in fascicles or more haphazardly. Typical myofibroblasts have elongated, tapered cytoplasmic processes, fine nuclear chromatin, and pinpoint nucleoli. Spindle cells may show *focal* pleomorphism in inflammatory myofibroblastic tumor. Scattered mitotic figures may be identified in the proliferating, mostly spindle-shaped cells; they may be frequent, but not atypical. There is also a fair number of chronic and occasionally acute inflammatory cells (*tick*) admixed with the neoplastic cells; the background usually contains a sparse inflammatory component. A prominent network of thin-walled blood vessels (*arrow*) in an edematous stroma with little to moderate collagen deposition is common in inflammatory myofibroblastic tumor

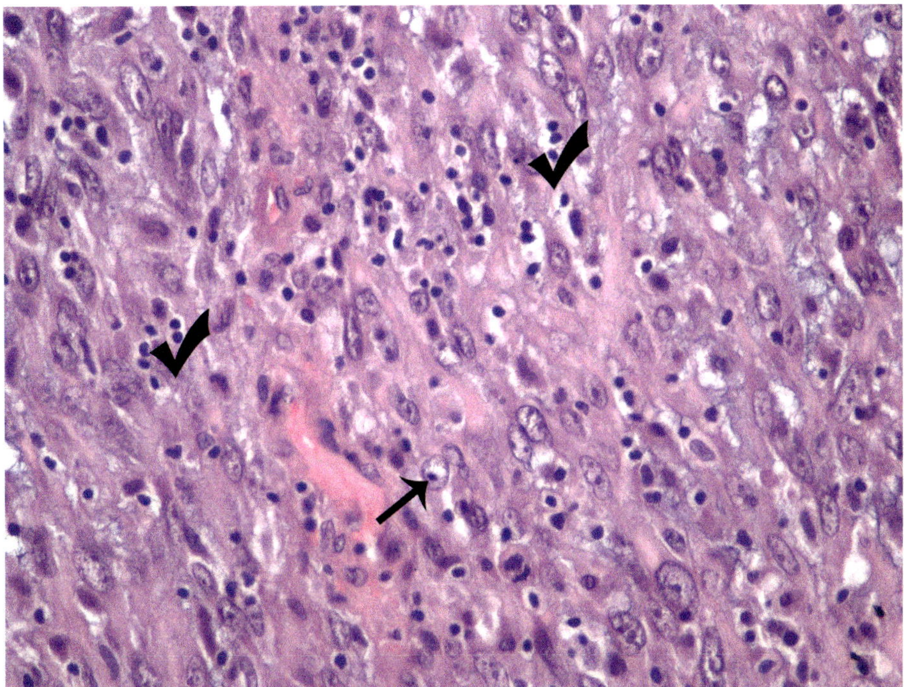

Fig. 2.121 (H-E, ×200) Focally, the neoplastic cells of this inflammatory myofibroblastic tumor show plumper morphology. In these areas the nuclei are vesicular, oval to round shaped, and enlarged, with prominent nucleoli (*arrow*). Scattered enlarged nuclei with macronucleoli can be encountered in myofibroblastic proliferations; however, the *chromatin* should be *fine* and *evenly dispersed*. Mononuclear inflammatory infiltrates are easily detected among the neoplastic population (*ticks*). Admixed inflammatory cells justify the synonymous terms "inflammatory myofibroblastic tumor/ inflammatory pseudotumor".

All the above morphological features are compatible with the diagnosis of an inflammatory myofibroblastic tumor (IMT). This is a locally aggressive mesenchymal neoplasm, practically never metastasizing. In contrast to sarcomatoid component of sarcomatoid urothelial carcinoma, in benign to borderline myofibroblastic proliferations such as inflammatory myofibroblastic tumor, chromatin should be fine and evenly dispersed, despite marked variation in nuclear size and scattered macronucleoli.

In the group of myofibroblastic proliferations, the postoperative spindle cell nodule is also included; relevant history is mandatory for this diagnosis

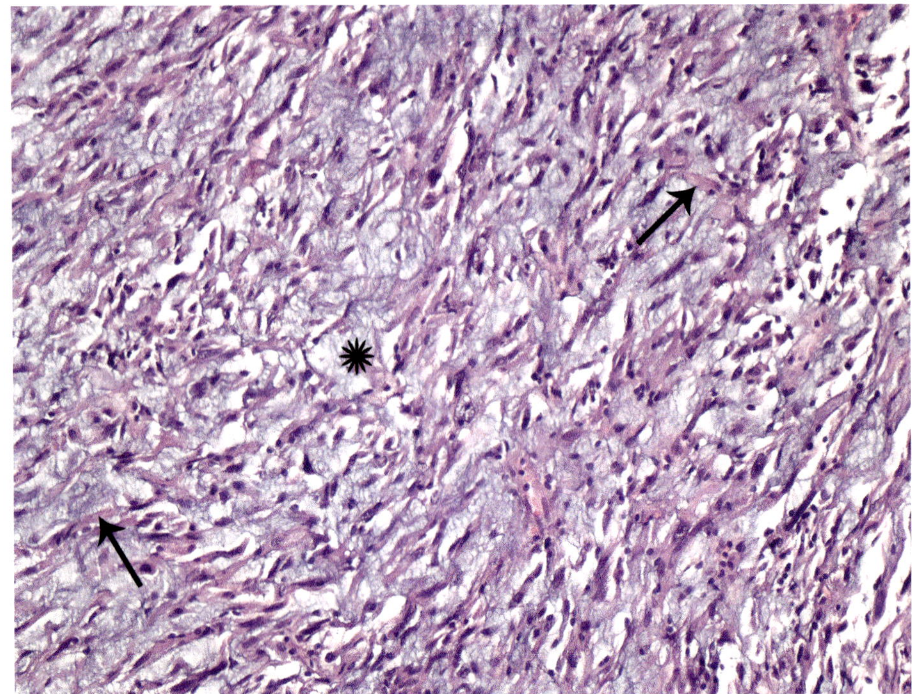

Fig. 2.122 (H-E, ×100) In inflammatory myofibroblastic tumor, individual myofibroblasts are commonly separated by myxoid stroma (*asterisk*). The stroma in some areas demonstrates prominent myxoid change with significantly lower cellularity suggesting a "tissue culture" appearance. Collagen bundles are also seen (*arrows*). Loose stellate cells, with myxoid background containing scattered inflammatory cells, can be noticed (nodular fasciitis-like pattern). These cells are stellate myofibroblasts with abundant eosinophilic cytoplasm and elongated nuclei.

A subset of sarcomatoid carcinomas have prominent myxoid stroma; the subtle degree of nuclear chromatin changes, as the above, favors a myofibroblastic lesion rather than the sarcomatoid component of a sarcomatoid carcinoma.

The myxoid variant of leiomyosarcoma should also be excluded. In such cases, immunohistochemistry may be of little help. Leiomyosarcomas exhibit smooth muscle morphology and strong h-caldesmon staining and, as a rule, are totally keratin-negative at least as far as HMW cytokeratins are concerned; a considerable number of leiomyosarcomas show some AE1/AE3 pancytokeratin expression, however. Necrosis at the tumor-smooth muscle interface (invading margin) and abnormal mitoses are the most reliable diagnostic features of a myxoid leiomyosarcoma that may lack significant nuclear pleomorphism. Doubtful cases are best considered low-grade neoplasms with a favorable outcome and treated accordingly.

Inflammatory myofibroblastic tumor is a rare myofibroblastic spindle cell neoplasm of the bladder with unknown neoplastic potential; actually, it is more common at other sites (the lung most common, followed by soft tissue, bone). It is similar to postoperative spindle cell nodule, but without a history of surgery, and it is characterized by spindle cell proliferation with characteristic fibro-inflammatory and pseudosarcomatous appearance. It may recur locally.

With regard to differential diagnosis between inflammatory myofibroblastic tumor and sarcomatoid urothelial carcinoma, the former lesion exhibits fine nuclear chromatin, smooth muscle actin (SMA) immunoreactivity, as well as ALK1 immunoreactivity; the latter varies widely, though. Cytokeratin expression in myofibroblastic cells is probably limited to LMW forms; as a rule, in contrast to sarcomatoid carcinoma, p63 and HMW cytokeratin are not expressed in inflammatory myofibroblastic

Fig. 2.122 (continued)

tumor. Sarcomatoid carcinomas lack both inflammatory background and network of thin-walled blood vessels. The present lesion was ALK1 immunonegative. Differentiating sarcomatoid carcinoma from inflammatory myofibroblastic tumor can be very difficult, especially when the tumor is ALK-1 negative. In the present tumor, however, no epithelial differentiation was detected, either morphologically after extensive sectioning or immunohistochemically (HMW cytokeratin and p63 were absolutely negative).

The typical immunophenotype of inflammatory myofibroblastic tumor is as follows (Pathology Outlines 2017):

Positive stains

- SMA, ALK1, vimentin, calponin
- Variable, aberrant cytokeratin expression

Negative stains

- EMA, myogenin, *p53*, h-caldesmon

In contrast to inflammatory myofibroblastic tumors, primary leiomyosarcomas expresses desmin *and* actin (myofibroblasts do not commonly coexpress desmin) and, above all, h-caldesmon. Cytokeratin expression may be only focally detected, and, when so, it is probably limited to low molecular weight forms in both myofibroblastic and smooth muscle tumors.

In the present case, SMA was diffusely positive as well as muscle-specific actin (MSA) and *p53*. CD34 and low molecular weight cytokeratin were focally positive. HMW cytokeratin and p63 were absolutely negative. Staining for h-caldesmon, desmin, S-100, and b-catenin were negative. *ALK-1* was negative, too.

Due to marked increased p53 protein accumulation in >60% of myofibroblasts' nuclei supporting a malignant nature, along with ALK-1 negative staining (i.e., two findings against the diagnosis of inflammatory myofibroblastic tumor), close patient's follow-up was recommended similar to that for patients with low-grade myofibroblastic sarcomas. Both entities (inflammatory myofibroblastic tumor and low-grade myofibroblastic sarcoma) are locally aggressively with a generally favorable outcome; nevertheless, low-grade myofibroblastic sarcoma rarely metastasizes. Among the suggested systems for sarcoma grading, the most accepted is according to "Federation Nationale des Centers de Lutte Contre le Cancer – FNCLCC," and it is currently adopted by the World Health Organization. This is a three-tiered grading system (grade 1 to grade 3) which takes into account three main parameters: differentiation, mitotic count, and necrosis. The present tumor shows myofibroblastic differentiation, very low mitotic rate, and no necrotic areas (apart from its ulcerated surface), thus corresponding to grade 1 sarcoma (low grade). The diagnosis of a low-grade myofibroblastic sarcoma was finally favored in this particular case.

To sum up, in most of the areas of an inflammatory myofibroblastic tumor, the neoplastic cells should exhibit morphological features resembling myofibroblasts; the nuclei should be elongated to spindle-shaped with minimal to moderate atypia. *Sparse* cells though showing higher degree of atypia with pyknochromatic, enlarged, and wavy nuclei, surrounded by an obviously collagenous matrix, may be encountered in inflammatory myofibroblastic tumor. Mitotic rate is often very low, and there are also moderately dense inflammatory infiltrates composed of mononuclear cells, mainly lymphocytes and some eosinophils. Additionally, there is increased vascularity including either thin-walled, slit-like elongated vessels or irregularly shaped ones

2.6.1.1 Clinical Commentary

Vasileios Spapis

Two cases of spindle cell neoplasms of urinary bladder are presented.

The first one is a muscle-invasive sarcomatoid urothelial carcinoma with heterologous osteosarcomatous differentiation and nodal metastases at the initial presentation. Increased incidence of bladder cancer after external beam radiation therapy has been reported (Nieder et al. 2008). Pure primary bladder sarcomas are not smoking related, but there is an association with pelvic radiation and systemic chemotherapy for other malignancies (Spiess et al. 2007). The most common subtype is leiomyosarcoma, whereas osteosarcoma is considered rare. Usually they are confined to the bladder and almost always are considered to be high grade. Detection of sarcomatoid or sarcomatous elements in a TUR specimen automatically places the patient in the highest-risk subgroup (Dotan et al. 2006; Rosser et al. 2003). Early cystectomy could be offered, even for nonmuscle-invasive bladder cancer (NMIBC) (Witjes et al. 2017a, b). If MIBC is diagnosed, radical cystectomy is the treatment of choice. Care should be taken to obtain a negative surgical margin because the local recurrence rate is 2.4 times higher in patients with a positive surgical margin (Dotan et al. 2006). Chemotherapy is not that effective, with doxorubicin, ifosfamide, and cisplatin being the most effective agents.

The second case is of an inflammatory myofibroblastic tumor with p53 protein overexpression a possible sign of malignancy, which necessitates close follow-up of the patient, analogous to that of a low-grade myofibroblastic sarcoma. An inflammatory myofibroblastic tumor (IMT) is a rare neoplasm consisting of myofibroblastic and fibroblastic spindle cells accompanied by infiltration of plasma cells, lymphocytes, and eosinophils (Fletcher et al. 2013). Care should be taken to distinguish this tumor from other malignant spindle cell tumors (sarcomatoid urothelial carcinoma, leiomyosarcoma). IMTs rarely occur in the urinary bladder. They have been associated with trauma and infection, but the majority of cases occur spontaneously. They are classified as intermediate (rarely metastasizing) tumors. Surgical resection is recommended, and complete resection is of great importance to avoid local recurrence.

Key Points

- Inflammatory myofibroblastic tumors, postoperative spindle cell nodules, and urothelial carcinomas may assume sarcomatoid growth patterns and be mistaken histologically for sarcomas. The distinction between benign and malignant tumors rests primarily on the nuclear pleomorphism, abnormal mitoses, and deep necrosis of the detrusor muscle, the latter characteristic of sarcomas.
- The term "sarcomatoid urothelial carcinoma" should be used for any biphasic malignant neoplasm that exhibits morphologic and/or immunohistochemical evidence of both epithelial and mesenchymal differentiation.
- Differentiation of sarcomatoid variant of urothelial carcinoma from pseudosarcomatous lesions is achieved by appreciating the presence of both malignant epithelial islands and malignant spindle cells. Extensive sectioning is required to identify a coexistent in situ or invasive epithelial component.
- Nuclear features are key to distinguish myofibroblastic proliferations from sarcomatoid carcinomas; the former are cured by conservative surgery.

References

Babjuk M, Böhle A, Burger M et al (2017a) EAU guidelines on non-muscle-invasive urothelial carcinoma of the bladder: update 2016. Eur Urol 71(3):447–461

Babjuk M, Burger M, Compérat E, et al (2017b) Non-muscle-invasive bladder cancer. In: European Association of Urology Guidelines. European Association of Urology. Available via https://uroweb.org/guideline/renal-cell-carcinoma. Accessed 05 July 2017

Balar AV, Galsky MD, Rosenberg JE et al (2017) Atezolizumab as first-line treatment in cisplatin-ineligible patients with locally advanced and metastatic urothelial carcinoma: a single-arm, multicentre, phase 2 trial. Lancet 389(10064):67–76

Bamias A, Aravantinos G, Deliveliotis C et al (2004) Docetaxel and cisplatin with granulocyte colony-stimulating factor (G-CSF) versus MVAC with G-CSF in advanced urothelial carcinoma: a multicenter, randomized, phase III study from the Hellenic Cooperative Oncology Group. J Clin Oncol 22:220–228

Bellmunt J, Théodore C, Demkov T et al (2009) Phase III trial of vinflunine plus best supportive care compared with best supportive care alone after a platinum containing regimen in patients with advanced transitional cell carcinoma of the urothelial tract. J Clin Oncol 27:4454–4461

Bellmunt J, von der Maase H, Mead GM et al (2012) Randomized phase III study comparing paclitaxel/cisplatin/gemcitabine and gemcitabine/cisplatin in patients with locally advanced or metastatic urothelial cancer without prior systemic therapy: EORTC Intergroup Study 30987. J Clin Oncol 30:1107–1113

Brierley JD, Gospodarowicz MK, Wittekind C (eds) (2017) TNM classification of malignant tumors, 8th edn. UICC International Union Against Cancer, Oxford

Burger M, Catto JW, Dalbagni G et al (2013) Epidemiology and risk factors of urothelial bladder cancer. Eur Urol 63(2):234–241

Cambier S, Sylvester R, Collette L et al (2016) EORTC Nomograms and risk groups for predicting recurrence, progression, and disease-specific and overall survival in non-muscle-invasive stage Ta-T1 urothelial bladder cancer patients treated with 1-3 years of maintenance bacillus Calmette-Guérin. Eur Urol 69(1):60–69

Cheng L, Cheville JC, Neumann RM et al (1999) Natural history of urothelial dysplasia of the bladder. Am J Surg Pathol 23(4):443–447

Cheng L, Montironi R, Davidson DD et al (2009) Staging and reporting of urothelial carcinoma of the urinary bladder. Mod Pathol 22:S70–S95

De Santis M, Bellmunt J, Mead G et al (2012) Randomized phase II/III trial assessing gemcitabine/carboplatin and methotrexate/carboplatin/vinblastine in patients with advanced urothelial cancer who are unfit for cisplatin-based chemotherapy: EORTC study 30986. J Clin Oncol 30:191–199

Dotan ZA, Tal R, Golijanin D et al (2006) Adult genitourinary sarcoma: the 25-year Memorial Sloan-Kettering experience. J Urol 176(5):2033–2038. discussion 2038–2039

Epstein JI, Amin MB, Reuter VR et al (1998) The World Health Organization/ International Society of Urological Pathology consensus classification of urothelial (transitional cell) neoplasms of the urinary bladder. Bladder Consensus Conference Committee. Am J Surg Pathol 22(12):1435–1448

Epstein JI (2005) The lower urinary tract and male genital system. In: Kumar V, Abbas AK, Fausto N (eds) Robbins and Cotran pathologic basis of disease, 7th edn. Elsevier Saunders, Philadelphia, pp 1030–1032

Epstein JI, Reuter VE, Amin MB (2010) Biopsy interpretation of the bladder. Lippincott, Williams & Wilkins, Philadelphia

Fernandez-Gomez J, Madero R, Solsona E et al (2009) Predicting nonmuscle invasive bladder cancer recurrence and progression in patients treated with bacillus Calmette-Guerin: the CUETO scoring model. J Urol 182(5):2195–2203

Fletcher CDM, Bridge JA, Hogendoorn P, Mertens F (2013) WHO classification of tumours of soft tissue and bone, vol 5. IARC Press, Lyon, pp 83–84

Franke EI, Misseri R, Cain MP et al (2011) Nephrogenic adenoma in the augmented bladder. J Urol 186(4 Suppl):1586–1589

Gabrilove JL, Jakubowski A, Scher H et al (1988) Effect of granulocyte colony-stimulating factor on neutropenia and associated morbidity due to chemotherapy for transitional-cell carcinoma of the urothelium. N Engl J Med 318:1414–1422

Galsky MD, Iasonos A, Mironov S et al (2007) Phase II trial of dose-dense doxorubicin plus gemcitabine followed by paclitaxel plus carboplatin in patients with advanced urothelial carcinoma and impaired renal function. Cancer 109:549–555

Hansel DE, Amin MB, Comperat E et al (2013) A contemporary update on pathology standards for bladder cancer: transurethral resection and radical cystectomy specimens. European Urol 63:321–332

Hoffman-Censits JH, Grivas P, Van Der Heijden MS et al (2016) IMvigor 210, a phase II trial of atezolizumab (MPDL3280A) in platinum-treated locally advanced or metastatic urothelial carcinoma (mUC). J Clin Oncol 34(Suppl 2S):Abstr 355

Jones S (2016) Non–muscle-invasive bladder cancer (Ta, T1, and CIS). In: Wein A, Kavoussi L, Partin A, Peters C (eds) Campbell-Walsh urology, 11th edn. Elsevier, Philadelphia, p 2205

Konety B, Carol LP (2013) Urothelial carcinoma: cancers of the bladder, ureter, & renal pelvis. In: McAninch J, Lue T (eds) Smith and Tanagho's general urology, 18th edn. McGraw-Hill, New York, pp 310–322

Lamm D (1992) Carcinoma in situ. Urol Clin North Am 1992 19(3):499–508

Lim M, Adsay NV, Grignon D et al (2009) Urothelial carcinoma with villoglandular differentiation: a study of 14 cases. Mod Pathol 22(10):1280–1286

Loehrer PJ, Einhorn LH, Elson PJ et al (1992) A randomized comparison of cisplatin alone or in combination with methotrexate, vinblastine, and doxorubicin in patients with metastatic urothelial carcinoma: a cooperative group study. J Clin Oncol 10:1066–1073

Lopez-Beltran A, Pacelli A, Rothenberg HJ et al (1998) Carcinosarcoma and sarcomatoid carcinoma of the bladder: clinicopathological study of 41 cases. J Urol 159:1497–1503

Milowsky MI, Nanus DM, Maluf FC et al (2009) Final results of sequential doxorubicin plus gemcitabine and ifosfamide, paclitaxel, and cisplatin chemotherapy in patients with metastatic or locally advanced transitional cell carcinoma of the urothelium. J Clin Oncol 27:4062–4067

Nieder AM, Porter MP, Soloway MS (2008) Radiation therapy for prostate cancer increases subsequent risk of bladder and rectal cancer: a population based cohort study. J Urol 180(5):2005–2009

Ozaki K, Kitagawa K, Gabata T et al (2014) A case of polypoid and papillary cystitis mimicking an advanced bladder carcinoma with invasion of perivesical fat. Urol Ann 6(1):72–74

PathologyOutlines.com website. http://www.pathologyoutlines.com/topic/bladderclearcell.html. Accessed 2 July 2017

Ramirez D, Gupta A, Canter D et al (2016) Microscopic haematuria at time of diagnosis is associated with lower disease stage in patients with newly diagnosed bladder cancer. BJU Int 117(5):783–786

Rosai, Ackerman (2007) Urinary Tract. In: Damjanov I, Nola M, Rosai J (eds) Rosai and Ackerman's surgical pathology review. Mosby Elsevier, Philadelphia, pp 237–238
Rosser CJ, Slaton JW, Izawa JI et al (2003) Clinical presentation and outcome of high-grade urinary bladder leiomyosarcoma in adults. Urology 61(6):1151–1155
Sauter G, Amin AF, Busch C et al (2004) Noninvasive urothelial neoplasias: WHO classification of noninvasive papillary urothelial tumors. In: Eble J, Epstein J, Sesterhenn I (eds) World Health Organization classification of tumors: pathology and genetics of tumors of the urinary system and male genital organs. IARC Press, Lyon, p 110
Semins MJ, Schoenberg MP (2007) A case of florid cystitis glandularis. Nat Clin Pract Urol 4(6):341–345
Sharma P, Retz M, Siefker-Radtke A et al (2017) Nivolumab in metastatic urothelial carcinoma after platinum therapy (Checkmate 275): a multicenter, single arm, phase II trial. Lancet Oncol 18(3):312–322
Smith AK, Hansel DE, Jones JS (2008) Role of cystitis cystica et glandularis and intestinal metaplasia in development of bladder carcinoma. Urology 71(5):915–918
Solsona E, Iborra I, Dumont R et al (2000) The 3-month clinical response to intravesical therapy as a predictive factor for progression in patients with high risk superficial bladder cancer. J Urol 164(3 Pt 1):685–689
Spiess PE, Kassouf W, Steinberg JR et al (2007) Review of the M.D. Anderson experience in the treatment of bladder sarcoma. Urol Oncol 25(1):38–45
Sternberg CN, de Mulder P, Schornagel JH et al (2006) Seven year update of an EORTC phase III trial of high-dose intensity M-VAC chemotherapy and G-CSF versus classic M-VAC in advanced urothelial tract tumours. Eur J Cancer 42:50–54
Strojan Flezar M (2010) Urine and bladder washing cytology for detection of urothelial carcinoma: standard test with new possibilities. Radiol Oncol 44(4):207–214
Takenaka A, Yamada Y, Miyake H et al (2008) Clinical outcomes of bacillus Calmette-Guérin instillation therapy for carcinoma in situ of urinary bladder. Int J Urol 15(4):309–313
Têtu B (2009) Diagnosis of urothelial carcinoma from urine. Mod Pathol 22(Suppl 2):S53–S59
von der Maase H, Hansen SW, Roberts JT et al (2000) Gemcitabine and cisplatin versus methotrexate, vinblastine, doxorubicin, and cisplatin in advanced or metastatic bladder cancer: results of a large, randomized, multinational, multicenter, phase III study. J Clin Oncol 18:3068–3077
von der Maase H, Sengelov L, Roberts JT et al (2005) Long-term survival results of a randomized trial comparing gemcitabine plus cisplatin, with methotrexate, vinblastine, doxorubicin, plus cisplatin in patients with bladder cancer. J Clin Oncol 23:4602–4608
Witjes AJ, Lebret T, Compérat EM et al (2017a) Updated 2016 EAU guidelines on muscle-invasive and metastatic bladder cancer. Eur Urol 71(3):462–475
Witjes J, Compérat E, Cowan N, et al (2017b) Muscle-invasive and metastatic bladder cancer. In: European Association of Urology Guidelines. European Association of Urology. Available via https://uroweb.org/guideline/renal-cell-carcinoma. Accessed 05 July 2017
Wright JL, Lin DW, Porter MP (2008) The association between extent of lymphadenectomy and survival among patients with lymph node metastases undergoing radical cystectomy. Cancer 112(11):2401–2408
Yafi F, Brimo F, Steinberg J et al (2015) Prospective analysis of sensitivity and specificity of urinary cytology and other urinary biomarkers for bladder cancer. Urol Oncol 33(2):66.e25-31
Zelefsky MJ, Housman DM, Pei X et al (2012) Incidence of secondary cancer development after high-dose intensity-modulated radiotherapy and image-guided brachytherapy for the treatment of localized prostate cancer. Int J Radiat Oncol Biol Phys 83(3):953–959

Prostate Gland Pathology

Maria Gkotzamanidou, Andreas C. Lazaris, Vasileios Spapis, Nikolaos Spetsieris, and Popi Tsagaraki

A. C. Lazaris (ed.), *Clinical Genitourinary Pathology*,
https://doi.org/10.1007/978-3-319-72194-1_3

A pathologic report for prostate biopsy specimens (core or transurethral prostate resection) should include the following information: histologic type of cancer; Gleason primary and secondary pattern and total score; total number of cores; number of involved cores; percentage of prostatic tissue involved by tumor (especially for needle biopsies, either in each core or total linear mm of carcinoma/total linear mm of each core tissue); presence of perineural, angiolymphatic, and periprostatic fat invasion and seminal vesicle invasion; presence of high-grade prostate intraepithelial neoplasia (PIN) (if no carcinoma is found, the number of cores involved and pattern of high-grade PIN should be reported); and therapy-related changes.

A pathologic report for prostatectomy specimens should include the following information: structures included in specimen [prostate (complete or not), seminal vesicles, vas deferens, bladder neck]; weight; size in three dimensions; histologic type and location of tumor (if any); Gleason pattern(s) and score; percentage of prostate involved by tumor (need not give exact tumor volume but an indication of minute vs. voluminous); presence of perineural invasion; presence of angiolymphatic invasion; presence of extraprostatic tissue invasion; presence of high-grade PIN; margin status; lymph nodes (number of involved lymph nodes, number of sampled lymph nodes; extranodal tumor extension is not related to survival) and diameter of largest metastasis; acute or chronic inflammation (which often doesn't correlate with clinical prostatitis); and presence of granulomatous prostatitis (which may elevate PSA and produce suspicious feeling gland).

3.1 Introduction to Prostate Gland Clinical Pathology

Popi Tsagaraki, Nikolaos Spetsieris, Vasileios Spapis, and Andreas C. Lazaris

The prostate and the breast have many similarities in health and disease. Their structure consists of glands producing fluid that is collected through ducts. Disorders of fluid production cause similar structural changes to these glands and ducts. Most prostate and breast cancers begin in the glands – these are the cancers best controlled by early detection through screening. The cancers originating in the major ducts are less common but more difficult to control (Tabar et al. 2013).

The prostate gland consists of four zones: anterior fibromuscular stroma, central zone, peripheral zone, and transition zone. The latter is a balloon-shaped component of the prostate that is located in the periurethral region. Most of the conventional prostatic acinar adenocarcinomas are of intermediate or high histological grade and develop in the peripheral zone just like their precursor lesion (i.e., high-grade prostatic intraepithelial neoplasia, HG PIN) and thus give no clinical symptoms. Some better differentiated acinar adenocarcinomas arise in the transition zone and are less likely to behave aggressively. The transition zone is the exclusive site of benign prostatic hyperplasia (BPH), a highly common lesion associated with obstructive or irritating symptoms. Needle biopsy mainly examines the peripheral zone, whereas surgical specimens (apart from radical prostatectomies, of course) mainly examine the transition zone.

The epithelium of the prostate is principally composed of three cell types: secretory (acinar) cells, basal cells, and several neuroendocrine cells.

With regard to glandular size and configuration, normal, hyperplastic, and PIN glands are medium to large sized and, as a rule, are characterized by intraluminal papillary-type projections/infoldings, while atrophic and cancerous glands are usually small sized with a smooth/sharp luminal border and no intraluminal projections/infoldings.

Prostate cancer (PCa) is the most commonly diagnosed cancer in men. The incidence of PCa diagnosis varies widely between different geographical areas, largely because of the use of prostate-specific antigen (PSA) testing and the aging population. PCa incidence is associated with family history and ethnicity (Cooperberg et al. 2013; Hemminki 2012; Jansson et al. 2012). However, true hereditary disease is rather uncommon (<9%). In these cases, disease onset is usually 6–7 years earlier than average, but clinical course is the same on all other aspects (Hemminki 2012). African men are under greater risk of suffering from the disease and seem to have higher mortality rates (Tan et al. 2016). A lot of exogenous factors have been discussed as being potential risk factors of progression from latent to clinical PCa, but, currently, no effective preventative dietary or pharmacological interventions can be made (Leitzmann and Rohrmann 2012).

Population screening for PCa remains the most controversial subject in urology because of the risk of over-detection and overtreatment. The use of prostate-specific antigen (PSA) revolutionized PCa diagnosis (Stamey et al. 1987). There are no universally accepted standards defined for measuring PSA (Semjonow et al. 1996). Generally, the higher the PSA levels, the higher the possibility of PCa. It should be noted though that there are no PSA levels that, beyond which the possibility of cancer is zero. Numerous attempts to refine PSA for cancer detection have been studied, the most common of them being:

- PSA density: PSA levels divided by the TRUS-determined prostate volume. The higher the PSA density, the more likely it is that the PCa is clinically significant.
- PSA velocity: the rate of change of serum PSA.
- PSA ratio: free/total PSA. Levels below 21% are considered suspicious for men with PSA levels between 4 and 10 ng/ml and negative digital rectal examination (DRE).

Prostate cancer tissue is of greater density than normal prostate tissue. This increased density makes the cancer tissue "harder" or more inelastic than normal tissue. This inelasticity is the reason that some of these tumors are palpable on the DRE.

The *ultrasound* evaluation of the prostate requires the determination of a number of factors including echogenicity and symmetry of the outer and of the inner gland and evaluation of periprostatic tissues ("capsule" and periprostatic fat), neurovascular bundles, seminal vesicles, apex of the prostate, ejaculatory ducts, and periprostatic lymph nodes (Rifkin et al. 1993).

The most obvious lesion seen in the prostate that represents prostate cancer is a *hypoechoic, peripherally oriented* lesion. These lesions are most often seen in the posterior portion of the prostate. Hypoechoic lesions are the most obvious and easiest to identify because they are adjacent to more echogenic tissue, the normal peripheral prostate.

A minority of prostate cancer cases arises in the inner gland, in the transition zone. The following may be helpful diagnostically:

1. Focal hypoechoic lesions within the inner gland, particularly if single and not multifocal, should raise the suspicion of cancer.
2. Irregularity of the normally sharply demarcated surgical capsule, which separates the enlarged (from BPH) inner gland from the compressed outer gland, should raise suspicion.
3. Multiple hypoechoic lesions scattered randomly throughout the enlarged inner gland suggest benignity, although malignancy cannot be definitively excluded.

4. Cysts within the enlarged inner gland are benign. Care must be taken to ensure that these lesions meet all of the criteria of a simple cyst.

The exact etiologies for different echogenic characteristics of prostate cancer are unclear. In fact, there is controversy regarding each possible etiology. The following have been suspected as reasons for different lesions having different acoustic reflectivity:

1. Histological grade and size of tumor: There have been conflicting reports regarding the importance of histological grade and tumor size on the ultrasound appearance of prostate cancer. Some researchers have felt that the larger the tumor, the more hyperechoic or acoustically mixed it will appear (Rifkin 1998). Others have suggested that larger tumors are more hypoechoic (Scardino 1988). The largest and most pathology-correlated studies [with ultrasound-guided biopsy and radical prostatectomy (RP) specimens] have shown that the larger the tumor, the more likely it may have hyperechoic elements, being either of mixed echogenicity or subtly hyperechoic (Rifkin et al. 1989).
2. Fibrosis: Research has shown that those cancers that have increased elements of subtle hyperechogenicity, either those of mixed or hyperechoic characteristics, are more likely to have a higher Gleason grade or fibrosis. Fibrosis in prostate cancer is specifically not a classic desmoplastic reaction that other cancers, e.g., breast or pancreatic cancer, may develop.
3. Crystalloid formation: Recent work has suggested that some cancers with subtle areas of increased echogenicity may have developed crystalloid bodies within the cancer (Hamper et al. 1990). This may be a reason for increased echogenicity.
4. Inhomogeneity of tissue: When one type of tissue mixes heterogeneously with another type of tissue, the result may be an increase in the number of interfaces. These interfaces are areas of adjacent tissue with differing acoustic characteristics, resulting in increased echogenicity.

The most difficult lesion to directly identify with ultrasound is the isoechoic lesion. As the terminology suggests, this lesion is of equal echogenicity as the surrounding normal tissue. Thus, it can be difficult to differentiate from the normal tissue because the intrinsic acoustic properties of both the normal and the abnormal are similar. This lesion is best identified by the secondary sonographic characteristics it may produce. These include the following:

1. Asymmetry: It is the most telling sign of the isoechoic lesion. Because there is no asymmetry in echogenicity, symmetry or lack of symmetry in architecture is of importance. Evaluation of the inner-outer gland interface and possible distortion may be useful in delineating an area of concern.
2. Periprostatic bulge. Bulging of periprostatic tissues is suggestive of a neoplastic process that is less elastic or compressible than normal tissue. This type of abnormality may be accentuated by the use of elastography. Those transducers can often demonstrate the "bulge" and incompressible tissue by pressing the transducer, under ultrasonic control, into the tissue of concern and notice the difference index in compressibility from normal tissue when compressed.
3. Periprostatic fat erosion. When the bright echogenic line representing the periprostatic fat is irregular and asymmetric, tumor invasion beyond the prostate "capsule" must be considered. Other pathologies, particularly post-inflammatory fibrosis, post-biopsy fibrosis, and actively inflamed tissue, must be considered.

Although echogenicity is an important feature in the analysis of the endorectal sonogram of the prostate, other characteristics may help in defining areas of concern. These include the following, regardless of the echogenicity of a lesion:

1. A focal lesion in the peripheral or outer gland regardless of echogenicity is of concern and warrants further evaluation.
2. Asymmetry in the architecture of the prostate in either the outer or inner gland, but particularly the outer gland, requires further consideration.
3. In terms of the capsule and pericapsular area, the pseudocapsule of the prostate is rarely defined on the endorectal sonogram. The periprostatic tissue, predominately the fat, is identified as a thin hyperechoic band surrounding the prostate. If this is *bulged* or *disrupted*, concern is raised.
4. Thickening of the neurovascular bundle(s) is not normal and should raise suspicion.
5. While nonvisualization of normal ejaculatory ducts is not uncommon, the inability to visualize them in a man with a marked elevation of PSA may raise concern.
6. Identification of periprostatic lymph nodes, regardless of size, is suspicious. Normal lymph nodes are rarely seen.

Early results suggested that up to 85% of men with prostate cancers >5 mm in size have visibly increased flow to the area of tumor involvement (Kelly et al. 1993). Later results have been less optimistic, i.e., about 50% of those patients with hypoechoic lesions representing cancer have increased flow (Cheng et al. 1996). Perhaps more importantly, hypervascularity can be seen in patients with the more difficult to identify isoechoic and hyperechoic lesions. Three different flow patterns have been identified in prostate cancer. All have low-resistance patterns:

1. Diffuse flow has been seen in patients with obvious hypoechoic lesions as well as those with less obvious grayscale findings.
2. Focal flow within a cancer may be punctate or scattered but is clearly identified as asymmetric flow, within a lesion, within the prostate.
3. Surrounding flow in the immediate periphery to a lesion may be identified in a small number of men.

During conventional prostate cancer diagnosis by rectal exam, blood test, or ultrasound evaluation, categorization of the disease is difficult because of its highly heterogeneous nature. Up till now, the role of histopathology is predominant in the *diagnosis* and *prognostic categorization* of prostate cancer, the latter being based on five-tiered grade groups according to Gleason's grading score.

3.2 Histological Diagnosis of Conventional Adenocarcinoma (Acinar Adenocarcinoma) of the Prostate: The Small Gland Pattern

Since the majority of prostatic carcinomas are diagnosed in needle biopsy material, the proper handling of this material is of vital importance. Two to three tissue cylinders should be put on each slide; three levels of sections should be examined under the microscope with some interface sections kept in case immunohistochemistry is needed in selected cases to confirm the diagnosis of cancer. Since the cytoplasm of cancer cells is frequently amphophilic, in order that it can be easily noticed in the hematoxylin-eosin (H-E) sections, the cytoplasm of normal prostate epithelial cells should appear pale or clear. Microscopic evaluation should initially be performed under low microscopy so that, after taking into account which zone of the prostate (central-transitional or peripheral) we examine, we evaluate the tissue architecture, the shape, and size of the glands as well as their luminal borders, their diversity, and any change in color. Dark staining (basophilic) lesions include inflammation and related changes; complete atrophy of prostate glands; prostatic intraepithelial neoplasia (PIN), the latter as far as medium- to large-sized glands of the peripheral zone of the prostate are concerned; and basal cell hyperplasia as far as glands of the transition prostate zone are concerned. There is no harmony in cancer; it frequently develops between and *around* normal glands. Cancerous glands are characterized by sharp luminal borders and frequently amphophilic cytoplasm. On higher magnification, we can estimate nuclear morphology, preferably by comparison of suspicious nuclei to those of prostate secretory (acinar) cells of adjacent glands which we are sure are non-neoplastic. When we examine nuclei of prostate epithelial cells, we evaluate their size and hyperchromasia and the presence of nucleoli and mitoses. Intraluminally, the detection of geometrically shaped structures (i.e., crystalloids), wispy, blue-tinged mucinous or pink amorphous, dense material favors the diagnosis of cancer. Prostate cancer cells usually possess a sufficient amount of cytoplasm or even abundant, occasionally foamy cytoplasm.

Pathologic diagnosis of prostatic carcinoma requires *a synthesis of a constellation of histological features* (architectural, nuclear, cytoplasmic, and intraluminal) that allows for a definitive diagnosis which must always be based on morphology (Amin 2010; Bostwick and Chen 2014; Epstein and Netto 2015; Fine and Humphrey 2013). Some individual features may also be seen in benign glands. An architectural major criterion of malignancy is the *infiltrative growth pattern* which commonly presents as the observation of small malignant glands either extending between and *around* larger, more complex (and often paler), benign glands or, less often, having a haphazard arrangement. These acinar adenocarcinomas are of intermediate differentiation/grade (Gleason pattern 3) and constitute the most common pattern recognized in needle biopsy; they exhibit individual and discrete glands. The infiltrative character of poorly differentiated/high-grade (Gleason patterns 4 or 5) prostatic carcinoma is typified by ragged invasion of fused microacinar, cribriform, or papillary masses; ill-defined glands with poorly formed, occasional, glandular lumina; and linkage of carcinoma cells into chains (Gleason pattern 4) or even sheets with or without comedo necrosis, cords, or single cells with essentially no glandular differentiation, despite the possible occasional presence of vacuoles (totally absent lumens, Gleason pattern 5). Rarely, in needle biopsy material, no infiltrative pattern is noticed; these appear to be well-differentiated/low-grade carcinomas (Gleason patterns 1 or 2) which are defined as well-circumscribed small gland proliferations, with smooth, mainly pushing margins, characteristically found in the transition zone of the prostate which is not typically targeted for needle biopsy but can be sampled in transurethral prostatectomy (TUR) specimens. In needle biopsies, Gleason patterns 1 and 2 (high differentiation/low grade) should not be reported as such, when encountered, but should be reported as Gleason pattern 3 (moderate differentiation/intermediate grade).

The second of the major criteria for diagnosis of adenocarcinoma is the *total absence of basal cells in an adequate number of atypical glands (no less than three glands).* The distinction of periglandular stromal fibroblasts from basal cells is quite challenging. Application of a basal cell-specific immunohistochemical stain for high molecular weight cytokeratin [such as 34βE12 (CK903), CK5/6] and/or p63 can be diagnostically advantageous only when combined with atypical morphology of prostate glands, since basal cells may be partially (or even completely, in exceptional cases) absent in scattered benign and especially atrophic glands; moreover, adenosis of the prostate – a noncancerous entity – is characterized by a fragmented basal cell layer. On rare occasions though, lesions that fully satisfy the histologic criteria for acinar adenocarcinoma may contain few cells stained positive for 34βE12, and this staining may indeed be specific. In the event of observing 34βE12-immunopositive cells, the diagnosis of carcinoma should be made with extreme caution.

Nuclear atypia in the form of nuclear enlargement and nucleolar enlargement is the third of the major criteria for diagnosis of prostate adenocarcinoma. When macronucleoli are absent, there should be significant nucleomegaly with or without nuclear hyperchromasia, to definitively diagnose carcinoma.

Minor diagnostic criteria are not sufficient for the diagnosis of carcinoma but are useful for defining the glands harboring these changes as suspicious for cancer. These criteria include intraluminal wispy blue-tinged mucin, pink amorphous secretions, mitotic figures, intraluminal crystalloids, adjacent HG PIN, amphophilic cytoplasm, and nuclear hyperchromasia.

Diagnostic features considered specific/pathognomonic for prostatic carcinoma [(a) perineural invasion, defined as cancer tracking all along or circumferentially around a nerve and which needs to be distinguished from benign glands abutting prostatic peripheral nerves; (b) collagenous micronodules, also known as mucinous fibroplasia; (c) glomeruloid intraglandular projections; (d) extraprostatic adipose tissue or seminal vesicle invasion] are observed less often in prostate needle biopsy compared to whole resected prostate glands with carcinoma.

A minimum of three cancerous glands is considered to be necessary for a definitive diagnosis of malignancy. A descriptive term that may be rendered if the histological and/or immunohistochemical findings are felt to be worrisome but not completely diagnostic of carcinoma is "atypical small acinar proliferation (ASAP)." ASAP is neither a precursor to carcinoma nor a pathologic entity; it's a term used when uncertainty is encountered on prostate needle (core) biopsy.

The most valuable adjunctive study for the confirmation of diagnosis of prostatic adenocarcinoma, particularly minimal adenocarcinoma, is immunohistochemistry with antibodies against basal cells (e.g., 34βE12 and p63) and alpha-methylacyl-CoA racemase (AMACR), the latter also known as P504S. Racemase is relatively specific for malignant prostatic epithelial cells in conjunction with negative basal cell markers, on condition that AMACR is not expressed by obviously benign epithelial cells. In poorly differentiated/undifferentiated carcinomas, establishing prostatic origin of the tumor may be necessary; so, immunostaining against prostate-specific antigen (PSA), prostate acid phosphatase (PAP), or prostate-specific membranous antigen (PSMA), among other newer, more specific immunomarkers (e.g., prostein, NKX3.1), is performed.

The most important attributes of adenocarcinoma in prostate needle biopsy that merit reporting are Gleason score and amount of tumor in needle biopsy tissue. The Gleason grading system is based on the architectural pattern of the tumor alone and constitutes a very powerful prognostic factor. In the Gleason system, the most prevalent and the second most prevalent pattern (if at least 5% of the tumor) are added together to obtain a Gleason score; it is important that the primary and secondary patterns always be recorded, followed by the Gleason score. If the tumor has only one pattern, the number of the pattern is simply doubled to obtain the Gleason score. At times, in addition to the primary and secondary patterns, a third pattern might be present; when this third or "tertiary" Gleason pattern is 4 or 5, it should be reported in addition to the Gleason score, even if, as "tertiary," it occupies less than 5% of the tumor (e.g., Gleason score 3 + 3 = 6, with tertiary pattern 4). In needle biopsy specimens, when this tertiary pattern corresponds to a higher grade of malignancy, it should be reported as secondary. Based on Gleason score, the following prognostic grade groups have recently been defined (in ascending order of biological aggressiveness):

- Grade group 1 [Gleason score < or = 6, well- and moderately differentiated (low- and intermediate-grade) carcinomas]
- Grade group 2 [Gleason score 3 + 4 = 7, moderately to poorly differentiated (intermediate- to high-grade) carcinomas]
- Grade group 3 [Gleason score 4 + 3 = 7, mainly poorly differentiated (mainly high-grade) carcinomas]
- Grade group 4 [Gleason scores 4 + 4 = 8, 3 + 5 = 8, 5 + 3 = 8, poorly differentiated (high-grade) carcinomas]
- Grade group 5 [Gleason scores 9–10, poorly differentiated (high-grade) to undifferentiated prostate carcinomas]

With regard to needle biopsy specimens, the lowest Gleason score which can be reported is that of 6 (3 + 3).

The most common benign mimickers of adenocarcinoma in prostate needle biopsy tissue are, in order of declining frequency, partial atrophy, crowded benign glands, benign glands, complete (simple) atrophy, radiation atypia, inflammatory atypia, adenosis, and basal cell hyperplasia. The absence of infiltrative growth, macronucleoli, and nucleomegaly, in combination with the presence of basal cells, is the factor with the greatest power in diagnosing benign atrophy and crowded benign glands. Atrophy is a lesion frequently, but not always retaining a lobular configuration in contrast to the ordinary type of prostate cancer. Glands with complete (simple) atrophy are small and dark staining (basophilic); however, on high magnification, we can see that their basophilia is due to the scanty amount of cytoplasm and not to nuclear enlargement. Furthermore, in atrophy, we will be unable to detect normal prostate glands among the atrophic ones (i.e., absence of infiltrative growth). When there is atrophy, *all* glands are atrophic. A rare exception to the above rule is the atrophic type of prostate carcinoma; in this case, however, under high magnification, nuclear atypia and prominent nucleoli will be detected, and, under low magnification, the infiltrative growth will be observed. In (benign) partial atrophy, the glands' architecture is distorted, and, in contrast to complete (simple) atrophy, the cytoplasm is not scanty; so, cancer has to be ruled out, particularly since there can be some degree of nuclear enlargement and visible – though not prominent – nucleoli. In cells with partial atrophy, the cytoplasm is mainly situated on the lateral aspect of the nucleus and not toward the luminal surface; the luminal border is not always sharp; adjacent, easily recognized, foci of complete atrophy are frequent.

Adenosis (atypical adenomatous hyperplasia) is a lesion related to hyperplastic glandular nodules of the prostate and thus is frequently detected in the transition region of the prostate where usual glandular hyperplasia occurs. This lesion is therefore mainly diagnosed in surgical specimens such as transurethral resection (TUR) specimens where features of adenosis can be compared with adjacent, benign, hyperplastic glands. In the rare cases where adenosis is present in needle specimens, there is no such possibility; so, morphology should be meticulously examined, particularly since immunohistochemistry can be misleading [focal AMACR (racemase) immunopositivity].

Basal cell hyperplasia is another small gland lesion of the transition zone of the prostate and thus frequently encountered in TUR specimens. Its characteristic basophilia is due to the hyperplastic basal cells which by definition have scanty cytoplasm and push the secretory (acinar) cells toward the lumen; the latter acquire some sort of atrophic morphology with possible reduction in their cytoplasm and thus become inconspicuous.

3.3 The Large Gland Pattern

This is the pattern of central zone normal prostate glands at the base of the prostate and of usual glandular epithelial hyperplasia of the prostate, as far as nonneoplastic entities are concerned.

With regard to neoplastic lesions, while rather uniform nuclear atypia is the hallmark of HG PIN, it is the low-power (4×) appearance of dark staining glands with acinar cells having basophilic to amphophilic cytoplasm and nuclear crowding and simultaneously having the overall size, shape, and tissue distribution of benign prostatic glands that is useful in identifying potential foci of HG PIN; a number of basal cells should be retained in PIN.

Identifying rounded or circumscribed masses of overtly malignant acinar cells with complex architecture and/or obvious nuclear atypia and a somehow preserved basal cell layer should raise the diagnostic possibility of intraductal carcinoma of the prostate, frequently being close to an invasive acinar adenocarcinoma which spreads along prostate glands/ducts.

A type of high-grade prostate adenocarcinoma composed of large glands lined by tall pseudostratified columnar cells is known as "ductal adenocarcinoma" of the prostate; basal cells may be retained.

The cribriform pattern of invasive acinar adenocarcinoma of the prostate, is always classified as high grade and, of course, is completely devoid of basal cells.

The treatment options of a newly diagnosed localized prostate tumor depend upon the risk stratification of the patient. Gleason score and the cancer extent in the biopsy specimen are pathological parameters of prognostic value in prostate cancer, along with other clinical and biochemical characteristics like digital rectal examination, radiographically determined clinical T stage, and serum PSA level (Gordetsky and Epstein 2016; Montironi et al. 2016). Especially the Gleason grading system is of great value in prostate cancer pathology and remains the most powerful prognostic tool for clinical decision-making. As previously mentioned, a new prostate cancer grading system was developed during the 2014 International Society of Urologic Pathology Consensus Conference, including five distinct grade groups based on the modified Gleason score groups: grade group 1 = Gleason score ≤ 6, grade group 2 = Gleason score 3 + 4 = 7, grade group 3 = Gleason score 4 + 3 = 7, grade group 4 = Gleason score 4 + 4 = 8, and grade group 5 = Gleason scores 9 and 10. These groups have been validated in predicting the possibility of cancer progression by two studies, reflecting prostate cancer biology accurately. Patients are assigned to a risk group based on PSA value, clinical T stage, and Gleason score. Low-risk parameters include stage T1–T2a and Gleason score ≤ 6 and PSA ≤10 ng/ml. Intermediate risk is determined by stage T2b and/or Gleason score 7 and/or PSA 10–20 ng/ml, while high-risk patients are characterized by a stage ≥T2c or Gleason score 8–10 or PSA > 20 ng/ml. Men with low-risk disease may opt for active surveillance of the cancer and intervention upon tumor progression. Radical prostatectomy (RP) or radiotherapy (external beam radiation therapy, brachytherapy) is recommended for patients with low- or intermediate-risk disease. Men with high-risk disease must undergo radical prostatectomy with pelvic lymphadenectomy (in order to better assess the extent of the disease) or external beam radiotherapy with hormone treatment. Neoadjuvant and concurrent androgen deprivation therapy (ADT) are recommended for men receiving radiotherapy for high-risk cancer, along with adjuvant ADT for 2–3 years, to better eradicate micrometastatic disease. The former could be considered for patients with intermediate-risk disease.

Relapse of prostate cancer after radical therapy is treated either with salvage radiotherapy, in the case of a PSA failure after radical prostatectomy, or with intermittent ADT, if the patient was initially treated with radiotherapy.

The main treatment options for metastatic, hormone-naïve disease are continuous ADT or ADT with docetaxel, in men fit enough to tolerate chemotherapy. Patients eventually progressing to castration-resistant prostate cancer without having received prior chemotherapy may be managed with abiraterone or enzalutamide (novel anti-androgens), sipuleucel-T (immunotherapy), or docetaxel. Radium-223 is a radiopharmaceutical agent indicated for patients with symptomatic castration-resistant prostate cancer bone metastases (without visceral metastatic lesions). In the post-chemotherapy setting, the management of the patient, depending on the performance status and treatment option tolerability, includes second-line chemotherapy with cabazitaxel or abiraterone, enzalutamide, and radium-223. In patients with bone metastases, denosumab and zoledronate are recommended, as they decrease skeletal-related events, while external beam radiation may provide symptomatic relief to patients with painful bone metastases. Special attention must be given toward the early detection and management of spinal cord compression (NCCN 2017; Parker et al. 2015).

3.4 Case 3.1: Benign Prostate Hyperplasia and Incidental Prostate Carcinoma

Case Study

Data Prior to Microscopy

A 70-year-old man complains of frequent urination, nocturia, inability to initiate and stop urinary flow, overflow dribbing, and painful micturition. From the patient's history, sudden, acute urinary retention had appeared and persisted until the patient received emergency catheterization.

Digital rectal palpation revealed an enlarged, nodular, symmetric, and rubbery prostate. This firm enlargement of the prostate was associated with a marginally increased serum PSA (8 ng/ml).

Due to medical therapy ineffectiveness, transurethral resection of the prostate (TURP) was performed. TURP is the surgical treatment of choice for benign prostatic hyperplasia (BPH).

The prostate "chips" weighed 45 g. Since minimal cancer was found in the first six cassettes, we performed additional partial sampling (1 block per 5 g of remaining tissue).

3.4.1 Microscopic Evaluation of the Prostate "Chips"

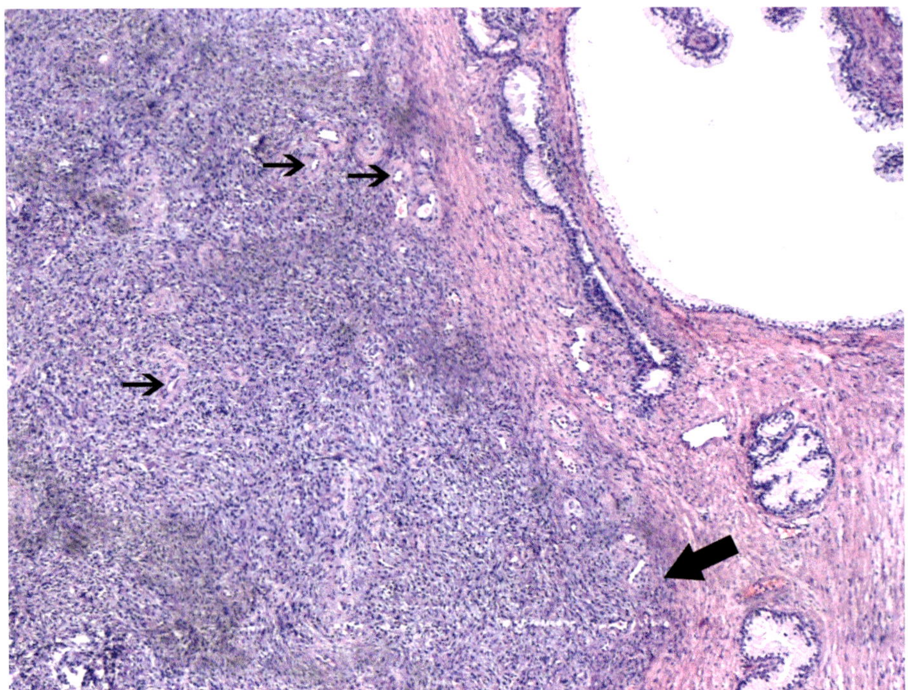

Fig. 3.1 (H-E, ×50) Fibromuscular stromal nodule of the prostate (left part of the image).The hyperplastic stromal component is composed of fibroblasts, vessels (*thin arrows*), and smooth muscle cells. It appears that stromal hyperplasia precedes and induces glandular hyperplasia.

Benign prostatic hypertrophy-hyperplasia (BPH)/nodular hyperplasia is a disease of the periurethral and transitional zones of the prostate, the peripheral zone being pushed aside. Microscopically, the hallmark of nodular hyperplasia is nodularity (*thick arrow*) due to fibrous or muscular proliferation of the stroma and/or to glandular proliferation or dilation.

It is recommended *not* to use the diagnosis of BPH on biopsies due to lack of correlation of histology with obstructive symptoms; however, the presence of stromal nodules does correlate with increased prostatic weight

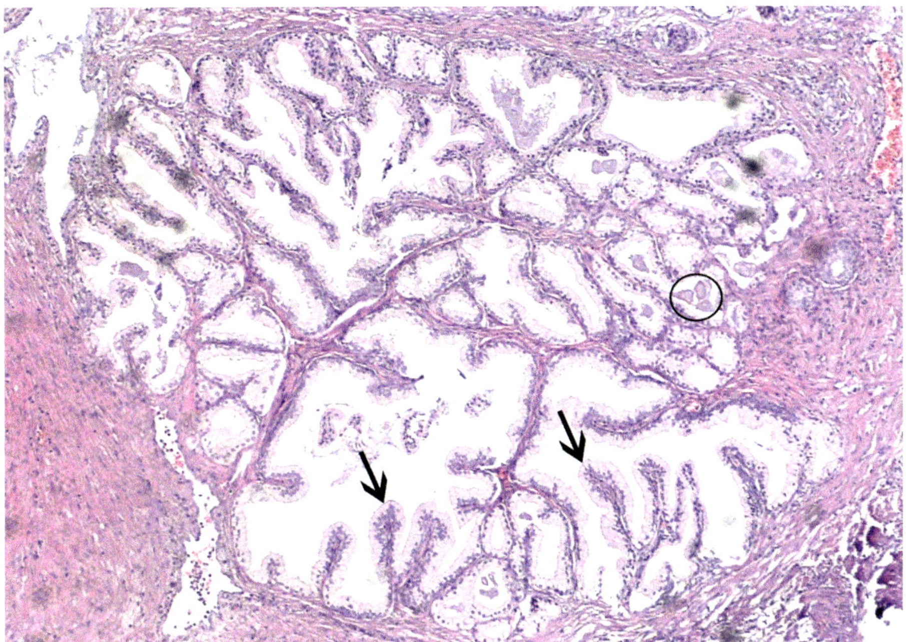

Fig. 3.2 (H-E, ×50) Nodular BPH. Irregularly shaped glands of medium or large size with a nonencapsulated nodular configuration.

[On the contrary, adenosis (atypical adenomatous hyperplasia) is mainly a small glandular proliferation]

Papillary infoldings and papillae with fibrovascular cores are evident in the glands' lumens (*arrows*). Although the epithelium is characteristically thrown up into numerous papillary buds and infoldings, this finding is not specific for nodular hyperplasia.

Corpora amylacea (amyloid bodies), i.e., well-circumscribed round to oval, pink-purple concretions with concentric lamellar rings (*ellipse*), are much more common in benign prostate glands than in cancerous prostate glands; they should be distinguished from pink dense amorphous acellular secretions which are considered an intraluminal secondary criterion of cancer.

On higher magnification, a double cell layer and focal pseudostratification of secretory cells may be observed.

The diagnosis of nodular hyperplasia cannot usually be made on needle biopsy material, as the histology of glandular or mixed glandular-stromal nodules of nodular hyperplasia cannot be appreciated on this limited sampling. Also, needle biopsies do not typically sample the transition zone where nodular BPH occurs

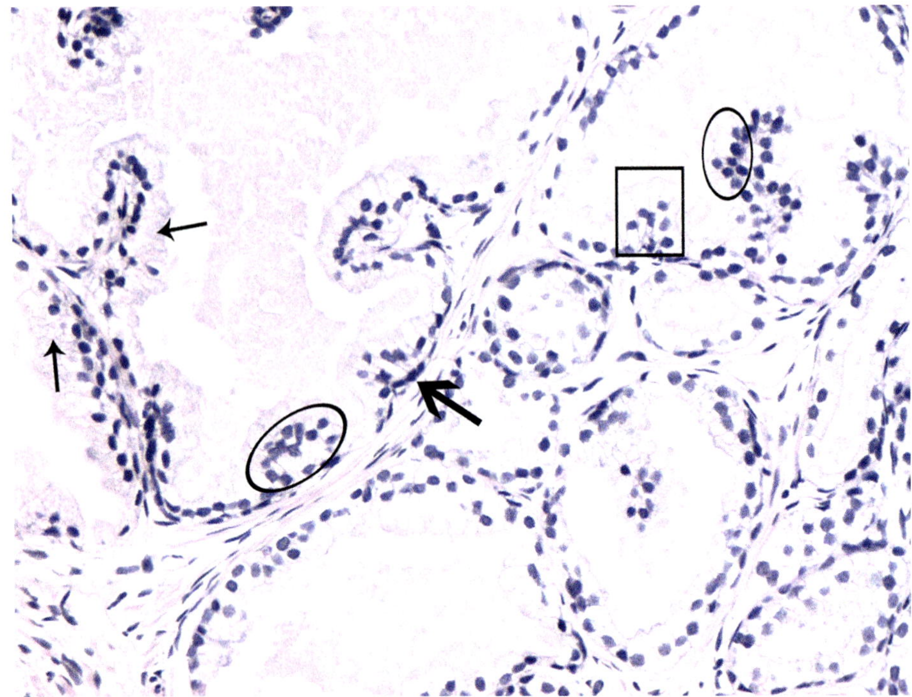

Fig. 3.3 (H-E, ×100) Glands with focal pseudostratification of secretory/acinar cells (*ellipses*) and a double cell layer (*thick arrow*).

Columnar, secretory/acinar cells have pale-staining, granular cytoplasm (*thin arrows*). Small papillary inbuddings (*square frame*) are common in normal prostate glands.

Situated beneath the secretory/acinar cells is the basal cell layer, composed of cells with scant cytoplasm and oval nuclei oriented horizontally, parallel to the basement membrane (*arrow*). It is of interest that scattered circumferential loss of basal cell immunostaining in morphologically benign glands (average, two to three glands) is not unusual and can be seen in 15–30% of cases

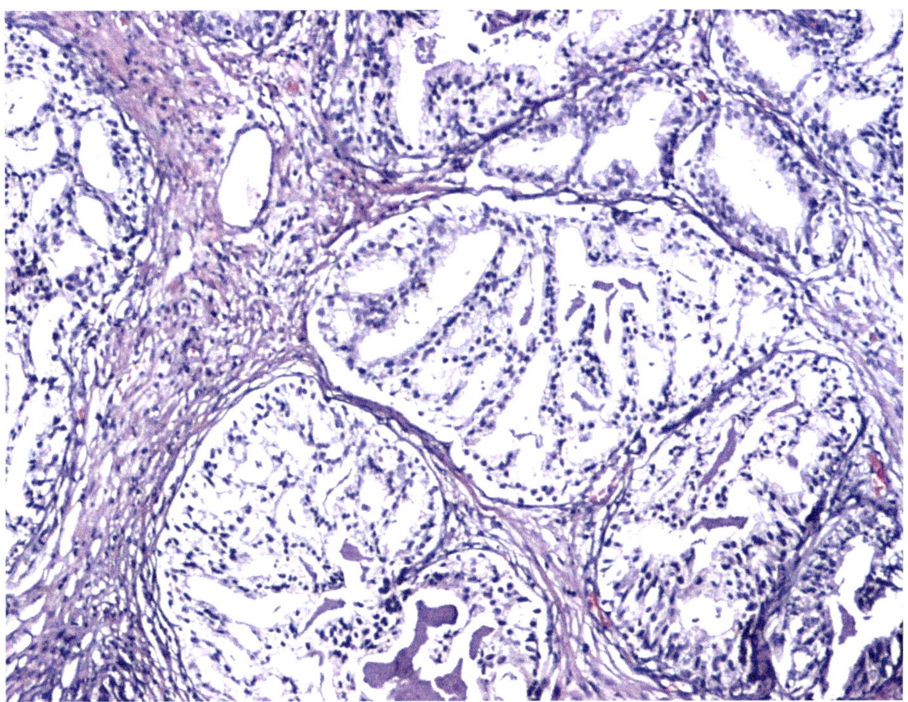

Fig. 3.4 (H-E, ×100) Cribriform structures may be encountered in normal glands/acini of the central zone, at the base of the prostate (large and complex acini with tall, pseudostratified nuclei, eosinophilic cytoplasm, no cytologic atypia), as well as in a benign condition entitled "clear cell cribriform hyperplasia." The latter is usually seen in the transition zone (and thus not found on needle biopsy) and is almost always associated with benign nodular hyperplasia. In *clear cell cribriform hyperplasia*, cytoplasm is distinctly clear, nuclei are small and hyperchromatic, and nucleoli are indistinct; basal cell layer is retained, of course, and is frequently prominent

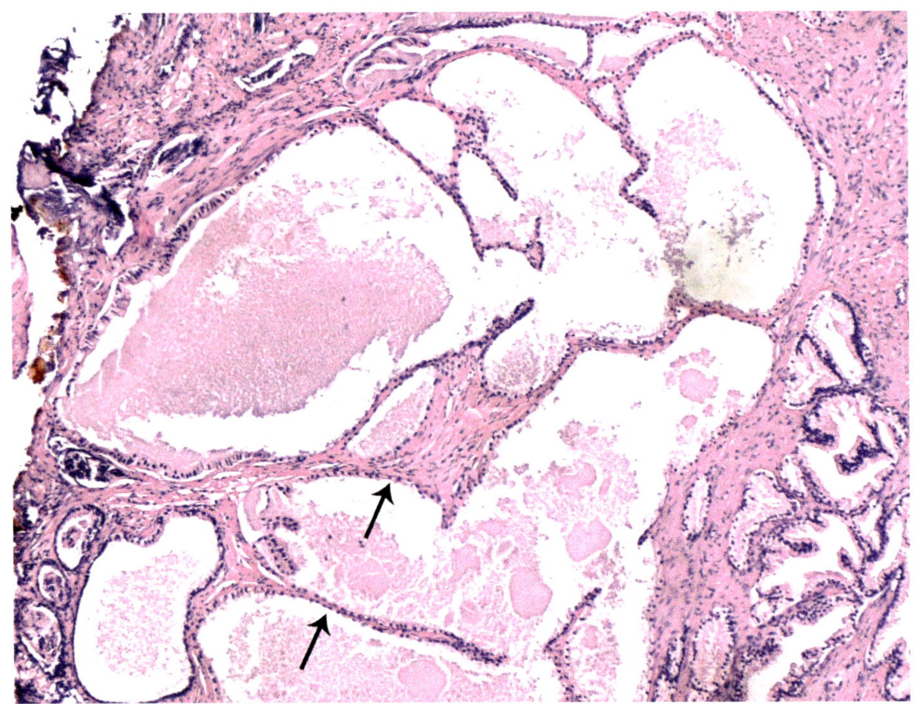

Fig. 3.5 (H-E, ×50) Cystically dilated glands/acini lined by flattened epithelium (*arrows*). A varying degree of acinar dilatation is seen in cystic atrophy which may coexist with BPH

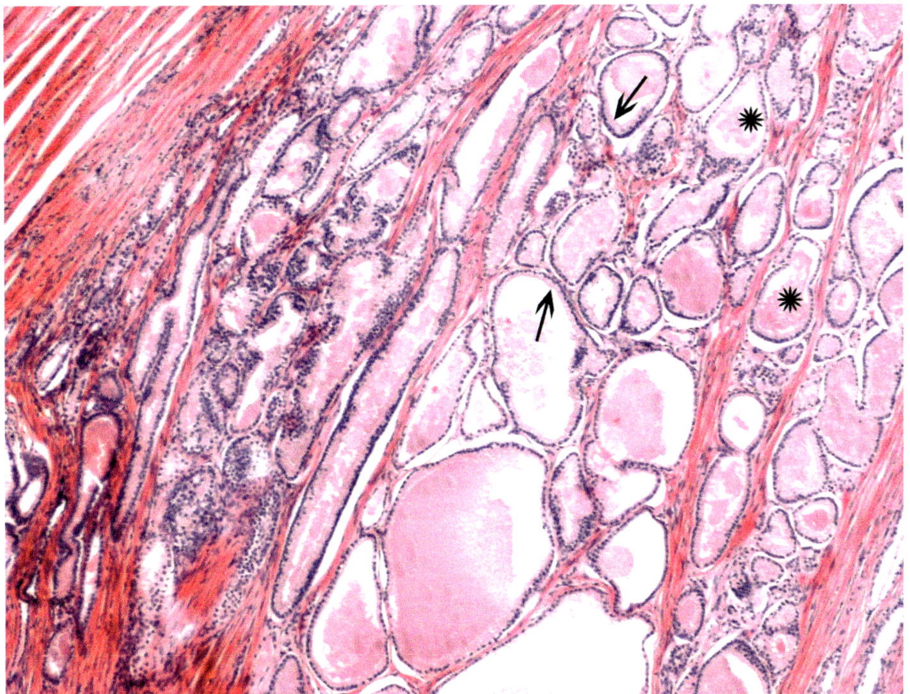

Fig. 3.6 (H-E, ×50) Hyperplastic nodule composed of cystically dilated large glands of non-atrophic type with a sufficient amount of cytoplasm (*arrows*); therefore, basophilia is generally lacking.

In this field, smooth luminal borders (*arrows*) and pink amorphous secretions (*asterisks*) are noticed; a closer inspection is thus necessary to rule out the presence of enlarged nuclei and numerous or prominent nucleoli and so exclude the possibility of pseudohyperplastic carcinoma, an unusual variant of prostate acinar adenocarcinoma, which may elsewhere be associated with typical intermediate-grade cancer, and can exhibit aggressive behavior. The nuclei of pseudohyperplastic adenocarcinoma are rounded, not pseudostratified, and harbor prominent nucleoli. The malignant glands should be more closely packed than benign glands. To diagnose cancer, basal cells should be *totally* absent; as always, racemase (AMACR) positivity will be taken into account as an indicator of cancer only if benign glands in the section we examine are AMACR-immunonegative.

Rarely, prostatic adenocarcinomas may resemble benign glands and be composed of numerous, crowded, large, open glands with a crisp, even luminal surface without papillary infoldings or ruffling. Straight luminal borders and abundant cytoplasm in large glands are considered as features indicative of cancer. Comparably sized, *benign* glands *either* tend to have papillary infolding and luminal undulations or ruffling of their luminal border *or* have atrophic cytoplasm. Nevertheless, even when large glands with rounded profiles have an atrophic appearance, the possibility of diagnosing the microcystic variant of acinar adenocarcinoma should be considered, and thus, nuclear features and presence of basal cells should be meticulously evaluated

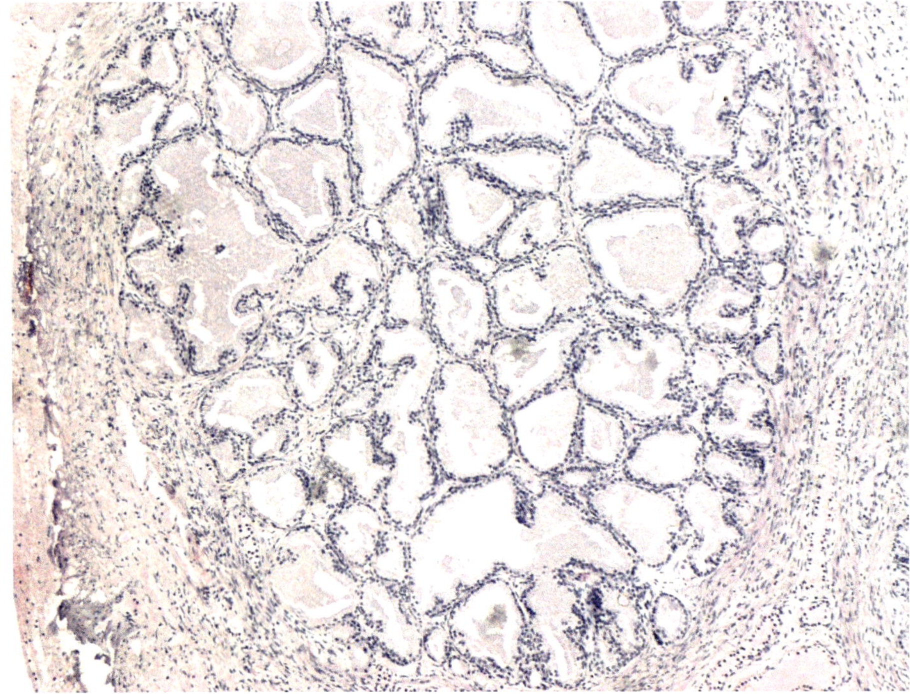

Fig. 3.7 (H-E, ×50) Well-circumscribed, nonencapsulated adenomatous nodule of BPH, composed of tightly packed hyperplastic epithelial components.

- Distinction from adenosis should be made. Adenosis is defined as a small- to medium-sized acinar proliferation usually forming a quite well-circumscribed nodule in the transition zone of the prostate, the acini of which have basal cell layer, at least focally (and do not fulfill cytological criteria of carcinoma). Compared with adenosis, BPH nodules are better circumscribed with no peripheral infiltration by glands; in BPH nodules, glands are larger with papillary infoldings and consistent double cell layer. Adenosis has a high density of small, closely packed glands; BPH glands are typically not as crowded.
- Differential diagnosis should also include well-differentiated/low-grade prostate acinar adenocarcinoma with similar architecture. In the pseudohyperplastic variant of prostate adenocarcinoma, two patterns on low-power microscopy have been described: either large acini (similar to those in Fig. 3.6) or crowded glands lined by truly pseudohyperplastic epithelium. In both patterns, high-power microscopy should show nucleomegaly and nucleolomegaly

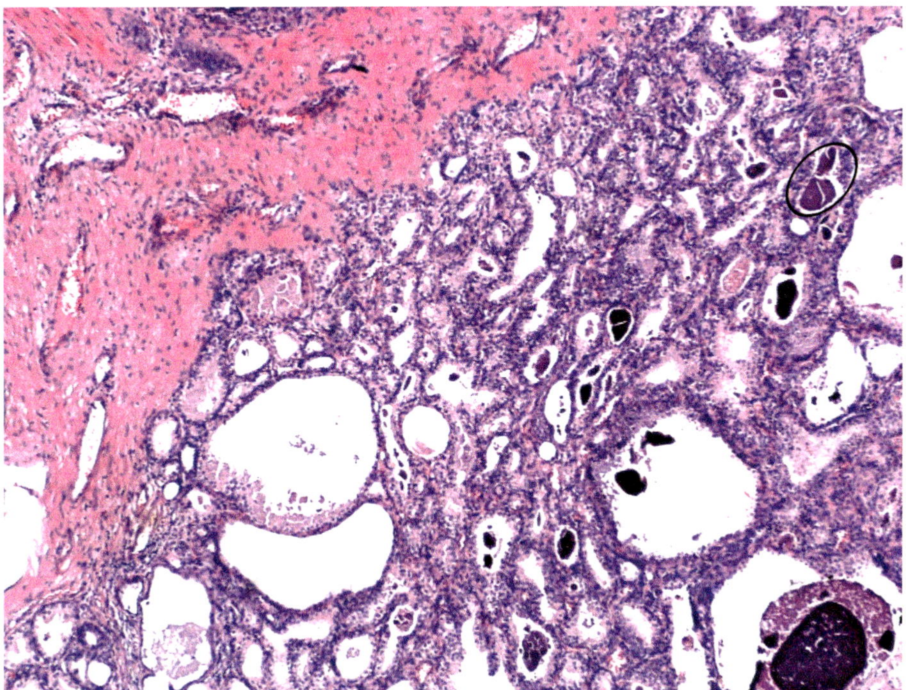

Fig. 3.8 (H-E, ×50) A focus of adenosis/atypical adenomatous hyperplasia in the present patient's TURP specimen.

Adenosis is defined as a localized proliferation of predominantly small, closely spaced glands within the prostate, arranged in a circumscribed cluster or nodule. The finding of crowded small glands is suspicious but not diagnostic of carcinoma.

Differential diagnosis from well-differentiated/low-grade prostate acinar adenocarcinoma with similar architecture should be made. Whereas one should be able to say with confidence when assessing a focus of adenocarcinoma of the prostate which are the benign glands and which are malignant, in adenosis, this distinction cannot be made.

Features of *adenosis* include:

Variably sized, predominantly small, crowded acini/glands admixed with similar, larger glands with luminal infolding. The variable size of acini/glands is a key low-power feature of adenosis; a more dilated "parent" gland may be centrally located. Small glands share cytoplasmic and nuclear features with intermixed larger benign glands.

Not so sharp luminal borders.

Corpora amylacea (*ellipse*) are often present (much less common in adenocarcinoma).

Pale-clear cytoplasm.

No nuclear or nucleolar enlargement. Macronucleoli (>3 μm) should not be present.

Glands with basal cells. Basal cell layer may be discontinuous and indistinct but is usually present in at least some glands. In a nodule of adenosis, glands that lack HMW CK staining are identical to adjacent HMW CK-immunoreactive glands of adenosis.

Focal (pseudo)infiltration at the periphery of adenosis is possible.

Adjacent, unequivocal adenocarcinoma may be present.

In contrast, features of *cancer* include:

Frequently pure population of small crowded glands.

Small glands differ from adjacent benign glands in cytoplasmic and/or nuclear features.

Cytoplasm may be amphophilic.

Basal cells are totally absent

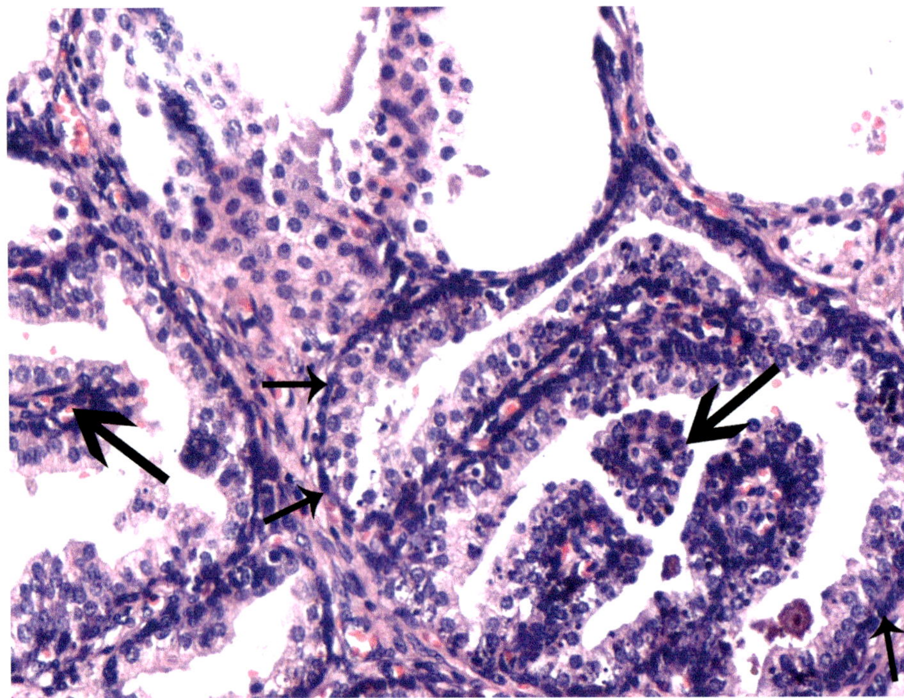

Fig. 3.9 (H-E, ×100) Within the nodule of adenosis of the previous image, we notice larger, more obviously benign glands with papillary infolding (*big arrows*) being admixed with *similar* smaller glands. Glands with basal cells (*small arrows*) which lie beneath the secretory/acinar cells can be noticed in adenosis, even in H-E sections. Basal cells' nuclei are cigar shaped or may resemble those associated with fibroblasts and are oriented parallel to the basement membrane.

We should bear in mind that in cases of obvious carcinoma, there may be cells that closely resemble basal cells but are, of course, negative for basal cell markers and are in fact fibroblasts closely apposed to the cancerous glands. Staining for a basal cell marker is therefore recommended.

True absence of basal cells has been described *only focally* in adenosis. A diagnosis of carcinoma should not be made based on identification of a few malignant-appearing cells in a background clearly demonstrating adenosis. In adenosis, basal cell layer should be focally present in at least some glands

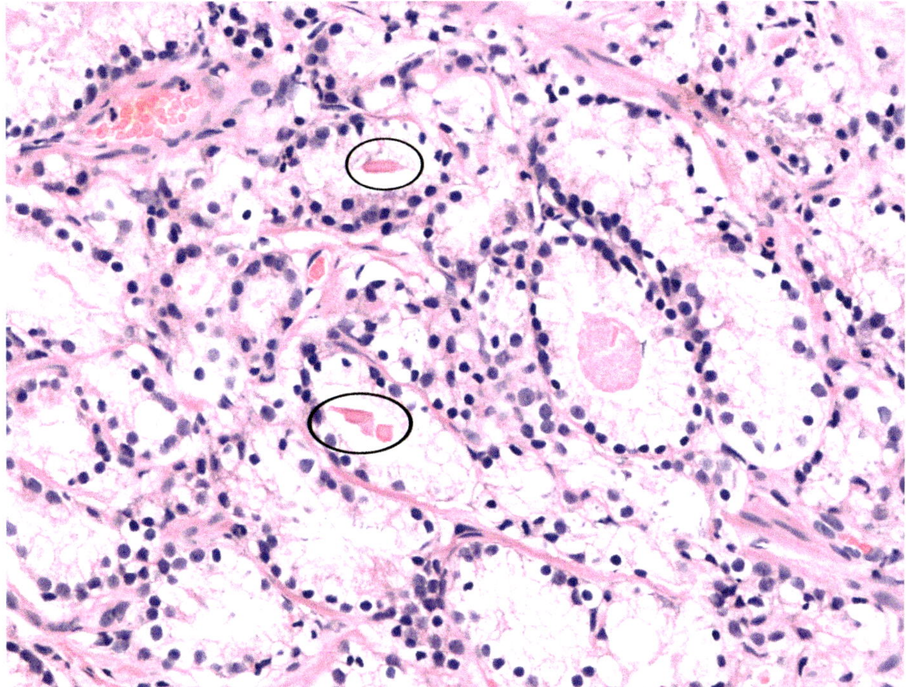

Fig. 3.10 (H-E, ×100) This focus of adenosis consists of a lobule of pale-staining glands.

Intraluminal crystalloids, i.e., eosinophilic, crystalline-like structures that appear in various geometric configurations (*ellipses*), are suggestive of prostate adenocarcinoma, low grade, in particular. However, they have been described in benign lesions such as those of adenosis. Actually, the only condition that mimics cancer and in which crystalloids are often seen is adenosis.

Adenosis occurs mostly within the transition zone, so it is relatively uncommon on needle biopsy. In needle biopsies, adenosis may be mistaken for adenocarcinoma of intermediate grade (Gleason pattern 3), but the latter has haphazard cancerous glands, often at right angles to each other, with no basal cells at all

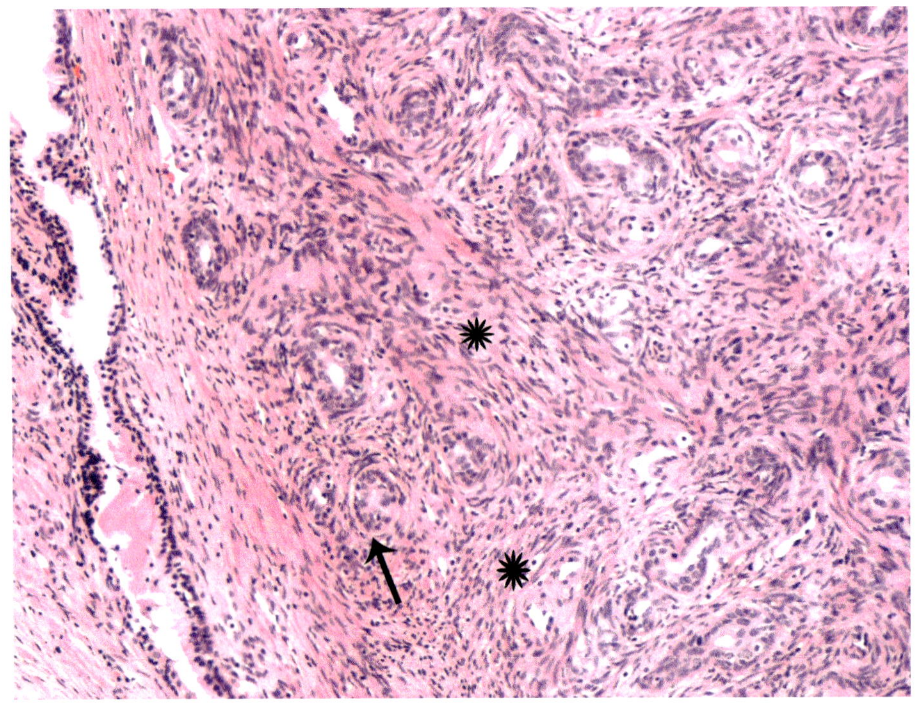

Fig. 3.11 (H-E, ×100) Sclerosing adenosis is a rare lesion commonly observed in the transition zone and thus detectable in surgical specimens.

A small, relatively localized, nodular mixture of well- and poorly formed glands, round or compressed/angulated, and possibly merging with cytologically similar cords and single cells within a cellular spindle cell component (*asterisks*).

A focally infiltrative pattern is possible.

Nucleoli are typically indistinct but may occasionally be fairly prominent.

The glands' double cell layer may be difficult to appreciate in H-E sections.

An eosinophilic hyaline sheath/paucicellular hyalinized stroma around some glands, probably corresponding to a thickened basement membrane (*arrow*), is supportive of this benign mimicker of cancer.

The distinctive cellular stromal component seen within sclerosing adenosis contains plump spindle cells arranged randomly or in fascicles (*asterisk*). In contrast, acinar adenocarcinomas of the prostate usually show no apparent stromal response.

Normal prostate does not contain any myoepithelial cells. In sclerosing adenosis, basal cells show myoepithelial metaplasia and expression of S100 protein. In case there is some degree of nuclear atypia, immunopositivity of cytokeratin 34βE12 in basal cells as well as of smooth muscle actin (SMA) and S-100 protein in basal *and* spindle cells confirms the diagnosis of this benign lesion of the prostate

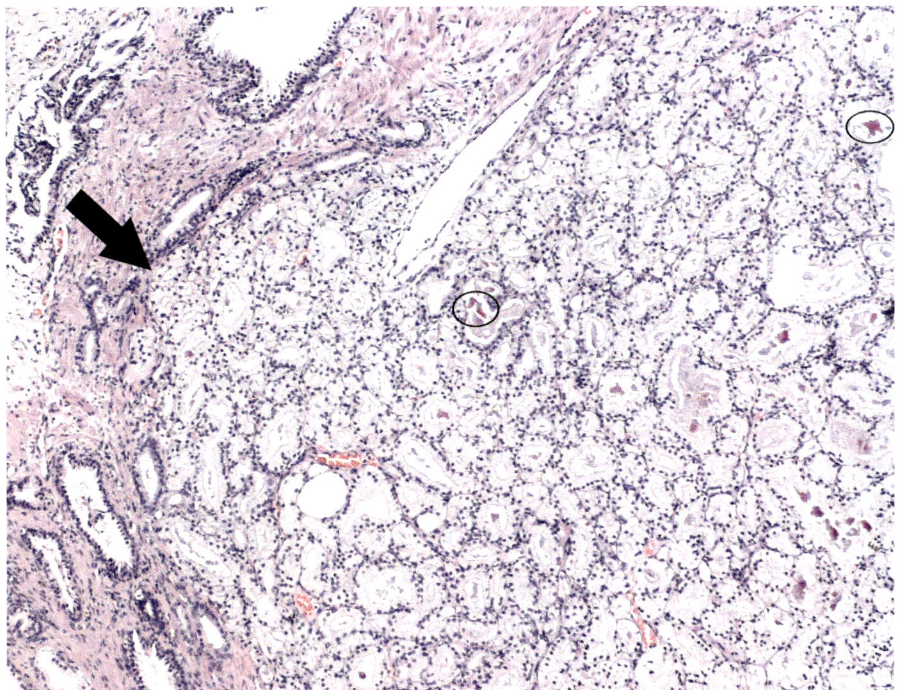

Fig. 3.12 (H-E, ×50) A focus of well-differentiated/low-grade prostate acinar adenocarcinoma, incidentally detected in few prostate "chips" of the present patient.

According to the Gleason grading system, prostate cancers are stratified into five patterns on the basis of glandular architecture as seen under low magnification.

Low grade/high differentiation (Gleason pattern 1) consists of crowded, separate glands, in a rounded mass with a fairly well-circumscribed border/pushing edge (*arrow*). Here's a circumscribed nodule with a uniform proliferation of round, closely packed, but not fused, similar glands, of small to intermediate size, lined by a single layer of rectangular epithelial cells. Low-grade prostate cancer (Gleason extremely rare score 1 + 1 = 2) consists of back-to-back, uniformly sized malignant glands, completely devoid of basal cells, of course. Glands contain eosinophilic intraluminal prostatic crystalloids (*ellipses*), a feature that is more commonly seen in cancer than in benign glands and more frequently seen in lower-grade than in higher-grade prostate cancer. Although the cytoplasm is not evaluated in the Gleason grading system, in Gleason patterns 1 and 2 cancer glands, it tends to be abundant and pale-clear as in the illustrated glands. Some nucleoli should be visible under ×100 magnification

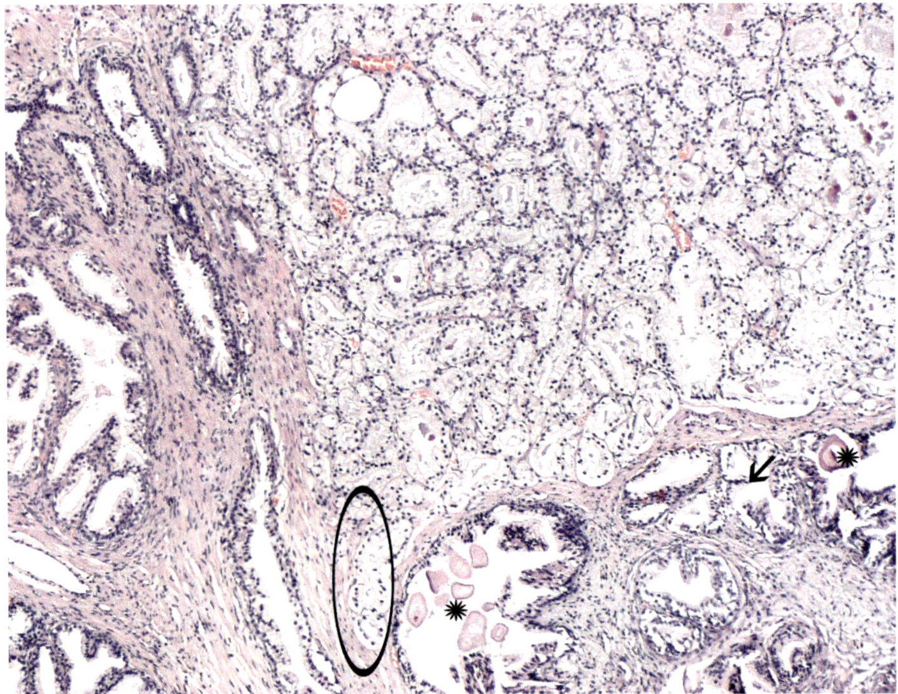

Fig. 3.13 (H-E, ×50) Well-differentiated/low-grade, incidental, prostate acinar adenocarcinoma with a tendency of only minimal infiltration into adjacent prostatic parenchyma (*ellipse*). Minimal invasion of cancer glands into surrounding tissue is compatible with Gleason pattern 2; so this focus could be assigned score 3 (=1 + 2).

Notice again the abundant pale cytoplasm of low-grade cancer cells.

Glands of low-grade adenocarcinoma stand out in sharp contrast to surrounding benign glands. Presence of amyloid bodies (*asterisks*) in benign, tumor neighboring, prostate glands with papillary infolding of their epithelium (*arrow*)

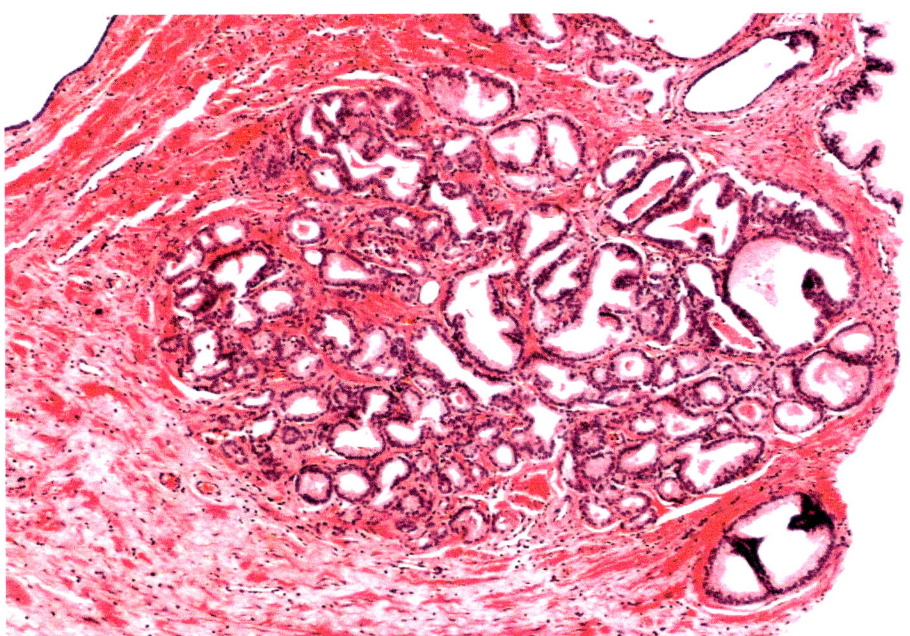

Fig. 3.14 (H-E, ×50) Another incidental limited focus of well-differentiated/low-grade, prostate acinar adenocarcinoma in prostate "chips".

Note this well – circumscribed nodule of small to medium sized, separate glands that do not infiltrate into adjacent tissue. By comparison to Gleason pattern 1, these glands are more variable in size and shape with a relatively loose arrangement, separated up to one gland diameter, with a somehow "loose" edge (Gleason pattern 2)

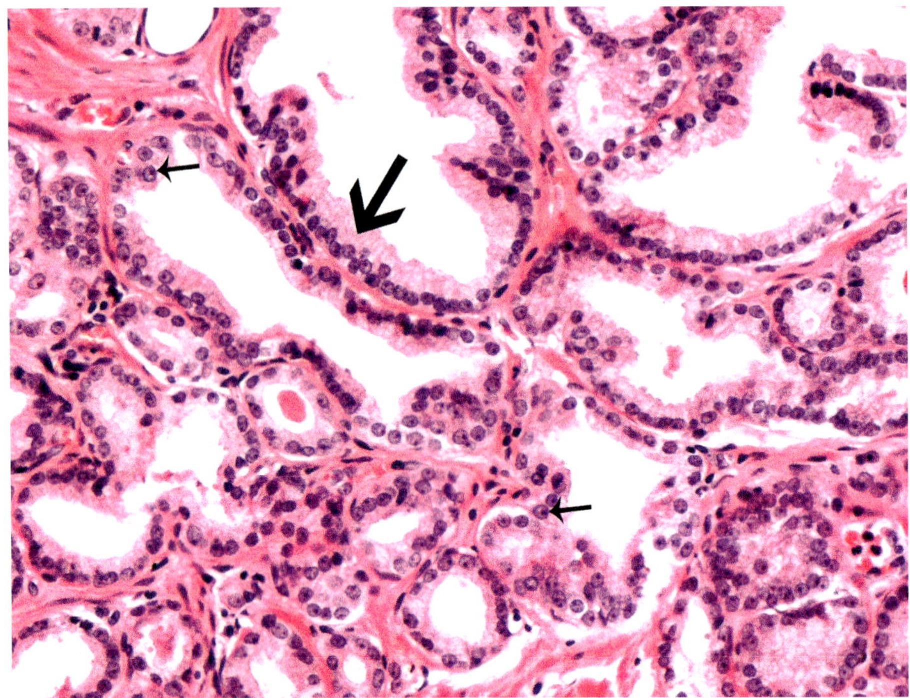

Fig. 3.15 (H-E, ×100) The previous well-differentiated/low-grade, incidental prostate acinar adenocarcinoma under ×100 magnification.

Abundant pale cytoplasm of cancer cells (*big arrow*), a common finding in well-differentiated acinar adenocarcinoma of the prostate. Distinct nucleoli (*small arrows*) under this magnification.

Gleason scores of 2 to 4 are typically found in small tumors within the transition zone and may lack prominent nucleoli. In surgical specimens such as TUR performed for symptoms of nodular hyperplasia, low-grade acinar adenocarcinomas are typically incidental findings and probably represent primaries within the transition zone. The diagnosis of low-grade adenocarcinoma, even if present in a small account of TUR material (< 5%), like in the present case, may set prostatectomy under consideration especially in *young* men.

Gleason scores 2–5 are no longer assigned on needle biopsy material and are only rarely assigned on other specimens (TUR, enucleation, radical prostatectomy) where they are discovered as incidental findings. In radical prostatectomies with higher cancer scores elsewhere in the gland, scores 2–5 are disregarded

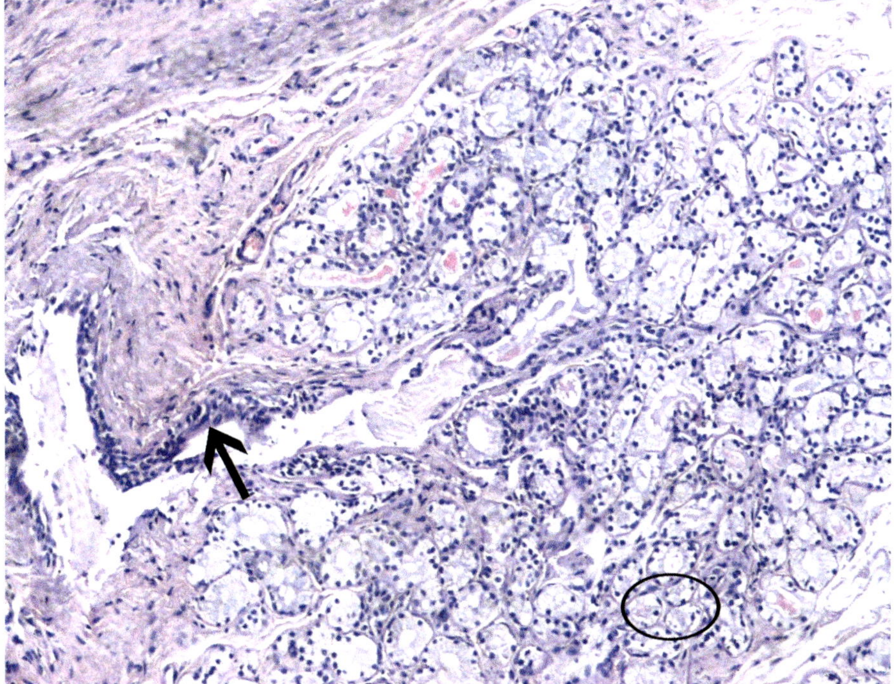

Fig. 3.16 (H-E, ×100) Cowper's bulbourethral glands. Normal Cowper's glands are extrinsic to the prostate and have the appearance of mucinous salivary glands embedded in skeletal muscle. Cowper's glands are characterized by lobular architecture, presence of excretory duct-like structures (*arrow*), and closely packed uniform glands with bland cytologic features and abundant apical mucus-filled cytoplasm to the extent that the lumina are almost occluded (*ellipse*). Because of Cowper's glands' proximity to the urethra, they may be inadvertently sampled by TUR or rarely by needle biopsy of the apex. The correct diagnosis lies in recognizing the dual population of acini *and* ducts often surrounded by skeletal muscle, as opposed to benign prostatic glands.

Immunohistochemistry for high molecular weight cytokeratin is positive in basal cells; furthermore, negativity for PSA and PAP can help in the differential diagnosis for prostate cancer. Additionally, with regard to the latter differential diagnosis, in foamy gland prostatic carcinoma, the glands are larger and the mucin stains are negative.

Another entity in the differential diagnosis is mucinous metaplasia which, however, is an *intra*prostatic process

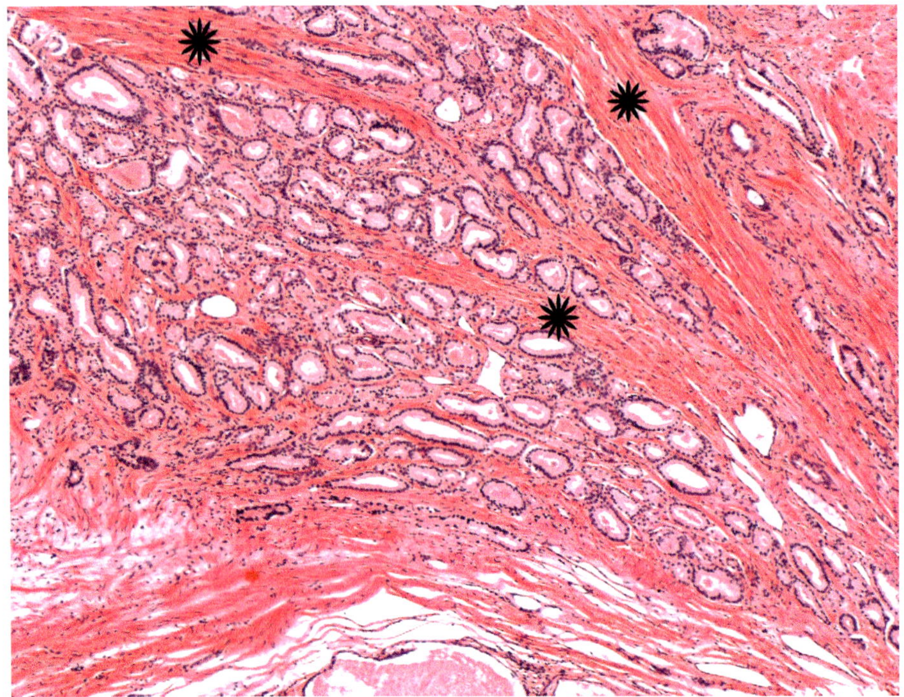

Fig. 3.17 (H-E, ×50) The diagnosis of moderately differentiated prostate carcinoma (Gleason pattern 3) in TUR specimens is primarily based on architectural growth pattern as seen at relatively low magnification: thick muscular bundles (*asterisks*) separate cancerous glands. Glands oriented perpendicular to each other and glands irregularly separated by bundles of smooth muscle are indicative of an infiltrative process. Concomitant nuclear enlargement, visible nucleoli, pink amorphous secretions, and intraluminal crystalloids *may* be observed, or they may be obscured by cautery artifacts.

Such moderately differentiated/intermediate-grade tumors of Gleason score 6 (=3 + 3) may represent primaries within the transition zone; however, there's a possibility of spread from the peripheral zone. High-grade tumors of Gleason score = or >7 in TUR specimens are the ones which certainly indicate spread from the peripheral zone.

With regard to staging, stage T1 refers to cancer found incidentally either on transurethral resection done for nodular hyperplasia symptoms (T1a and T1b depending on the extent and tumor grade) or on needle biopsy, typically performed for elevated PSA levels with unremarkable DRE (stage T1c; see case 3.2)

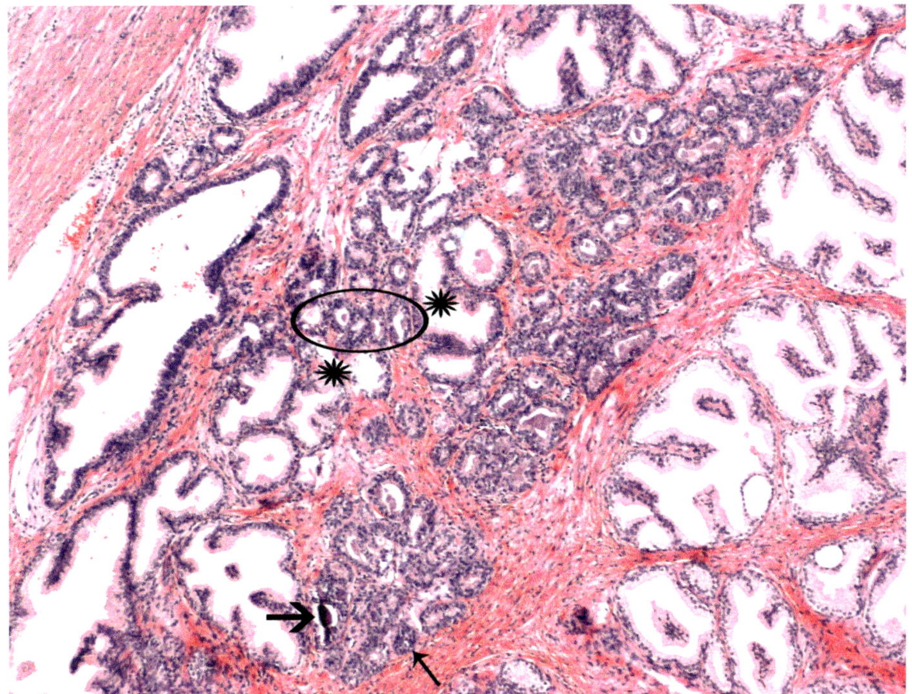

Fig. 3.18 (H-E, ×50) Basal cell hyperplasia: a lesion usually seen in the transition zone of the prostate.

Basal cell hyperplasia is the expansion of the basal cells within the prostatic acini, and it may mimic prostate adenocarcinoma, especially when prominent nucleoli and indications of invasion are present. Although more common in TURP specimens, basal cell hyperplasia can also be seen in needle biopsies and radical prostatectomies.

At low magnification, basal cell hyperplasia is characterized by a basophilic appearance of its small glands due to multilayering of the hyperplastic basal cells which have scant cytoplasm, blue nuclei, and, possibly, nucleolomegaly. In contrast, conventional prostate cancerous glands are rarely basophilic due to the generally sufficient or abundant cytoplasm of prostate secretory/acinar cancer cells.

Basal cell hyperplasia can form solid nests (*thin arrow*), back-to-back glands (*ellipse*), or pseudocribriform glands. Coarse calcifications (*thick arrow*) and intracytoplasmic eosinophilic inclusions are often noticed. Basal cell hyperplasia is actually one of the few prostatic entities that contain well-formed lamellar calcifications in up to half of the cases.

Basal cell hyperplasia is typically an incidental finding in TUR specimens, often seen together with typical benign nodular hyperplasia. Basal cell lesions in the prostate form a spectrum of disease behavior that is typically benign. Basal cell hyperplasia should exhibit contained growth and lack invasive features. The well-defined, small solid nests or glandular structures of basophilic basal cells may, however, have an infiltrative architecture, as here implied. Intermingling of the small glands of basal cell hyperplasia with normal prostate glands (*asterisks*) makes a suspicious architectural pattern which possibly warrants immunohistochemical investigation. Despite this architectural distortion, no malignancy has been proved here. Immunohistochemical confirmation of basal cells by their positive staining for HMW CK 34βE12 ruled out prostatic acinar adenocarcinoma. Nevertheless, it should be taken into account that cases of basal cell carcinoma and cribriform basal cell tumors with signs of malignancy have been described in the prostate gland.

By the way, another entity also with possibly infiltrative appearance which should be differentiated from infiltrating prostatic acinar adenocarcinoma is mesonephric remnant hyperplasia, characterized by the presence of a dense, eosinophilic luminal substance; immunohistochemically, mesonephric remnant hyperplasia is PSA- and PAP-negative

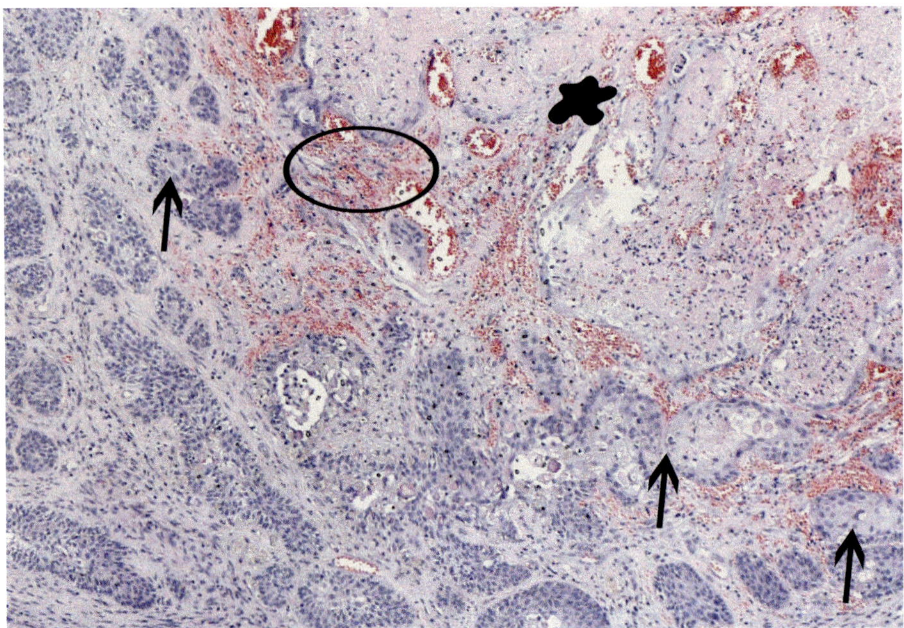

Fig. 3.19 (H-E, ×100) Ischemic coagulative necrosis, typically occurring in a background of nodular hyperplasia (about 20% of cases of BPH). As the prostate expands within its capsule, it is not surprising that interstitial pressure rises; this may compress the vascular supply to the nodules. Prostatic infarcts range in size from a few millimeters to 5 cm. An acute infarction is shown here with central coagulative necrosis (*blob*) of prostate gland and stroma, with surrounding hemorrhage (*ellipse*).

Infarcts quite commonly elicit reactive as well as metaplastic changes (*arrows*) in adjacent ducts/glands, typically of the early squamous type. Squamous metaplasia at the periphery of the infarct should not be confused with squamous cell carcinoma. The squamous nests of prostatic infarct rarely show keratinization; their lack of pleomorphism, and the localized nature of the process to the area immediately adjacent to the infarct, easily exclude squamous cell carcinoma (which rarely may affect the prostate gland).

In remote infarction, a central fibrous scar with hemosiderin is observed instead of the necrotic area

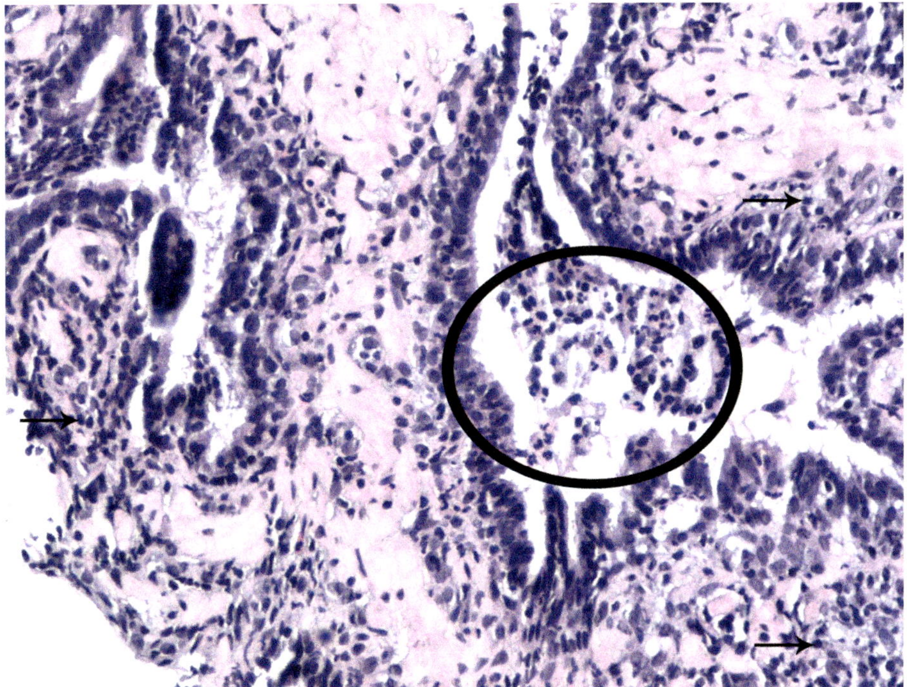

Fig. 3.20 (H-E, ×200) Acute and chronic inflammation of the prostate is either of bacterial pathogenesis or not; the latter most commonly encountered. Within areas of nodular hyperplasia, one often finds nodules or diffuse stromal infiltrates of lymphocytes and plasma cells in a periglandular distribution. Here's a basophilic area of chronic active inflammation disrupting prostatic glands. Abscess formation (*ellipse*) with concomitant periglandular lymphocytic presence (*arrows*). Neutrophils are usually confined to the glands. The prostatic stroma is usually infiltrated by lymphocytes, macrophages, and plasma cells.

It is preferable to diagnose inflamed prostate specimens as having acute or chronic inflammation than as acute or chronic prostatitis (i.e., the latter are clinical diagnoses related to the duration of symptoms).

Minimal nuclear atypia in prostate epithelial cells can be justified by inflammation. A diagnosis of malignancy should be rendered with great caution in the setting of inflammatory infiltrates

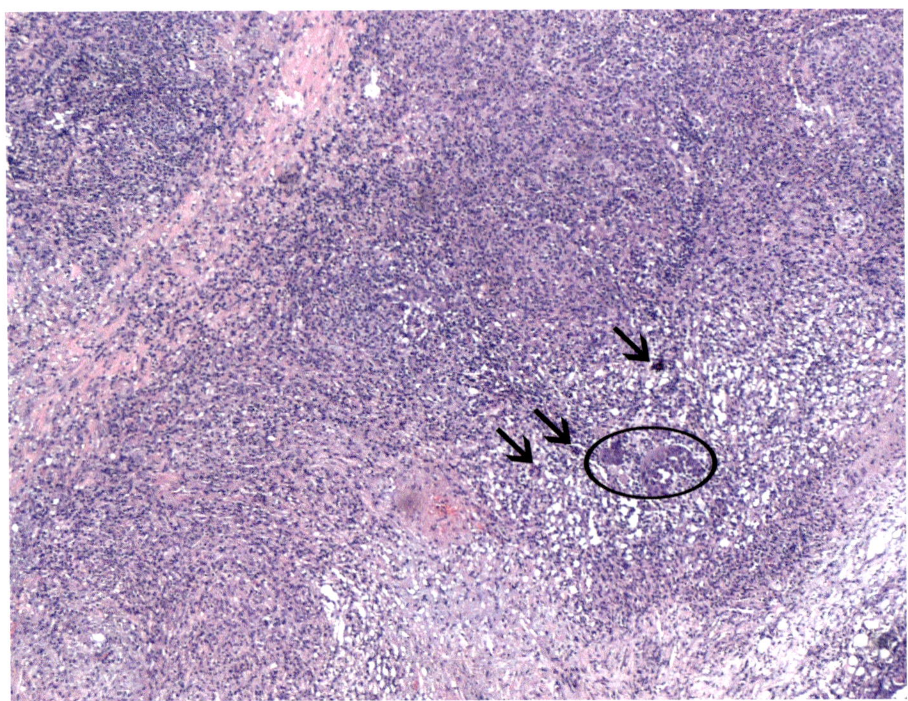

Fig. 3.21 (H-E, ×50) This is a case of another patient, 60 years old, with obstructive symptoms due to nonspecific (idiopathic) granulomatous prostatitis. Nonspecific granulomatous prostatitis is a rare disorder, but it is the most common granulomatous prostatitis seen on needle biopsy. It is defined as an immune-mediated, foreign-body inflammatory reaction to prostate secretions released into the prostate tissue by ruptured, obstructed ducts; therefore, it is most commonly seen in nodular hyperplasia/BPH of the prostate.

Nonspecific granulomatous prostatitis consists of noncaseating, lobular dense infiltrates of lymphocytes, plasma cells, and macrophages/histiocytes; many of the latter have a foamy appearance. The nodules of inflammation tend to obscure and efface ductal and acinar components (*ellipse*). The defining criterion for nonspecific granulomatous prostatitis is a prominent macrophage infiltration with the presence, in some instances, of multinucleated giant cells (*arrows*). Neutrophils and eosinophils make up a smaller component of the inflammatory infiltrate. Nonspecific granulomatous prostatitis tends to resolve spontaneously.

Nonspecific granulomatous prostatitis may clinically mimic carcinoma since prostate on palpitation can be firm, nodular, and indurated. Serum PSA can be significantly increased. Microscopically, an admixture of various types of inflammatory cells arranged in sheets is seen around ruptured ducts and acini. Inflammatory cell infiltrate is unusual in adenocarcinoma; however, sometimes it is difficult to distinguish prominent, cholesterol-laden macrophages or epithelioid histiocytes from a small focus of Gleason pattern 4/high-grade adenocarcinoma. The key feature to avoid a misdiagnosis of cancer is the recognition of a mixed inflammatory infiltrate and multinucleated giant cells. In case a high-grade adenocarcinoma is suspected, immunopositivity for histiocytic markers (e.g., CD68) combined with immunonegativity for epithelial markers (i.e., pancytokeratins) excludes malignancy.

Other types of granulomatous prostatitis include post-bacillus Calmette-Guerin (BCG) therapy (tuberculous involvement of the prostate), post-transurethral or post-biopsy pathogenesis (composed of a central region of fibrinoid necrosis surrounded by palisading epithelioid histiocytes), infectious etiology (special histochemical stains are recommended so that causative organisms are identified), and malakoplakia; in the latter, Michaelis-Gutmann bodies are highlighted by special histochemical stains, too

3.4.1.1 Clinical Commentary

Vasileios Spapis

This is a case of benign prostate hyperplasia (BPH) with focal inflammatory infiltrates and an incidentally diagnosed, low to intermediate grade, prostate acinar adenocarcinoma of Gleason score 5 and pT1a stage, in a 70-year-old patient, with a serum PSA value of 8 ng/ml.

BPH is very common among men. At the age of 75, about 50% of men mention a decrease in the force and caliber of their urinary stream (Cooperberg et al. 2013). Obstructive (hesitancy, decreased force and caliber of stream, double voiding, straining to urinate, etc.) and irritative symptoms (urgency, frequency, nocturia) could be both present. Several questionnaires have been proposed to assess the quality of life (QoL) of these patients, the most common of them being the IPSS which is recommended for all patients before the initiation of therapy. Physical examination, digital rectal examination (DRE), ultrasound examination of the whole urinary tract before and after urination, and focused neurologic examination should be performed on all patients. BPH usually results in a smooth, firm, elastic enlargement of the prostate. The size of the prostate gland does not correlate closely with the degree of obstruction or with clinical symptoms.

Most prostate carcinomas (PCas) are located in the peripheral zone and may be detected by DRE when their volume is >0.2 mL. In about 18% of cases, PCa is detected by suspect DRE alone, even when PSA levels are low. After all, there is no level of PSA below which prostate cancer risk falls to zero. Suspect DRE in patients with PSA level < 2 ng/mL has a positive predictive value of 5–30% (Carvalhal et al. 1999). Abnormal DRE is also associated with an increased risk of higher Gleason score when PCa is diagnosed. PSA level between 4 and 10 ng/ml has a positive predictive value of approximately 20–30% (Gosselaar et al. 2008; Okotie et al. 2007).

The first line of BPH treatment traditionally includes the use of a-blockers or 5-aRIs. When symptoms progress, surgery (TURP or open enucleation prostatectomy) is the next step. In cases where PCa is diagnosed through pathology report, patients are categorized in risk groups. A patient like the one of this case presentation, with T1a disease ("normal" DRE, tumor incidental histological finding in 5% or less of tissue resected), PSA < 10 ng/ml, and Gleason score < 7, is considered to be in the low-risk group. That means that no additional imaging for staging purposes is needed (Mottet et al. 2017).

Radical prostatectomy (RP) remains the gold standard for all cases of localized PCa in men with life expectancy of more than 10 years, offering excellent results regarding cancer-specific survival (CSS). However, analysis of men like the one herein (with low-risk PCa) showed that RP did not significantly reduce all-cause mortality or death from PCa at 10 years compared with deferred treatment [active surveillance (AS) or watchful waiting (WW)] (Mottet et al. 2017). Deferred treatment aims to reduce overtreatment of PCa. AS is recommended for low-risk patients with more than 10 years life expectancy; its goal is to minimize treatment-related toxicity without compromising survival. Patients remain under close surveillance. Treatment is dictated by predefined thresholds indicative of potentially life-threatening disease. WW, on the other hand, can apply to patients in all stages and has palliative intent. Another option for definitive treatment is external beam radiation therapy (EBRT) which can be offered to all risk groups of nonmetastatic PCa, especially when combined with neoadjuvant androgen deprivation therapy (ADT) (Mottet et al. 2017).

Key Messages

- Transurethral specimens consist of tissue from the transition zone, the urethra, periurethral tissues, bladder neck, and anterior fibromuscular stroma, whereas most needle biopsy specimens consist chiefly of tissue from the peripheral zone.
- Nodular hyperplasia is confined to the transition and periurethral zones, peripheral zone tissue being compressed as the nodules expand. The transition zone is the most common site for benign prostatic hyperplasia and adenosis.
- The Gleason grading system is based on the glandular pattern of the tumor as identified at relatively low magnification. Grading is of particular importance in prostatic cancer because it is the best marker, along with the stage, for predicting prognosis. Gleason scores of 2 to 4 indicate a low malignant potential and are often of transition zone origin. Tumors of the transitional zone are less aggressive than those of the peripheral zone.
- The term "prostatitis" should be reserved for those cases in which the clinical features encountered are due to the presence of the inflammation rather than for prostatic tissue in which a few aggregates of inflammatory cells are seen.

3.5 Case 3.2: Prostate Needle Biopsy Specimens

Case Study

The histologic diagnosis of prostate cancer on needle biopsy specimens can be challenging. In part, the difficulty stems from the scant amount of tissue available for histologic examination removed by the needle biopsy; biopsy often samples only a few malignant glands among many benign glands. In general, the diagnosis is made on the basis of a *constellation* of architectural, cytological, and ancillary (immunohistochemical) findings. Up to 5% of prostate needle biopsies may have small foci suspicious for, but not diagnostic of, adenocarcinoma which cannot be resolved by using immunohistochemistry. This finding warrants a second biopsy.

In the following five cases, prostate gland needle biopsies were obtained from five men with familial predisposition for prostate cancer, due to a gradual increase of their PSA values and/or an abnormal free to total PSA ratio. Digital examination of the prostate was unremarkable in all presented cases. Transrectal ultrasound (TRUS) guided the placement of the needle biopsies to thoroughly sample the gland.

The cores obtained contain various types of prostate glands in some of which certain criteria for the diagnosis of neoplasia are fulfilled. The question is whether their combination is adequate for a definite diagnosis of malignancy.

3.5.1 Microscopic Evaluation of the Biopsy Material

First Case

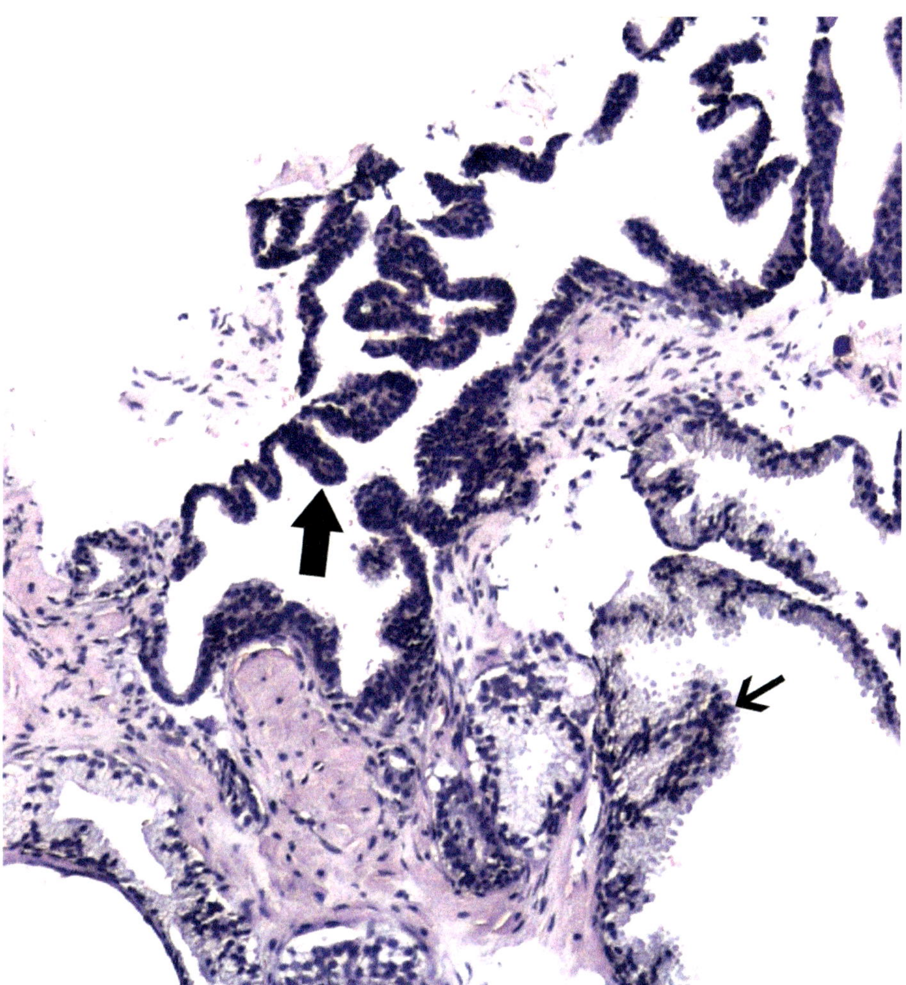

Fig. 3.22 (H-E, ×100) Prostatic intraepithelial neoplasia (PIN) is a term used to describe cellular dysplasia of the acinar/secretory prostatic epithelium. High-grade prostatic intraepithelial neoplasia (HG PIN) is most commonly found in medium- or large-sized acini/glands of the peripheral zone of the prostate. HG PIN is characterized by a neoplastic proliferation of acinar/secretory cells showing nuclear changes generally resembling those seen in cancer, within pre-existing ducts and acini with intraluminal papillary projections/infoldings (*thick arrow*), similar to adjacent, nonbasophilic, benign prostate glands (*thin arrow*). HG PIN tends to have a *basophilic* appearance, due to a combination of features, including enlarged nuclei, hyperchromasia, overlapping/pseudostratification of the nuclei, and epithelial hyperplasia; so it attracts our attention under *low* magnification.

PIN is a lesion of the peripheral zone and thus it is frequently encountered in needle biopsy material, like moderately to poorly differentiated prostate acinar adenocarcinoma of which HG PIN is the precursor lesion.

PIN does not elevate PSA but increases the risk of prostate cancer. Only high-grade PIN (not low-grade PIN) has been associated with an increased incidence of adenocarcinoma in follow-up biopsy (30%, if HG PIN is found in only one core; up to 75%, if HG PIN is found in more than three cores).

Low-grade PIN should not be mentioned in pathology reports

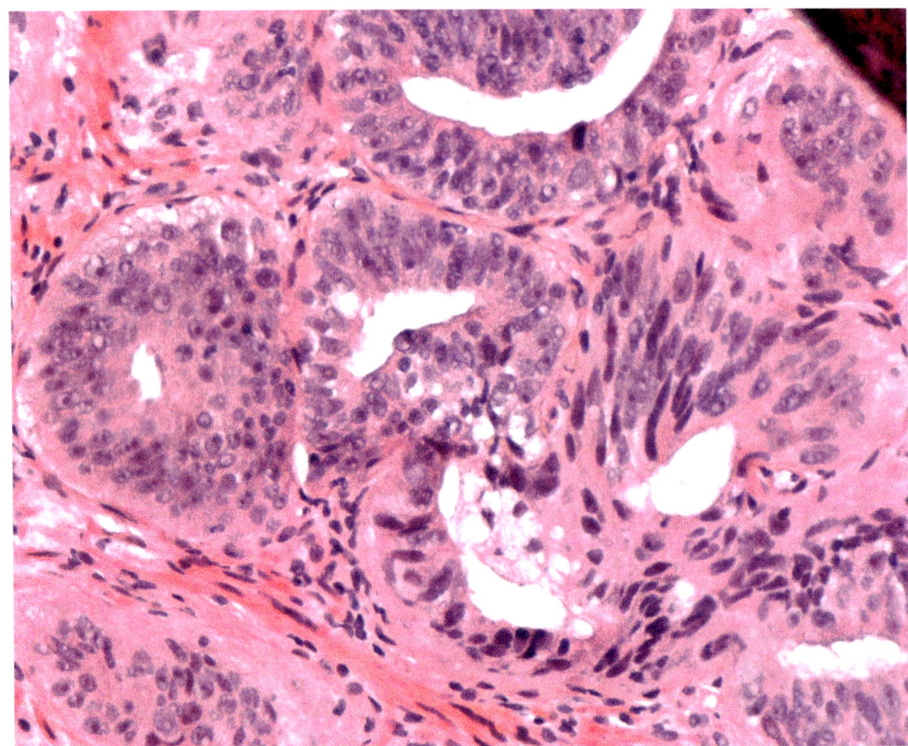

Fig. 3.23 (H-E, ×200) PIN-like (invasive) prostate acinar adenocarcinoma. This image is from another case in which simple, non-cribriform, medium-size glands are lined by two or more layers of evidently malignant non-columnar secretory/acinar cells with rounded nuclei (mainly on the left part of the figure) and columnar cells of ductal morphology with ovoid/cylindrical nuclei (on the right part), with either prominent nucleoli or nuclear hyperchromasia. The whole configuration resembles flat HG PIN, but these glands totally lack basal cells by immunohistochemistry.

It is noteworthy that a few prostate adenocarcinomas may have stratified epithelium and may form medium- to large-sized (PIN-like) glands resembling flat or tufted HG PIN. PIN is usually detected in single glands or small groups of glands with a lobular configuration. When numerous large glands are too crowded and back-to-back, immunodetection of basal cells will rule out a PIN-like acinar adenocarcinoma. Positive high molecular weight cytokeratin staining of basal layer elements distinguishes HG PIN from PIN-like carcinoma. If basal cells are not at all detected in a sufficient number of glands, the diagnosis of cancer can be made

Limited data shows that a component of PIN-like adenocarcinoma with either acinar or ductal epithelial features has behavior akin to Gleason pattern 3 acinar adenocarcinoma; so, PIN-like ductal adenocarcinoma should be differentiated from traditional ductal adenocarcinoma due to differences in biological behavior and grade (see Case 3.6)

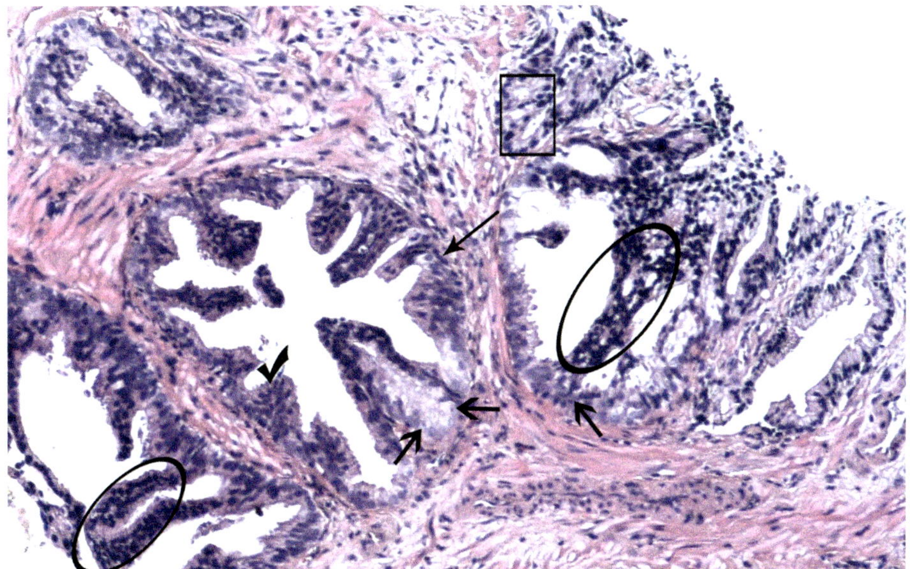

Fig. 3.24 (H-E, ×100) HG PIN. Basophilic, medium- to large-sized, branched glands with intra-acinar proliferations of cells that demonstrate uniform nuclear anaplasia, mainly basally. Nuclei are enlarged, elongated, and pseudostratified, with focally to diffusely detected, visible nucleoli (*short arrows*). Some degree of nuclear enlargement of acinar/secretory cells, orientated basally, perpendicular to the basement membrane (*short arrows*), is observed.

Diagnosis of HG PIN should be made conservatively (cells must ideally show both nucleomegaly and nucleolomegaly). Nuclear atypia in HG PIN consists of loss of polarity, numerous visible eccentric nucleoli, and quite uniform atypia in acinar/secretory cells (i.e., cuboidal cells with round nuclei) close to the basement membrane. At least some basal cells (*long arrow*) should be present in PIN. It is noteworthy that, occasionally, basal cells show prominent nucleoli, mimicking HG PIN.

Within HG PIN epithelial projections, the nuclei toward the center of the gland sometimes tend to have a more bland cytologic appearance compared with the nuclei peripherally, located up against the basement membrane (maturation phenomenon). Note that acinar/secretory cells toward the center (*ellipses*) exhibit nuclei with more benign morphology compared to the basally orientated acinar/secretory cells (by which PIN grading should be made); this maturation phenomenon can be observed in HG PIN. This phenomenon, when present, along with the quite uniform atypia of acinar/secretory cells discriminates HG PIN from intraductal carcinoma of the prostate.

The commonest architectural pattern of PIN is the tufted one (*tick*); other patterns [i.e., flat, micropapillary, cribriform, inverted] frequently coexist. Complex architecture with bridges and occasional cribriform formations may be occasionally encountered in PIN glands (*square frame*). It can be difficult to differentiate between HG PIN with cribriform architecture and invasive adenocarcinoma of Gleason pattern 4. Basal cells should be found in PIN, albeit potentially decreased in number and partly disconnected from each other. As far as Gleason pattern 5 is concerned, as a rule, in HG PIN, central comedo necrosis is totally absent or very limited and focal, in contrast to Gleason pattern 5 acinar and ductal prostate adenocarcinomas.

The grade of PIN is assigned based on assessment of the nuclei peripherally located up against the basement membrane rather than the often more bland-appearing nuclei toward the center of the gland, as previously mentioned. In contrast to Gleason's grading, HG PIN is defined *cytologically* by the presence of macronucleoli, regardless of architecture. The safest hallmark distinguishing low-grade and high-grade PIN is the presence of prominent nucleoli

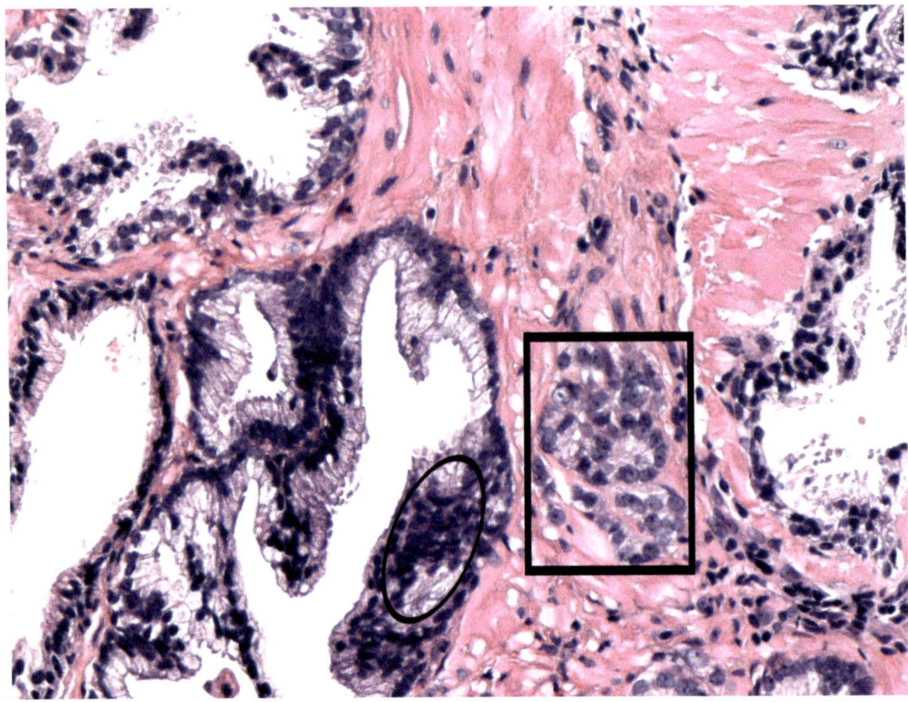

Fig. 3.25 (H-E, ×100) PIN with high degree of crowding/stratification (*ellipse*) and adjacent small atypical glands with distinct nucleoli (*square frame*) suspicious for cancer. The latter may represent a minute focus of invasive prostate carcinoma or tangential sectioning of a HG PIN gland with its basally orientated acinar/secretory cells having enlarged, atypical nuclei. Early stromal invasion, the earliest evidence of carcinoma, can occur at sites of acinar outpouching and basal cell disruption of acini/glands with HG PIN. In foci of HG PIN with budding/tangentially sectioned glands, the atypical glands may fuse with HG PIN on levels, but the absence of fusion should *not* be taken as evidence supporting a diagnosis of invasive carcinoma.

In this PIN gland and these few, right-adjacent atypical glands (PIN-ATYP), immunohistochemistry would not be particularly useful. Racemase (AMACR) would be expectedly expressed both in the PIN focus and in the adjacent small atypical glands. At least some basal cells would be identified in HG PIN focus and perhaps in the small glands nearby; in the latter case, diagnosis of malignancy would be excluded. In case the small atypical glands were completely devoid of basal cells, the uncertainty would remain because the small atypical glands are too close to the HG PIN gland to be considered invasive. Meticulous examination of this biopsy material in its entirety is mandatory, of course, so that invasive cancer developing elsewhere is not overlooked.

We should bear in mind that the diagnosis of cancer cannot be safely made if *a few* PIN-adjacent, small atypical glands (PIN-ATYP) lack basal cells, even completely. Negative staining for high molecular weight cytokeratin (34βE12) in such PIN-ATYP glands foci has not been helpful in predicting risk of cancer on repeat biopsy, either

Second Case

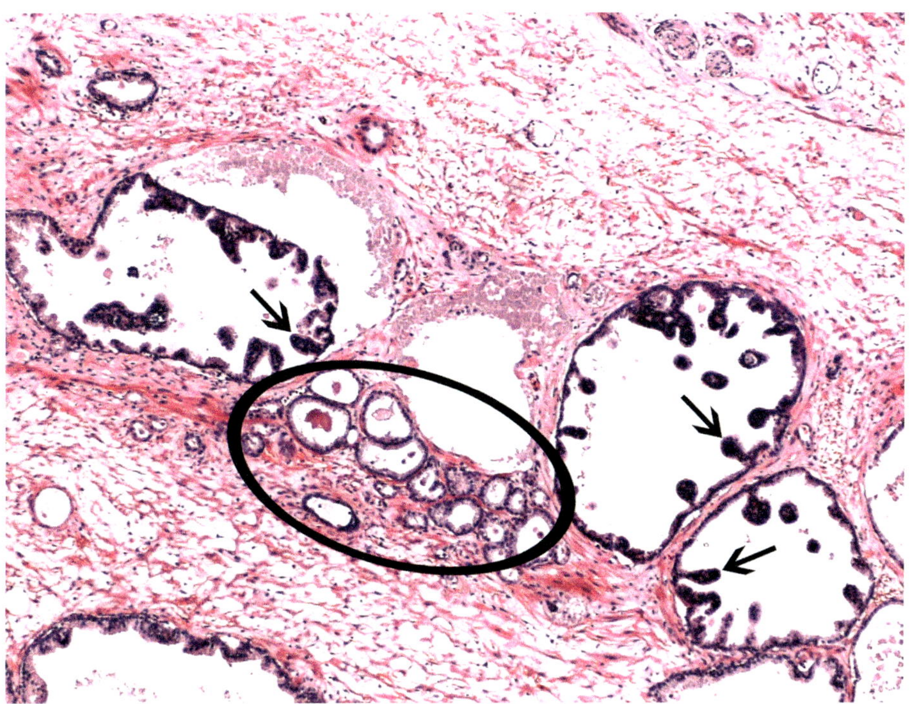

Fig. 3.26 (H-E, ×50) Development of prostate acinar adenocarcinoma (small-sized cancerous glands) adjacent to HG PIN of the micropapillary type (*arrows*).

HG PIN consists of widely separated, larger branching glands with papillary infolding; in contrast, invasive cancer is typically characterized by small, crowded glands with straight luminal borders (*ellipse*). Cytologically, the two processes may be identical; furthermore, they both predominate in the peripheral zone.

HG PIN is a low-power diagnosis. Basophilic appearance at low power is due to enlarged hyperchromatic nuclei and amphophilic cytoplasm. It is possible to diagnose PIN in the absence of prominent nucleoli, based on nuclear pleomorphism, marked hyperchromasia (as in this case and in Fig. 3.22), and/or mitotic figures.

In this field, glands of cancer (*ellipse*) have probably budded from HG PIN. Their *number* and their *considerable distance* from HG PIN foci are sufficient to make a diagnosis of prostate acinar adenocarcinoma, since all these small glands are unlikely to represent outpouchings of HG PIN. Infiltrative carcinoma between HG PIN glands can be diagnosed if the small infiltrating glands are too numerous or too far away (> 0.4 mm) from the HG PIN glands

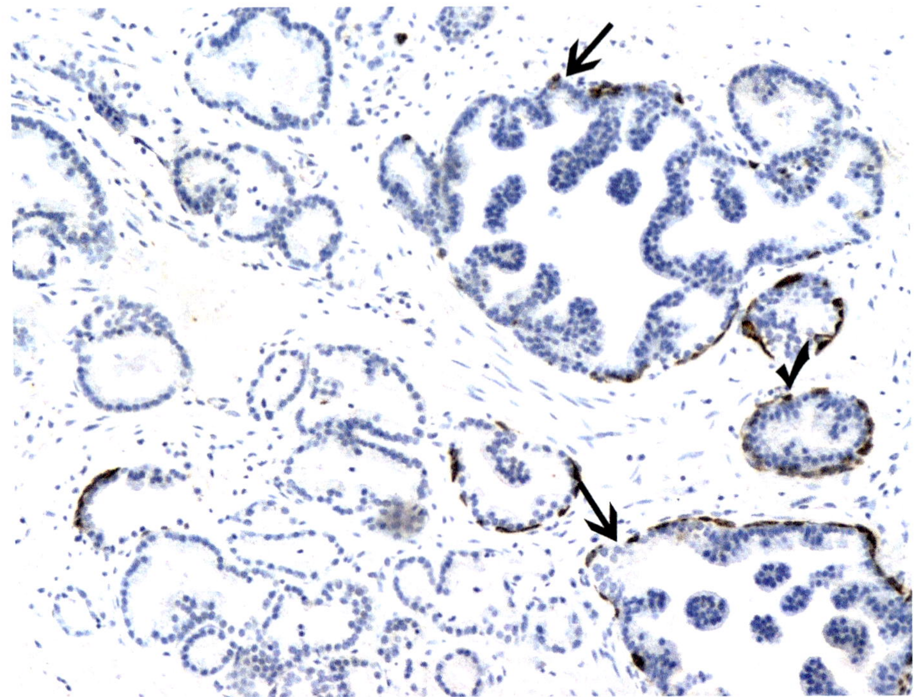

Fig. 3.27 [Immunohistochemistry for HMW CK (34βE12), ×100] Immunohistochemistry results of the previous lesion. PIN and adjacent carcinoma of Gleason pattern 3, score 6(=3 + 3), budding off HG PIN.

PIN retains an intact or fragmented (*arrow*) basal cell layer, whereas cancer does not. Basal cells are present in PIN glands but may be attenuated. Remnants of the thin basal cell layer are observable both in PIN glands (*arrow*) and their outpouchings (*tick*), while, in this field, an *adequate number* of glands are *completely* immunonegative for the basal cell immunomarker (about 20 cancerous glands). Remember that in order to diagnose cancer, a sufficient number of glands (at least three) should be completely devoid of basal cells

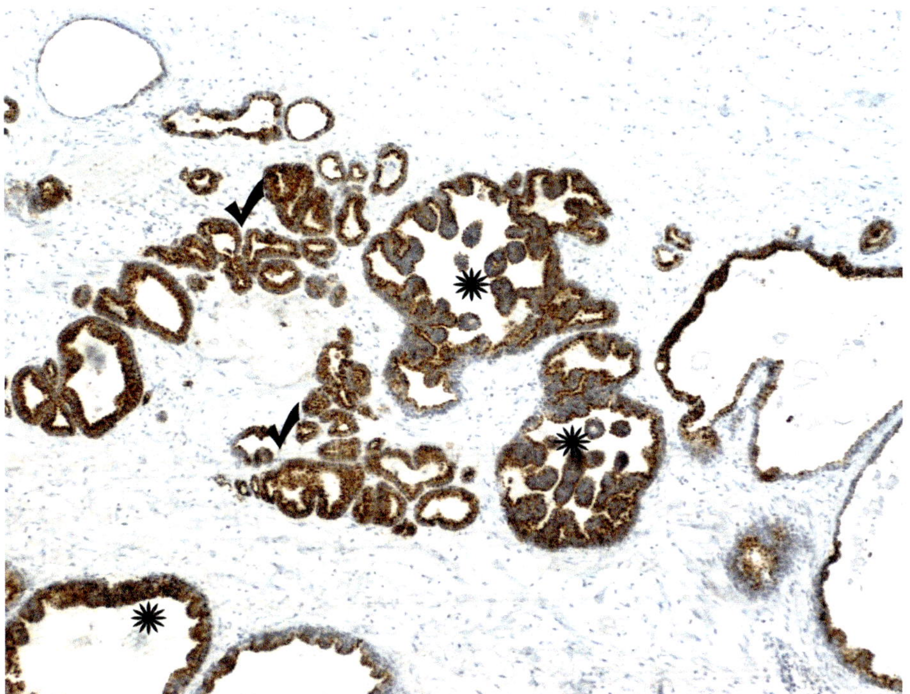

Fig. 3.28 [Immunohistochemistry for AMACR (racemase), ×50] AMACR is useful for staining of the dysplastic acinar/secretory cells of PIN.

It has been reported that HG PIN adjacent to carcinoma is more likely to show AMACR expression (56%) than HG PIN distant from carcinoma (14%); those cases with any HG PIN gland that is AMACR-positive are 5.2x more likely to show carcinoma on repeat biopsy than completely AMACR-negative HG PIN.

Here, AMACR is strongly expressed both in HG PIN glands (*asterisks*) and in adjacent cancerous glands (*ticks*). HG PIN is known to be often AMACR-positive; this staining is arguably more apical and granular and less intense than that of carcinoma. In any case, AMACR cannot distinguish between non-invasive and invasive neoplastic epithelium; so, it is of no use in the diagnosis of acinar adenocarcinoma adjacent to HG PIN.

Third Case

Needle biopsies are taken from the prostate of a middle-aged man with a mild, though gradual, increase in his serum PSA values up to 6.7 ng/ml (the "gray zone" for PSA increased values is between 4 and 10 ng/ml). A reduced free to total PSA ratio (i.e., lower than 0.20) is found; so, multiple biopsies are taken, even though digital examination of the prostate and TRUS have been unremarkable.

After the pathology report, the patient's close follow-up is considered necessary

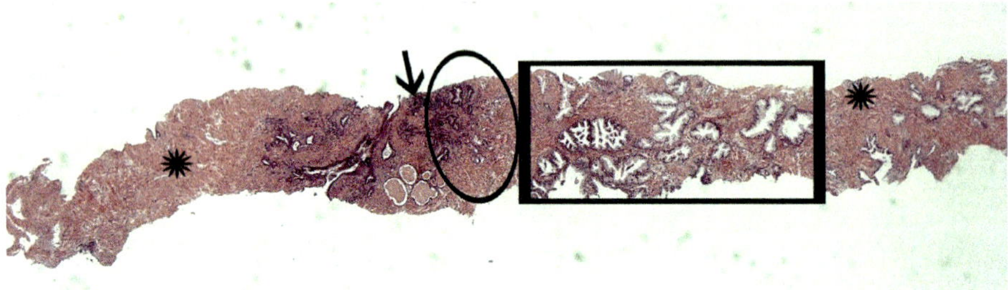

Fig. 3.29 (H-E, ×20). Under low magnification, we notice prostate glands of medium/large and small size (*square frame* and *ellipse*, respectively), some basophilic areas (*arrow*), and the fibromuscular prostate stroma (*asterisks*).

As previously stated, the epithelium of noncancerous prostate glands consists of basal cells [which are immunoreactive to high molecular weight cytokeratins such as 34βE12 and CK5/6) and p63] and luminal acinar/secretory cells. With regard to their luminal border, noncancerous prostate glands frequently demonstrate micropapillary projections/folds, unless they are atrophic

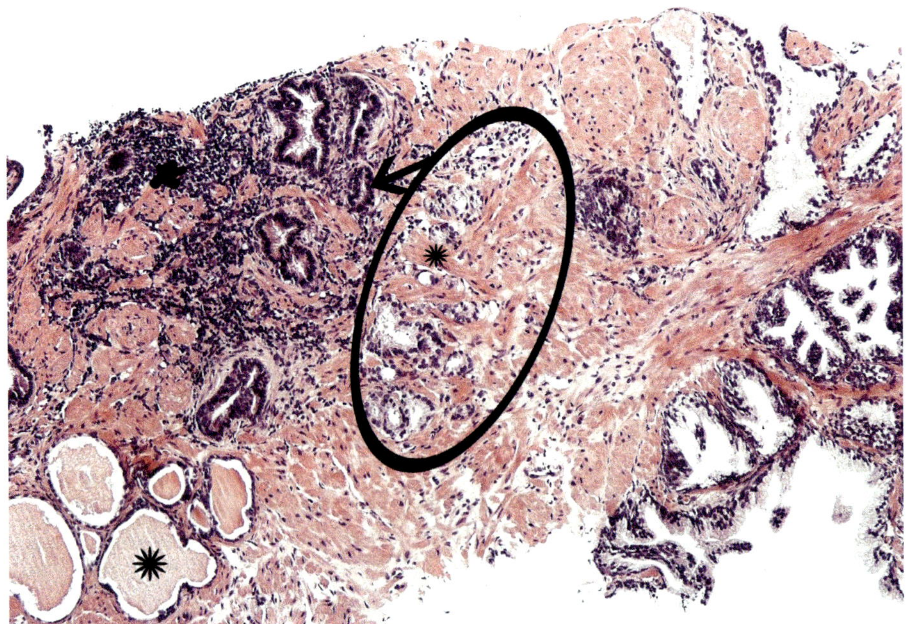

Fig. 3.30 (H-E, ×100). Under medium magnification, we notice that the focally basophilic appearance of the fibromuscular stroma is due to lymphocytic aggregates (*blob*)

Fig. 3.30 (continued)

The conventional, acinar type of adenocarcinoma usually consists of small-sized glands. There are three types of small-sized prostate glands in the present field:

(a) The more basophilic ones (*arrow*) may show either reactive atypia (due to inflammation), complete (simple) atrophy, or basal cell hyperplasia (the latter condition, however, is mainly observed in the transition zone of the prostate gland, and thus it is not likely to be detected in needle biopsy specimens which are mainly taken from the peripheral zone of the gland).
(b) The glands with microcystic dilation (*big asterisk*) are probably atrophic.
(c) The central ones (*ellipse*) which are vertically orientated alongside the biopsy are suspicious for cancer. The cells in the latter glands contain a sufficient amount of cytoplasm, in contrast to the atrophic ones. Furthermore, the suspicious glands interrupt the muscular bundles of the prostate stroma (*small asterisk*)

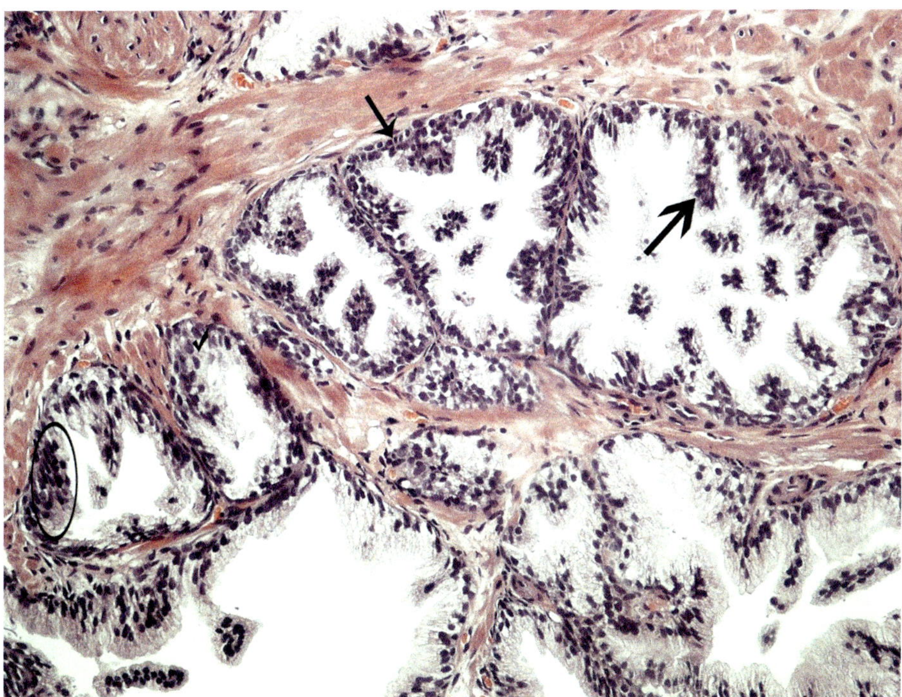

Fig. 3.31 (H-E, ×100). Nearby, we notice prostate glands of a larger size with luminal micropapillary folds (*big arrow*) and of a slightly basophilic appearance due to focal crowding of nuclei (*ellipse*).The size of the glands and their folded luminal border are against the diagnosis of invasive malignancy. Furthermore, basal cells are probably present in these glands (*small arrow*). As far as acinar cells are concerned, no uniform atypia (consistent with HG PIN) is noticeable. Focally, a nucleus located rather close to the basement membrane (*tick*) is of bigger size by comparison to other nuclei toward the center of the lumen. This implies some sort of maturation which could be indicative of PIN; nevertheless, it is not so consistently detected in the above glands, so the diagnosis of HG PIN cannot be safely made in this H-E field. This morphology might imply low-grade PIN, a lesion which should not be reported in the pathologic examination since it is of ambiguous clinical significance. To sum up, these large glands should finally be considered as normal, not dysplastic

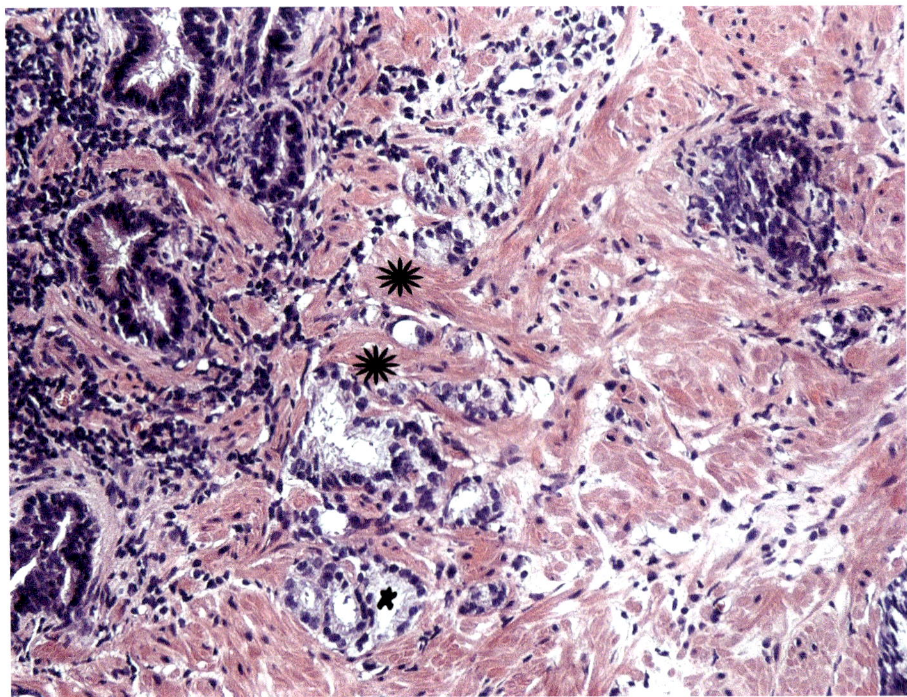

Fig. 3.32 (H-E, ×100). Let's have a closer look at the suspicious glands in the center of this image. Note their vertical orientation, the interruption of muscular bundles (*asterisks*), the sufficient amount of cytoplasm, and their sharp luminal borders (*blob*).

In addition to the suspicious glands, on the left side, we notice the basophilic, small-sized, atrophic glands surrounded by inflammation

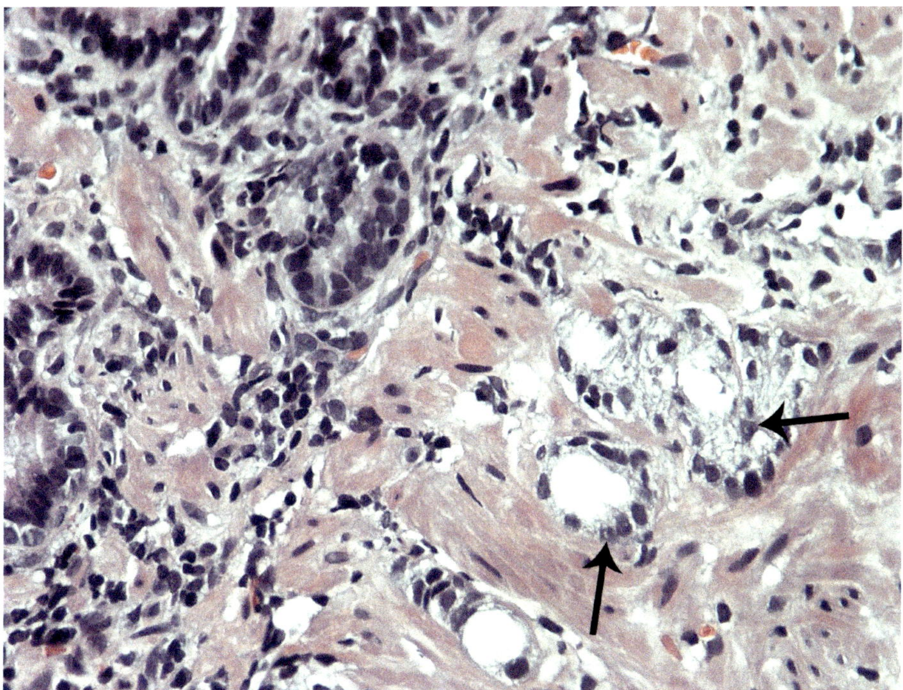

Fig. 3.33 (H-E, ×200) Conspicuous nucleoli (*arrows*) in the nuclei of suspicious glands.

Neighboring basophilic atrophic glands are surrounded by some inflammatory cells. Minimal nuclear atypia in prostate epithelial cells can be justified by inflammation.

In some glands with sharp luminal borders, epithelial cells' nuclei have visible and occasionally conspicuous nucleoli (*arrows*). Prominent nucleoli favor the diagnosis of prostate adenocarcinoma. Moreover, some of the nuclei in the suspicious glands are hyperchromatic. Since elements of the basal cell layer are not always easy and safe to identify in H-E sections, immunohistochemistry with specific markers against basal cells [i.e., high molecular weight cytokeratins, HMW CK (e.g., 34βE12, CK5/6)] is performed

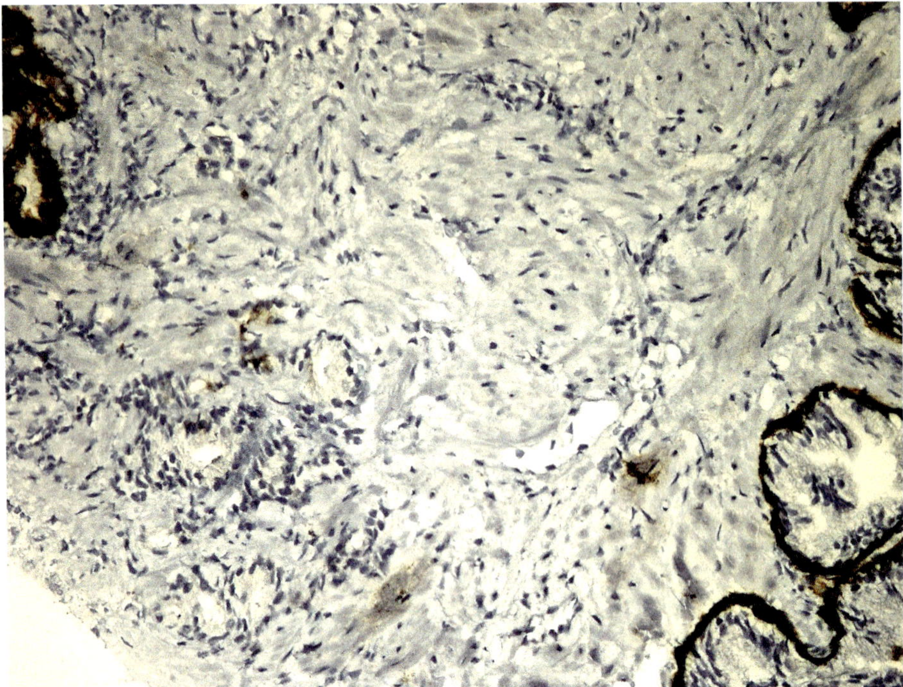

Fig. 3.34 (HMW CK immunohistochemistry, ×100). An intact HMW CK-immunoreactive, basal cell layer is noticed in normal prostate glands at the right side. Relatively increased immunoreactivity is noticed in the small-sized glands at the left side by comparison to the other benign prostate glands at the right side. The glands on the left correspond to the basophilic, small-sized, atrophic glands we noticed in the previous H-E sections (Figs. 3.30, 3.32, and 3.33); glands with complete (simple) atrophy are indeed basophilic in H-E sections, and since their luminal cells frequently appear somehow atrophic, the HMW CK-immunoreactive, intact basal cells do predominate, as in this field

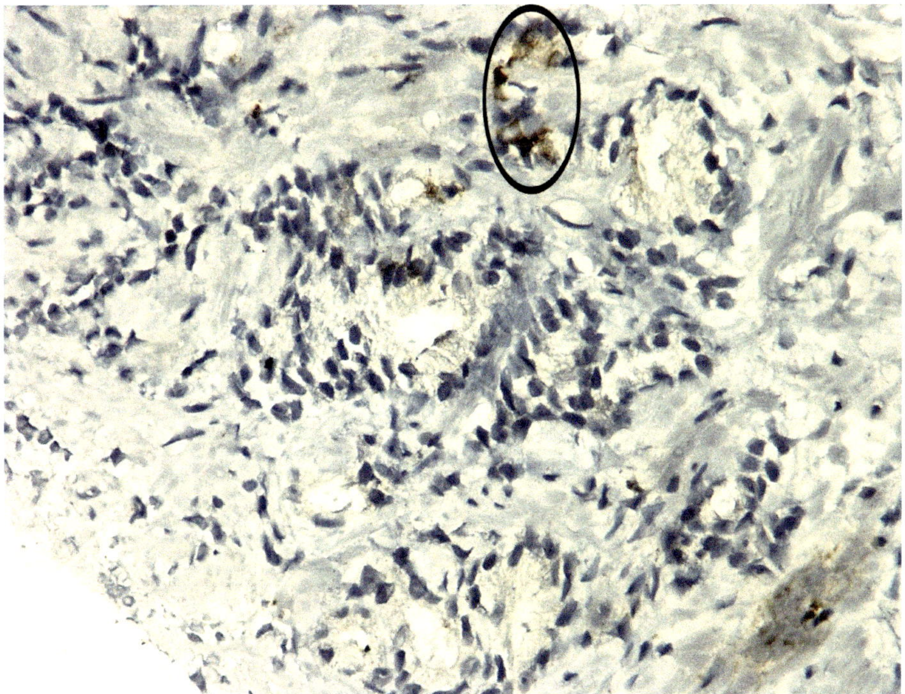

Fig. 3.35 (HMW CK immunohistochemistry, ×200). With regard to the suspicious glands, no specific immunostaining against basal cells is observed; so, these glands appear to lack basal cells, not entirely though. A minimal immunostaining, possibly aberrant, is detectable in one or two glands (*ellipse*). We cannot be sure whether this represents remnants of the basal cell layer or not. In order to make a diagnosis of prostate cancer with certainty, we shouldn't be able to observe any basal cells at all; otherwise, the diagnosis of cancer should be made with extreme caution

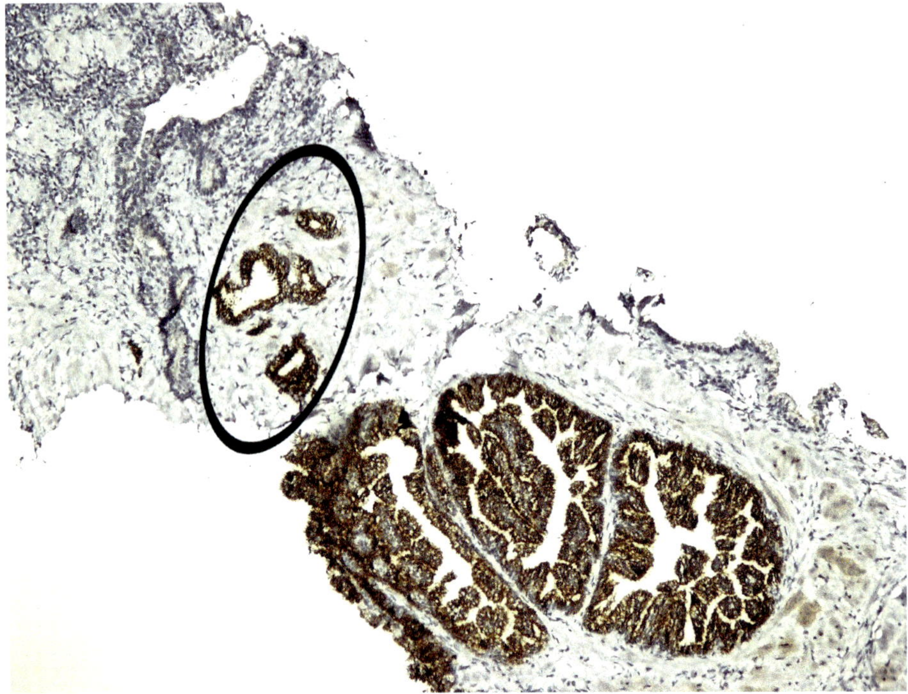

Fig. 3.36 (AMACR-racemase immunohistochemistry, ×50). Additional immunohistochemistry is performed, this time against AMACR (racemase). As previously mentioned, this enzyme is mainly detected in neoplastic prostatic epithelium. We can see that this marker is strongly expressed both in the small-sized suspicious glands (*ellipse*) and in the larger prostate glands which we had considered of almost normal morphology. When AMACR is expressed in normal glands, it loses its specificity as a prostate cancer marker.

The small-sized, benign basophilic glands with complete atrophy and prominent basal cells (left side) are AMACR-immunonegative, since basal cells do not express AMACR.

In conclusion, as far as the present biopsy specimen is concerned, there is some evidence that a prostate acinar adenocarcinoma of intermediate grade [Gleason score 6 (3 + 3), prognostic group 1 out of 5] has developed in only one of the cylinders and to a limited extent. All the rest of the patient's material was unremarkable with regard to prostate neoplasia. Since, however, the pathologist may not be fully convinced due to ambiguous immunohistochemical results, the term "atypical small acinar proliferation (ASAP) favoring malignancy" can be used in the pathology report.

Taking into account that PSA values are below 10 ng/ml and that this presumptive limited prostate carcinoma has no high-grade component, surgery is not necessary; a close follow-up of the patient seems adequate.

The histologic features that most often preclude a definitive diagnosis of malignancy are the small size of the focus (70% of cases), disappearance on step levels (61%), lack of significant cytologic atypia such as nucleolomegaly (55%), and presence of associated inflammation, either acute or chronic (9%), raising the possibility of one of many mimics of adenocarcinoma, such as atrophy or reactive acini/glands.

The following images are derived from prostate gland biopsies of two patients (Figs. 3.37, 3.38, 3.39, 3.40, 3.41 and 3.42, respectively) in which the diagnosis of limited prostate carcinoma was made

Fourth Case

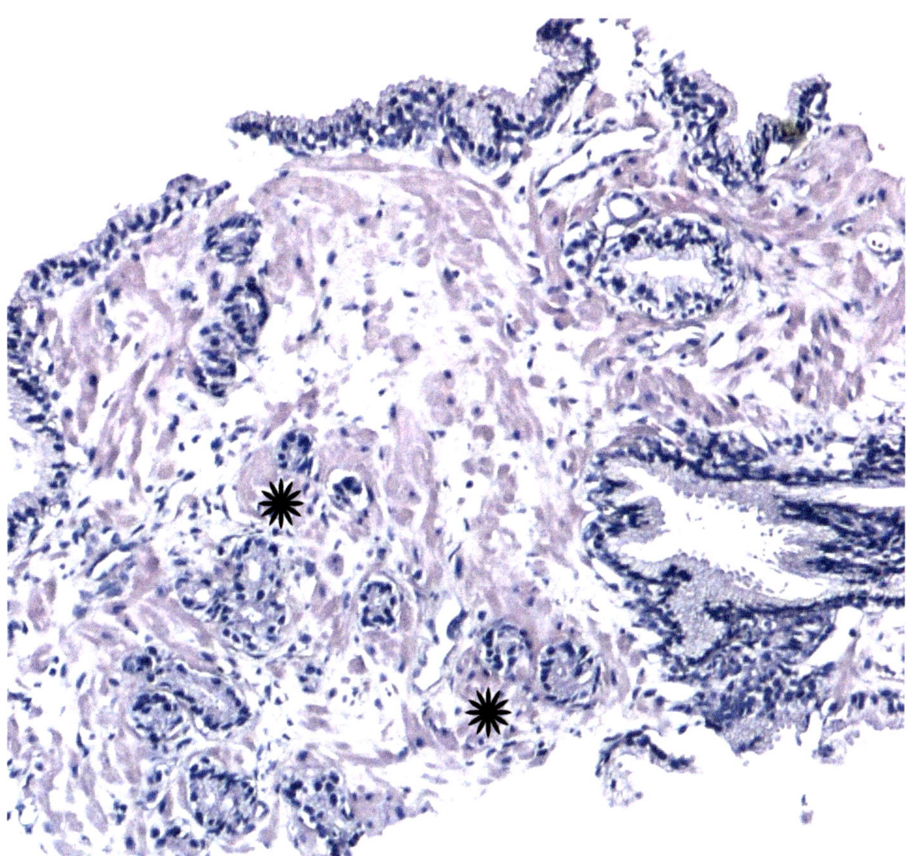

Fig. 3.37 (H-E, ×100) It is uncommon for a diagnosis of limited tumor to be based solely on the architectural pattern without some definitive cytological features of malignancy. The nuclei in these small glands appear hyperchromatic; however, it's the small gland's haphazard arrangement in relation to the fibromuscular stroma (*asterisks*) that justifies their immunohistochemical investigation

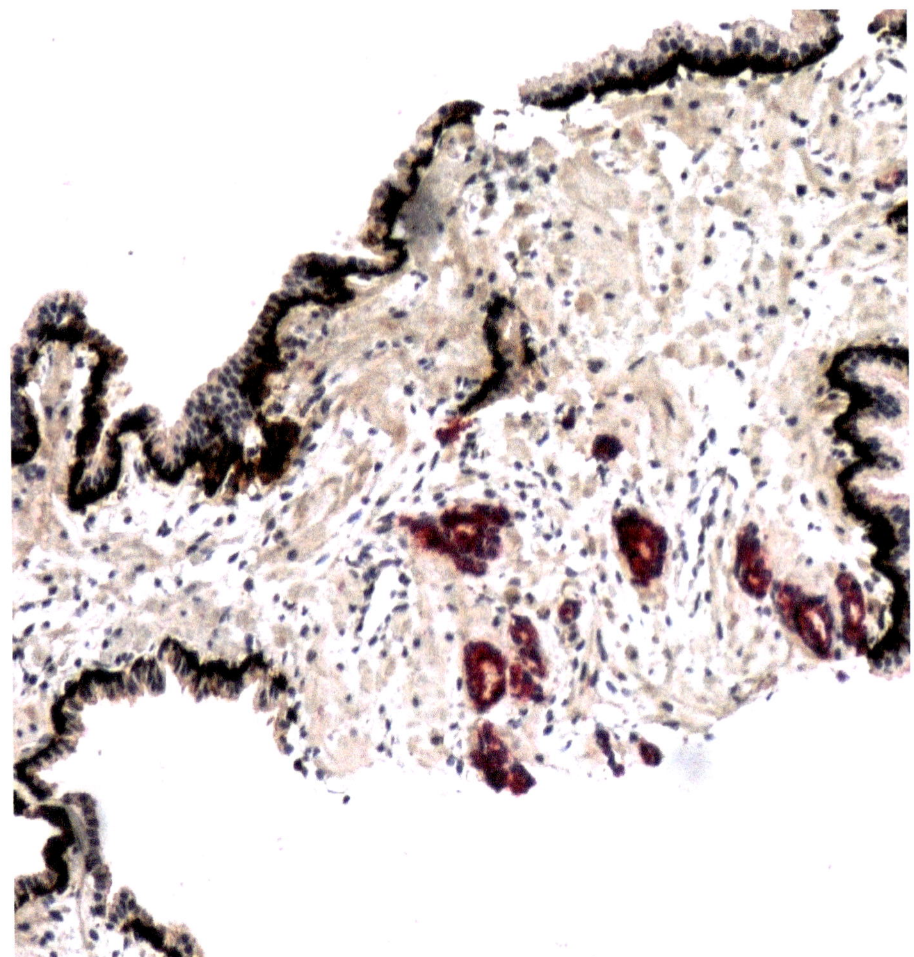

Fig. 3.38 [Double immunohistochemistry for HMW CK 34βE12(*brown color*) and AMACR (*red color*), ×100] Dual chromogen antibody cocktails utilize two chromogens, red for AMACR and brown for basal cell marker; positive marker AMACR complements negative basal cell marker in carcinoma.

The complete absence of basal cells (morphologically and immunohistochemically) in an adequate number of glands in conjunction with AMACR selective immunopositivity does favor the diagnosis of prostate adenocarcinoma, here of a Gleason score 6 (=3 + 3).

The small amount of cancerous tissue has nothing to do with its grading according to Gleason system.

Also remember that the lowest Gleason score which can be diagnosed in needle biopsy material is that of 6 (=3 + 3)

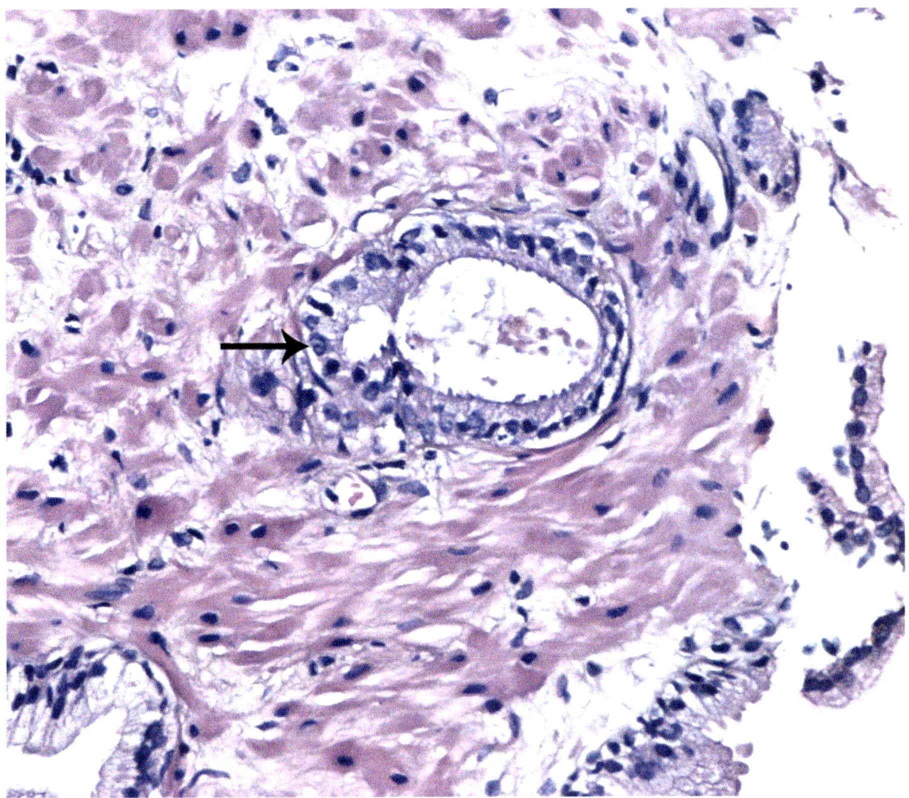

Fig. 3.39 (H-E, ×200) Another minimal focus of a suspicious small gland in the material of the previous patient. Visible nucleolus (*arrow*), sharp luminal border, intraluminal pink amorphous secretion

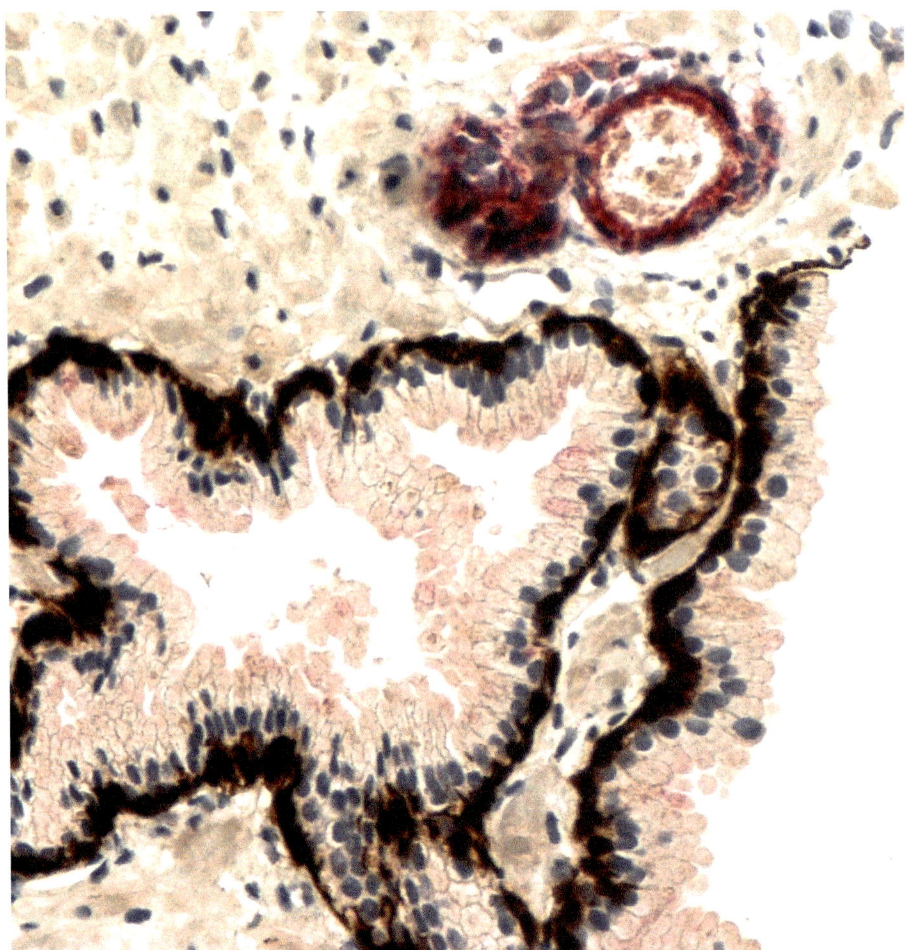

Fig. 3.40 [Double immunohistochemistry for HMW CK 34βE12 (*brown color*) and AMACR (*red color*), ×200] Dual chromogen antibody cocktails utilize two chromogens, red for AMACR and brown for basal cell marker. Positive marker AMACR again complements negative basal cell marker in minimal carcinoma glandular elements.

If this was the only lesion in the cores, despite the AMACR overexpression (*red*) and lack of basal cell markers (*brown*), typical of carcinoma, this would be regarded as "ASAP suspicious for focal adenocarcinoma," given the presence of only two glands.

Of importance, negative staining for HMW CK in only a few glands suspicious for cancer is not a proof of their malignancy; loss of basal cells per se is nonspecific/non-pathognomonic for carcinoma and may be observed in benign, pseudoneoplastic conditions, partial atrophy, in particular.

Specific AMACR (racemase) immunostaining can be quite helpful in the confirmation of malignancy as far as ordinary, moderately differentiated prostate acinar adenocarcinoma is concerned. On the other hand, negative staining with AMACR in suspicious foci does not necessarily indicate a benign diagnosis

Fifth Case

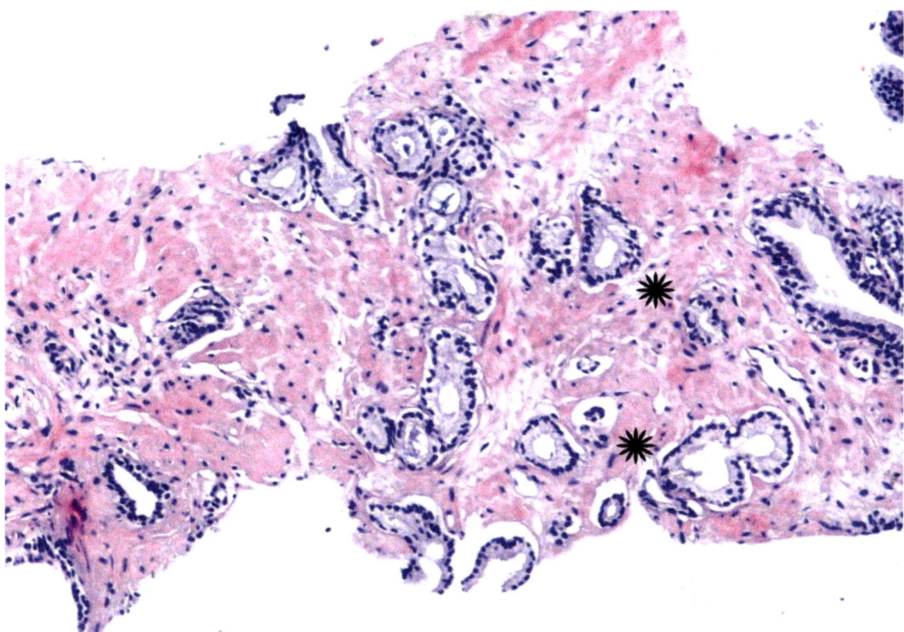

Fig. 3.41 (H-E, ×100) Linear row of small glands spanning the width of the core combined with their adjacent haphazard arrangement interrupting the stroma (*asterisks*) is evidence of invasion of prostate fibromuscular stroma by cancerous glands. Lack of stromal reaction is usual in prostate acinar adenocarcinoma. Blue wispy mucin is detected in the lumens of some cancerous glands

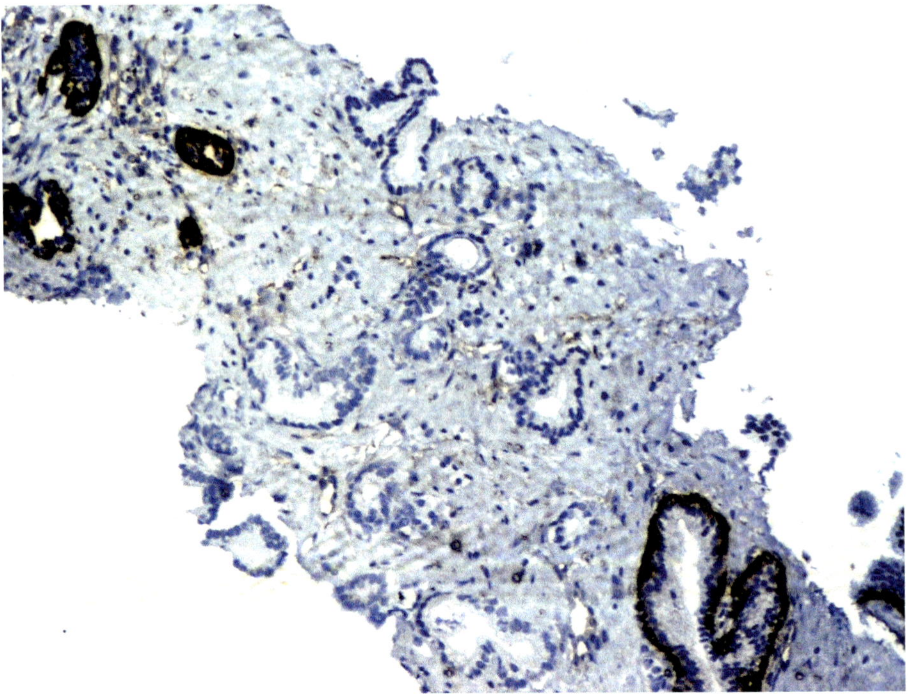

Fig. 3.42 [Immunohistochemistry for HMW CK 34βE12, ×100].

High molecular weight cytokeratin (CK34βE12) immunoreactivity in basal cells of noncancerous prostate glands, either normal with papillary infolding (down, right side) or atrophic (up, left side).

Complete lack of basal cells in cancerous glands at the center, evidenced by negative immunostaining against high molecular weight cytokeratin 34βE12.

Here are four more pictures of minimal prostate acinar adenocarcinoma from four other patients, the first two of Gleason score 6 (=3 + 3), grade group 1, and the remaining two of Gleason score 8 (=4 + 4), grade group 4.

Let's point out again that low tumor burden on needle biopsy does not necessarily indicate low-volume, low-stage cancer

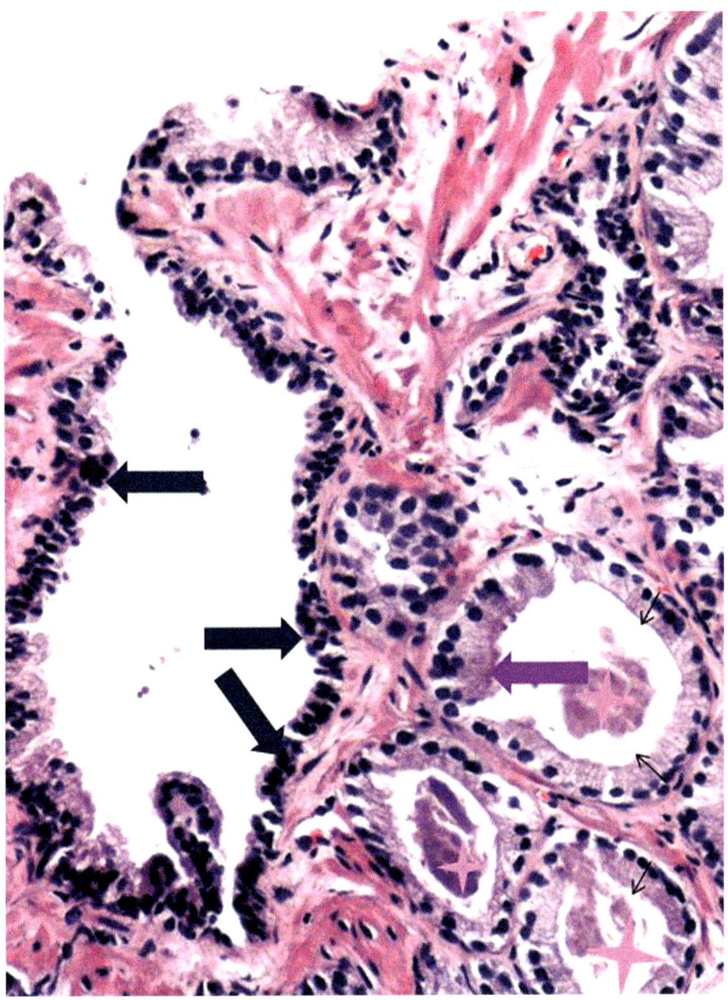

Fig. 3.43 (H-E, ×200) Cancerous glands adjacent to an atrophic gland. Abundant, amphophilic cytoplasm of cancerous glands (*purple arrow*) in contrast to the little amount of cytoplasm in the remaining basophilic basal cells (*dark blue arrows*) of an adjacent, benign gland with complete (simple) atrophy. In cancerous glands, the abundant cytoplasm is noticed over (and not among) the nuclei, up to their sharp luminal borders (*thin black arrows*). Intraluminal pink amorphous secretions are noticed in cancerous glands with sharp luminal borders (*pink asterisks*)

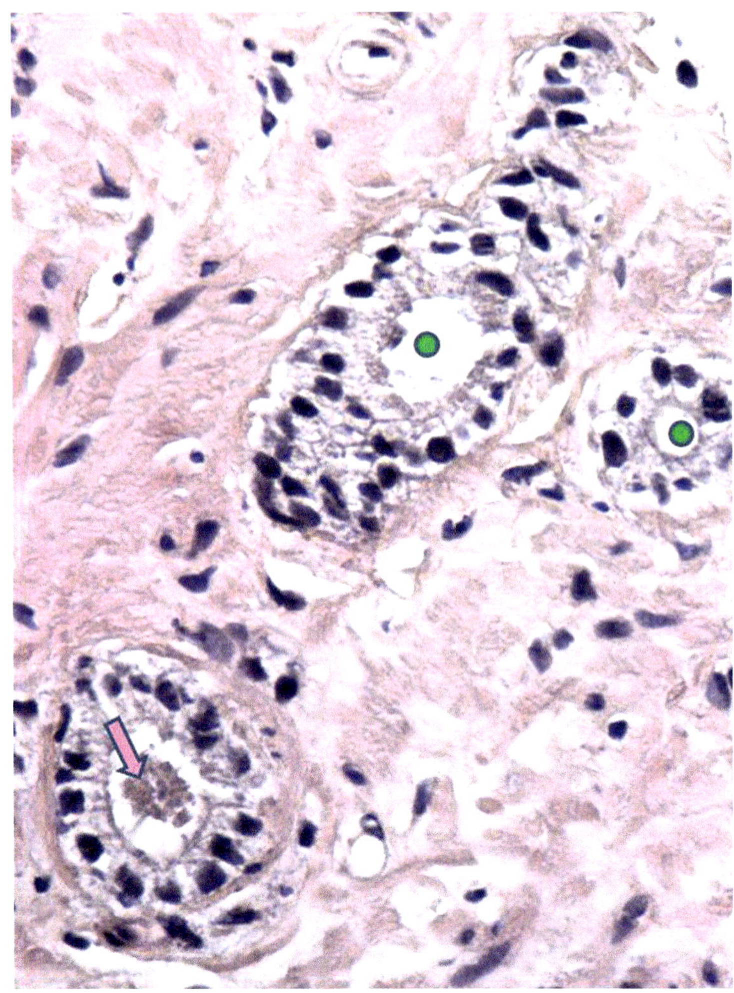

Fig. 3.44 (H-E, ×200) Minimal adenocarcinoma (only three cancerous glands). Nuclear enlargement and hyperchromasia. Sharp luminal border (*green circles*). Pink amorphous secretion (*pink arrow*)

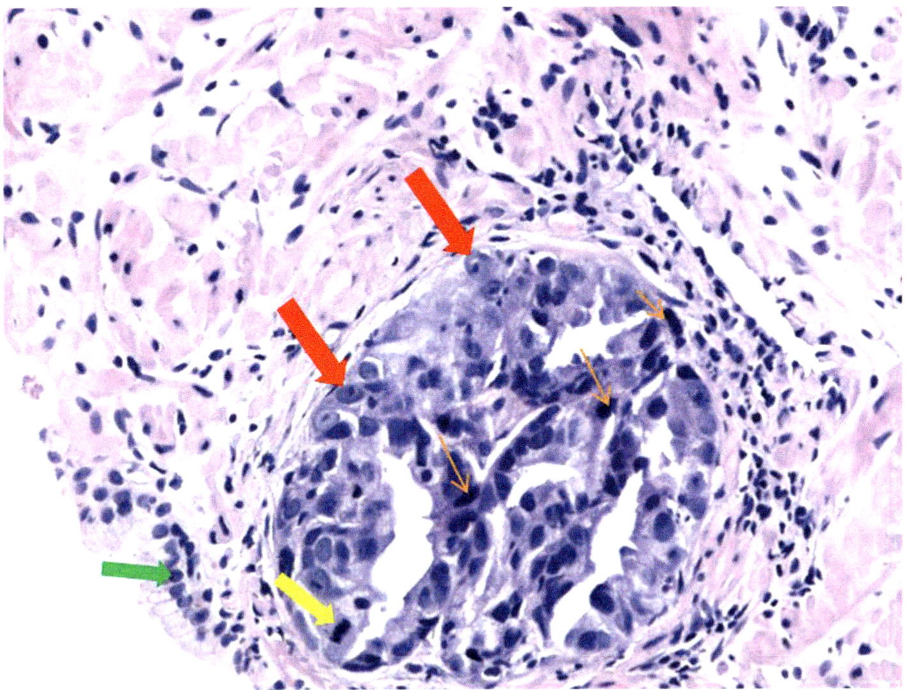

Fig. 3.45 (H-E, ×200) Frankly malignant nuclear features of fused glandular structures, under intermediate magnification. Malignant cells' features are better estimated when compared with features of normal adjacent prostate acinar/secretory (not basal) cells (*green arrow*). Nuclear enlargement is here easily appreciated even when a comparison to adjacent normal prostate cell nuclei would not be possible. Nuclear hyperchromasia (*thin orange arrows*). Prominent nucleoli which would have been identifiable even with the 10X lens (*red arrows*). Mitotic activity (*yellow arrow*)

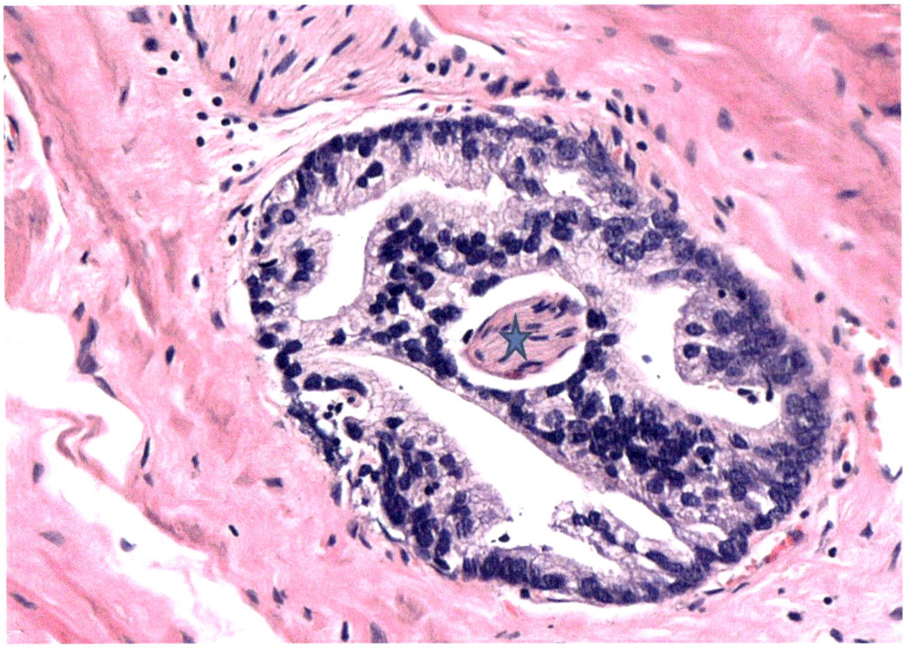

Fig. 3.46 (H-E, ×200) Conventional acinar adenocarcinoma of the prostate with merging cancerous glands resulting in cribriform architecture (Gleason pattern 4). Concomitant atypical acinar/secretory cell morphology. Perineural invasion (*asterisk*) is pathognomonic of cancer and definitively rules out the diagnosis of HG PIN.

Perineural invasion should be combined with atypical cellular morphology. For perineural involvement to be used as the key diagnostic feature to establish malignancy in a given case, complete circumferential growth around the nerve must be evident, particularly when the glands have cytological and architectural features more typically associated with benign glands.

Often, partially perineural glandular tissue per se is not indicative of malignancy as the presence of benign glands in perineural spaces (perineural indentation) has been described; benign prostate glands can be seen partially wrapping around, abutting, and, less commonly, within a nerve.

If the diagnosis of cancer is established based on *other* criteria, then the diagnosis of perineural invasion for prognostic purposes in needle biopsy material can be made with less stringent criteria, including perineural tracking, intraneural involvement, and less than total circumferential growth.

The finding of perineural invasion *on needle biopsy* has been shown to have over a 95% association with capsular penetration in the corresponding radical prostatectomy specimen (stage pT3) and is thus worth searching for and recording when diagnosing adenocarcinoma in needle biopsy samples

3.5.1.1 Clinical Commentary

Vasileios Spapis

These are cases of HG PIN, atypical small acinar proliferation (ASAP), and minimal prostate acinar adenocarcinoma either of intermediate or high grade, all diagnosed through prostate needle biopsy.

Transrectal ultrasound (TRUS)-guided biopsy of the prostate is now the standard of care for the diagnosis of prostate cancer, although some urologists may prefer a perineal approach. Both techniques arguably have similar results. Prostate biopsy is indicated when serum PSA is elevated, DRE is suspicious, or a combination of the two (Cooperberg et al. 2013). Limited PSA elevation alone should not lead to an immediate prostate biopsy. PSA level should be verified a few weeks later under standardized conditions (Eastham et al. 2003). Before performing a prostate biopsy, patient's overall health, comorbidities, and life expectancy should be taken into consideration. When the decision is made, a 12-core TRUS-guided biopsy is considered to be the preferred technique (Bjurlin et al. 2013). Biopsies are usually taken through the peripheral zone of the prostate, with optional additional sampling of any abnormal areas found on US or DRE. Local anesthesia and antibiotic prophylaxis are highly recommended (Mottet et al. 2017). Complications are not rare, the most common of them being hematospermia (37.4%), hematuria (14.5%), rectal bleeding (2.2%), prostatitis (1.0%), and fever >38.5 °C (0.8%) (Mottet et al. 2017).

Presence of HG PIN is detected in about 4–5% of the prostate biopsies (Epstein and Herawi 2006). HG PIN is a precursor lesion to many peripheral, intermediate- to high-grade adenocarcinomas of the prostate. When a repeat biopsy is performed (within a year), the mean risk of cancer is about 26%, which is not much higher than the risk reported in the literature for repeat biopsy following a benign diagnosis (Epstein and Herawi 2006). When only unifocal HG PIN is detected, a repeat biopsy within a year is not considered necessary. A mere suggestion is made to perform a repeat biopsy within 3 years following a diagnosis of HG PIN on a single core on needle biopsy (Godoy et al. 2011). Presence of HG PIN on more than one core is correlated with a significantly higher risk of subsequent prostate cancer, and a re-biopsy within 12 months is suggested (Abdel-Khalek et al. 2004; Merrimen et al. 2009; Merrimen et al. 2010). If a repeat prostate needle biopsy is performed, it should sample the entire prostate with relatively increased sampling of the initial sextant site where the HG PIN was found (Epstein and Herawi 2006).

About 5% of needle biopsy pathology reports contain the "diagnosis" of "atypical glands suspicious for carcinoma" (Epstein 2016) or, synonymously, "atypical small acinar proliferation (ASAP) (favoring malignancy)." These cases have the highest likelihood of being changed upon expert review, and the use of consultation is suggested in an attempt to resolve the diagnosis as definitively benign or malignant before considering a re-biopsy. ASAP "diagnosis" is followed by an average risk of cancer of approximately 40%. There are no clinical or pathological parameters that could help us predict which men with such a "diagnosis" will have cancer on repeat biopsy. Repeat biopsy should include increased sampling of the initial atypical site. All men with an ASAP "diagnosis" should undergo re-biopsy within 3–6 months (Epstein and Herawi 2006).

Presence of a few malignant cells/glands in the prostate biopsy should be co-evaluated with serum PSA levels and a DRE, since that low tumor burden on needle biopsy does not necessarily indicate low-volume, low-stage cancer. In fact, understaging is not that rare in prostate biopsies. Patients with up to three positive cores with <50% cancer involvement in each positive core, PSA < 10 ng/ml, and Gleason score 6 could benefit from active surveillance (AS) instead of definitive treatment. If this option is chosen, re-biopsy within 6–12 months to exclude sampling error is mandatory, and a close follow-up based on serial DRE (at least once per year), PSA (at least once every 6 months), and repeated biopsy (at a minimum interval of 3–5 years) (Mottet et al. 2017) is appropriate.

Key Messages

- Basophilic appearance of prostate epithelium may correspond to Prostate Intraepithelial neoplasia (PIN) when medium to large glands are involved; when small-sized glands are concerned, basal cell hyperplasia and complete (simple) atrophy must be considered.
- Presence of high-grade PIN mandates re-biopsy since high-grade PIN is considered a premalignant condition. Clinical significance of low-grade PIN is unclear, and thus low-grade PIN should not be diagnosed.
- In needle biopsy specimens, a vertical orientation of small-sized glands interrupting the muscular bundles of prostate stroma, a sufficient amount of cytoplasm, and a sharp luminal border and conspicuous nucleoli are in favor of the diagnosis of acinar adenocarcinoma of the prostate.
- Immunohistochemistry is a valuable *complementary* tool for the diagnosis of prostate cancer; immunostaining results should be interpreted with caution and always in relation to morphology of routine, H-E-stained sections. Diagnosis of carcinoma requires complete absence of basal cell markers in all atypical glands in suspicious foci. A negative high molecular weight keratin is only diagnostic of adenocarcinoma if there is a high H-E suspicion of carcinoma; one must also see staining of obviously benign glands as internal control.

3.6 Case 3.3: Moderately to Poorly Differentiated Prostate Carcinoma

Case Study

Data Prior to Microscopy

This is a case of a prostate acinar adenocarcinoma from an asymptomatic patient in which the finding of a hard nodular prostate on digital rectal examination in combination with elevated serum PSA level and TRUS findings aroused the suspicion of carcinoma.

Needle core biopsy was performed via TRUS guidance, using an 18 gauge needle. Cancer was found in all cores. The percentage of cancerous tissue in each core ranged from 20% to 60%; a general Gleason score of 7 (=3 + 4) was assigned with the percentage of secondary Gleason pattern 4 among all cancer tissue being estimated at 20% (Gleason pattern 3 occupied the remaining 80% of cancerous tissue).

3.6.1 Microscopic Evaluation of the Needle Biopsy Specimen

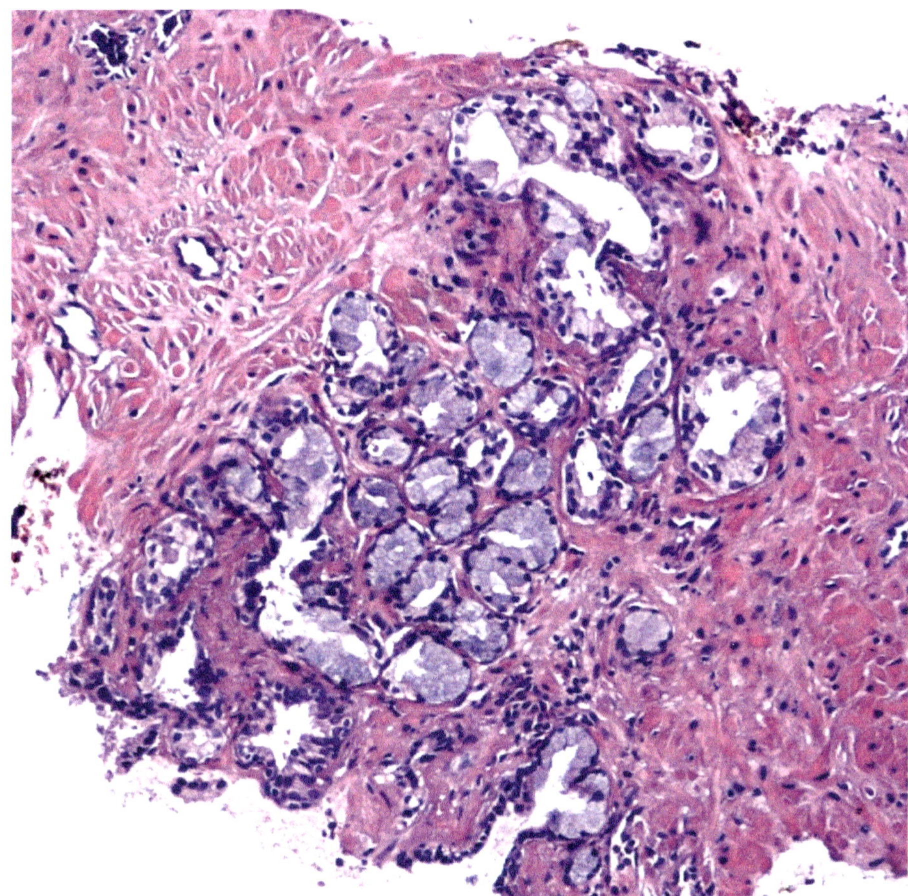

Fig. 3.47 (H-E, ×100) Mucinous metaplasia. In these acini/glands, the majority of acinar/secretory cells are metaplastic cells with small, dark, basally oriented, bland nuclei and abundant mucin-filled, foamy cytoplasm. Lobular architecture is retained in this small group of acini/glands.

However, similar glands with tall, mucin-filled cells can be haphazardly scattered; immunohistochemical detection of intact basal cells can rule out carcinoma and especially foamy gland prostate acinar adenocarcinoma in such an instance. Another prostate malignancy, much less likely to be considered in the differential diagnosis, is previously designated "hypernephroid" adenocarcinoma of Gleason pattern 4 which shows nests of optically clear cells resembling renal cell carcinoma with small, hyperchromatic nuclei; fusion of acini into more solid sheets with the appearance of back-to-back glands without intervening stroma certainly rules out benign entities.

In the rare case of complete involvement of a lobular aggregate of acini/glands with mucinous metaplasia, Cowper's glands should be taken into consideration in the differential diagnosis.

Prostatic xanthoma can also enter in the differential diagnosis. Xanthoma lacks glandular formation and its cells are positive for CD68 and KP-1 and negative for pancytokeratin, PSA, and PAP

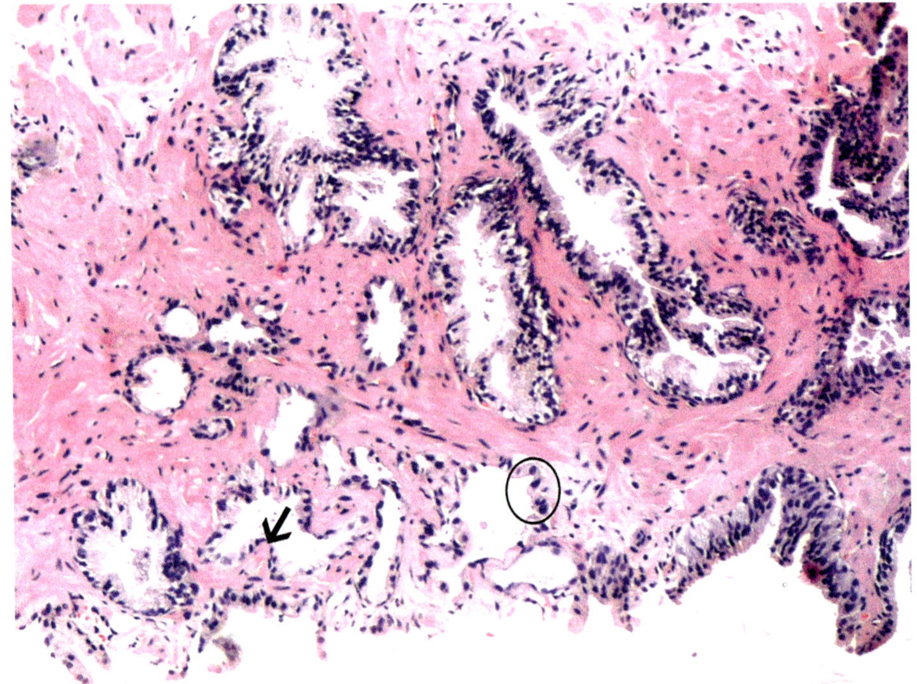

Fig. 3.48 (H-E, ×100) All forms of atrophy are characterized by the presence of well-formed glands that exhibit a reduction in cytoplasmic volume of luminal epithelial cells. Partial atrophy lacks the basophilic appearance of simple, fully developed (complete) atrophy, because the nuclei are more spaced apart (in partial atrophy). Although the glands may appear infiltrative, lobular architecture is often implied as the benign atrophic glands appear quite circumscribed as a group, without infiltration of individual glands between benign, non-atrophic glands. In this image, benign small glands with atrophic features (lower left part) are located on one side (not both sides) of benign, bigger prostate glands.

Benign atrophic glands may have a focally pseudoinfiltrative architecture and thus may mimic atrophic-type adenocarcinoma of Gleason pattern 3, score 6 (=3 + 3). The benign small glands of partial atrophy appear similar to adjacent larger benign glands; the small glands of partial atrophy have pale to clear, attenuated cytoplasm with small, somewhat crinkly or irregular, or possibly enlarged nuclei, often with visible small nucleoli. The loss of luminal cytoplasm with preserved lateral cytoplasm which makes nuclei frequently reach full height (*ellipse*) is characteristic of partial atrophy and is against carcinoma; in contrast to cancerous glands, in partially atrophic glands, cytoplasm is situated between nuclei (*ellipse*) and not from the nuclei up to the luminal surface (see Figs. 3.43 and 3.55). Other benign features of partial atrophy include pale-clear cytoplasm, relatively bland nuclear features without prominent nucleoli, and an undulating luminal surface (*arrow*). One or two immunoreactive basal cells per gland in at least some of the partially atrophic glands – provided that there is sufficient number of them – are noticed by basal markers' immunohistochemistry. While some glands with partial atrophy may be entirely negative for basal cells, focal patchy positive staining should exclude atrophic-type acinar adenocarcinoma of the prostate. The total absence of basal cells, however, may apply to this benign mimicker of cancer, especially when few glands with partial atrophy are there to be examined. Stromal alterations, such as fibrosis and sclerosis, may also be present.

On the other hand, atrophic pattern adenocarcinoma glands may resemble benign atrophic glands, but atrophic cancer glands should intermingle with larger benign glands (evidence of invasiveness).

Fig. 3.48 (continued)

Despite this infiltrative growth pattern, it may be difficult to establish a diagnosis of malignancy when most nuclei are flattened such that prominent nucleoli or nuclear enlargement may not be evident everywhere. In general, cytological features are often crucial for the correct diagnosis of prostate carcinoma and should be meticulously investigated, especially in small biopsies, in small tumor foci, and in unusual histological subtypes (e.g., adenocarcinoma with atrophic features, pseudohyperplastic prostatic adenocarcinoma). The key morphologic features to reach a diagnosis of atrophic cancer in needle biopsies include huge nucleoli, infiltrative growth between benign glands without atrophy, and the adjacent presence of conventional-type acinar adenocarcinoma component.

Small malignant acini or even single malignant cells are also encountered in residual, *treated* prostate adenocarcinoma (which should not be Gleason graded)

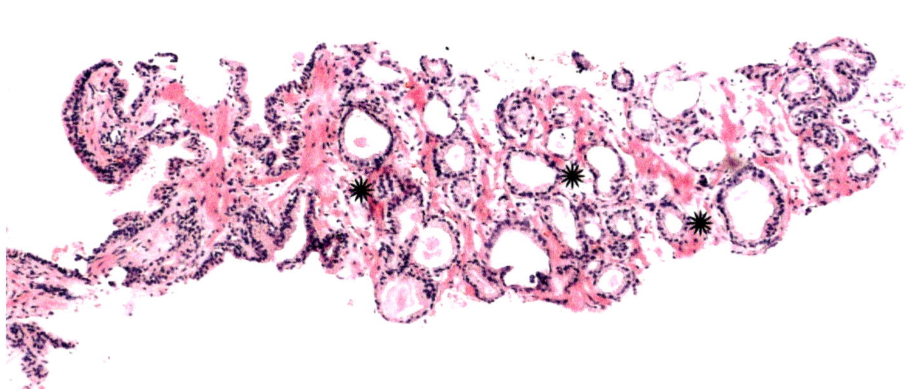

Fig. 3.49 (H-E, ×50) Moderately differentiated prostate acinar adenocarcinoma. Under the Gleason grading system, cytological features are not important. This is Gleason pattern 3 (i.e., intermediate grade/differentiation): variably sized, mainly small, discrete, more widely dispersed (than Gleason patterns 1 and 2) glandular units infiltrating prostate fibromuscular stroma (*asterisks*), here with a haphazard distribution; note that in prostate cancer of intermediate or poor differentiation, infiltrates are not always noticed around or among nonneoplastic acini/glands (left side of this image).

When the tumor has the same Gleason pattern throughout, its score is obtained by doubling the Gleason pattern. So, if this was the only cancerous tissue in the biopsy specimen, it would be assigned a score of 6 (=3 + 3). We also have to report the percentage of cancerous tissue over the total area of each cylinder involved

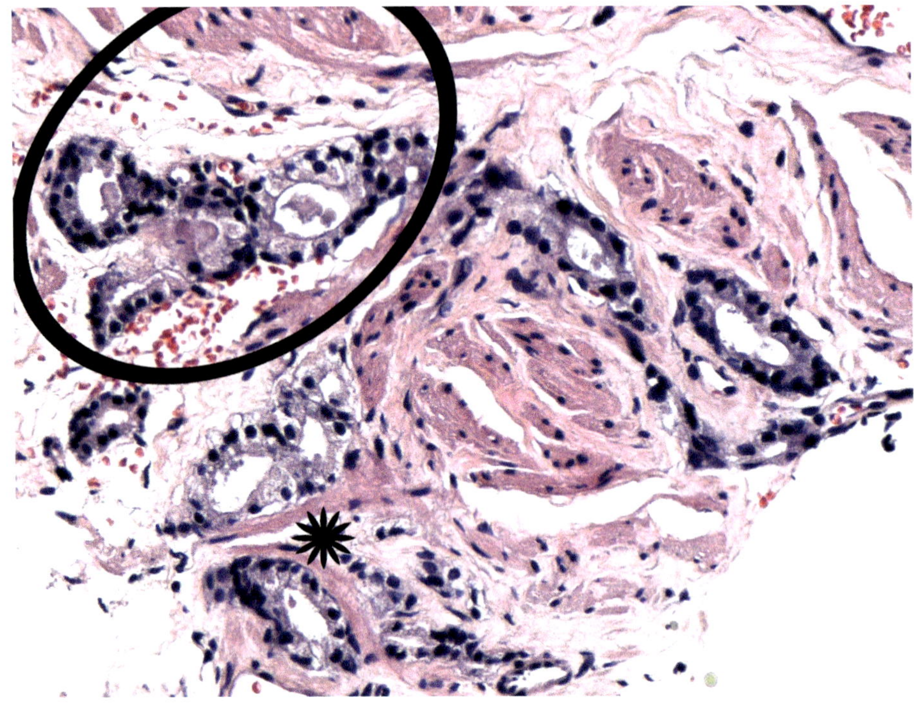

Fig. 3.50 (H-E, ×200) Clear invasion of prostate fibromuscular stroma by separate cancerous glands. Stroma elements being interrupted by cancerous glands (*asterisk*). Lack of stromal reaction is usual in acinar adenocarcinoma of the prostate. Nuclear hyperchromasia, sharp luminal borders, and intraluminal pink amorphous secretions (*ellipse*)

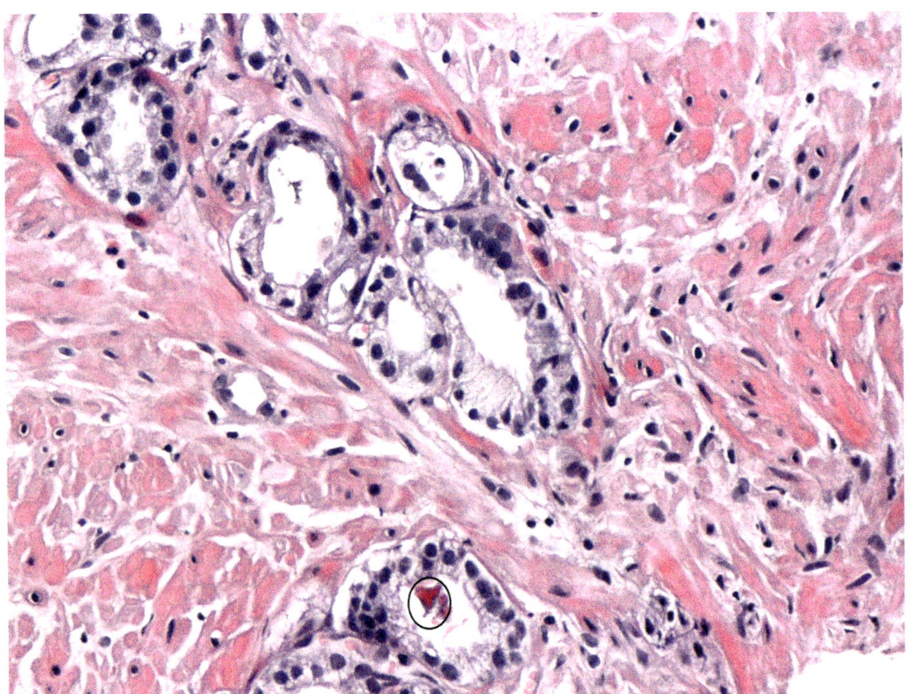

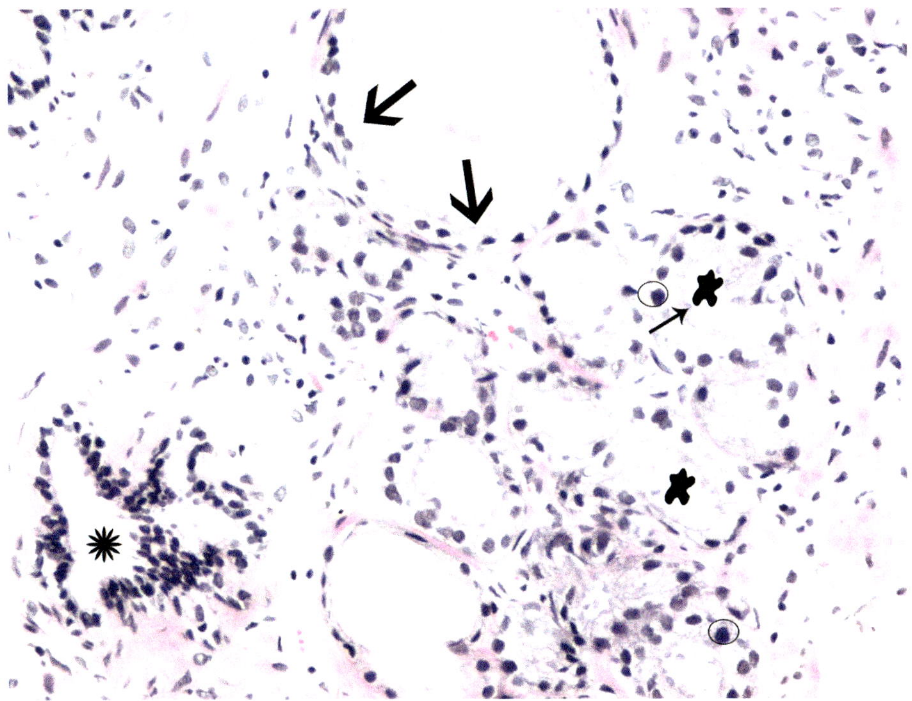

Fig. 3.52 (H-E, ×200) Usual appearance of cancerous prostate glands of intermediate grade. Abundant cytoplasm in most cancerous glands (*small arrow*) as opposed to an adjacent, completely atrophic (and thus basophilic) gland (*asterisk*). Nuclear enlargement and hyperchromasia (*ellipses*) and sharp luminal borders in cancerous glands (*big arrows*). Microprotrusions in the lumen (*blobs*) do *not* mean that the luminal border is undulating or has papillary infoldings; the latter two characteristics are frequently encountered in benign glands and only rarely in cancerous glands

Fig. 3.51 (H-E, ×200) Intraluminal crystalloid in cancerous gland lumen (*ellipse*).

Sometimes cancer does not occupy the cylinder tissue continuously but grows as scattered microscopic foci. The diameter of the cancerous foci may be measured in millimeters and reported. If the normal tissue located between the cancer foci is less than 5 mm, instead of mentioning the maximum diameter of each cancerous focus and the length of the whole cylinder, we can report the percentage of cancerous tissue over the total cylinder area

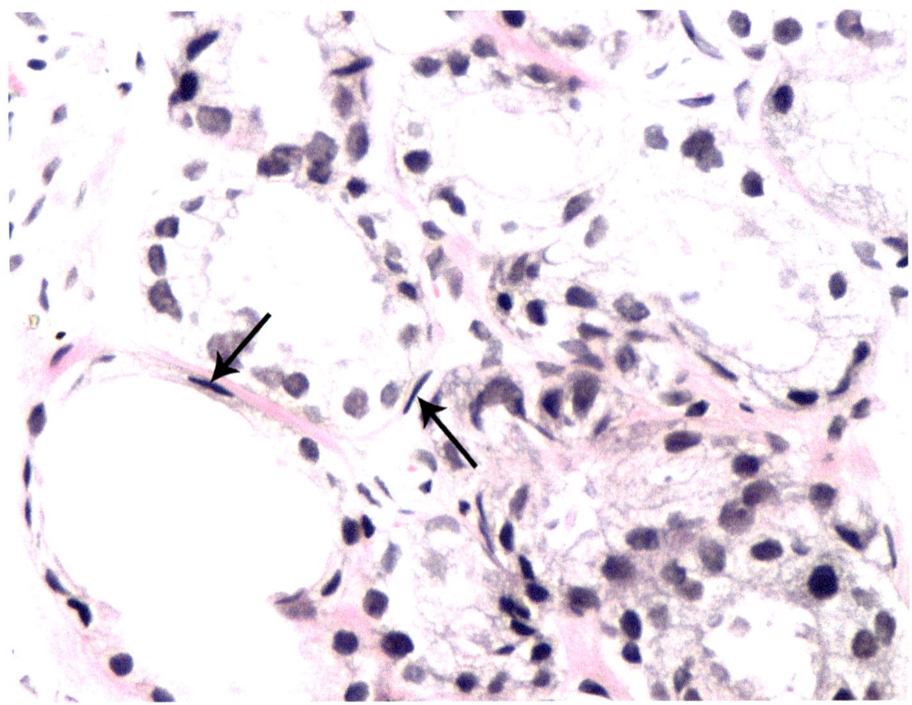

Fig. 3.53 (H-E, ×400) Thin, hyperchromatic, characteristically elongated nuclei of fibroblasts of prostate stroma (*arrows*), with basal "location," mimicking basal cells of normal prostate glandular epithelium. Prostate cancer should be entirely devoid of basal cells. The presence of fibroblasts in close proximity with cancerous glands can occasionally be confusing; in such cases, immunohistochemistry provides significant help

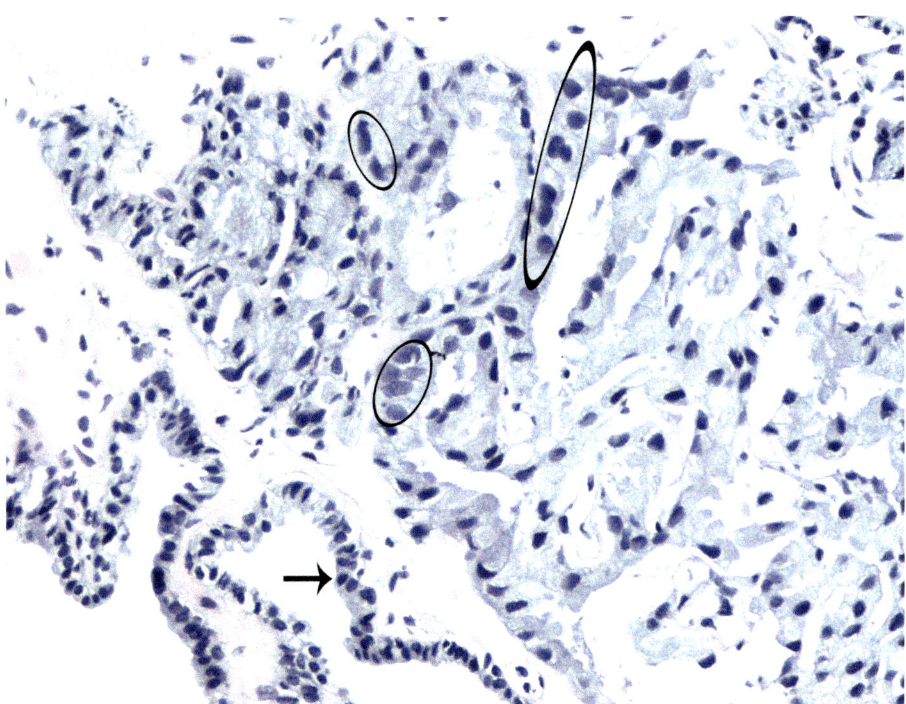

Fig. 3.54 (H-E, ×200) Evaluation of malignant nuclear features. Nuclear enlargement in cancerous cells (*ellipses*) can be properly evaluated when compared to the size of benign nuclei of neighboring acinar/secretory cells (*arrow*). Often, only significant nuclear enlargement discriminates cancer from the surrounding benign glands

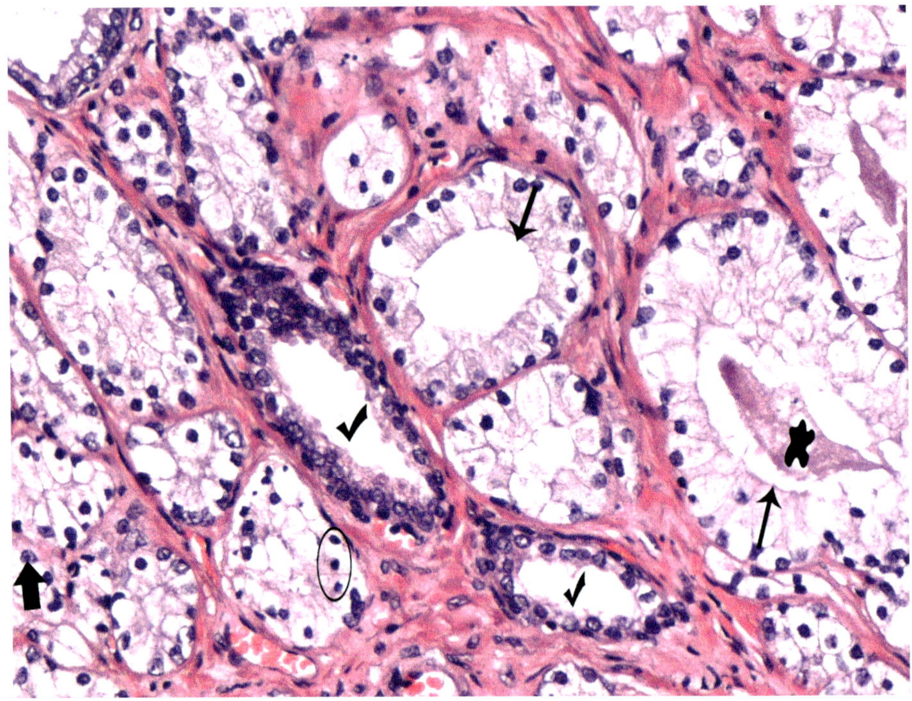

Fig. 3.55 (H-E, ×200) Cancerous glands, under high magnification, with abundant (here rather foamy/xanthomatous) cytoplasm, *surrounding* two atrophic glands (*ticks*) (*infiltrative* pattern) with basophilic appearance of fully developed atrophy. Gleason pattern 3 is assigned based on architecture, as always.

Note that in cancerous glands, the abundant cytoplasm is mainly noticed over the nuclei, up to the sharp luminal border (*thin arrows*) and not so much among the nuclei. A lateral location of cytoplasm with regard to nuclei is consistent with partial atrophy, the before mentioned benign entity, which is often confused with cancer.

Malignant nuclear features are not always present, as nuclei may be small and pyknotic (*ellipse*). In fact, nuclei of foamy gland adenocarcinoma are often pyknotic (small, round, and densely hyperchromatic), without nuclear enlargement or prominent nucleoli; conspicuous nucleoli can be focally detected in this field though (*thick arrow*). Pink, eosinophilic homogeneous intraluminal secretions (*blob*) are common in foamy gland adenocarcinoma

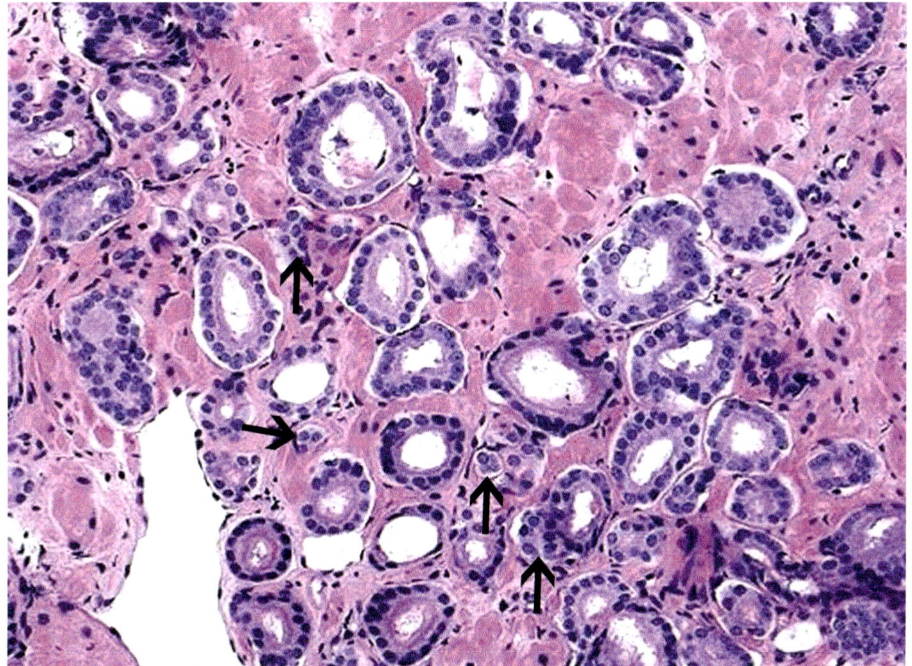

Fig. 3.56 (H-E, ×200) The neoplastic glands of Gleason pattern 3 are typically smaller than benign glands and are lined by a single uniform layer of cuboidal or low columnar epithelium. The cytoplasm of the tumor cells ranges from pale to clear, as is seen in benign glands, to a distinctive amphophilic appearance, evident here.

Gleason pattern 3, the most common prostate cancer pattern, consists of variably sized, often angular, typically small, individual glands that are well-formed and discrete units. Tangentially sectioned pattern 3 glands may mimic fused pattern 4 glands, and this is a common cause of overgrading. In this field, we notice only a few glands with no obvious lumens (*arrows*), probably due to tangential cutting; this is compatible with Gleason pattern 3.

If, on the other hand, there are too many glands with poorly formed or absent lumens and the lack of well-defined gland formation is visible at low magnification, a diagnosis of Gleason pattern 4 should be made. Accurate recognition of Gleason pattern 4 prostate carcinoma on needle biopsy is critical for patient management and prognostication. "Poorly formed glands" are the most common Gleason pattern 4 subpattern. Grading Gleason pattern 4 "poorly formed glands" and the criteria to distinguish them from tangentially sectioned Gleason pattern 3 glands challenge pathologists in their daily practice.

Cancer glands with no or rare lumens, elongated compressed glands, and elongated nests are considered "poorly formed glands." Poorly formed glands immediately adjacent to other well-formed glands regardless of their number and small foci of ≤5 poorly formed glands regardless of their location are not graded as Gleason pattern 4 but as Gleason pattern 3. In contrast, large foci of >10 poorly formed glands that are not immediately adjacent to well-formed glands are graded as Gleason pattern 4 (Zhou et al. 2015)

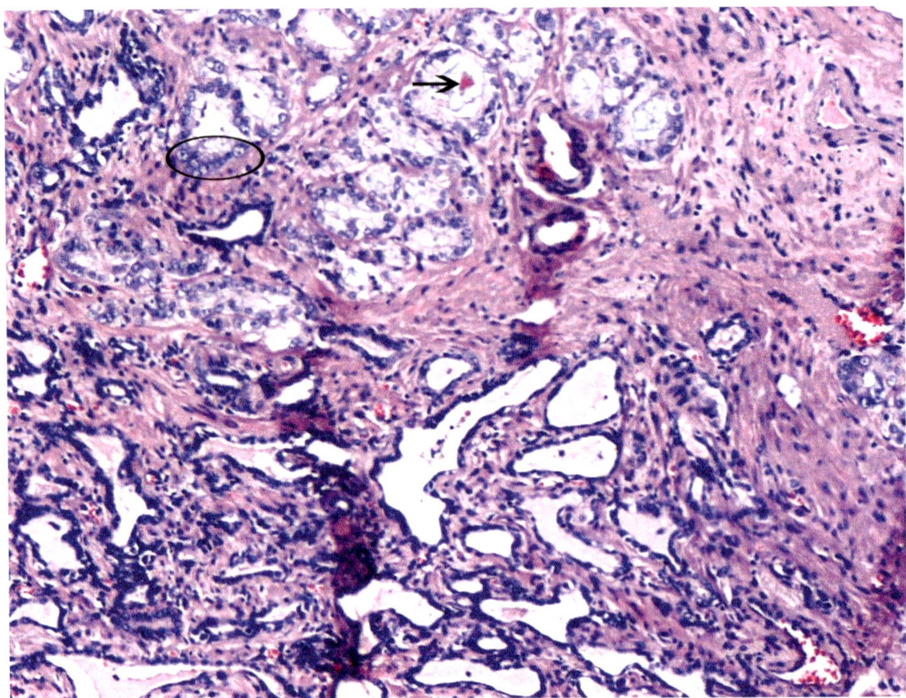

Fig. 3.57 (H-E, ×100) Gleason pattern 3 cancerous acini/glands between benign glands with simple atrophy (upper left part). Basophilic glands with simple atrophy occupy the lower half of the image. Prominent nucleoli in cancer cells (*ellipse*). Intraluminal crystalloid in cancerous acinus/gland (*arrow*). Two cancerous glands may be situated tightly adjacent to each other; when even tiny amounts of stroma are recognizable between them and/or two separate rows of nuclei are observed, each row belonging to each cancerous gland, the Gleason pattern is still 3 (not 4).

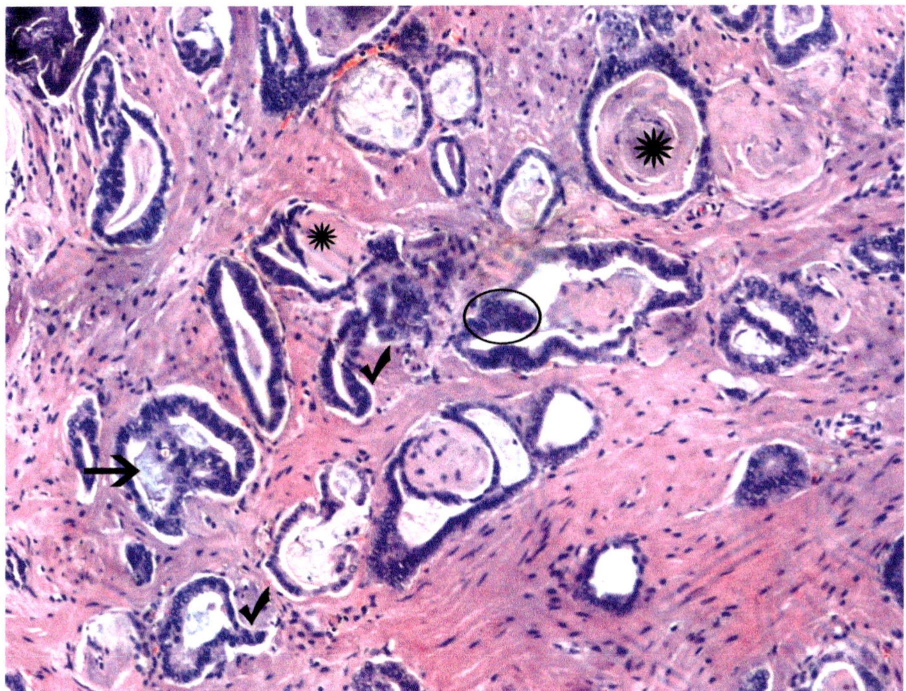

Fig. 3.58 (H-E, ×100) A mucinous fibroplasia/collagenous micronodule is one of the pathognomonic findings for prostatic acinar adenocarcinoma. Mucinous fibroplasia consist of delicate loose fibrous tissue with an ingrowth of fibroblasts (*asterisks*) often associated with intraluminal, blue-tinged mucinous secretions (*arrow*). In early collagenous micronodules, the fibrous tissue is scant, and more mucin is seen. Mucinous fibroplasia are typically assigned a 6 (=3 + 3) Gleason score. Mucinous fibroplasia/collagenous micronodules may mimic another pathognomonic feature of prostate cancer, complete (or near complete) nerve encirclement; S-100 protein immunonegativity of the central structures excludes perineural invasion.

Small cancerous acini/glands of Gleason pattern 3 often have irregular contours (*ticks*). Gleason pattern 3 glands may rarely be of medium to large size with papillary configuration (*ellipse*)

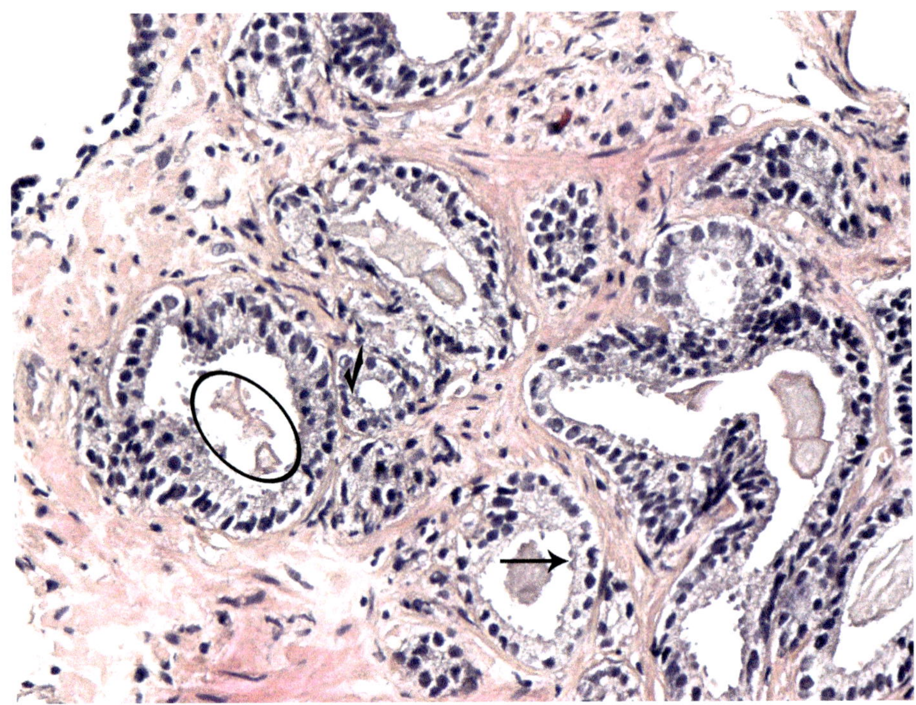

Fig. 3.59 (H-E, ×100) Cancerous prostate glands of Gleason pattern 3. Sharp luminal border, focally (*arrow*). Intraluminal crystalloids (*ellipse*). Prominent nucleoli, noticeable even under the ×100 magnification (*tick*). Although the presence of prominent nucleoli is important in the diagnosis of cancer, it should not be the sole criterion used to establish the diagnosis, since prominent nucleoli may be seen in various mimickers of cancer and are certainly not seen in all cases of prostate cancer on needle biopsy.

Using basal cell immunomarkers, it is worth investigating whether the large-sized gland with papillary infolding on the right side corresponds to HG PIN or is cancerous. A PIN-like adenocarcinoma, by definition being composed entirely of discrete glands, is assigned a Gleason pattern 3

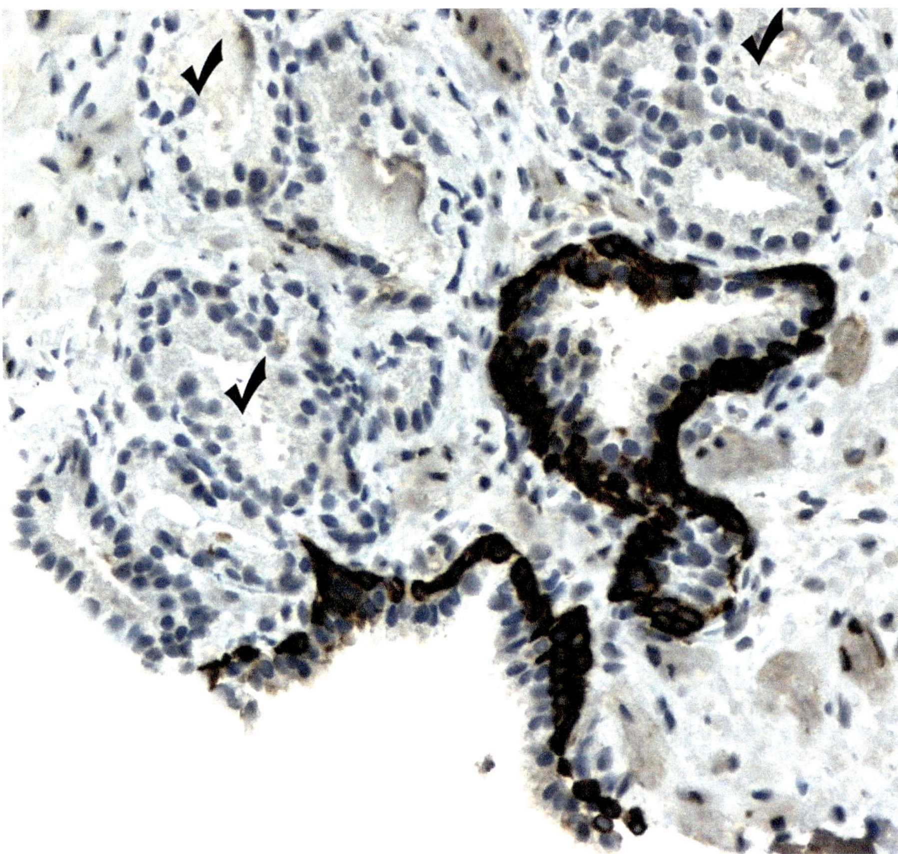

Fig. 3.60 [HMW CK (34βE12) immunohistochemistry, ×200] Immunohistochemical confirmation of invasive cancerous acini/glands. Complete absence of basal cells is expected in a sufficient number of cancerous prostate glands (*ticks*). Consequent complete lack of HMW CK immunoreactivity in this suspicious, atypical glandular focus is supportive of carcinoma diagnosis

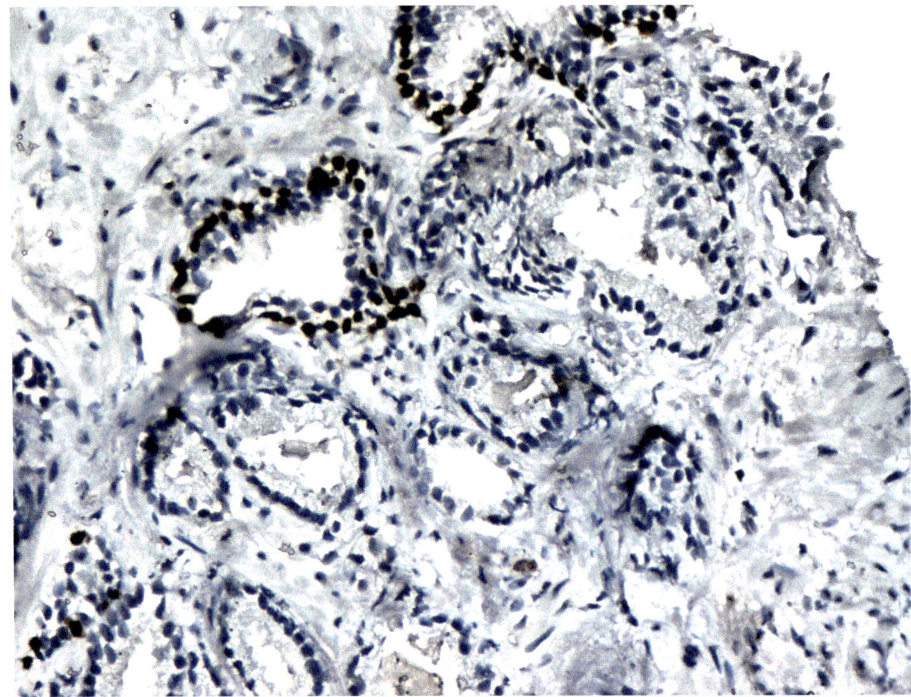

Fig. 3.61 (p63immunohistochemistry, ×200) A nuclear basal cell immunomarker. All morphologically atypical glands must be identified by H&E, and corresponding glands on immunohistochemical slide should be completely p63-negative. Benign glands serve as an internal positive control (upper part).

We should bear in mind, however, that rare, aberrant nuclear p63 staining may occur in malignant acinar/secretory cells of a conventional acinar adenocarcinoma (!)

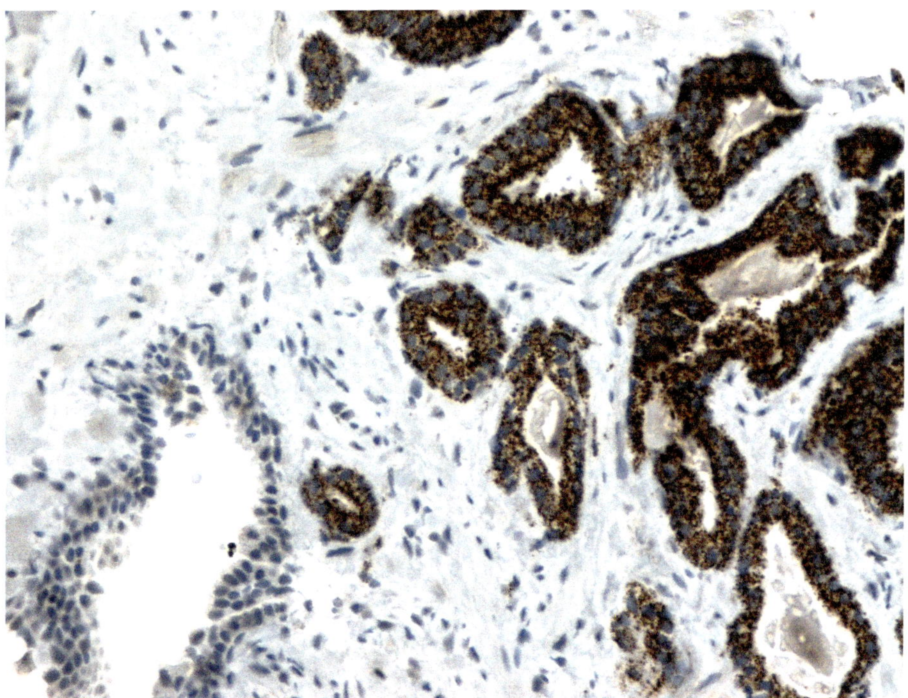

Fig. 3.62 (AMACR-racemase immunohistochemistry, ×200) Specific, granular, intense AMACR (racemase) immunostaining, sometimes with luminal accentuation, can be quite helpful in the confirmation of malignancy as far as ordinary, moderately differentiated acinar prostate adenocarcinoma is concerned. The use of monoclonal antibody P504S is recommended. Note the intense specific immunostaining of racemase (AMACR) in cancerous glands with simultaneous negative expression in nonmalignant, adjacent gland at the lower left part of the image.

AMACR is less useful in evaluating metastases because many tumors in other organs are immunopositive

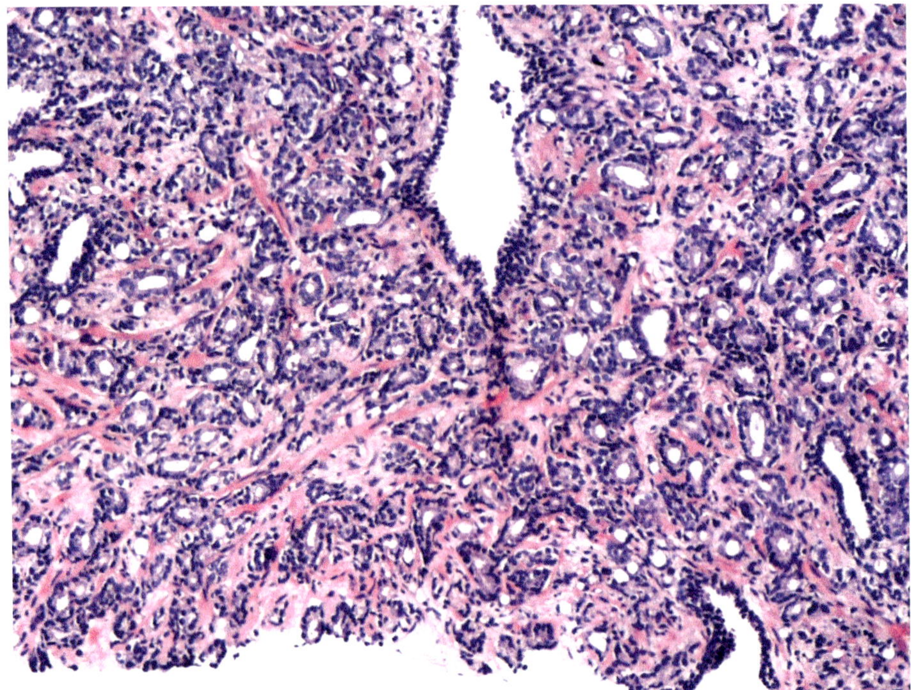

Fig. 3.63 (H-E, ×50) The initial grading of prostate carcinoma should be performed under low to medium magnification; if necessary, the ×20 objective may then be used to verify the grade.

In this field of the same case, clusters of clearly poorly formed or fused glands (where tangential section of Gleason pattern 3 glands cannot account for this histology) are seen and graded as Gleason pattern 4. This pattern is detectable in few cores and so is the secondary Gleason pattern as far as the whole material of the present needle biopsy is concerned

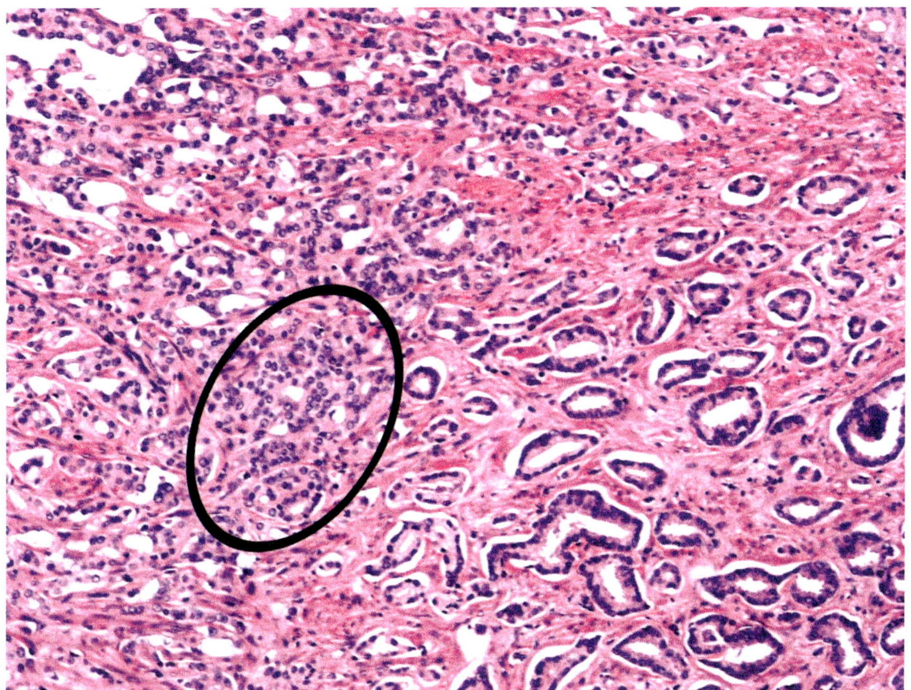

Fig. 3.64 (H-E, ×100) Intermediate and poor differentiation of prostate acinar adenocarcinoma. Cancerous glands on the right half of the picture are separate (Gleason pattern 3, intermediate differentiation/grade). The rest of the glands are obviously fused (*ellipse*) (Gleason pattern 4, poor differentiation/high grade).

High cancer burden on needle biopsy, as the present case, is strongly suggestive of large-volume high-stage cancer.

Most tumors contain more than one pattern, in which case one assigns a primary grade to the dominant pattern and a secondary grade to the subdominant pattern. The two numeric grades are then added to obtain a combined Gleason score with the dominant pattern cited first. This case is assigned a Gleason score 7 (3 + 4), grade group 2, which portends better prognosis than 4 + 3, grade group 3.

For needle biopsies and radical prostatectomy specimens in which the highest score is Gleason score 7, it is recommended that the *Gleason pattern 4 percentage of the total cancerous tissue* be reported along with the overall score for the case

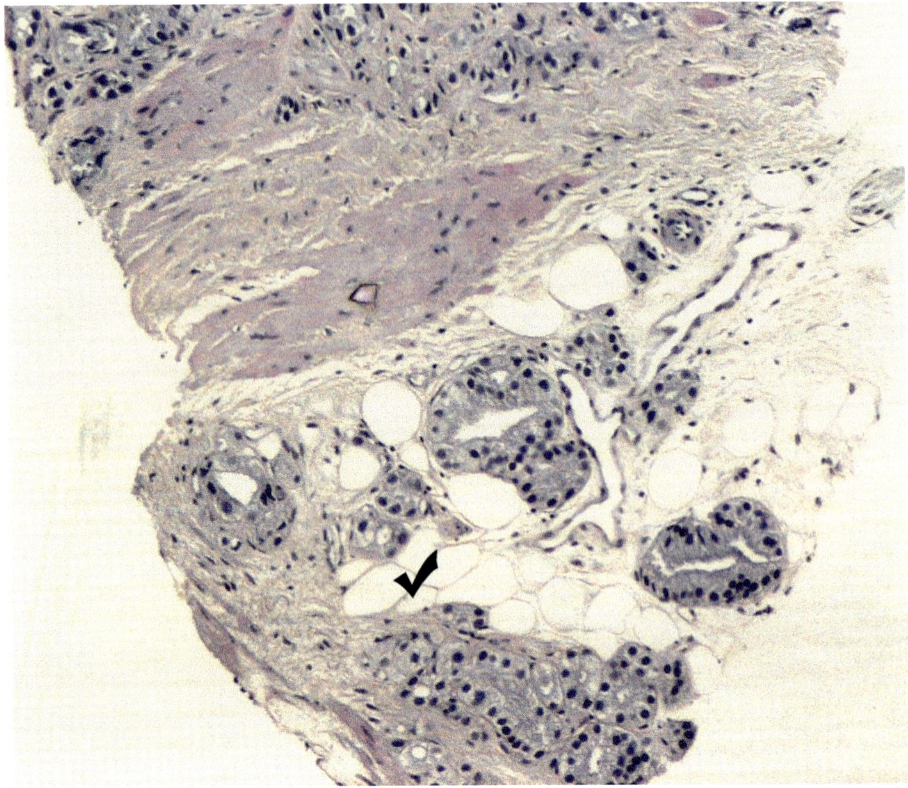

Fig. 3.65 (H-E, ×100) This image comes from another tumor-positive needle biopsy. Infiltration of periprostatic adipose tissue (*tick*) by malignant glands is a pathognomonic finding of cancer which can occasionally be diagnosed in needle biopsies and should be assigned as *pathologic* stage *p*T3, since intraprostatic fat is exceedingly rare.

Patients with *clinical* (not pathologic) T3 disease are usually not surgical candidates; 50% have nodal metastases at diagnosis, 50% develop metastases at 5 years, and 75% die of prostate carcinoma within 10 years

3.6.1.1 Clinical Commentary

Vasileios Spapis

This is a case of a clinically perceivable prostate carcinoma with sufficient amount of cancerous tissue in all cores and a Gleason score of 7 (=3 + 4), grade group 2.

In a prostate needle biopsy, the percentage of malignant tissue, as assessed in the pathology report, is a strong predictor of positive surgical margins and non-organ-confined disease (Cooperberg et al. 2013; Freedland et al. 2002). PSA levels usually increase with tumor stage but cannot be used for accurate prediction of the final pathologic stage (Partin et al. 1990). When the tumor is palpable, it is automatically classified as T2 in the TNM classification system, but if extraprostatic extension is detected, then it is classified as T3 or T4. This means that, regardless of PSA level and Gleason score, the patient is considered to belong in the high-risk group for biochemical recurrence of localized and locally advanced prostate cancer, defined according to the EAU classification (Mottet et al. 2017).

Imaging for high-risk patients is of great importance in order to detect presence of distant metastases or lymph node involvement. In fact, risk of nodal metastases is 20–45%, when any core has a predominant Gleason 4 pattern or >3 cores have any Gleason 4 pattern (Mottet et al. 2017). CT and MRI scans are usually used but have low sensitivity detecting LN invasion in patients with a Gleason score < 8, PSA < 20 ng/mL, or localized disease. Bone scanning (BS) is also needed and is found positive in about 49.5% of men with locally advanced cancers. PET/CT and mpMRI seem to be more accurate than BS; the clinical benefit of detecting bone metastases at an earlier time using more sensitive techniques remains unclear in the initial staging setting. Bone scan is therefore usually preferred (Mottet et al. 2017).

Patients with high-risk PCa have a greater risk of PSA failure, metastatic progression, and death from PCa. However, not all high-risk patients have a poor prognosis after RP (Yossepowitch et al. 2007). RP is a reasonable solution for selected high-risk, well-informed patients, with small tumor volume and long life expectancy. Extended lymphadenectomy (LND) should be performed in all these cases, as the risk of LN involvement is high (LE 2a, GR A) (Mottet et al. 2017). Retrospective studies show that surgery (as part of a multimodal approach) can offer more than 70% overall survival (OS) at 10 years to these patients (Ward et al. 2005; Hsu et al. 2007; Joniau et al. 2015). Radiotherapy (RT) can also offer increased OS, but it should always be combined with long-term androgen deprivation therapy (ADT). Pelvic lymphatics should also be irradiated. The duration of ADT has to take into account WHO performance score, comorbidities, and the number of poor prognostic factors (Mottet et al. 2017). Patients unwilling or unfit to undergo RP or radiotherapy (RT) could benefit from ADT alone, either immediately or after symptomatic progression or occurrence of serious complications (watchful waiting).

Key Messages

- Increased serum PSA level and abnormal digital rectal examination are the main indications for prostate needle biopsy.
- The diagnosis of cancer should always be based on a constellation of features rather than relying on any one criterion alone. Of course, when pathognomonic features of cancer are indeed present, the diagnosis is much easier.
- Small glands infiltrating haphazardly in the stroma or crowded between and around normal, atrophic, or dysplastic glands are indicative of cancer even if the small glands lack cytological atypia.

3.7 Case 3.4: Radical Prostatectomy-pT3 Prostate Carcinoma

Case Study

Data Prior to Microscopy

A 60-year-old man with an increased serum PSA value of 15 ng/ml. Involvement of posterior aspects o f the peripheral zone of the prostate gland had rendered a tumor palpable on digital rectal examination. Needle biopsies revealed an acinar adenocarcinoma of Gleason score 7 (=4 + 3) in five cylinders of both lobes, with a mean occupancy percentage of 40%, a predominant Gleason pattern 4 percentage of 55%, and focal perineural involvement. Upper and lower abdomen CT scan and bone scan were unremarkable.

Radical prostatectomy, the most common treatment for localized prostate cancer (PCa) when life expectancy is >10 years, was performed.

Macroscopically, firm, gritty, solid tumor areas, yellowish in color, are noticed within the prostate parenchyma; the tumor borders can be determined only under microscopic examination though. The surrounding, nonneoplastic prostate has a spongy appearance.

3.7.1 Microscopic Evaluation of the Radical Prostatectomy Specimen

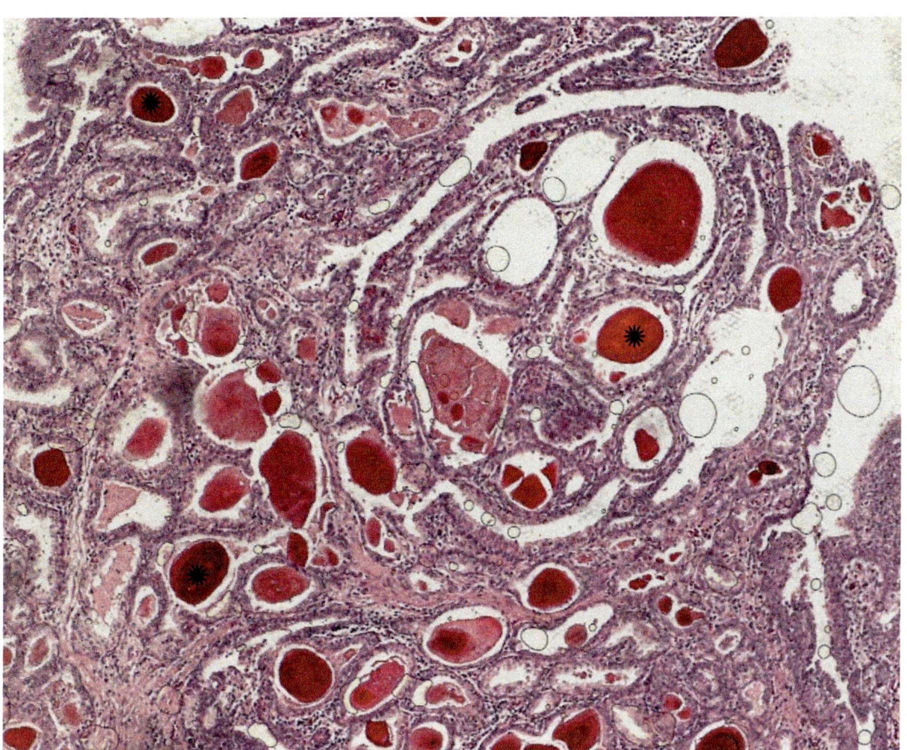

Fig. 3.66 (H-E, ×50) Verumontanum mucosal gland hyperplasia: an incidental finding in 14% of radical prostatectomy specimens. It is an uncommon lesion in prostate needle biopsies, and it is almost never seen in transurethral resection of prostate specimens, since the verumontanum is spared in this procedure.

The verumontanum protrudes from the posterior wall of the distal prostatic urethra into its lumen. The verumontanum contains closely apposed, small- to medium-sized glands of varying caliber, with luminal undulation; verumontanum mucosal glands often contain corpora amylacea (like benign prostate glands) or distinctive orange-brown luminal concretions (*asterisks*).

The verumontanum mucosal glands retain a lobular architecture and lack the infiltrative and haphazard arrangement of glands typically found in the commonest type of prostatic acinar adenocarcinoma [i.e., intermediate-grade (moderately differentiated), Gleason pattern 3]. Differential diagnosis from low-grade, Gleason pattern 2, prostate acinar adenocarcinoma is sometimes necessary due to the small size and crowded nature of verumontanum mucosal glands. There are numerous dark staining bodies and distinctive orange concretions in the verumontanum glands' lumen (*asterisks*). A preserved basal cell layer excludes cancer

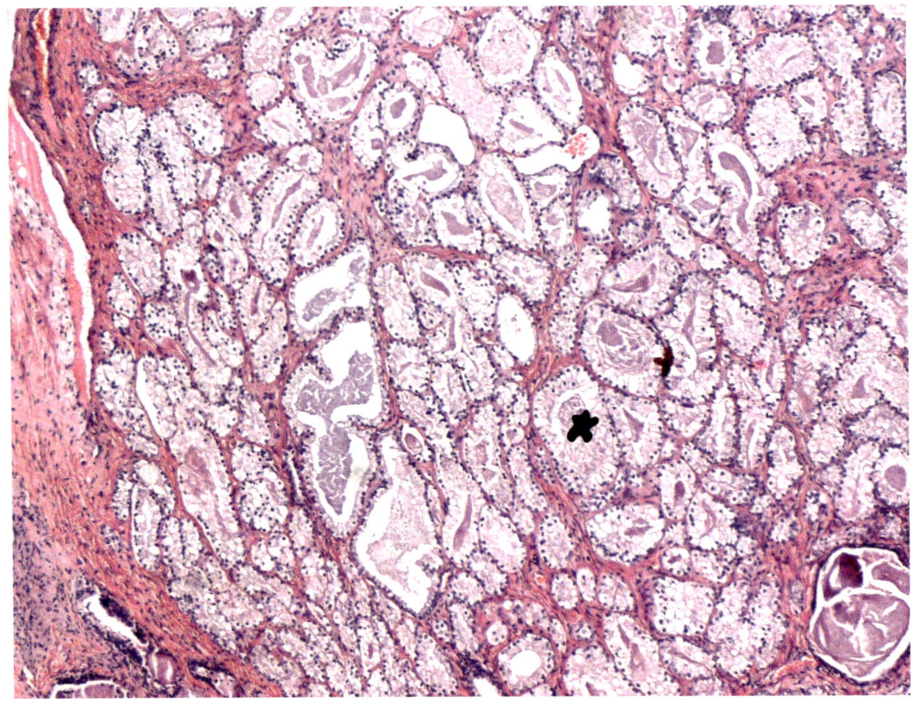

Fig. 3.67 (H-E, ×50) Here's an unusual variant of prostate malignancy which involves cancers with voluminous xanthomatous cytoplasm in which nuclei are small and often show no or minimal atypia; intraluminal pink homogeneous secretions are often present (*blob*). Basally oriented nuclei and prominent luminal cytoplasm are suggestive of malignancy. There is no hint of a basal cell layer as compared with neighboring normal glands; this rules out adenosis.

The diagnosis of foamy gland prostate carcinoma is based on its architectural pattern of crowded and/or infiltrative glands, abundant foamy cytoplasm, and frequent, intraluminal, dense, pink, acellular secretions. This variant, when of low grade, as here, may be underdiagnosed on needle core, but it is usually associated with easily recognizable, higher Gleason score, prostate acinar adenocarcinoma. Gleason scores 2–5 are never assigned on biopsy, and, actually, they are assigned only rarely on other prostate specimens, when higher scores are absent.

This low-grade, Gleason score 5 (=2 + 3), foamy gland adenocarcinoma is histologically characterized by cells with abundant foamy cytoplasm and bland nuclei. Since much more extensive cancer of higher Gleason score is detected in other parts of the prostatectomy specimen, this cancer focus is disregarded in Gleason scoring in the pathology report.

As mentioned in case 3.1, low-grade carcinomas (in TUR specimens or prostatectomy) probably represent primaries within the transition zone and often have "clear cell" features with optically clear cytoplasm. The cytoplasm of the malignant glandular prostate epithelium is usually finely granular but may sometimes have a foamy appearance due to the accumulation of neutral fat. These low-grade clear cell adenocarcinomas of the transition zone do not have high rates of dissemination. In contrast, high-grade, large-volume carcinomas of the peripheral zone that involve the transitional only once they are quite advanced, have high rates of dissemination

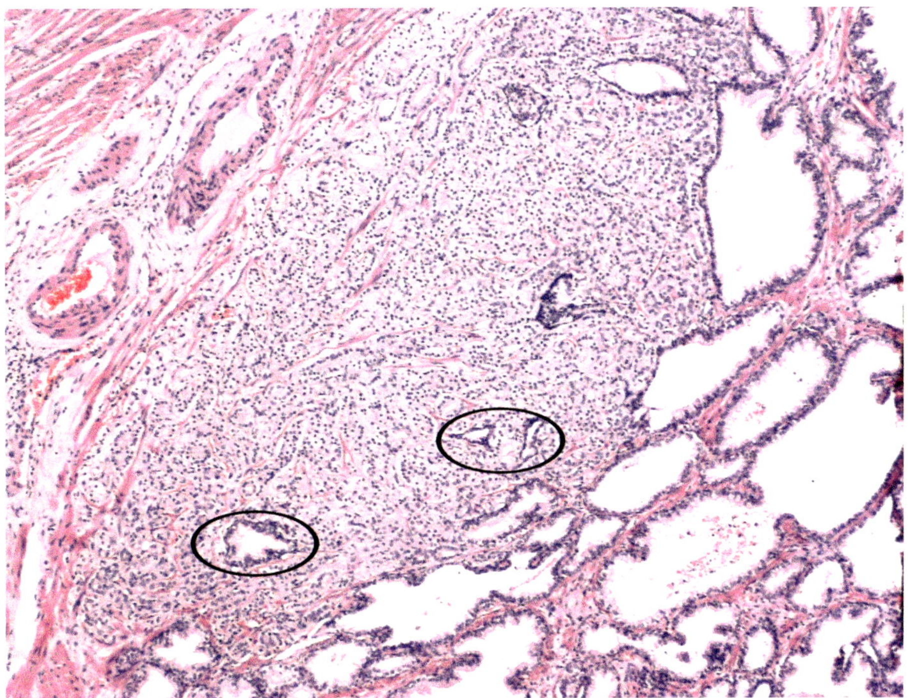

Fig. 3.68 (H-E, ×50) Most prostatic adenocarcinomas are multifocal. Here we observe another cancerous focus of different morphology, entrapping benign prostate glands (*ellipses*)

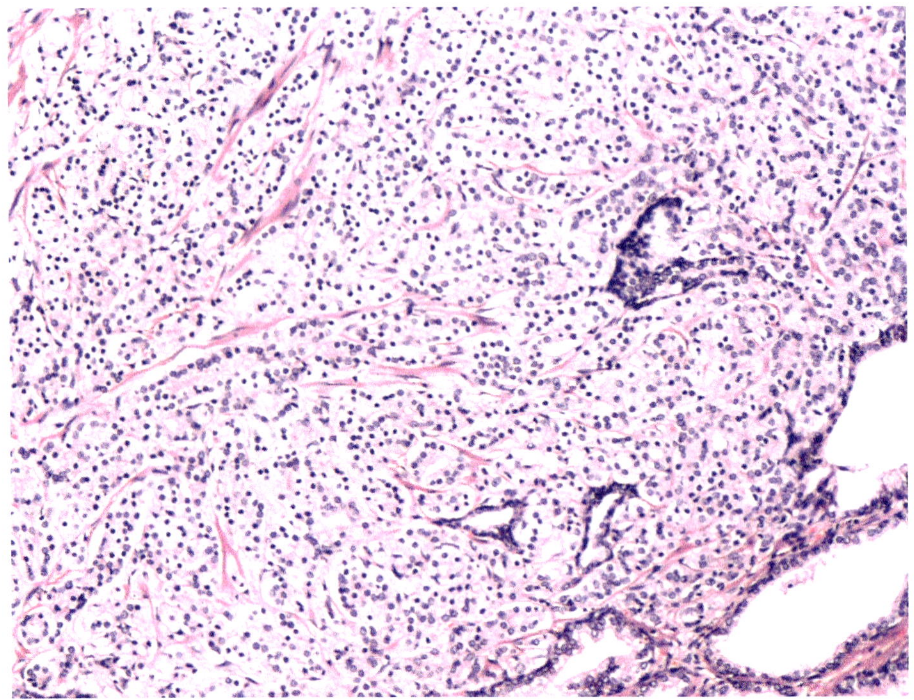

Fig. 3.69 (H-E, ×100) Fused and poorly formed cancerous glands with rare lumens justify the assignment of Gleason pattern 4 (high grade, poor differentiation) in this cancerous focus, despite its partially smooth margin, evident at the upper left side of the previous image

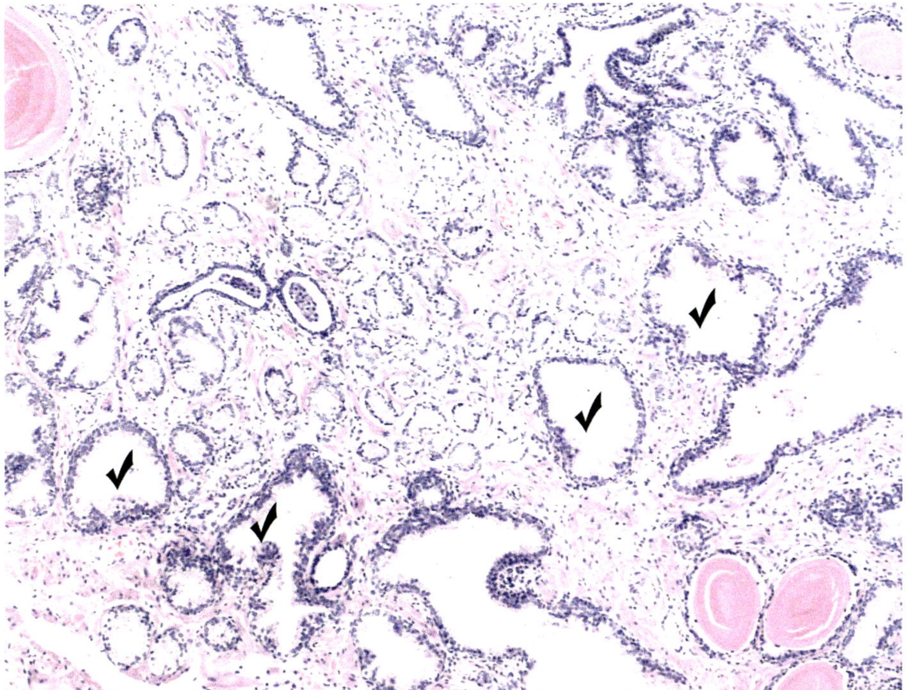

Fig. 3.70 (H-E, ×50) Here's another cancerous focus in the prostatectomy specimen. Small cancerous prostate glands among benign prostate glands, often of larger size (*ticks*), characterize Gleason pattern 3 (intermediate grade/moderate differentiation)

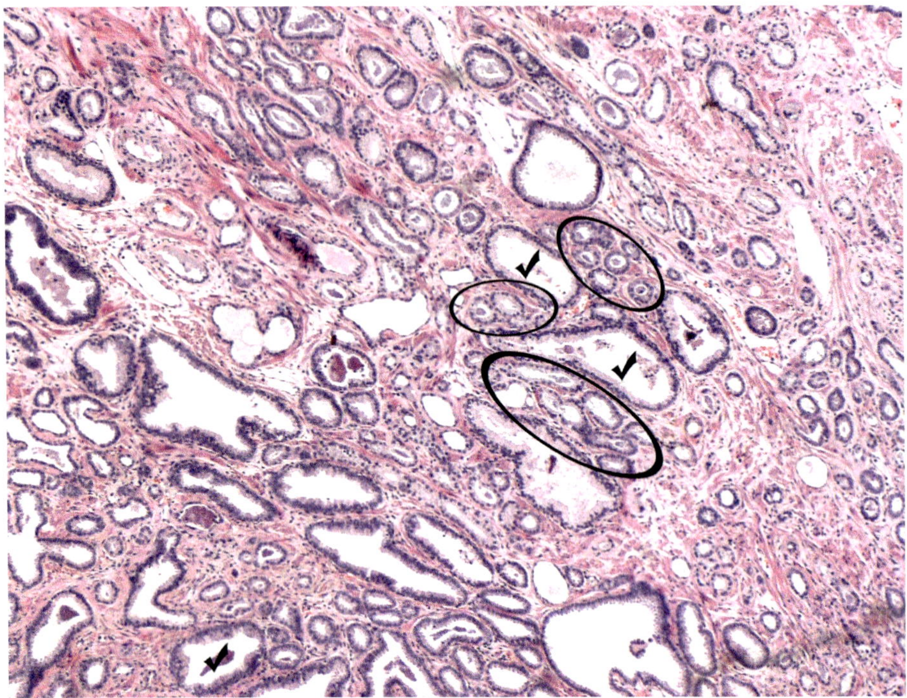

Fig. 3.71 (H-E, ×50) Gleason pattern 3/intermediate differentiation of prostate acinar adenocarcinoma: the commonest type of prostate cancer.

Under low magnification, there is a much wider separation of the individual cancerous glands by comparison to low-grade Gleason patterns (i.e., 1 and 2). Cancerous glands of small size (*ellipses*) extend irregularly into the stroma and surround bigger, nonneoplastic glands (*ticks*). Small atypical glands between and *around* (*on both sides*) benign glands constitute a characteristic architectural feature of Gleason pattern 3 in any tissue material (needle biopsy, TUR, or open surgery)

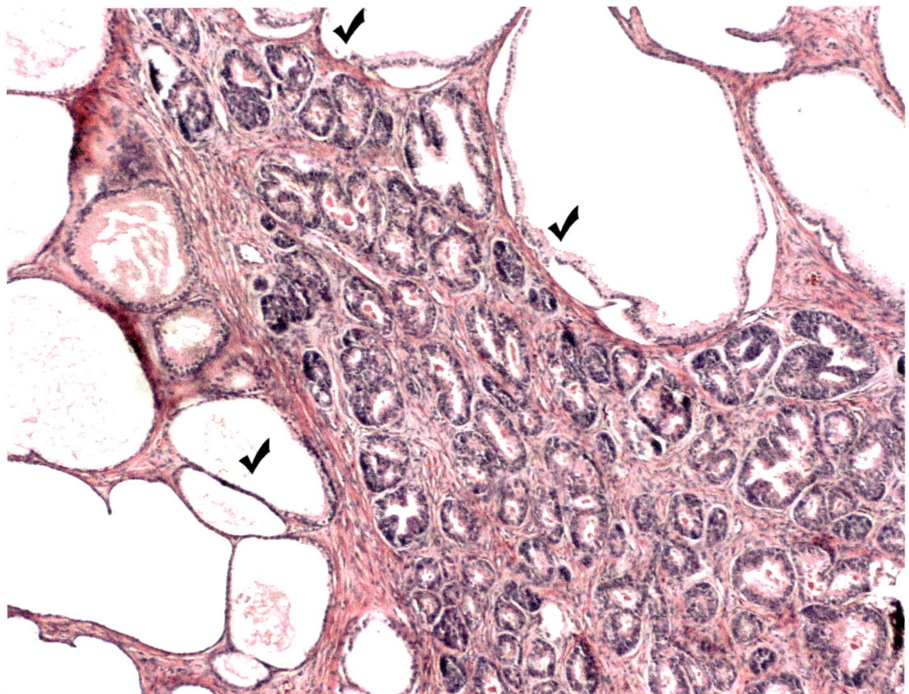

Fig. 3.72 (H-E, ×100) Infiltrative architecture of cancer. Notice these small to medium-sized basophilic glands located between larger, cystically dilated ones (*ticks*). Can it be basal cell hyperplasia?

Pseudostratification of malignant nuclei, typical for PIN-like adenocarcinoma, is responsible for the basophilic appearance of these particular cancerous glands; this basophilic appearance is an infrequent finding as far as prostate cancerous glands are concerned. Despite the somewhat basophilic appearance of the small glands – which, though not characteristic of cancer, can be rarely noticed when malignant nuclei appear somehow stratified – their infiltrative architectural pattern is certainly indicative of cancer.

Complete lack of basal cells can be immunohistochemically confirmed.

In general, because of the difficulty in distinguishing basal cells from fibroblasts, and because of problems with stratification of neoplastic nuclei due to tangential sectioning or thick sections and observation of pyknotic carcinoma nuclei that can simulate basal cells, immunohistochemistry is often necessary to more definitively identify basal cells

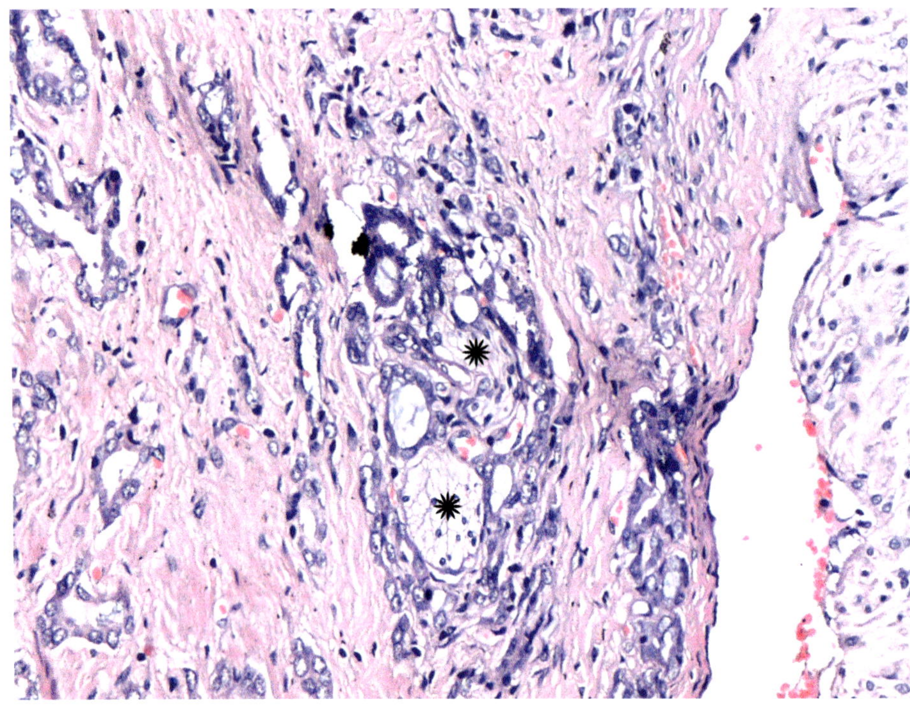

Fig. 3.73 (H-E, ×200) Circumferential perineural invasion (*asterisks*) by cancerous glands. A cancer-specific (pathognomonic) finding.

In contrast to needle biopsy specimens, in radical prostatectomy specimens, perineural invasion is not associated with outcome; therefore, the reporting of perineural invasion in these specimens is not necessary

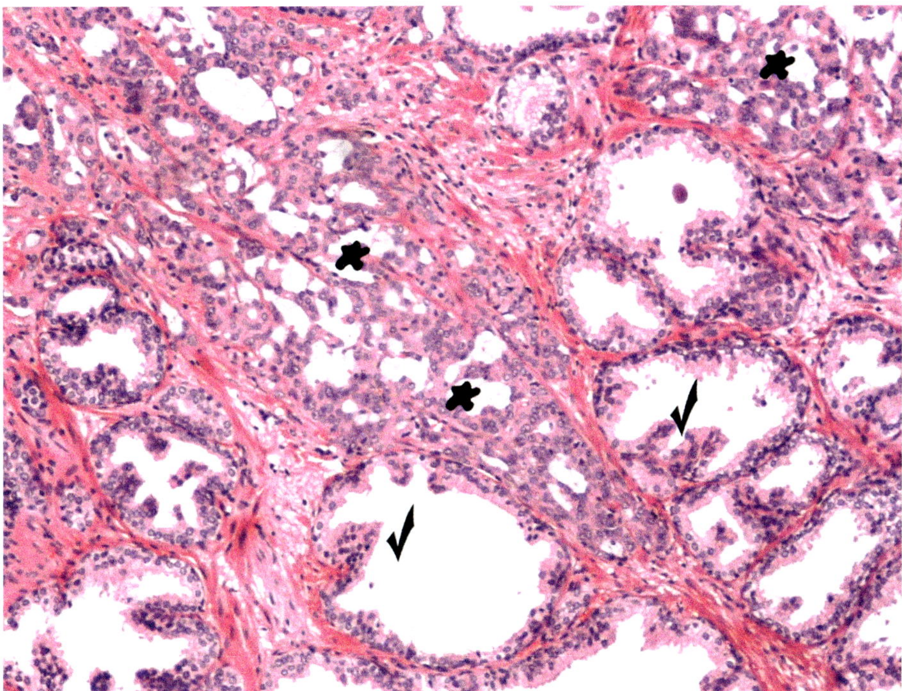

Fig. 3.74 (H-E, ×100) Poorly differentiated/high-grade prostate acinar adenocarcinoma. Fused, poorly formed cancerous glands (*blobs*) of Gleason pattern 4 invading prostatic parenchyma [larger, benign glands with papillary projections (*ticks*)].

The percentage of the radical prostatectomy sections involved by carcinoma should be reported for the quantitation of tumor size. The predominant poorly differentiated tumor component of this case should also be quantified and reported

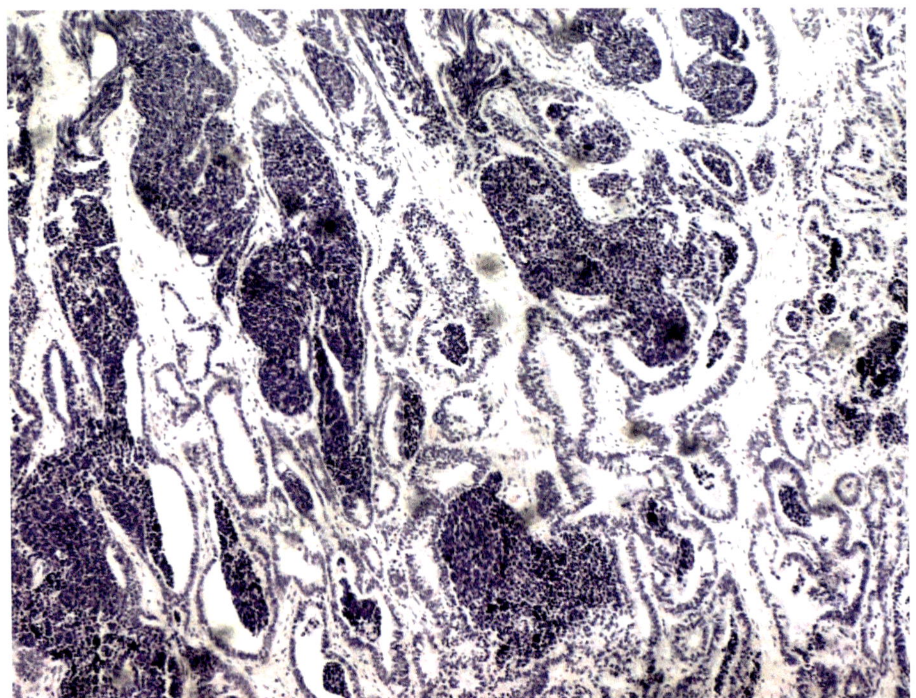

Fig. 3.75 (H-E, ×50) Basophilic areas of neuroendocrine differentiation within the prostatic acinar adenocarcinoma.

Such areas can range from "carcinoid (when well-differentiated) to small cell or large cell (when poorly differentiated)" appearance as distinct components (not just scattered cells) within an associated, usual, intermediate grade, prostate acinar adenocarcinoma. Neuroendocrine differentiation has been described in 10–33% of otherwise typical acinar adenocarcinomas of the prostate. Chromogranin and synaptophysin immunopositivity can confirm the neuroendocrine differentiation of this cancer cell subpopulation. Since CD57 can be expressed by benign prostate epithelium and many prostatic adenocarcinomas, it does not seem to indicate neuroendocrine differentiation reliably.

The most aggressive variant of prostate cancer is pure small cell neuroendocrine carcinoma; its differential diagnosis includes metastatic small cell carcinoma from the bladder or lung and non-Hodgkin lymphoma. Clinical history is important

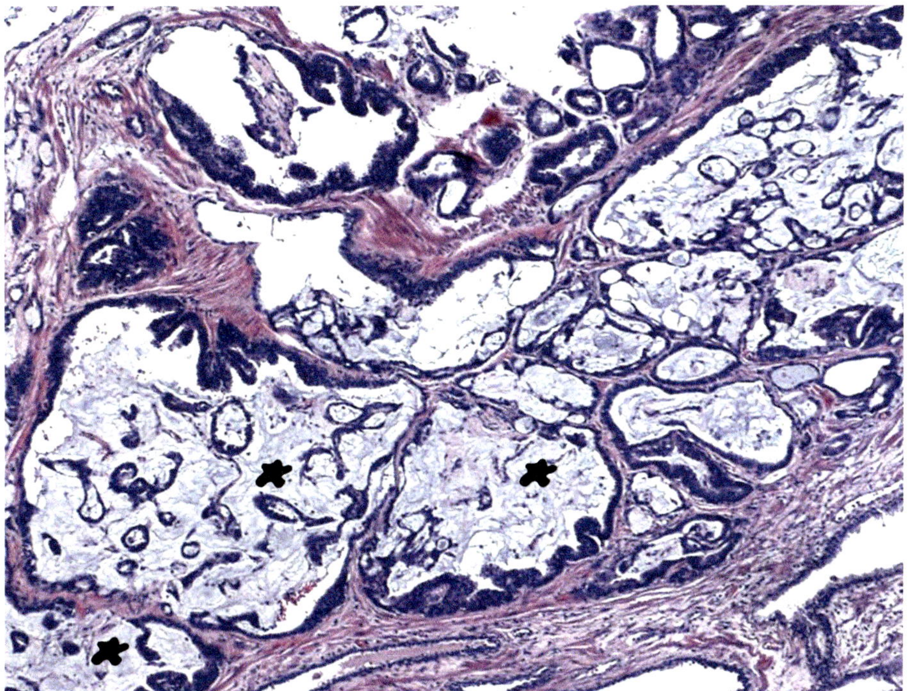

Fig. 3.76 (H-E, ×50) Focal mucinous areas within the prostate acinar adenocarcinoma. Extracellular mucin is secreted in sufficient quantity to result in lakes (*blobs*). Neoplastic cells and glands float within lakes of abundant extracellular mucin.

When this finding is seen exclusively in a needle biopsy, confirmation of prostatic origin by immunostains is necessary so that metastasis from another primary site is excluded.

In the prostate, a cutoff point of 25% has been used for the diagnosis of mucinous (colloid) prostatic adenocarcinoma; of course, this diagnosis can be made reliably only on radical prostatectomy specimens. This variant of prostate adenocarcinoma is associated with aggressive biologic behavior. Grade is determined by ignoring the mucin and applying the usual Gleason criteria to the underlying architecture

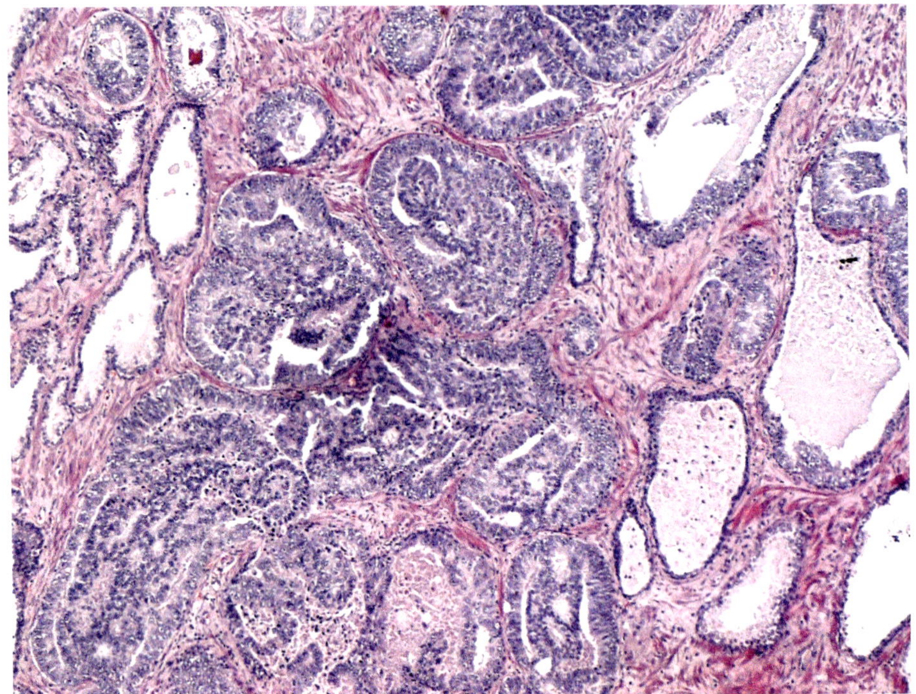

Fig. 3.77 (H-E, ×50) Confluent, extensive, complex, cribriform structures of an intraductal carcinoma of the prostate gland.

Intraductal carcinoma of the prostate is defined as a proliferation of prostate acinar/secretory carcinoma cells that is within and may significantly expand the native prostatic ducts and acini, with the basal cell layer at least partially preserved.

Intraductal carcinoma of the prostate should not be factored into the grading of a carcinoma

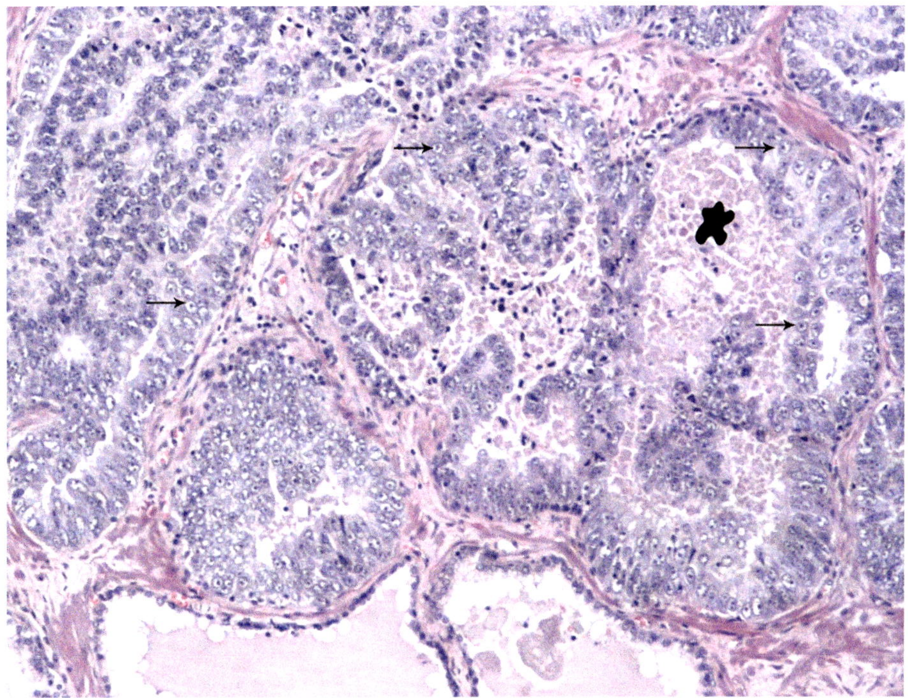

Fig. 3.78 (H-E, ×100) Comedo necrosis is evident (*blob*) in intraductal carcinoma. No maturation phenomenon is observed in intraductal carcinoma.

Differential diagnosis between intraductal carcinoma and ductal adenocarcinoma of the prostate is often challenging. Whereas intraductal carcinoma of the prostate has high-grade, *acinar/secretory cuboidal cells with round nuclei* (*arrows*), ductal adenocarcinoma has tall pseudostratified columnar epithelium with cylindrical nuclei; in some cases there is histomorphological overlap, however

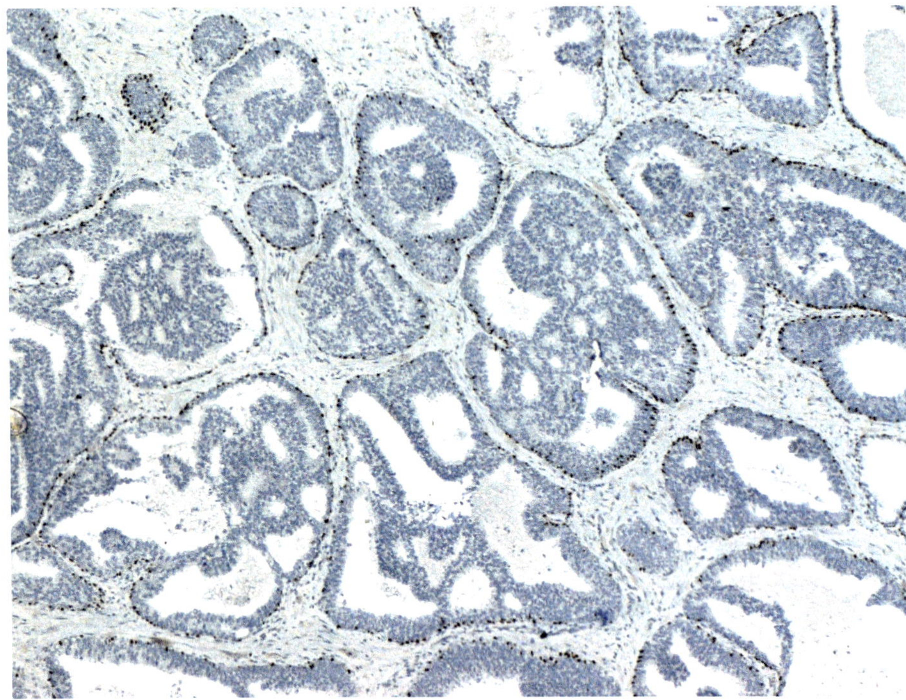

Fig. 3.79 (p63 immunohistochemistry for demonstration of basal cells, ×50) Basal cells are preserved in intraductal carcinoma of the prostate; so, apart from ductal prostatic adenocarcinoma, HG PIN should be excluded.

To clarify things, the diagnosis of "intraductal" prostate carcinoma mainly depends on the type of cell morphology.

An intraductal lesion retaining basal cells and exhibiting atypical *ductal cell morphology* is *distinct* from that of atypical *acinar/secretory cell morphology.*

- The former is characteristic of ductal adenocarcinoma (irrespective of the presence or absence of basal cells)
- The latter is characteristic:

either of HG PIN which is the precursor of acinar adenocarcinoma *or*, when atypical morphology is beyond what is acceptable for a HG PIN diagnosis, of intraductal spread of an (already) invasive neighboring, acinar adenocarcinoma; intraductal carcinoma of the prostate is thus a late event in the evolution of prostate neoplasia

So we can understand the critical importance of separating HG PIN from intraductal carcinoma of the prostate in needle biopsy. High-grade PIN is less often associated with invasive disease and, by itself, of course has a better prognosis (Pickup and van der Kwast 2007).

The most common criteria associated with intraductal carcinoma are the following:

1. Expanded, often markedly distended, yet circumscribed intraductal foci with dense cribriform to solid masses (more solid than cribriform) with too complex architecture, often with nonfocal comedo necrosis (> 1 duct showing comedo necrosis)
2. Marked, rather nonuniform, nuclear atypia (enlargement, hyperchromasia, and pleomorphism), well beyond that of HG PIN, absence of maturation phenomenon (Fig. 3.78 contrasts with Fig. 3.24), and presence of mitotic figures
3. ERG nuclear staining and cytoplasmic loss of PTEN (Roberts et al. 2013)

With regard to differential diagnosis of intraductal carcinoma from urothelial cancer, intraductal carcinoma of the prostate is positive for prostate-specific markers but negative for urothelial markers

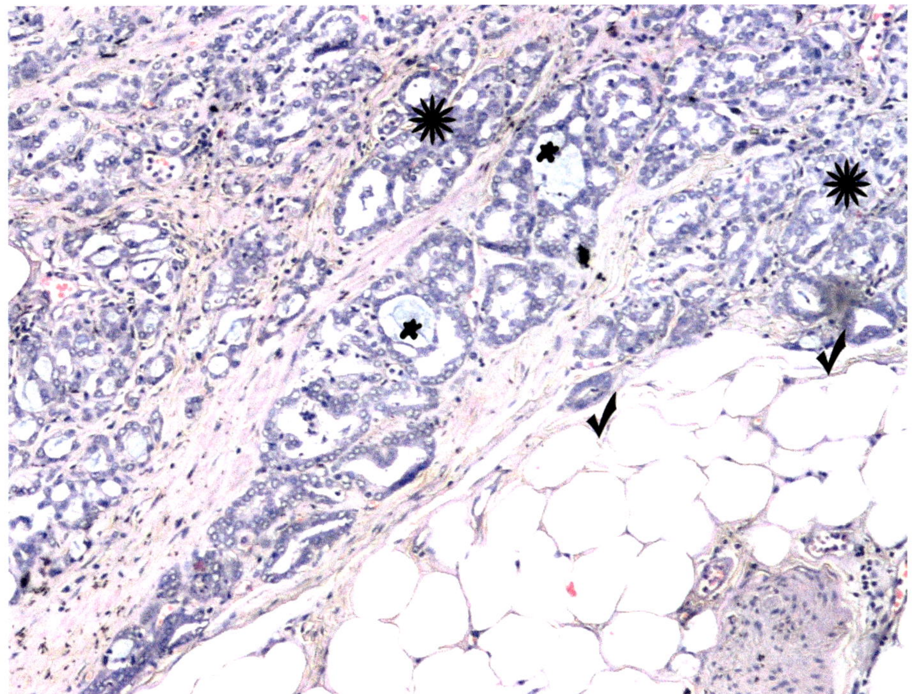

Fig. 3.80 (H-E, ×100) Imminent extracapsular extension/invasion of prostate cancer. Malignant prostate acini/glands in direct contact with periprostatic adipose tissue (*tick*). In cases with no direct contact to fat, tumor can be seen in loose connective tissues in plane of fat.

Wispy blue-tinged mucin in the lumen of malignant glands (*blobs*) constitutes a minor criterion in the diagnosis of prostate cancer. Fused glands (*asterisks*) are compatible with Gleason pattern 4

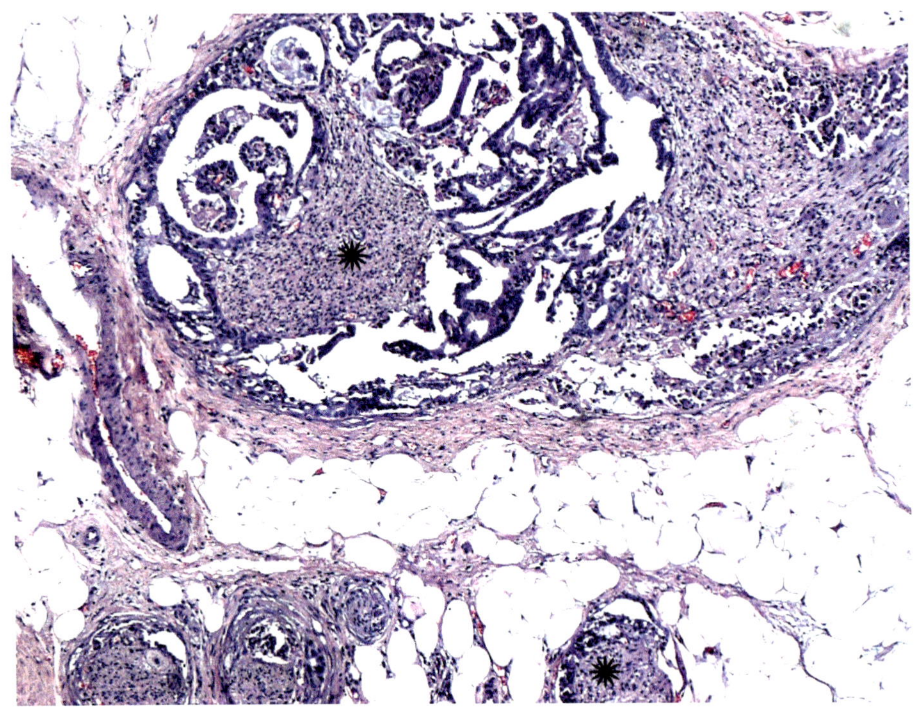

Fig. 3.81 (H-E, ×50) The infiltration of periprostatic fat is clear evidence of extraprostatic extension (pT3a). Adenocarcinomas of the prostate have a tendency to extend out of the prostate via perineural space invasion (*asterisks*). Peri–/intraneural invasion can be observed within or in plane of fat.

Extraprostatic extension is mainly defined as tumor involvement of adipose tissue; intraprostatic fat is exceedingly rare. There are three criteria for extraprostatic extension, depending on the site and composition of the extraprostatic tissue: cancer in adipose tissue, cancer in perineural spaces of the neurovascular bundles, and cancer in anterior muscle wall.

The extent of capsular penetration/extraprostatic extension varies from only a few cancerous glands outside the prostate (focal capsular penetration: < 1 high-power field and not in >2 sections) to cases with more extensive extraprostatic spread (established, nonfocal capsular penetration).

A comment should be made if there is a positive margin at the site of extraprostatic extension. In *this* case, a positive margin would show carcinoma transected at extraprostatic extension and would suggest lack of complete excision of extraprostatic tissue around extraprostatic extension

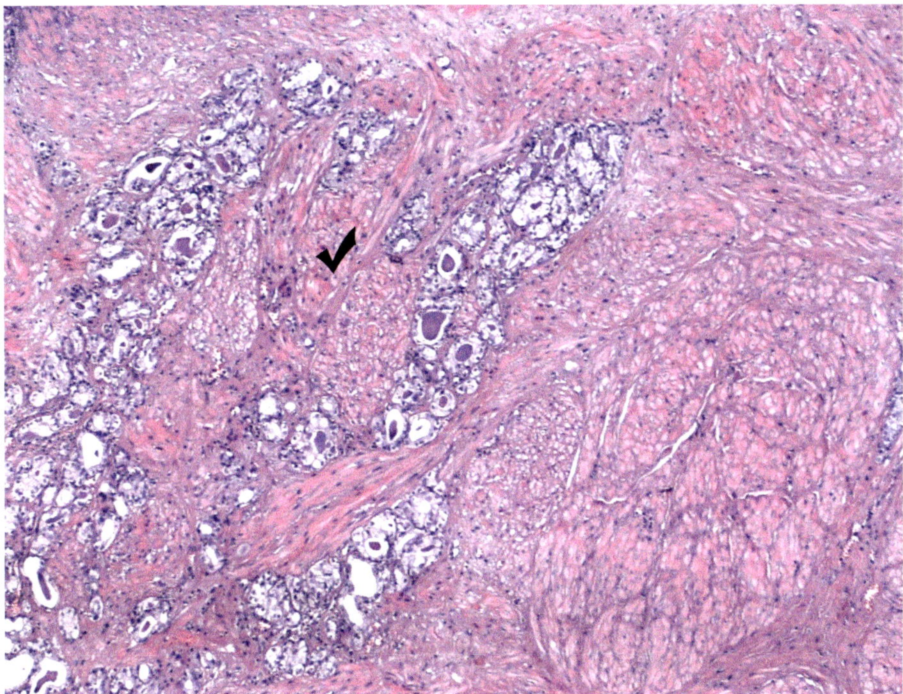

Fig. 3.82 (H-E, ×50) Microscopically detected extension of tumor into bladder neck thick *smooth muscle* bundles (*tick*) (stage pT3a); this usually correlates with extensive tumor and a high progression rate following radical prostatectomy.

With regard to *skeletal* muscle fibers, though mostly exterior to the prostate gland, they may extend into its peripheral portion; consequently, the finding of a few benign-appearing prostatic glands admixed with skeletal muscle fibers does not indicate that the glands are neoplastic, and the finding of adenocarcinoma of the prostate admixed with skeletal muscle fibers is likewise not diagnostic of extra-prostatic extension by carcinoma, except for anterior muscle involvement which corresponds to pT3a.

Stage T2 is organ-confined cancer. Stage T3a and T3b tumors show extraprostatic extension, with and without seminal vesicle invasion, respectively

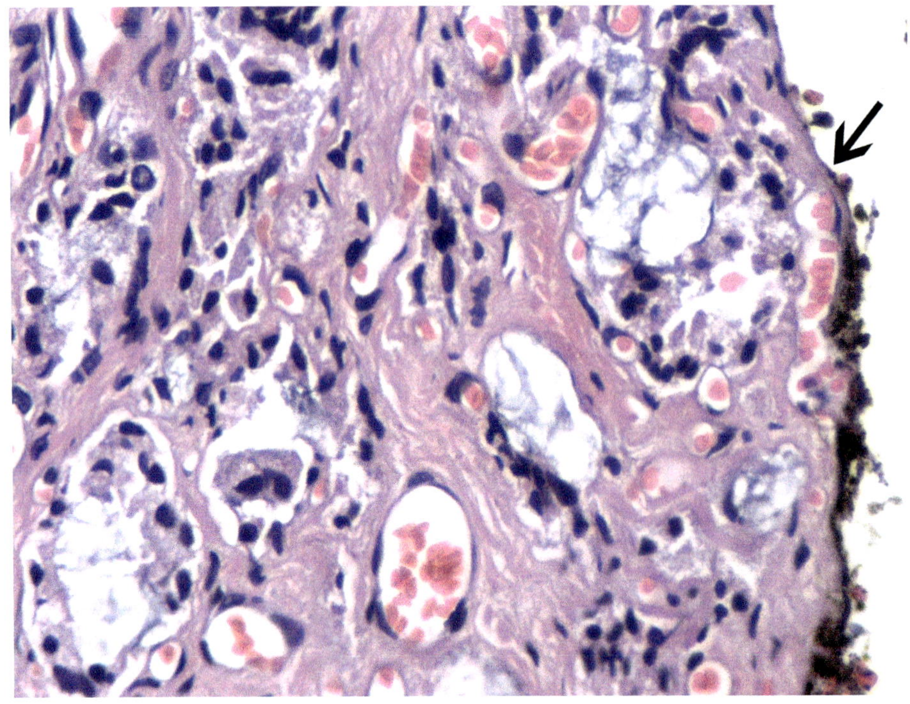

Fig. 3.83 (H-E, ×200) Evaluating inked margins of resection in radical prostatectomy specimens, irrespective of pT staging. Close margins (< 1 mm) are considered adequate for prostate.

The inked edge of the prostate physiologically acts as a fairly effective barrier. The prostate surface should be inked to facilitate distinction of the surgical resection margin from any artifactual margins resulting from gross dissection in the laboratory. The right and left surface of the gland should be separately examined to enable the identification of tumor laterality. Positive margins, when found, may be classified as focal or extensive, correlating with prognosis.

Cancer here almost makes contact with the inked surface which, in this field, is identical to the prostate "capsule," with no presence of any extraprostatic tissue (surgical incision of the prostate). This capsular margin, when considered tumor-positive, would show prostate cancer transected within the prostate parenchyma with no evidence of extracapsular extension (stage pT2 R+/R1 or pT2x). This type of positive margin most often occurs at the posterolateral aspect of prostate where parenchyma is inadvertently transected during dissection and preservation of the neurovascular bundle for potency sparing. Capsular invasion is quite common, but it should *not* be confused with extracapsular/extraprostatic extension, i.e., infiltration of extraprostatic tissue (pT3 stage). The smooth, rounded surface of the prostate (*arrow*) indicates that the tumor has not penetrated the capsule; in the latter case, a shaggy, irregular surface of the gland would have been observed. Even in these cases, however, if there is only a scant amount of benign soft tissue separating the tumor from the ink (arguably less than 0.25 mm), the margin should still be considered negative

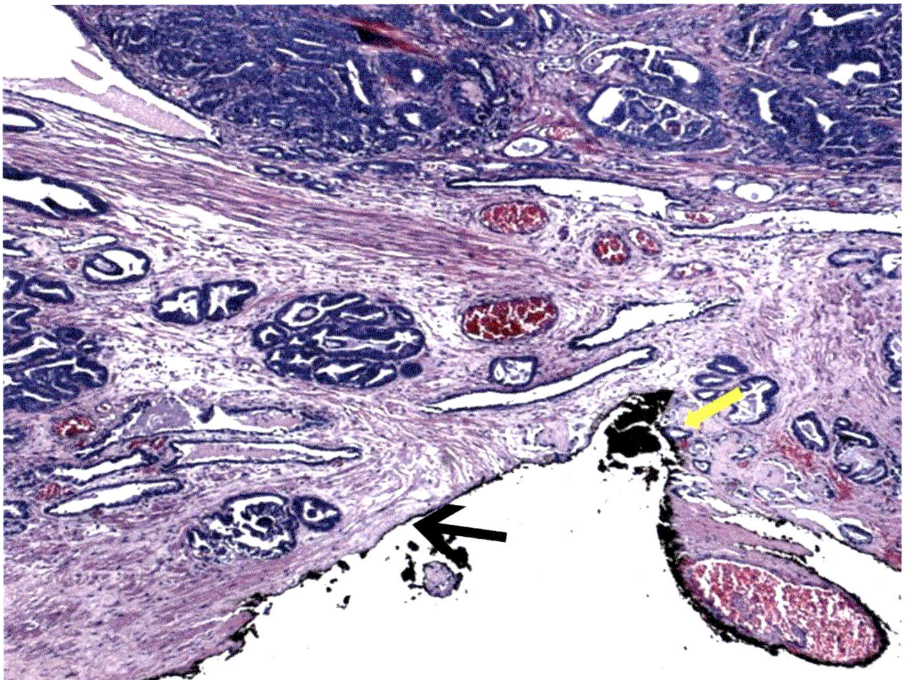

Fig. 3.84 (H-E, ×50) Another case of radical prostatectomy is shown in the next three images (Figs. 3.84, 3.85 and 3.86). Positive surgical margin is here defined as cancer glands that touch the inked surface of the prostate (*yellow arrow*). A margin is positive if tumor cells touch the ink; extent of positive margin in mm and its location should be reported. Surgical margins are *not* included in pathologic staging and are separately mentioned in the pathology report.

The prostate has a fibromuscular pseudocapsule that is discontinuous at its apex, bladder base and anteriorly, so the "capsule" is not relevant in staging prostate cancer. This fibromuscular layer is most prominent along the base and posterior portion of the lateral borders and is an inseparable component of the prostatic stroma.

There are two types of *positive margins*:

- Iatrogenic or capsular incision (pT2+, pT2 R1, or pT2x): tumor transected within the prostate.
- Noniatrogenic: tumor transected at extraprostatic extension (pT3a, as in this figure). Tumor induces here a desmoplastic stromal response and a *protuberance to the capsular surface* (*black arrow*). Extraprostatic extension is common and is often, but not always, defined as tumor in contact with extraprostatic fat. Extraprostatic extension, in addition to infiltration of periprostatic fat, may be recognized by the presence of tumor-associated desmoplastic stroma bulging beyond the prostatic contour in desmoplastic tissues beyond fat or beyond condensed prostatic smooth muscle. The best way of assessing whether capsular penetration has occurred is to look at the adjacent prostatic capsule on scanning magnification where there is no tumor and follow the edge of the gland to the area in question to see whether the normal rounded contour of the gland has been altered by a *protuberance* corresponding to *extension of tumor into periprostatic tissue*.

Positive surgical margins in a prostatectomy specimen correlate with tumor progression; their status is dependent on both the tumor volume and the surgical technique. Prostate apex is the most frequent site of positive margin. Positive margins at the base usually indicate extensive disease. Tumor at the anterior region margin is usually considered extraprostatic extension because it is usually exterior to the prostate. In case of extensive, multifocal positive margins, urologists elect to administer postoperative adjuvant therapy

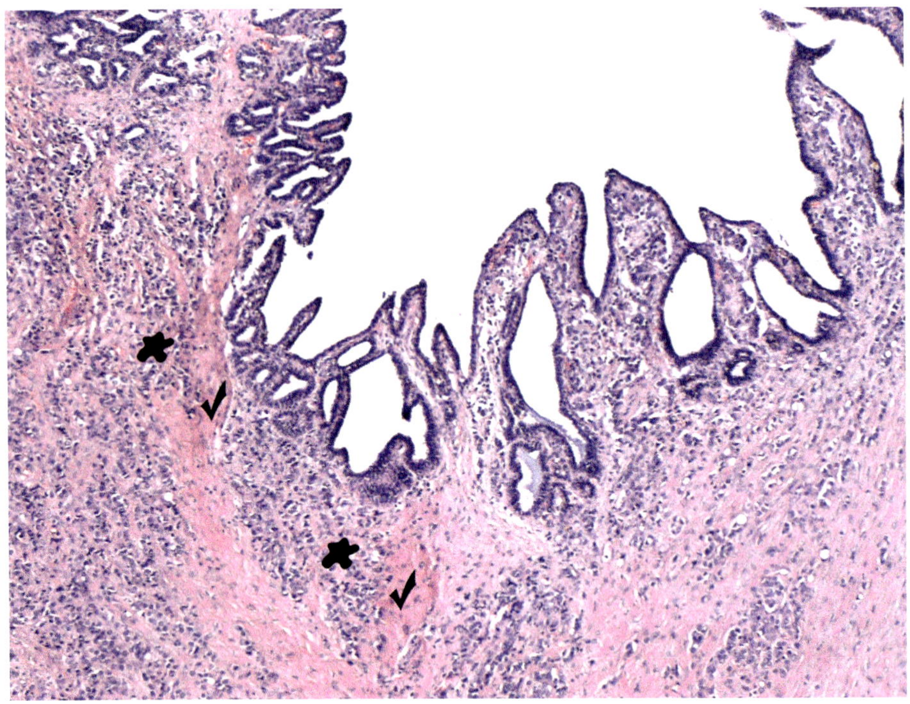

Fig. 3.85 (H-E, ×50) Seminal vesicle smooth muscular coat (*ticks*) invaded by high-grade prostatic adenocarcinoma (*blobs*) (stage pT3b). A diagnosis of seminal vesicle invasion requires infiltration of the muscular wall of the extraprostatic portion of the seminal vesicle

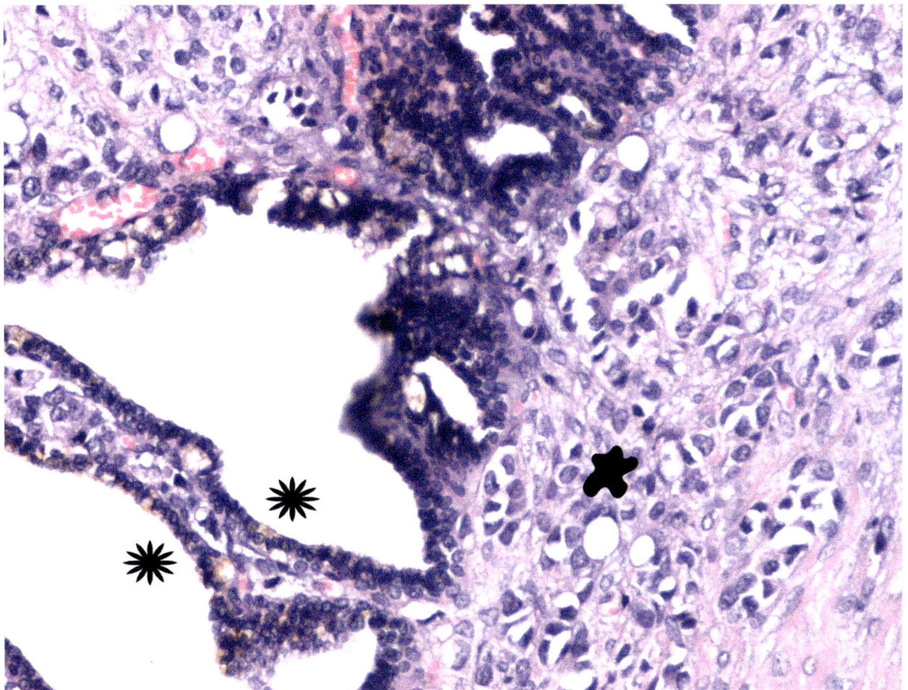

Fig. 3.86 (H-E, ×200) High-grade cancerous elements (*blob*) extending into the seminal vesicles (*asterisks*).

The incidence of invasion of the prostate "capsule" as well as of seminal vesicle involvement and distant metastases correlates very positively with total tumor volume and with the percentage of high-grade tumor (Gleason patterns 4 and 5)

3.7.1.1 Clinical Commentary

Vasileios Spapis

This is a case of a surgically resected, quite extensive prostate acinar adenocarcinoma, mainly of high grade (grade group 3), with nonfocal extraprostatic extension, staged as pT3a in the radical prostatectomy specimen, and with free margins of resection.

Radical prostatectomy (RP) specimens should be totally embedded in order to assess tumor multifocality, location, and heterogeneity. Partial embedding could be considered for larger prostates with comparable results (detection 98% of PCa, 96% accurate staging) (Sehdev et al. 2001; Stamey et al. 2000).

Grading using the Gleason score of the conventional prostatic adenocarcinoma system is the strongest prognostic factor for clinical behavior and treatment response. Nomograms using Gleason score predict disease-specific survival (DSS) after prostatectomy (Partin et al. 2001).

Extraprostatic extension (EPE) is defined as carcinoma mixed with periprostatic adipose tissue. Location and extent of EPE should always be reported as it is related to recurrence risk (Magi-Galluzzi et al. 2011). It should be noted though that in the urinary bladder neck, microscopic invasion of smooth muscle fibers is entirely different than bladder wall invasion (the latter staged as pT4) because the former does not carry independent prognostic significance for PCa recurrence (Aydin et al. 2004; Ploussard et al. 2010) and should thus be recorded as EPE (pT3a).

PCa volume in RP specimens has not yet been established as an independent prognostic factor (Epstein et al. 2005). 0.5 ml is used as a limit to distinguish clinically significant from insignificant tumors (Stamey et al. 2000).

Positive surgical margin is also an independent risk factor for biochemical recurrence (BCR). A positive margin is not necessarily evidence of EPE (Mottet et al. 2017). There are not enough data to prove a relationship between margin extent and recurrence risk (Marks et al. 2007). However, multifocality, extent of margin positivity, or number of blocks with positive margin involvement should be reported (Sammon et al. 2013).

Extracapsular invasion (pT3) and positive surgical margins (i.e., R1 or R+) are associated with a risk of local recurrence, which can be close to 50% after 5 years (Hanks 1988). For those patients, especially the ones that present with postoperative PSA < 0.1 ng/mL, two options can be offered: either immediate adjuvant radiotherapy (ART) to the surgical bed or clinical and biological monitoring followed by salvage radiotherapy (SRT) before the PSA exceeds 0.5 ng/mL (Mottet et al. 2017)

Key Messages

- Prostatic carcinoma is typically multifocal, and gross examination usually underestimates the extent of disease.
- Proven prognostic factors in prostate carcinoma include the preoperative PSA level, the stage of prostate carcinoma, Gleason score, status of surgical margins, and volume of the tumor (particularly high-grade cancer volume, a fact that fully justifies its quantification).

- Intraductal carcinoma of the prostate exhibits much greater architectural and/or cytological atypia than HG PIN and is associated with high-grade, high-stage carcinoma.
- Accurate pathological staging is possible only when the whole prostate has been removed by radical prostatectomy.
- Invasion into the prostatic apex or into (but not beyond) the prostatic "capsule" is classified as pT2, not pT3.
- Extraprostatic extension (pT3) should be quantitated as focal (< 1 HPF on 1–2 sections) or nonfocal.
- Determine extraprostatic extension in radical prostatectomy specimens by comparing the presence of tumor to the normal edge of the prostate gland.
- Seminal vesicle invasion means tumor invades its muscular coat, seen first at the base of the seminal vesicles.
- pT3 can have positive or negative margins.
- Margins are important, and margin status is independent of pT classification; classify positive margins as either focal or extensive based on the length of involvement of the inked line of resection.

3.8 Case 3.5: Metastatic Prostate Carcinoma

Case Study

Data Prior to Microscopy

A 75-year-old man complains of back pain. On physical examination, lower extremity edema is noticed.

Serum PSA value of 45 ng/ml is counted. Digital rectal examination of the prostate is highly suspicious for cancer. A needle biopsy is performed and confirms the presence of a Gleason score 9 cancer.

Enlarged external and internal iliac nodes are detected by CT scan, a finding that certainly precludes radical prostatectomy. Moreover, there is an increase in serum alkaline phosphatase concentration due to osteosclerotic metastatic deposits in lumbar vertebrae, confirmed by bone scintigraphy.

3.8.1 Microscopic Evaluation of the Needle Biopsy Specimen

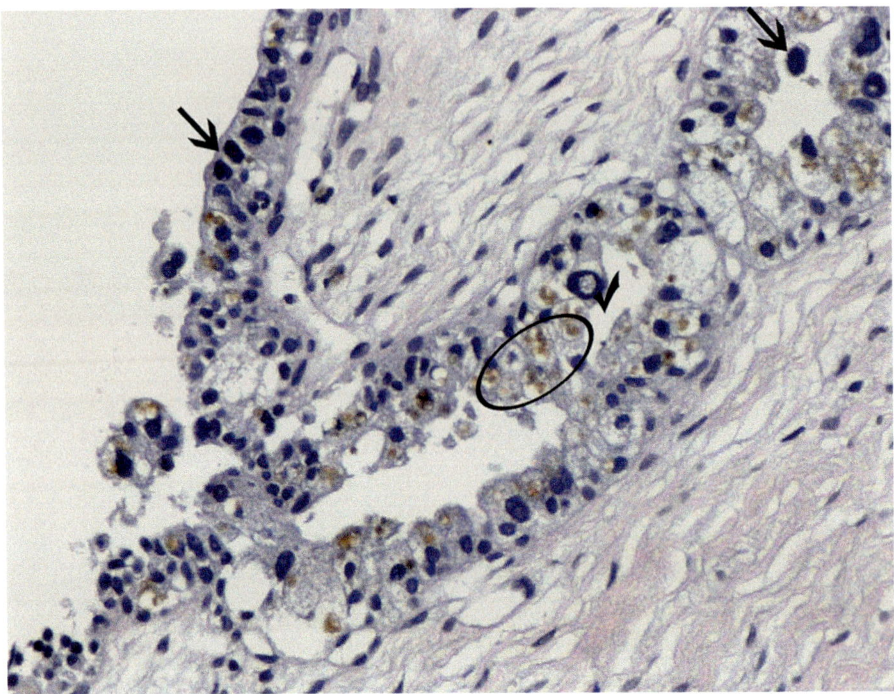

Fig. 3.87 (H-E, ×200) Seminal vesicles/ejaculatory duct segment included in the needle biopsy material.

A common finding on needle biopsy of the seminal vesicle is to see at the tip or at the edge of the core of tissue an irregular row of glandular epithelium that represents the lining of the central dilated seminal vesicle lumen, since the core of tissue fractures at this interface.

The epithelium of seminal vesicle and of ejaculatory duct may be mistaken as neoplastic, particularly when the outpouching from the seminal vesicle epithelium gives origin to clusters of small glands that mimic prostate cancer. The majority of cells are tall; scattered cells showing prominent nuclear pleomorphism (large "monstrous" cells, *arrows*) and also exhibiting hyperchromasia (*arrows*) often obscuring nuclear details are a common feature of the seminal vesicle/ejaculatory duct epithelium and should not be confused with malignancy. These cells lack mitotic activity and commonly appear degenerated in nature, similar to what is seen in radiation atypia. Even in poorly differentiated prostatic carcinoma, which lacks glandular differentiation, one rarely sees the severe atypia that is present within scattered seminal vesicle epithelial cells. Intranuclear inclusions are another hallmark of seminal vesicle epithelium (*tick*). Gold-brown lipochrome pigment (lipofuscin) is noticed in the cytoplasm (*ellipse*). Lipofuscin yellow-brown to gray-brown granules measure 1–3 microns in diameter and are supposed to have a predominantly subnuclear location. The presence of prominent lipofuscin granules within seminal vesicle epithelium is an important diagnostic aid; prostate carcinoma typically lacks lipofuscin pigment. One should be aware, though, that normal prostate glands may also demonstrate lipofuscin pigment or, more frequently, refractile red-brown granules corresponding to lysosomes. The presence of this pigment and the absence of mitoses are quite helpful to exclude the possibility of neoplasia (i.e., PIN or cancer). In the absence of the pigment, monoclonal PSA antibody and PAP antibody immunonegative staining will confirm the different histogenesis of these structures. Secretory cells' nuclei of seminal vesicles are strongly

Fig. 3.87 (continued)

pax-2(+) and basal cells are positive for basal cell markers. To sum up, the key to the differential diagnosis is in recognizing the degenerative nuclear atypia, the characteristic yellow pigment, and the nearby seminal vesicle epithelium; immunohistochemistry for pax-2 (or MUC6) can help, if necessary.

The ejaculatory ducts lack a well-formed smooth muscle wall and are entrenched by a band of loose fibrovascular/collagenous substrate. In contrast to seminal vesicles, invasion of the ejaculatory ducts by cancerous cells in needle biopsy material is not a contraindication of radical prostatectomy since it does not indicate extraprostatic extension; on the contrary, seminal vesicle involvement indicates high-stage disease (pT3b)

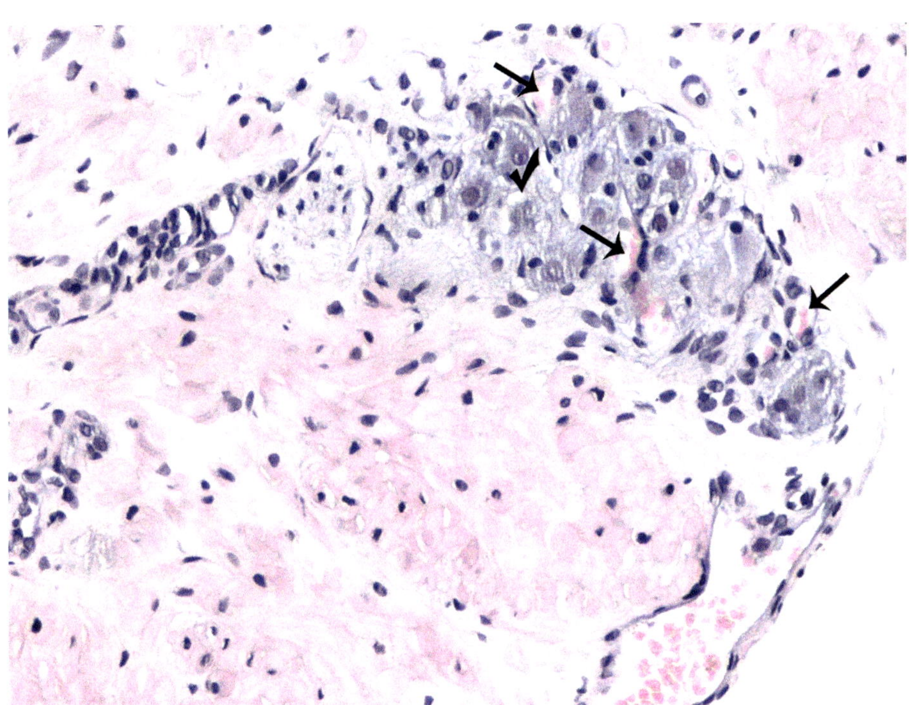

Fig. 3.88 (H-E, ×200) Paraganglion tissue cells (group of *neuroendocrine* cells derived from neural crest) can rarely be seen in TURP or needle biopsy specimens and be misdiagnosed as high-grade prostate acinar adenocarcinoma. In radical prostatectomy specimens, the misinterpretation of extraprostatic paraganglial tissue potentially leads to overstaging.

Notice this group of cells with vacuolated or amphophilic cytoplasm and a delicate blood vessel meshwork (*arrows*). Cytoplasm may also be clear. Nuclei may show prominent nucleoli (*tick*) or degenerative, endocrine-type atypia. Prominent nucleoli are very useful in the diagnosis of prostate cancer but they are not among the cancer-specific criteria. Here prominent nucleoli are observed in the nuclei of ganglion cells within the prostate stroma. Remember that, on everyday practice, diagnosis of prostate cancer should be based on a *combination* of histological findings

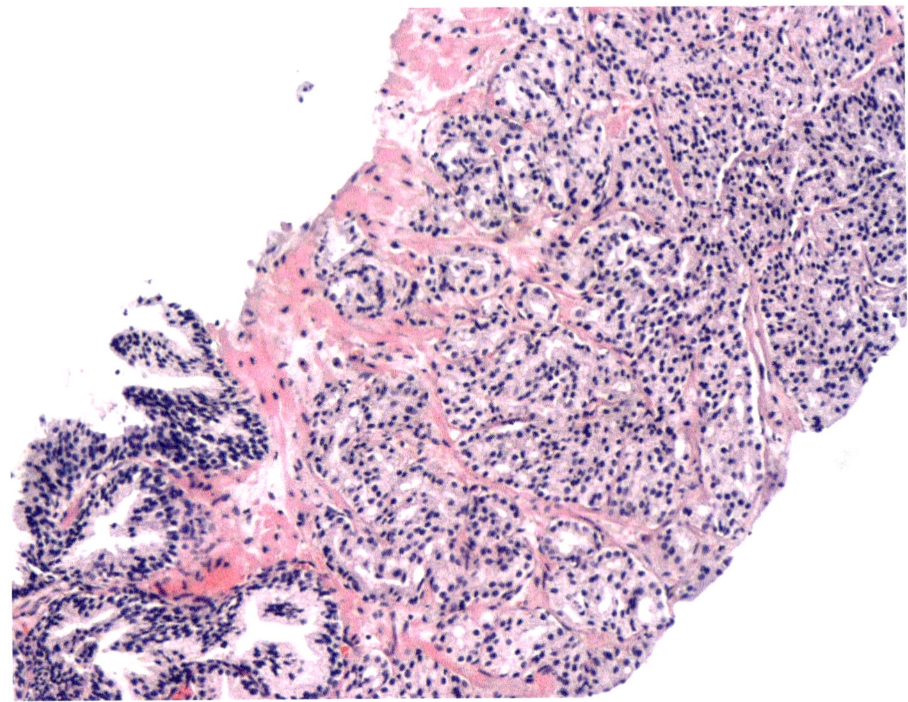

Fig. 3.89 (H-E, ×50) Gleason pattern 4 – poor differentiation/high grade. Fused, poorly formed cancerous glands invading prostate fibromuscular stroma. Lumens are barely noticeable
Gleason scores 8 to 10 represent poorly differentiated, highly aggressive adenocarcinomas

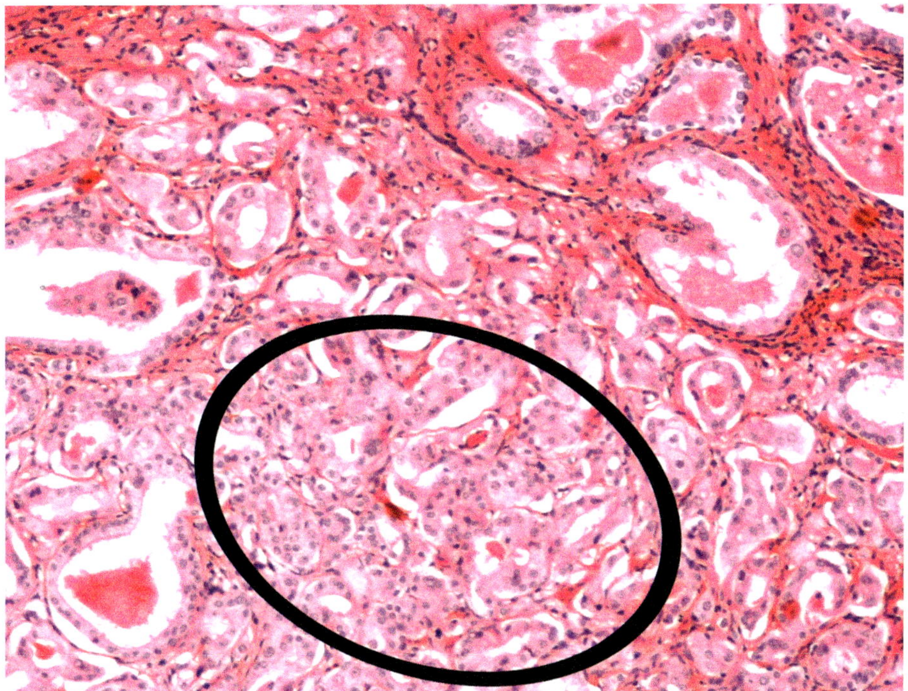

Fig. 3.90 (H-E, ×100) Loss of ability to form smooth surfaces against stroma (*ellipse*) is compatible with Gleason pattern 4.
These cancer cells have abundant amphophilic cytoplasm

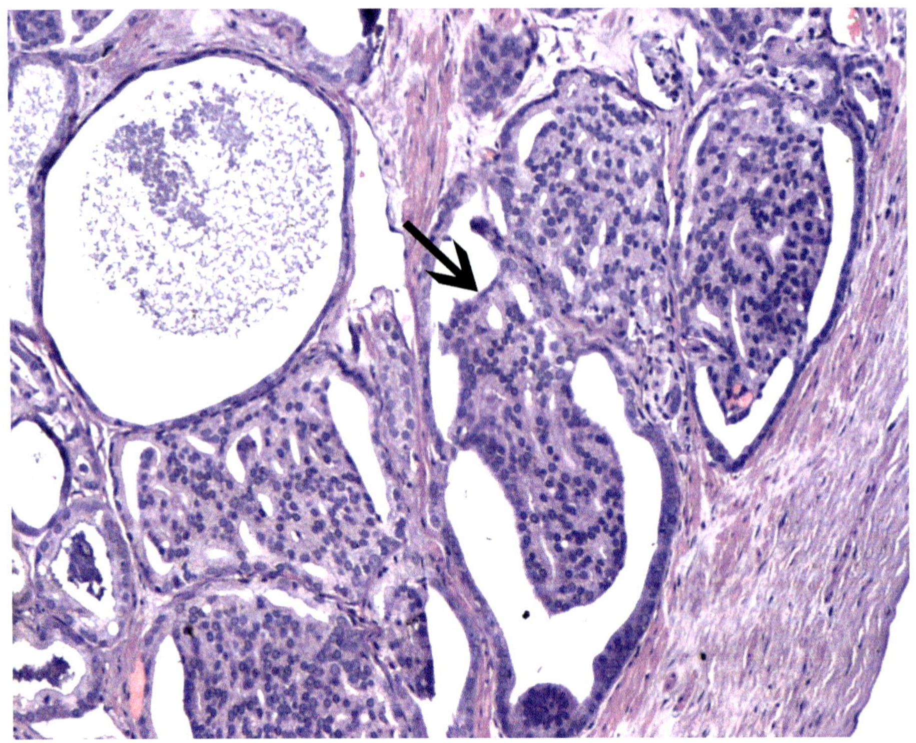

Fig. 3.91 (H-E, ×200) Glomeruloid bodies/glomerulations, a pathognomonic finding for prostatic acinar adenocarcinoma, are part of Gleason pattern 4. Glomerulations consist of glands where cribriform formations are attached to only one edge of the gland (*arrow*), resulting in a structure superficially resembling a glomerulus

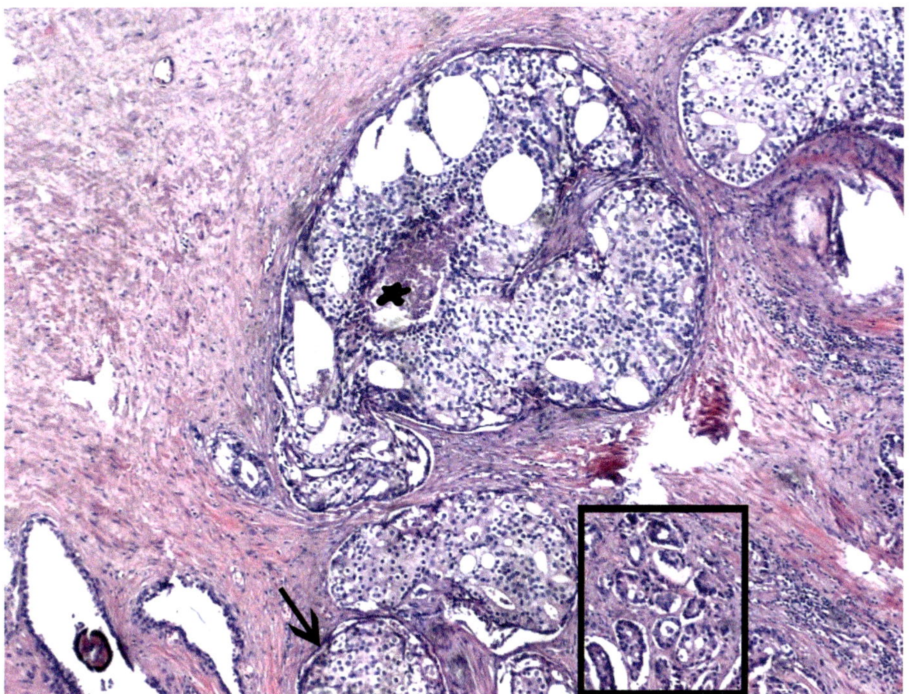

Fig. 3.92 (H-E, ×50) Cribriform pattern of high-grade prostate acinar adenocarcinoma. As the majority of prostate acinar adenocarcinomas, this is a lesion of the peripheral zone of the prostate, frequently accompanied by separate, small-sized infiltrating glands of Gleason pattern 3 (*square frame*). It is generally important to be able to separate pattern 3 from pattern 4 because this separation usually distinguishes Gleason score 6 from Gleason score 7, the latter having a significantly worse prognosis.

Note the regular round to oval nuclei of the acinar cell cribriform pattern (acinar cell type) – as opposed to the tall columnar cells with large elongated hyperchromatic nuclei making up the cribriform ductal adenocarcinoma we are going to examine in the next case. *Complete loss of basal cell layer* favors the diagnosis of invasive prostate carcinoma over intraductal carcinoma and HG PIN.

The cribriform glands of pattern 4 are either large cribriform glands, including cribriform sheets, or smaller cribriform glands often with irregular infiltrating borders. The cribriform glands of Gleason pattern 4 may have irregular/infiltrating *or* regular borders. It should be stressed that in cribriform pattern (always classified as pattern 4, at least), the cribriform proliferations may be rather small, rounded (*arrow*), and not crowded together. Rounded, well-circumscribed glands having the same size as normal glands as well as evenly spaced lumina and cellular bridges of uniform thickness are now considered in Gleason pattern 4 category.

(Central) Comedo necrosis, defined by intraluminal necrotic cells and/or karyorrhexis (*blob*), is classified as pattern 5, even when present in cribriform glands. Any necrosis of the tumor epithelium automatically assigns a tumor to Gleason pattern 5.

In the setting of high-grade cancer on needle biopsy or radical prostatectomy, lower-grade patterns should be ignored if they occupy <5% of the area of the tumor

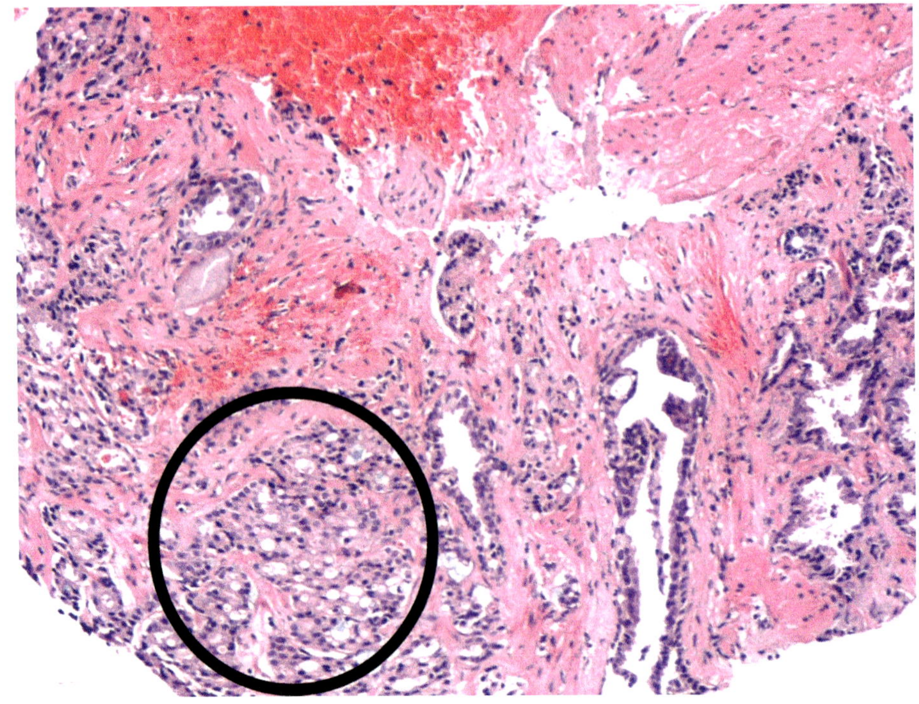

Fig. 3.93 (H-E, ×50) The underlying architecture of poorly formed glands with vacuolated cells (*circle*) is that of Gleason pattern 4

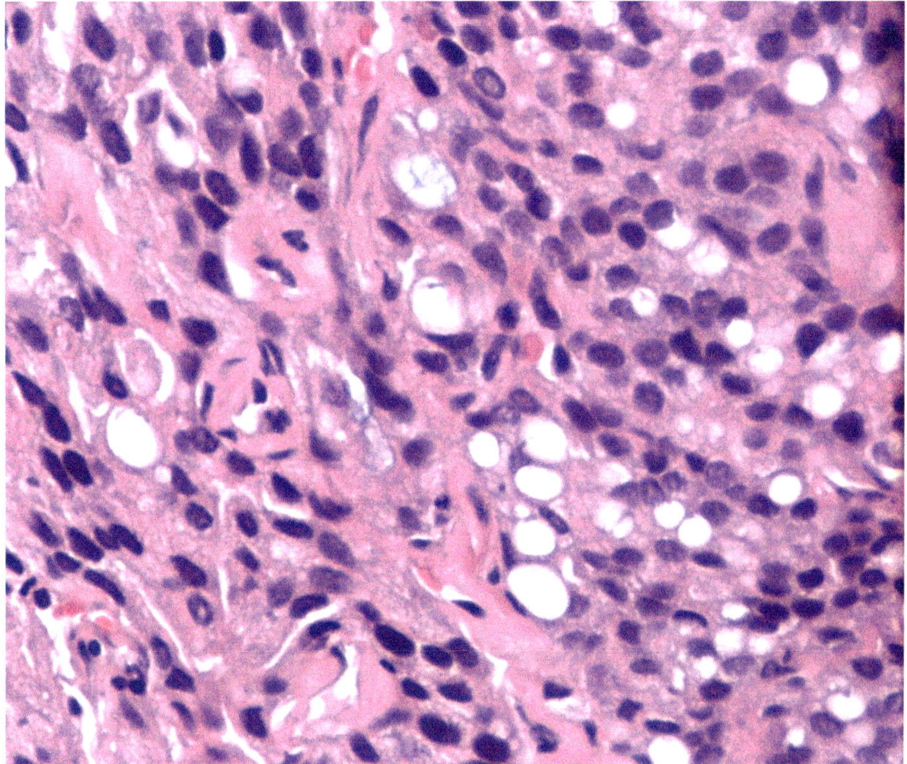

Fig. 3.94 (H-E, ×200) Vacuoles merely suggest adenocarcinoma but they are *not* evidence of lumen formation. Optically clear vacuoles can displace the nuclei peripherally. It is recommended to discount the vacuoles while assigning a grade

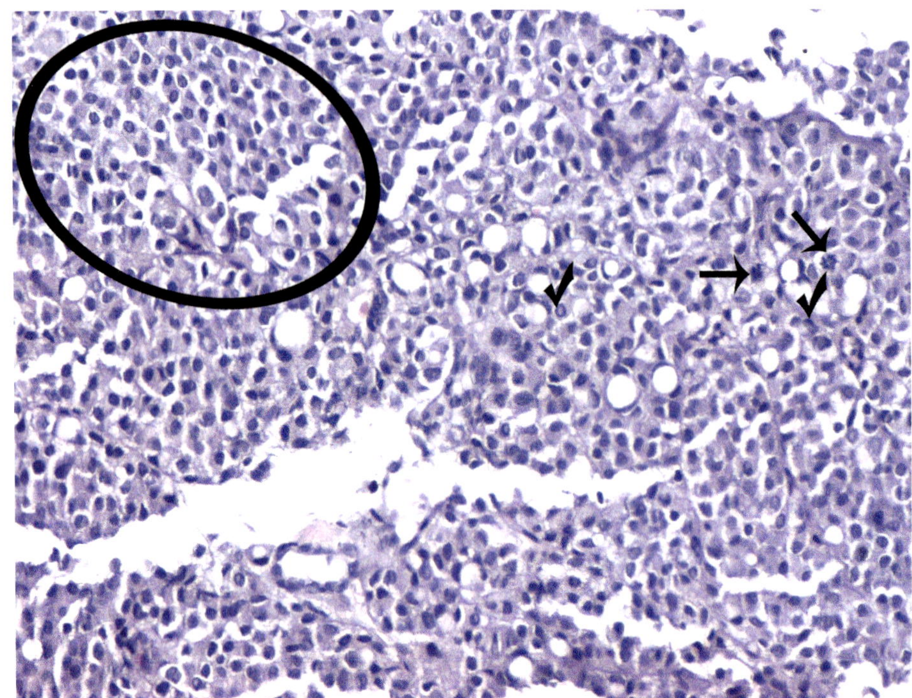

Fig. 3.95 (H-E, ×100) High-grade prostate cancer, Gleason pattern 5, composed of sheets of malignant cells predominantly lacking luminal formation/glandular differentiation (*ellipse*).

Cancer nuclei, even in poorly differentiated cancers, show little variation in size and shape. Mitoses (*arrows*) and apoptotic bodies are observable. Mitoses are a helpful feature of malignancy, but they are rarely present in prostate cancer, as far as limited carcinomas with a Gleason score of 6 and low-grade tumors are concerned; mitotic figures are more common in the setting of high-grade cancer, as here. In any case, mitoses are highly suggestive of malignancy, if present.

When vacuoles are seen in single cells of Gleason pattern 5 (*ticks*), the tumor may resemble a true signet ring cell carcinoma; nevertheless, unlike signet ring cells, these cells have empty vacuoles that lack intracellular mucin. For the diagnosis of a signet ring-like cell carcinoma in the prostate, the tumor must demonstrate a "great majority of cells, i.e., 25% or more" with signet ring-like morphology; this special subtype is basically an adenocarcinoma of small ducts and acini of high grade. Secondary involvement of signet ring carcinoma from the gastrointestinal or urothelial tract should be excluded

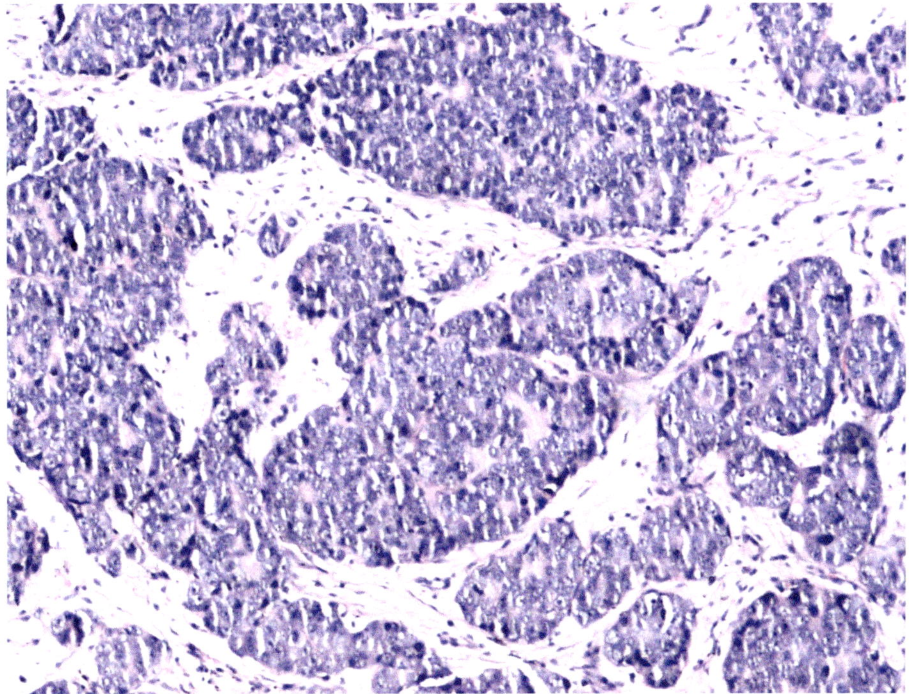

Fig. 3.96 (H-E, ×100) High-grade tumors of Gleason pattern 5 tend to grow in individual cells, cords, solid nests, linear arrays, and sheets. Totally fused cancerous glands and solid structures invading prostate fibromuscular stroma are shown here. Solid infiltrating cancerous structures are assigned Gleason pattern 5 (poorly differentiated/undifferentiated carcinoma). Gleason pattern 5 should totally lack glandular differentiation and lumen formation

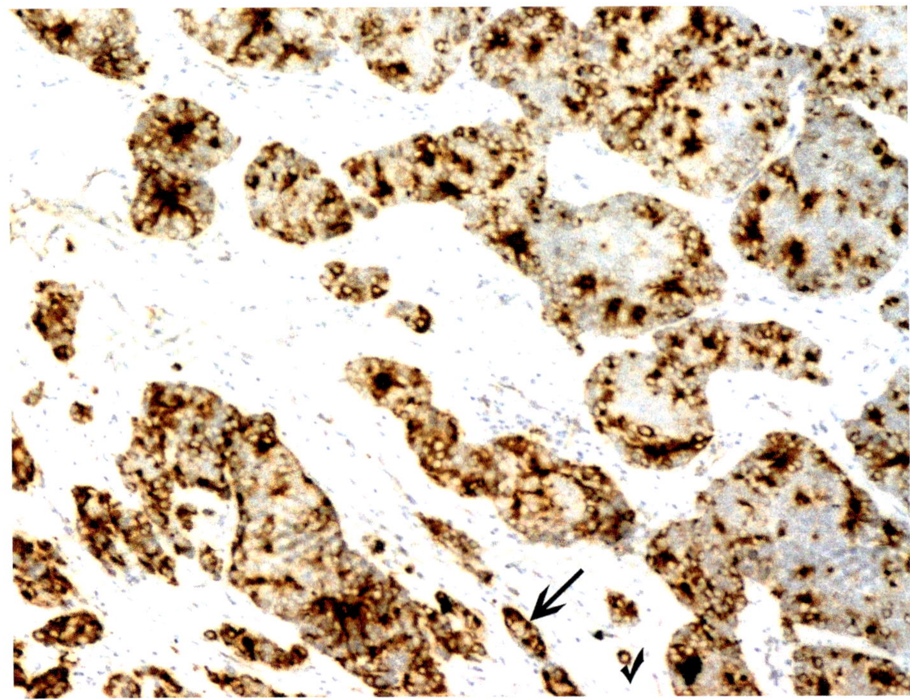

Fig. 3.97 (PSMA immunohistochemistry, ×100) Gleason pattern 5. Fusion of glands occurs with tumor cells joining up to form cords (*arrow*). Single cancer cells are also detected (*tick*). Immunohistochemical confirmation of prostatic origin [e.g., PSA, prostate-specific membrane antigen (PSMA), and androgen receptor (AR) positivity] is frequently necessary, especially in metastatic sites

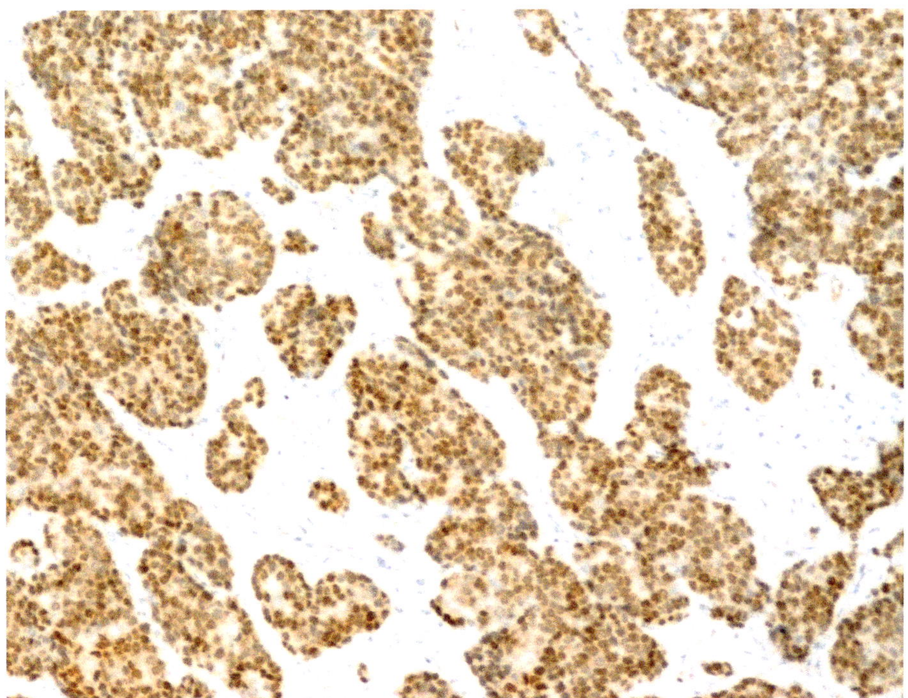

Fig. 3.98 (AR immunohistochemistry, ×100) Almost all prostatic carcinomas show nuclear expression of androgen receptors (and many of the expression of estrogen receptors-β).

Since PSA and PAP expression can be decreased after androgen deprivation therapy, newer immunomarkers such as prostein and NKX3.1 can be of use in metastatic cases, the latter marker arguably being highly specific for prostatic adenocarcinoma

3.8.1.1 Clinical Commentary

Maria Gkotzamanidou

This is a case of Gleason score 9, prostate acinar adenocarcinoma with symptoms of metastatic disease. The diagnosis of high-grade prostate cancer was confirmed by histologic findings in the needle biopsies taken, as analyzed above.

The median age at diagnosis of carcinoma of prostate is 66 years (Siegel et al. 2017). Prostate cancer is a leading cause of death due to cancer, after lung and colorectal cancer, in men. The diagnosis of prostate cancer is based on symptoms, an abnormal digital rectal examination (DRE) or, more frequently, a change in or an elevated serum PSA. Unlike other common malignancies, aging men have a high rate of asymptomatic prostate cancer.

Regarding the diagnostic workout, the clinical examination (DRE) is the initial evaluation. Ultrasound is the standard imaging tool to assess the prostate and assist in the guidance of needles for directed tissue biopsies to establish a diagnosis with the sensitivity of TRUS-guided biopsies reaching 70%. Computerized tomography (CT) scans of the pelvis are commonly used, but they possess limited capabilities in the detection of intraprostatic disease and quantification of extraprostatic extension and seminal vesicle involvement. MRI arguably provides the most optimal imaging to appreciate the prostate anatomy.

The diagnosis of metastatic disease should be completed by radionuclide bone scan evaluating the presence of osseous metastases. Bone scan is unnecessary and not recommended in patients with low-risk prostate cancer due to low yield. The staging system for prostate cancer follows the TNM (tumor, node, metastasis) system. The disease may be cured when localized, with local disease (T1 or T2) showing a 5-year survival rate of 100%. However, the rate of tumor growth varies from very slow to moderately rapid, and some patients may have prolonged survival even after the cancer has metastasized to distant sites. The preference of metastatic spread in prostate cancer is lymph node, bone, like in our case, with osteoblastic lesions being far more common than osteolytic lesions – but mixed, blastic/lytic lesions do exist – and also visceral metastases.

The prognosis or probability of recurrence after definitive therapy can be based on nomograms (Partin tables) with the clinical tumor stage, biopsy, Gleason score, and PSA being the parameters to predict pathologic stage (Partin et al. 2001). Other parameters that have been reported to predict outcomes include the apoptotic index/rate of programmed cell death, the proliferation rate measured by Ki67, p53, DNA ploidy, p16, p27, E-cadherin, microvessel density, bcl-2, bax, and others that should be further validated. Circulating tumor cells have recently been studied in prostate cancer, and the FDA has approved testing from a specific manufacturer (Veridex).

The approach to treatment of prostate cancer is influenced by age and coexisting medical problems (Nelson et al. 2003). For patients with low- and intermediate-risk prostate cancer observation, external beam radiation therapy (EBRT), brachytherapy, or radical prostatectomy (RP) with pelvic lymph node dissection are therapeutic options based on the expected life survival, the presence of lymph node metastases, etc. RP is recommended only for patients with clinically localized prostate cancer (cT1–T3a, N0 or Nx, M0 or Mx) and a life expectancy of 10 or more years. Because of the risk inherent in major surgery, RP should be reserved for patients with little or no systemic comorbidity. For patients with high-risk prostate cancer (T3, high Gleason score, or PSA > 20 ng/ml), EBRT in combination with androgen deprivation therapy (ADT) and brachytherapy and radical prostatectomy with pelvic lymph node dissection (PLND) constitute the recommended treatments. ADT in conjunction with radiotherapy is routinely recommended for patients with locally advanced prostate cancer. Regarding the hormonal therapy, two major classes of agents are FDA-approved and currently in use in advanced prostate cancer (LHRH analogues and antiandrogens) with different profiles of activity and toxicity. Abiraterone, an androgen biosynthesis inhibitor, recently received an FDA approval, showing a high activity in metastatic *castration-resistant* prostate cancer (De Bono et al. 2011). Finally, bisphosphonates have an important role in therapy of metastatic prostate cancer, reducing the skeletal-related events and contributing significantly in palliative treatment. Mitoxantrone, docetaxel, and cabazitaxel are chemotherapeutic options for metastatic prostate cancer (NCCN Guidelines 2017). Many novel agents are currently under investigation and patients with prostate cancer should be encouraged to enroll in clinical trials.

Key Message

- Prostatic adenocarcinoma, especially when of high grade, has a propensity to metastasize to the lymph nodes and bone.

3.9 Case 3.6: Prostate Ductal Adenocarcinoma

Case Study

Data Prior to Microscopy

A patient presented with hematuria and urinary obstruction symptoms, the latter not justifiable by the size of the prostate gland. Normal digital rectal examination.

Cystoscopy showed a polypoid lesion with extension into the prostatic urethra. Transurethral biopsies were taken, and after a diagnosis of malignancy, radical prostatectomy was performed.

3.9.1 Microscopic Evaluation of the Radical Prostatectomy Specimen

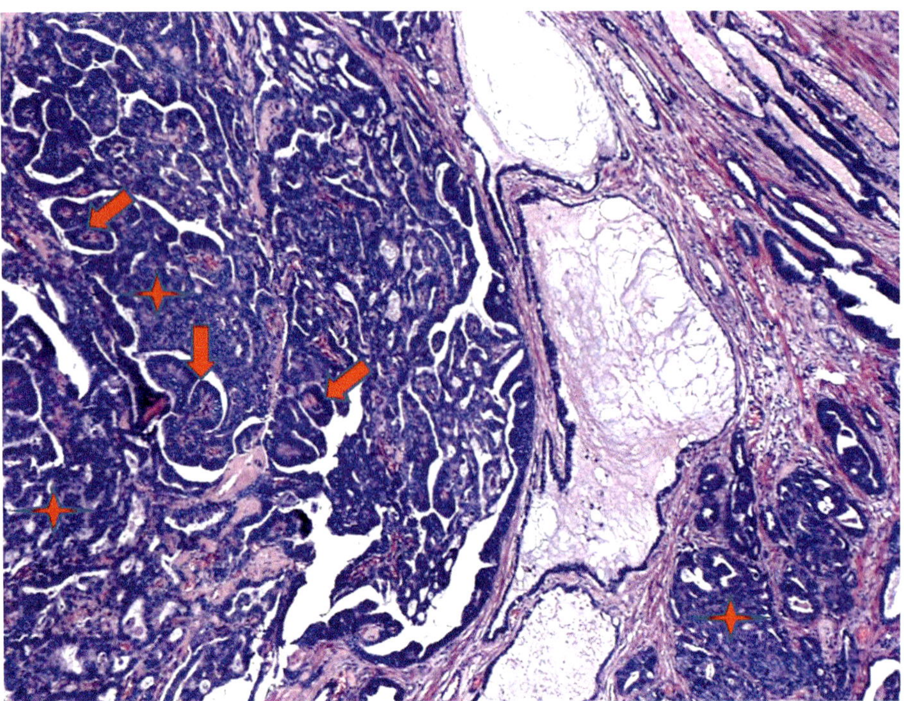

Fig. 3.99 (H-E, ×50) Prostate ductal adenocarcinoma. Prostate adenocarcinomas may also arise from prostatic ducts. Ductal adenocarcinomas are commonly located in the periurethral area, arising from the verumontanum and often extending into the periphery of the prostate.

We notice too large glandular structures of various sizes with distorted and complex architecture (solid, papillary, cribriform). Pseudostratified columnar cells. The glandular architecture is more complex than that of acinar adenocarcinoma.

True fibrovascular fronds are seen in the malignant papillary infoldings (*arrows*). Papillary architecture of cancer, when found, is a useful diagnostic feature. In the papillary pattern of ductal adenocarcinoma, the papillae are supported by fibrovascular cores; these cores are absent in the papillae of PIN.

The cribriform to solid pattern (*asterisks*) is not specific. Prostatic ductal adenocarcinomas may also invade as single glands lined by *tall columnar* epithelial cells, unlike the cuboidal cells that characterize typical acinar prostatic adenocarcinoma

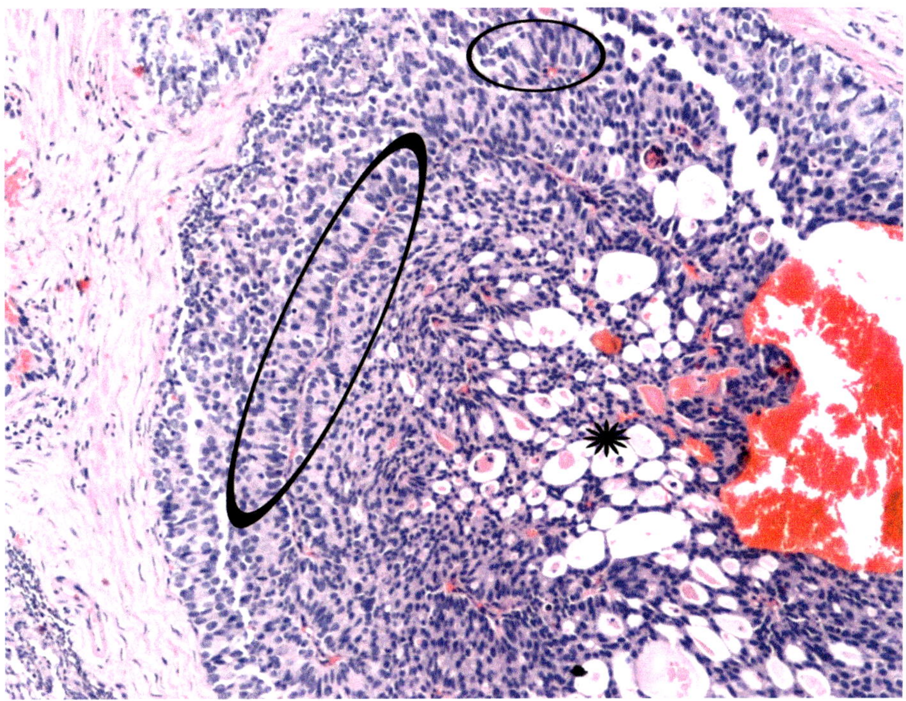

Fig. 3.100 (H-E, ×100) Ductal prostatic adenocarcinoma. Large, partially cribriform (*asterisk*) cancerous formation of a ductal adenocarcinoma of the prostate. *Tall columnar* pseudostratified cells (*ellipses*), resembling prostatic ductal cells, with high-grade nuclei and usually amphophilic cytoplasm

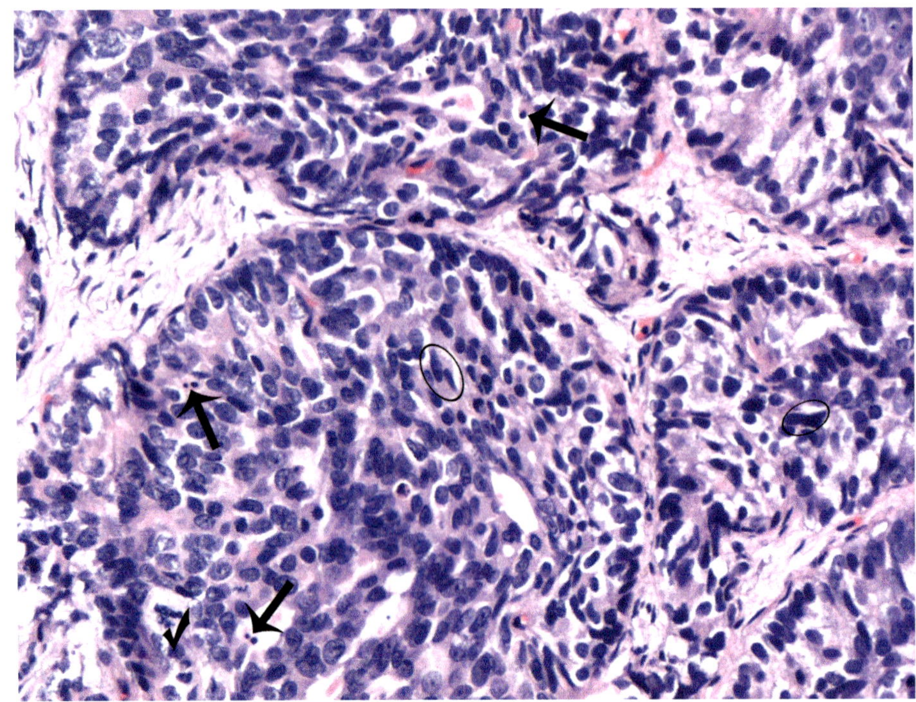

Fig. 3.101 (H-E, ×200) Ductal prostatic adenocarcinoma. Mitotic figures (*tick*), apoptotic bodies (*arrows*), and stromal fibrosis are common.

Ductal adenocarcinoma spreads along primary or secondary prostatic ducts, frequently retaining basal cells in a discontinuous or continuous manner, as can be evidenced by 34βE12 immunoreactivity. It is noteworthy that these carcinomas, retaining basal cells, should be regarded as ductal adenocarcinomas, since they progress as invasive ductal adenocarcinomas.

Distinction from HG PIN which is the precursor lesion to invasive prostate acinar adenocarcinoma is indeed important and depends on the fact that ductal adenocarcinomas with possibly preserved basal cells are architecturally more complex than HG PIN and cytologically different [predominance of rather *tall, columnar* cells with *elongated, cylindrical nuclei* (*ellipses*) instead of round to oval nuclei of the acinar type; atypical mitoses are encountered in ductal adenocarcinoma]. HG PIN typically does *not* have the same degree of glandular crowding, confluent growth pattern, true fibrovascular cores, prominent comedo necrosis, and high-grade nuclear features as ductal adenocarcinoma.

It is well known that invasive acinar adenocarcinoma has the capacity to spread along ducts and acini and form the cribriform pattern of intraductal carcinoma with preservation of basal cells; in this case, carcinoma cells retain the cytologic characteristics of acinar cells (i.e., cuboidal cells with round nuclei) and only seldom acquire the columnar cell features with the increased cytologic anaplasia of ductal adenocarcinoma.

[As regards the distinction of intraductal carcinoma from HG PIN, let it be pointed out again that the diffusely, markedly malignant, less uniform (than observed in HG PIN) nuclear morphology and the too complex architecture in such intraductal carcinomas, with atypical acinar cell-type morphology, should rule out the diagnosis of HG PIN (see Figs. 3.77, 3.78 and 3.79). This is the lesion which truly corresponds to "intraductal prostate carcinoma" and is almost always associated with neighboring invasive acinar adenocarcinoma]

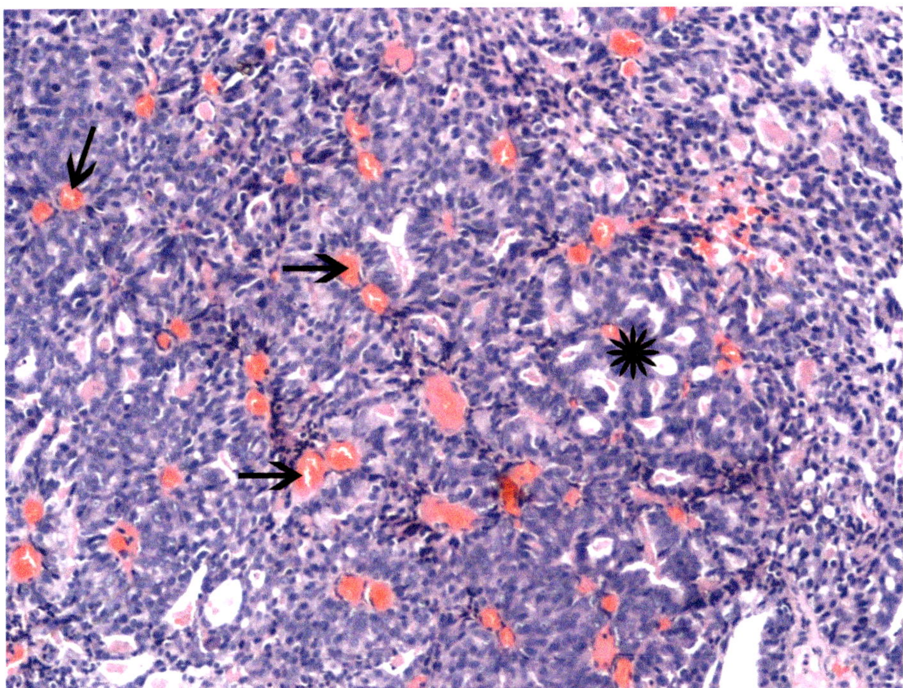

Fig. 3.102 (H-E, ×100) Prostate ductal adenocarcinoma. Distorted and complex architecture . Invasion of the prostatic stroma is usual.

Papillary architecture is not always easily recognizable. Solid papillary (*arrows* pointing to vascular cores of the papillae, which in this case appear solid) combined with cribriform-like architecture (*asterisk*)

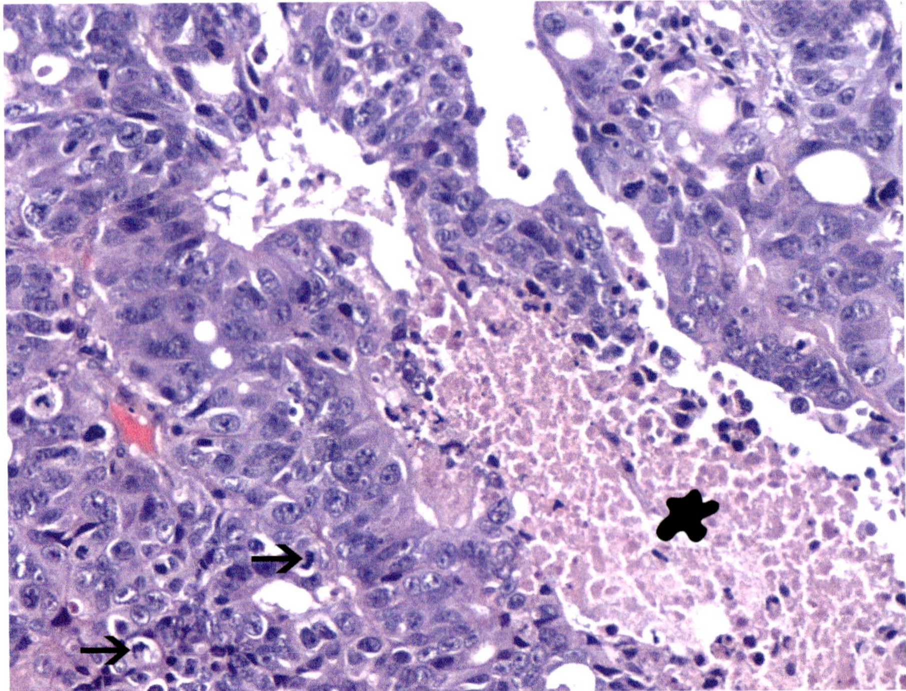

Fig. 3.103 (H-E, ×200) Prostate ductal adenocarcinoma. Mitotic figures (*arrows*) are common in *this type* of adenocarcinoma. Comedo necrosis is seen here (*blob*), and thus Gleason pattern 5 is assigned. Cribriform and papillary ductal adenocarcinoma of Figs. 3.99, 3.100, 3.101 and 3.102 is assigned Gleason pattern 4, but ductal adenocarcinoma with necrosis is Gleason pattern 5

In conclusion.

- Prostate adenocarcinoma characterized by tall columnar cells (resembling prostatic ductal cells) with high-grade nuclei is defined as ductal adenocarcinoma; on the contrary, prostate acinar adenocarcinoma is composed of cuboidal cells with round to oval nuclei, characteristic of prostate acini/glands.
- Prostate ductal adenocarcinoma is classified as Gleason pattern 4 and when comedo necrosis is present, Gleason pattern 5.
- Most, but not all, prostate ductal adenocarcinomas are distributed around the prostatic urethra.
- The assessment of invasion is occasionally difficult when the tumor mass invades in an expansile manner. However, ductal adenocarcinoma is commonly intermingled with usual prostate acinar adenocarcinoma; ductal adenocarcinomas admixed with acinar adenocarcinoma of Gleason pattern 3 are arguably considered more aggressive than Gleason score 7 purely acinar adenocarcinomas, if the ductal component of the former equals or exceeds 10% of the tumor mass.
- Ductal adenocarcinoma cells are always positive for PSA and PAP; this is particularly helpful in the differential diagnosis of urothelial or colon carcinoma involving the prostate. Urothelial cells are PSA (−) (unless they show glandular metaplasia).

The following images (Figs. 3.104, 3.105 and 3.106) derive from another tumor involving the periurethral ducts, which should be considered in the differential diagnosis of ductal adenocarcinoma of the prostate

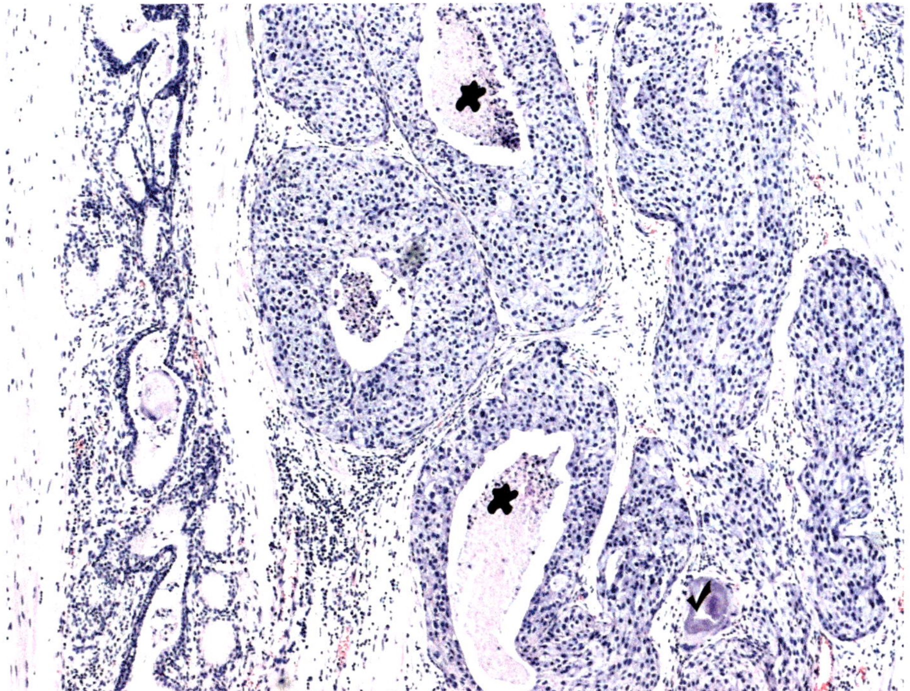

Fig. 3.104 (H-E, ×100) Involvement of periurethral ducts by urothelial carcinoma.

The proximal portion of the prostatic ducts is lined by urothelium, similar to the urethra. Urothelial metaplasia may be defined as the presence of urothelium within the distal portion of prostatic ducts and prostatic acini/glands, i.e., beyond the normal transitional-columnar junction; this junction is variable in location, creating difficulty on distinguishing metaplasia from normal urothelium in fragmented specimens such as TUR and needle biopsies. Prostatic acini may thus show urothelium mixed with cuboidal and columnar epithelium. In general, urothelial metaplasia poses little diagnostic difficulty, because it is composed of bland metaplastic urothelial cells.

Prostatic urethral polyps, benign polypoid intraurethral growths, consist of broad papillae being lined by either cytologically bland prostatic epithelial or urothelial cells with no atypia; their cores contain prostatic stroma and often prostatic glands. Cribriform growth patterns are absent.

On the right two thirds of the image, we notice high-grade malignant urothelium confined within expanded prostatic ducts or acini. Invasion into stroma should be meticulously ruled out in a urothelial carcinoma involving prostatic ducts and acini. Neoplastic urothelial morphology (significant nuclear pleomorphism, mitoses) combined with central comedo necrosis (*blobs*) is evident here; so a urothelial carcinoma is involving the epithelium of prostatic periurethral ducts, here without an infiltrative component, and thus there is no accompanying desmoplastic response. Concomitant involvement of the prostatic urethra is the rule. Typically, there is a history of carcinoma in situ (CIS) of the urinary bladder which has been treated conservatively. In CIS due to intraductal spread from CIS in the bladder, prostatic ducts and acini are filled with malignant urothelial cells, often with central necrosis, like here. Remaining amyloid bodies are observed in some prostate ducts/acini (*tick*). Urothelial neoplastic cells lack glandular differentiation. Basal cells may be identified

Fig. 3.104 (continued)

The most common tumor to secondarily involve the prostate is urothelial cancer. Two distinct patterns of involvement exist. Large, invasive urothelial cancers can directly invade from the bladder wall into the stroma of the prostate parenchyma; the latter situation dramatically worsens the prognosis of urothelial carcinoma of the bladder. Alternatively, urothelial CIS of the bladder can extend into the prostatic urethra and down into the prostatic ducts and acini, as is the case here; these patients have a history of carcinoma in situ of the bladder and have been treated over a period of months to years conservatively with intravesical topical therapy. Such patients should undergo periodic deep transurethral biopsies of the prostatic urethra and underlying prostate. Primary urothelial carcinoma of prostatic urethra, ducts, or acini is rare.

Pronounced nuclear pleomorphism, atypia, and overlapping, as well as increased mitotic rate, are hallmarks of high-grade urothelial cancer involving prostatic ducts or acini; glandular formation is often absent in urothelial cancer at this location.

Differential diagnosis of urothelial cancer includes HG PIN (which, however, is a lesion of the peripheral zone and uncommonly affects periurethral ducts), ductal adenocarcinoma, high-grade prostatic acinar adenocarcinoma, or intraductal carcinoma of the prostate. The urothelial immunomarkers GATA3, uroplakin III, and p63, high molecular weight cytokeratins, and the prostate markers PSA, PAP, prostein, and NKX3.1 provide diagnostic aid

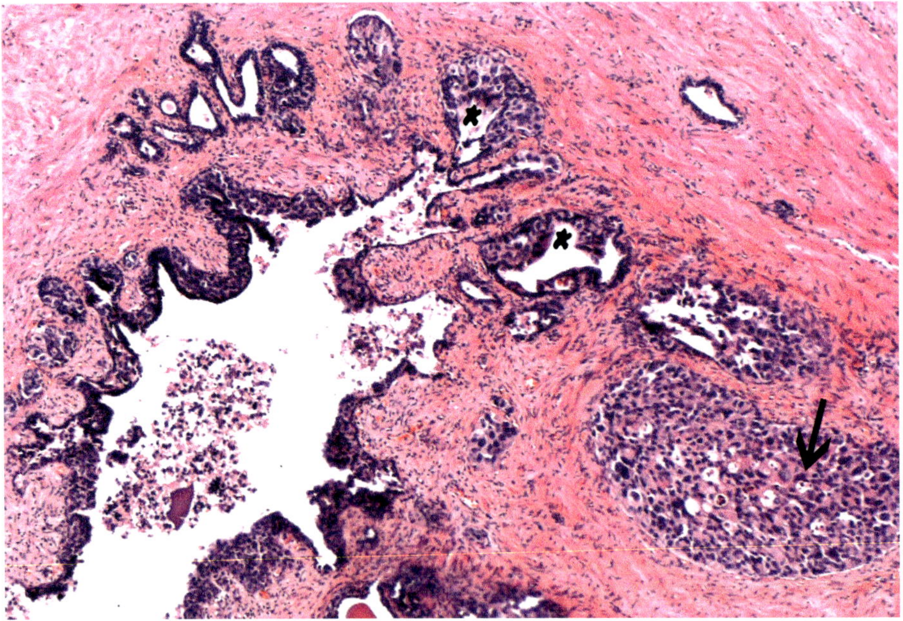

Fig. 3.105 (H-E, ×50) Urothelial carcinoma secondarily involving seminal vesicles' epithelium (*blobs*). Both CIS and invasive urothelial carcinoma can show *intraepithelial spread* along ejaculatory ducts into the seminal vesicle. Significant cellular pleomorphism and mitotic activity favor urothelial carcinoma, again. Cytoplasm is densely eosinophilic and may show squamoid features (*arrow*)

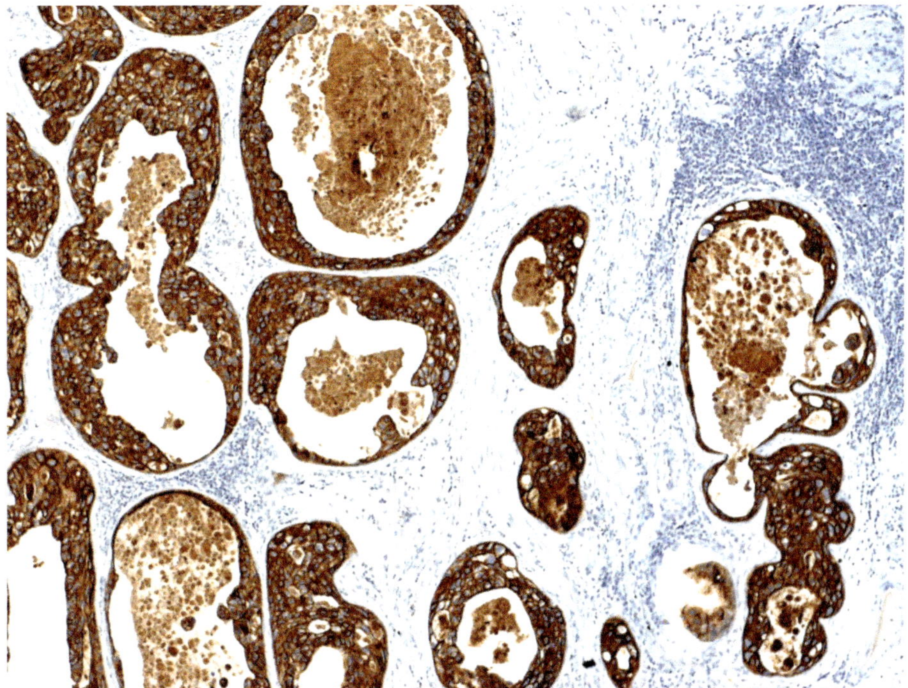

Fig. 3.106 (Uroplakin III immunohistochemistry, ×50) Uroplakin III immunoreactivity confirms the urothelial nature of this periurethral carcinoma.

More widely used immunomarkers such as CK7 and CK20 can also be helpful in differentiating prostatic adenocarcinoma from urothelial carcinoma only for those tumors that show either both markers positive (urothelial carcinoma) or both markers negative (prostate carcinoma). It is noteworthy that primary urinary bladder urothelial carcinomas may occasionally show immunoreactivity for PAP and PSA as the tumor spreads into the prostate. The latter immunoreaction is likely induced by the prostatic stroma through the mechanism of mesenchymal-epithelial interaction.

The rare primary urothelial carcinoma of the prostate cannot usually be differentiated morphologically or immunohistochemically from urothelial carcinoma of the urinary bladder or urethra spreading into the prostate. However, in most cases it is possible clinically to determine the origin of the tumor. Also, primary urothelial carcinoma of the prostate does not demonstrate "umbrella cells" which low-grade urothelial carcinoma of the bladder may do

3.9.1.1 Clinical Commentary

Vasileios Spapis

This is a case of a (high-grade) prostate ductal adenocarcinoma arising in periurethral ducts and visible in the prostatic urethra as a polypoid lesion, causing obstructive symptoms. The diagnosis was made by transurethral biopsy.

Less than 1% of prostatic adenocarcinomas arise exclusively from the prostatic ducts (Epstein and Woodruff 1986; Christensen et al.1991). Both ductal and acinar differentiations are found in about 5% of prostatic carcinomas. It is not rare for ductal adenocarcinomas to grow in the prostatic urethra arising in the large primary periurethral prostatic ducts and thus cause obstructive symptoms or hematuria, as in the present case. Care should be taken not to underestimate these tumors in spite of possibly normal DRE and serum PSA levels (Cooperberg et al. 2013). Tumors originating from peripheral prostatic ducts may present exactly like ordinary acinar adenocarcinomas of the prostate and may thus be diagnosed on needle biopsy (Brinker et al. 1999).

Typically, ductal adenocarcinomas are classified as Gleason pattern 4 [score 8 (=4 + 4)] because of their common morphologic architectural features with prostatic acinar adenocarcinoma Gleason score 8, and have a similar prognosis (Brinker et al. 1999). An exception is the detection of PIN-like *ductal* adenocarcinoma which is considered to be of Gleason pattern 3 (Tavora and Epstein 2008). Another exception is finding ductal adenocarcinoma with comedo necrosis, which is assigned a Gleason pattern 5, as in the present case. However, there is no sufficient data so far to prove whether a ductal adenocarcinoma Gleason pattern 4 (or pattern 5 if accompanied by comedo necrosis) is associated with a worse prognosis than a comparably graded acinar adenocarcinoma (Samaratunga et al. 2010; Seipel et al. 2013).

Since ductal adenocarcinomas are considered by definition to be poorly differentiated tumors, RP is an option that should be discussed carefully with the patient, especially in cases with no obstruction of the prostatic urethra. The rest of the treatment options seem to be equally effective as with acinar adenocarcinomas of the prostate.

Key Messages

- Ductal prostate adenocarcinoma is a subtype of prostatic adenocarcinoma with large glands lined by tall pseudostratified columnar cells. It is mainly located in the larger periurethral prostatic ducts and is usually found in association with conventional, acinar-type adenocarcinoma of the prostate.
- Ductal adenocarcinoma is by definition a high-grade carcinoma [Gleason patterns 4 or 5 (the latter, if comedo necrosis is present)].
- The optimal combination of prostatic and urothelial immunohistochemical markers could improve the ability to differentiate prostate adenocarcinoma from urothelial carcinoma pathologically, since common urothelial carcinoma expresses CK34βE12, CK7, CK20, p63, uroplakin III, and thrombomodulin and, as a rule, is simultaneously immunonegative for traditional prostate tissue immunomarkers (i.e., PSA, PSMA). Prostatic and urothelial markers, including PSA, NKX3.1 (for prostate) and p63, thrombomodulin, and GATA3 (for urothelium), are indeed very useful for differentiating prostate adenocarcinoma from urothelial carcinoma.

References

Abdel-Khalek M, El-Baz M, Ibrahiem E-H (2004) Predictors of prostate cancer on extended biopsy in patients with high-grade prostatic intraepithelial neoplasia: a multivariate analysis model. BJU Int 94:528–533
Amin MB (ed) (2010) Diagnostic pathology. Genitourinary. AMIRSYS, Salt Lake City
Aydin H, Tsuzuki T, Hernandez D et al (2004) Positive proximal (bladder neck) margin at radical prostatectomy confers greater risk of biochemical progression. Urology 64(3):551–555
Bjurlin MA, Carter HB, Schellhammer P et al (2013) Optimization of initial prostate biopsy in clinical practice: sampling, labeling and specimen processing. J Urol 189:2039–2046
Bostwick DG, Chen L (eds) (2014) Urologic surgical pathology. MOSBY Elsevier, Amsterdam
Brinker DA, Potter SR, Epstein JI (1999) Ductal adenocarcinoma of the prostate diagnosed on needle biopsy: correlation with clinical and radical prostatectomy findings and progression. Am J Surg Pathol 23:1471–1479
Carvalhal GF, Smith DS, Mager DE et al (1999) Digital rectal examination for detecting prostate cancer at prostate specific antigen levels of 4 ng./ml. or less. J Urol 161:835–839
Chen M, Rifkin M, Vo T et al (1996) Does color Doppler increase the ability to identify prostate cancer? In: Proceedings of the 44th Annual Meeting of the Association of University Radiologists. Birmingham, Alabama, p 65
Christensen WN, Steinberg G, Walsh PC et al (1991) Prostatic duct adenocarcinoma: findings at radical prostatectomy. Cancer 67:2118–2124
Cooperberg M, Prest J, Shinohara K, Caroll P (2013) Neoplasms of the prostate gland. In: McAninch J, Lue T (eds) Smith and Tanagho's general urology, 18th edn. McGraw-Hill, New York, pp 350–379
De Bono JS, Logothetis CJ, Molina A et al (2011) Abiraterone and increased survival in metastatic prostate cancer. N Engl J Med 364(21):1995–2005
Eastham JA, Riedel E, Scardino PT et al (2003) Variation of serum prostate-specific antigen levels: an evaluation of year-to-year fluctuations. JAMA 289:2695–2700
Epstein J (2016) Pathology of prostatic neoplasia. In: Wein R, Kavoussi L, Partin A, Peters C (eds) Campbell-Walsh urology, 11th edn. Elsevier, Philadelphia, pp 2593–2600
Epstein JI, Amin M, Boccon-Gibod L et al (2005) Prognostic factors and reporting of prostate carcinoma in radical prostatectomy and pelvic lymphadenectomy specimens. Scand J Urol Nephrol Suppl 216:34–63
Epstein JI, Herawi M (2006) Prostate needle biopsies containing prostatic intraepithelial neoplasia or atypical foci suspicious for carcinoma: implications for patient care. J Urol 175:820–834
Epstein JI, Netto GJ (2015) Biopsy interpretation of the prostate, 5th edn. Wolters Kluwer Health, Philadelphia
Epstein JI, Woodruff JM (1986) Adenocarcinoma of the prostate with endometrioid features: a light microscopic and immunohistochemical study of ten cases. Cancer 57:111–119
Fine SW, Humphrey PA (2013) Modern prostate needle biopsy interpretation. Short course # 22, syllabus. United States & Canadian Academy of Pathology
Freedland SJ, Csathy GS, Dorey F, Aronson WJ (2002) Percent prostate needle biopsy tissue with cancer is more predictive of biochemical failure or adverse pathology after radical prostatectomy than prostate specific antigen or Gleason score. J Urol 167:516–520
Godoy G, Huang GJ, Patel T et al (2011) Long-term follow-up of men with isolated high-grade prostatic intra-epithelial neoplasia followed by serial delayed interval biopsy. Urology 77:669–674
Gordetsky J, Epstein J (2016) Grading of prostatic adenocarcinoma: current state and prognostic implications. Diagn Pathol 11:25
Gosselaar C, Roobol MJ, Roemeling S et al (2008) The role of the digital rectal examination in subsequent screening visits in the European randomized study of screening for prostate cancer (ERSPC), Rotterdam. Eur Urol 54:581–588
Hamper U, Sheth S, Walsh P, Epstein J (1990) Bright echogenic foci in early prostatic carcinoma: sonographic and pathologic correlation. Radiology 176:339–343
Hanks GE (1988) External-beam radiation therapy for clinically localized prostate cancer: patterns of care studies in the United States. NCI Monogr 7:75–84
Hemminki K (2012) Familial risk and familial survival in prostate cancer. World J Urol 30:143–148

Hsu CY, Joniau S, Oyen R et al (2007) Outcome of surgery for clinical unilateral T3a prostate cancer: a single-institution experience. Eur Urol 51(1):121–128

Jansson KF, Akre O, Garmo H et al (2012) Concordance of tumor differentiation among brothers with prostate cancer. Eur Urol 62:656–661

Joniau S, Spahn M, Briganti A et al (2015) Pretreatment tables predicting pathologic stage of locally advanced prostate cancer. Eur Urol 67(2):319–325

Kelly IM, Lees WR, Rickards D (1993) Prostate cancer and the role of color Doppler US. Radiology 189:153–156

Leitzmann MF, Rohrmann S (2012) Risk factors for the onset of prostatic cancer: age, location, and behavioral correlates. Clin Epidemiol 4:1–11

Magi-Galluzzi C, Evans AJ, Delahunt B et al (2011) International Society of Urological Pathology (ISUP) consensus conference on handling and staging of radical prostatectomy specimens. Working group 3: extraprostatic extension, lymphovascular invasion and locally advanced disease. Mod Pathol 24(1):26–38

Marks RA, Koch MO, Lopez-Beltran A et al (2007) The relationship between the extent of surgical margin positivity and prostate specific antigen recurrence in radical prostatectomy specimens. Hum Pathol 38(8):1207–1211

Merrimen JL, Jones G, Srigley JR (2010) Is high grade prostatic intraepithelial neoplasia still a risk factor for adenocarcinoma in the era of extended biopsy sampling? Pathology 42:325–329

Merrimen JL, Jones G, Walker D et al (2009) Multifocal high grade prostatic intraepithelial neoplasia is a significant risk factor for prostatic adenocarcinoma. J Urol 182:485–490, discussion 490

Montironi R, Santoni M, Mazzucchelli R et al (2016) Prostate cancer: from Gleason scoring to prognostic grade grouping. Expert Rev Anticancer Ther 16(4):433–440

Mottet N, Bellmunt J, Briers E et al (2017) Prostate cancer. In: European Association of Urology Guidelines. European Association of Urology. Available via https://uroweb.org/guideline/renal-cell-carcinoma. Accessed 17 Apr 2017

National Comprehensive Cancer Network Clinical Practice Guidelines in Oncology (NCCN Guidelines) (2017) Prostate Cancer, Version 2. 2016 & 2.2017. Available via https://www.nccn.org/professionals/prostate. Accessed 20 April 2017

NCCN Clinical practice guidelines in Oncology-Prostate Cancer, Version 1.2018 (2017) Available via https://www.nccn.org/professionals/physician_gls/pdf/prostate.pdf. Accessed February 2018

Nelson WG, De Marzo AM, Isaacs WB (2003) Prostate cancer. N Engl J Med 349(4):366–381

Okotie OT, Roehl KA, Han M et al (2007) Characteristics of prostate cancer detected by digital rectal examination only. Urology 70:1117–1120

Parker C, Gillessen S, Heidenreich A et al (2015) Cancer of the prostate: ESMO clinical practice guidelines for diagnosis, treatment and follow-up. Ann Oncol 26(suppl 5):v69–v77

Partin AW, Carter HB, Chan DW et al (1990) Prostate specific antigen in the staging of localized prostate cancer: influence of tumor differentiation, tumor volume and benign hyperplasia. J Urol 143(4):747–752

Partin AW, Mangold LA, Lamm DM et al (2001) Contemporary update of prostate cancer staging nomograms (Partin tables) for the new millennium. Urology 58(6):843–848

Pickup M, Van der Kwast TH (2007) My approach to intraductal lesions of the prostate gland. J Clin Pathol 60:856–865

Ploussard G, Rotondo S, Salomon L (2010) The prognostic significance of bladder neck invasion in prostate cancer: is microscopic involvement truly a T4 disease? BJU Int 105(6):776–781

Rifkin MD (1998) Prostate cancer: the diagnostic dilemma and the place of imaging in detection and staging. World J Urol 16(1):76–80

Rifkin M, McGlynn E, Choi H (1989) Echogenicity of prostate cancer correlated with histologic grade and stromal fibrosis: Endorectal US studies. Radiology 170:549–552

Rifkin M, Sudakoff G, Alexander A (1993) Color Doppler imaging of prostate : Techniques, results and potential applications. Radiology 186:509–513

Roberts JA, Zhou M, Park YW et al (2013) Intraductal carcinoma of the prostate: a comprehensive and concise review. Korean J Pathol 47(4):307–315

Samaratunga H, Duffy D, Yaxley J et al (2010) Any proportion of ductal adenocarcinoma in radical prostatectomy specimens predicts extraprostatic extension. Hum Pathol 41:281–285

Sammon JD, Trinh QD, Sukumar S et al (2013) Risk factors for biochemical recurrence following radical perineal prostatectomy in a large contemporary series: a detailed assessment of margin extent and location. Urol Oncol 31(8):1470–1476
Scardino RT (1988) The appearance of stage A prostate cancer on transrectal ultrasonography: correlation of imaging and pathologic examination. In: Third international symposium on transrectal ultrasound in the diagnosis and management of prostate cancer, Chicago, pp 64–66
Sehdev AE, Pan CC, Epstein JI (2001) Comparative analysis of sampling methods for grossing radical prostatectomy specimens performed for nonpalpable (stage T1c) prostatic adenocarcinoma. Hum Pathol 32(5):494–499
Seipel AH, Wiklund F, Wiklund NP et al (2013) Histopathological features of ductal adenocarcinoma of the prostate in 1,051 radical prostatectomy specimens. Virchows Arch 462:429–436
Semjonow A, Brandt B, Oberpenning F et al (1996) Discordance of assay methods creates pitfalls for the interpretation of prostate specific antigen values. Prostate Suppl 7:3–16
Siegel RL, Miller KD, Jemal A (2017) Cancer statistics, 2017. CA Cancer J Clin 67(1):7–30
Stamey TA, Yang N, Hay AR et al (1987) Prostate-specific antigen as a serum marker for adenocarcinoma of the prostate. N Engl J Med 317:909–916
Stamey TA, Yemoto CM, McNeal J et al (2000) Prostate cancer is highly predictable: a prognostic equation based on all morphological variables in radical prostatectomy specimens. J Urol 163(4):1155–1160
Tabar et al (2013) Prostate and breast: brother and sister organs 3D book series, vol II. Tabar Foundation, Sweden
Tan DS, Mok TS, Rebbeck TR (2016) Cancer genomics: diversity and disparity across ethnicity and geography. J Clin Oncol 34:91–101
Tavora F, Epstein JI (2008) High-grade prostatic intraepithelial neoplasia-like ductal adenocarcinoma of the prostate: a clinicopathologic study of 28 cases. Am J Surg Pathol 32:1060–1067
Ward JF, Slezak JM, Blute ML et al (2005) Radical prostatectomy for clinically advanced (cT3) prostate cancer since the advent of prostate-specific antigen testing: 15-year outcome. BJU Int 95(6):751–756
Yossepowitch O, Eggener SE, Bianco FJ Jr et al (2007) Radical prostatectomy for clinically localized, high risk prostate cancer: critical analysis of risk assessment methods. J Urol 178(2):493–499
Zhou M, Li J, Cheng L et al (2015) Diagnosis of "poorly formed glands" Gleason pattern 4 prostatic adenocarcinoma on needle biopsy: an interobserver reproducibility study among urologic pathologists with recommendations. Am J Surg Pathol 39(10):1331–1339

Neoplastic Testicular Pathology

*Konstantinos Charitopoulos, Danai Daliani,
Maria Gkotzamanidou, Andreas C. Lazaris,
Argyris Siatelis, Vasileios Spapis, and Nikolaos Spetsieris*

A. C. Lazaris (ed.), *Clinical Genitourinary Pathology*,
https://doi.org/10.1007/978-3-319-72194-1_4

A pathologic report for radical orchiectomy specimens with tumors should include the following information: serum tumor markers [alpha-fetoprotein (AFP), human chorionic gonadotropin (HCG), lactic acid dehydrogenase (LDH)], specimen laterality, tumor focality, tumor size, macroscopic extent of tumor, histologic type of tumor, margin status, microscopic tumor extension, lymph-vascular invasion, pTNM including S status, and additional pathologic findings [i.e., germ cell neoplasia in situ (GCNIS), atrophy]. As far as tumor sampling is concerned, 1 cm^2 sections for every centimeter of maximum tumor diameter should be taken, including normal macroscopic parenchyma (if present), albuginea, and epididymis, the latter two with selection of suspected areas. The most important stain for testicular cancer histologic diagnosis is hematoxylin-eosin (H-E); immunohistochemistry is particularly useful in histologic typing of tumors with extensive necrosis, poor fixation, or ambiguous morphology as well as in metastatic tumors. In the microscopic examination of tumor specimens, the presence or absence of peritumoral venous and/or lymphatic vascular invasion should be carefully investigated and reported. It should be stressed that the diagnosis of choriocarcinoma requires the identification of mononucleated cytotrophoblastic cells. In stage 1 seminomas, the presence or absence of invasion of the rete testis should be reported. With regard to microscopic evaluation of tumors with mixed histology, the individual components should be specified, and their amount should be estimated as a percentage.

In experienced hands, guided fine needle cytology and/or core biopsy can be valuable tools for the morphological diagnosis of retroperitoneal and mediastinal manifestations of malignant germ cell tumors.

A pathologic report for retroperitoneal lymphadenectomy specimens should include the following data: pre-lymphadenectomy treatment, serum tumor markers, specimen site(s), number of nodal groups present, size of largest metastatic deposit in lymph node, histologic viability of tumor, histologic type of metastatic tumor, pN status, nonregional lymph node metastasis (M1a).

4.1 Introduction to Clinical Testicular Neoplastic Pathology

Konstantinos Charitopoulos, Vasileios Spapis, Nikolaos Spetsieris, and Andreas C. Lazaris

The testis is composed of seminiferous tubules and interstitium; the former are composed of germ cells, in varying stages of differentiation or maturation, supported by Sertoli cells attached to basal lamina. Germ cells mature from base to center of lumen and are divided into different stages based on their levels of maturation (spermatogonia, primary spermatocytes, secondary spermatocytes, spermatids, and spermatozoa). Interstitium is divided into intertubular and peritubular regions; the former contain blood vessels, lymphatics, nerve, and testosterone-producing Leydig cells, while the latter contain basement membranes and thin lamina propria.

Testicular cancer is the most common malignancy of the scrotum, and it makes up to 1% of all malignancies in men (Siegel et al. 2016). *Testicular germ cell tumors* (GCTs) are, however, the most frequent solid tumor malignancy in 15–34-year age group (Silverberg 1982) with a rising incidence over the past two decades (SEER 2016), while non-germ cell tumors are considered quite rare.

Germ cell neoplasia in situ (GCNIS) is the precursor of the vast majority of invasive testicular germ cell tumors, excluding spermatocytic seminoma and all prepubertal testicular germ cell tumors, and it is identified adjacent in about 90% of cases. GCNIS is a large primitive atypical element, twice the size of normal germ cells, with large nuclei and large clear cytoplasm enriched of glycogen. These cells lie along the thickened basement membrane of atrophic seminiferous tubules.

Numerous classification systems have been proposed for germ cell tumors of the testis. Classification by *histologic type* appears to be the *most useful* with respect to *treatment*. There are two major divisions, seminoma and nonseminomatous germ cell tumors (NSGCTs), which include embryonal cell carcinoma, teratoma, yolk sac tumor, choriocarcinoma, and mixed tumors. *Non-germ cell tumors of the testis* include Leydig cell tumors, Sertoli cell tumors, etc.; *tumors of the testicular adnexa* are a separate category (Amin 2010; Bostwick and Chen 2014; Moch et al. 2016).

Seminoma is the most common testicular germ cell tumor. Grossly, seminomas are firm with homogenous nodular appearance. Microscopically, nested seminomatous cells are separated by thin fibrovascular trabeculae infiltrated by reactive T cell lymphocytes. Seminomatous cells are large, uniform, with distinct cell membranes. Granulomatous reactions are frequently observed, resulting sometimes in obscuring neoplastic component. In some seminomas, larger cells with particularly high nuclear/cytoplasmic ratio, more than three mitoses per high-power field and relative lack of lymphocytes are noticed; these tumors may be typified as "seminomas with atypia." Necrotic areas can be quite prominent in some cases. Among other immunomarkers, KIT (CD117) is valuable in the diagnosis of seminoma.

Embryonal carcinoma (EC) is present as a component in 80% of mixed testicular germ cell tumors. Differently from seminoma, EC occurs as a poorly demarcated mass with large foci of hemorrhage and necrosis. Typically, CD30 is a sensitive immunohistochemical marker for EC, but it is frequently lost in metastasis after chemotherapy.

Teratomas are composed of different tissues deriving from one or more germinal endodermal, mesodermal, and ectodermal layers. The behavior of testis teratomas depends on patient age, prepubertal testis pure teratoma being invariably benign and postpubertal teratoma invariably malignant; in the margin of the latter, GCNIS is frequently encountered as its precursor intratubular malignant lesion. In postpubertal testis, pure teratomas are at risk of metastasis, despite their often mature histology.

Yolk sac tumor (YST) represents a frequent component of mixed germ cell tumors in adults. Microscopically, YST is characterized by different patterns of growth, among which the reticular-microcystic is the commonest. Alpha-fetoprotein (AFP) immunostaining is commonly observed in YST.

Among trophoblastic tumors, choriocarcinoma is absolutely the most frequent; it consists of variable amounts of two cell components, syncytiotrophoblast and cytotrophoblasts.

Useful immunomarkers for the differential diagnosis of testicular germ cell tumors include Oct3/4, SALL4, placenta-like/placental alkaline phosphatase (PLAP), KIT (CD117), podoplanin, CD30 (BerH2), SOX2, α-fetoprotein (AFP), glypican-3, human chorionic gonadotropin (HCG), and human placental lactogen (HPL).

The most common symptom of testicular germ cell neoplasms is a painless, gradual enlargement of the testis; the patient or his partner typically identifies a lump or a swelling of the testicle. The typical delay in treatment from the initial recognition of the lesion by the patient to definitive therapy (orchiectomy) ranges from 3 to 6 months and correlates with the incidence of metastases (Presti 2013). It is not entirely uncommon for testicular cancer to present itself with pain (approximately 10% of cases) (Khan and Protheroe 2007) which may be the result of intratesticular hemorrhage or infarction. Another 10% of patients present with symptoms related to metastatic disease. Back pain is the most common, while the others being cough, dyspnea, anorexia, nausea, bone pain, etc. (Presti 2013).

Diagnostic evaluation remains the same regardless of the histologic type of the primary tumor. Pre- and post-orchiectomy half-life kinetics of serum tumor markers [lactic acid dehydrogenase (LDH), alpha-fetoprotein (AFP), β subunit of human chorionic gonadotropin (HCG)], abdominopelvic computed tomography (CT) scan, chest CT, and bilateral testis ultrasound are highly recommended for all patients (Gr A). Placental alkaline phosphatase (PLAP) is an optional marker in monitoring patients with pure seminoma, but it is not recommended in smokers. LDH levels are elevated in approximately 20% of low-stage GCTs. As a nonspecific marker for GCTs, its main use is in the prognostic assessment of GCTs at diagnosis. The serum half-life of LDH is 24 h. HCG levels are elevated in approximately 15% of seminomas. Levels greater than 5000 IU/L are usually associated with NSGCT. The half-life of HCG is 24–36 h. Seminomas do not produce AFP. Patients with pure seminoma in the primary tumor with an elevated serum AFP value are considered to have NSGCT. The half-life of AFP is 5–7 days. Bone and brain scanning should be performed in case of symptoms. Fertility investigations [total testosterone, semen analysis, luteinizing hormone (LH), follicle-stimulating hormone (FSH)] could be performed (Gr B), and sperm banking should be discussed with all men before starting treatment for testicular cancer (Albers 2016).

While many clinical staging systems for testicular cancer have been proposed over the years, most of them are variations of the original system proposed by Boden and Gibb (1951). According to that system, a stage A lesion is confined to the testis, stage B demonstrates regional lymph node spread, and stage C is spread beyond retroperitoneal lymph nodes (Presti 2013). At the time of diagnosis, the proportion of patients with clinical stage I disease (confined to the testis) is about 85% (Stephenson and Gilligan 2012). In 1997, the International Germ Cell Cancer Collaborative Group (IGCCCG) defined a prognostic factor-based staging system for metastatic testis tumors based on identification of clinically independent adverse factors. This staging system has been incorporated into the TNM classification and uses histology, location of the primary tumor, location of metastases, and pre-chemotherapy marker levels in serum as prognostic factors to categorize patients into "good," "intermediate," or "poor" prognosis. For seminomas, good prognosis tumors are considered those which derive from any primary site, with normal AFP, any HCG and LDH, and have no non-pulmonary visceral metastases, while those of intermediate prognosis have non-pulmonary visceral metastases. There are no seminomas of poor prognosis. NSGCTs, on the other hand, are considered of good prognosis when their primary site is the testis or the retrop9ritoneum and have no non-pulmonary visceral metastases and S1 tumor markers (AFP < 1000 ng/mL, HCG < 5000 IU/L, LDH $< 1.5 \times$ ULN, post-orchiectomy). Intermediate prognosis NSGCTs also have the testis or the retroperitoneum as their primary site and have no non-pulmonary visceral metastases but S2 tumor markers (AFP 1000–10,000 ng/mL or HCG 5000–50,000 IU/L or LDH 1.5–10 × ULN, post-orchiectomy). The mediastinal primary tumors, those with non-pulmonary visceral metastases and S3 tumor markers (AFP $> 10{,}000$ ng/mL or HCG $> 50{,}000$ IU/L or LDH > 10 X ULN, post-orchiectomy), are considered as poor prognosis NSGCTs.

The mainstay of exploration for a possible testis tumor is the inguinal exploration with cross-clamping of the spermatic cord vasculature and delivery of the testis into the field. If cancer cannot be excluded, radical orchiectomy is warranted. Scrotal approaches and open testicular biopsies should not be performed in order to avoid tumor dispersion. Further therapy depends on the histologic characteristics of the tumor as well as the clinical stage (Presti 2013).

The basic treatment option for stage I *seminoma* is radical inguinal orchiectomy alone, with a disease specific survival approaching 100%. In order to prevent relapse in certain patients, post-surgery management includes active surveillance, radiotherapy, or carboplatin-based chemotherapy (Oldenburg et al. 2013). Patients with metastatic seminoma could be treated with cisplatin-based chemotherapy or radiotherapy, depending on the stage of the disease. After chemotherapy, all patients are evaluated and classified according to the presence of residual mass and serum tumor markers levels. Patients with no residual mass or residual mass of 3 cm or less, with normal markers, are scheduled for surveillance. If a residual mass greater than 3 cm is observed, with normal tumor marker levels, PET scan must be performed approximately 6 weeks after chemotherapy, in order to assess the viability of the residual tumor. In the case of a negative PET scan, the patient should be scheduled for follow-up. Patients with a positive PET scan must undergo either retroperitoneal lymph node dissection (if technically possible) or second-line chemotherapy. Standard second-line chemotherapy regimens include four cycles of TIP (paclitaxel, ifosfamide, cisplatin) or four cycles of VeIP (vinblastine, ifosfamide, cisplatin). They are administered to patients with favorable prognostic factors, i.e., complete response to first-line therapy, low levels of post-orchiectomy serum tumor markers, and low-volume disease. Unfavorable prognostic markers include incomplete response to first-line therapy, elevated serum tumor markers, bulky disease, and extratesticular primary tumor. Patients with unfavorable prognostic markers are candidates for high-dose chemotherapy regimens supported by autologous stem cell transplant. High-dose regimens include high-dose carboplatin plus etoposide followed either by autologous stem cell transplant or paclitaxel and ifosfamide followed by autologous stem cell transplant. For patients failing conventional second-line chemotherapy, high-dose chemotherapy is suggested, while for patients with unfavorable prognosis and late relapses without response to second-line high-dose chemotherapy, treatment options include palliative chemotherapy or participation in a clinical trial (Bahrami et al. 2007; Albers 2016).

NSGCTs are not radiosensitive. Stage I tumors after orchiectomy are treated with surveillance, nerve-sparing retroperitoneal lymph node dissection (RPLND), or adjuvant chemotherapy. In cases of metastatic disease, there is a general consensus that treatment should start with initial chemotherapy in all advanced cases of NSGCTs except for stage IIa NSGCT disease and pure teratoma without elevated tumor markers, which can be managed by primary RPLND or surveillance to clarify stage. Following first-line BEP (bleomycin, etoposide, cisplatin) chemotherapy, only 6–10% of residual masses contain viable cancer, 50% contain mature teratoma, and 40% contain necrotic-fibrotic tissue. Residual tumor resection is mandatory in all patients with a residual mass > 1 cm in the short axis at cross-sectional CT imaging. The role of surgery is debated in patients with retroperitoneal residual lesions <1 cm. There is still a risk of residual cancer or teratoma although the vast majority of patients (>70%) harbor fibronecrotic tissue. If necrotic debris or mature teratoma is found, patients require further surveillance, while if embryonal carcinoma, yolk sac tumor, choriocarcinoma, and seminoma elements are found, the patient must undergo chemotherapy (Albers 2016).

All patients with testicular cancer require regular follow-up care. Usually, they are followed at 3-month intervals for the first 2 years, then every 6 months until 5 years, and then yearly. Follow-up visits should include careful physical examination, investigation of serum tumor markers (LDH, AFP, HCG), and a plain chest radiography. Abdominopelvic, chest, and brain CT scans are used less frequently (Albers 2016; Presti 2013).

Sex cord stromal tumors of the testis are neoplasms that have features of Leydig (interstitial) cells, Sertoli cells, granulosa cells, or, rarely, theca cells. Inhibin immunoreactivity is generally useful in the diagnosis of these tumors. All sex cord stromal tumors may be positive for Melan-A (MART-1), most frequently expressed in Leydig cell tumors.

The most common *tumor of testicular adnexa* is adenomatoid tumor, a benign tumor of mesothelial cell origin, which has a variety of growth patterns, including glands, cysts, tubules, cords, or isolated cells.

4.2 Normal Spermatogenesis

- *Normally, in appropriate spermatogenesis, all* differentiation stages of the seminiferous epithelium must be distinguished simultaneously, and *mature (elongated) spermatids* should be noticed *in the vast majority* of correctly oriented seminiferous tubules of the biopsy material (not necessarily in all). The number of these late spermatids correlates best with sperm counts.

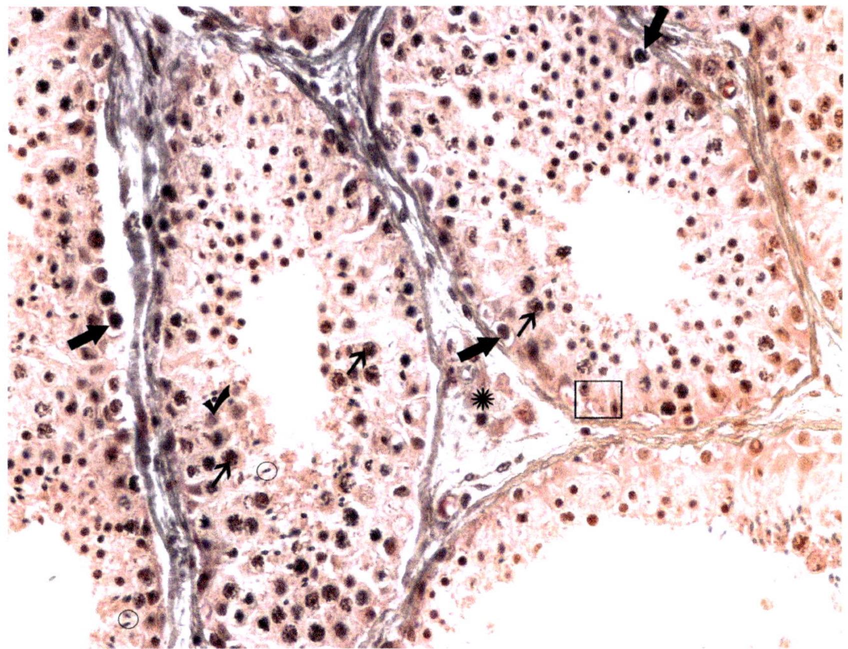

Fig. 4.1 (H-E, ×400) Spermatogenesis may be histologically thought of in a linear fashion, beginning with a pale spermatogonium and finishing with an elongated, late spermatid and, possibly, with spermatozoa. Seminiferous tubules with complete spermatogenesis are defined as the presence of spermatogonia (located close to the basement membranes, *thick arrows*), spermatocytes (*thin arrows*), and spermatids, both immature with round nuclei (*tick*) and mature (late) with elongated nuclei (*circles*). Sertoli cells (*square frame*) are noticed among germ cells. In the interstitium, Leydig cells form small intertubular clusters (*asterisk*)

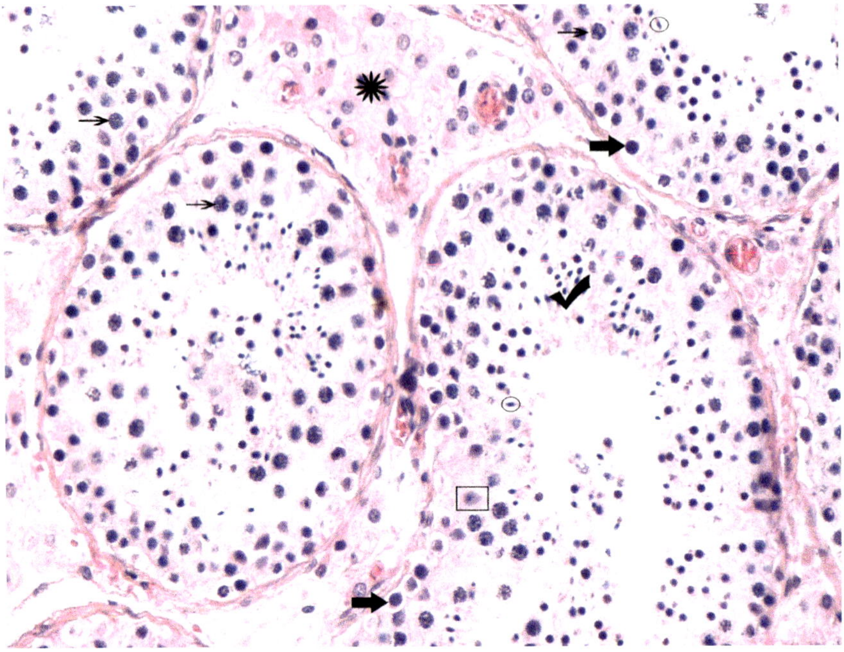

Fig. 4.2 (H-E, ×400) Spermatogenesis may be histologically thought of in a linear fashion, beginning with a pale spermatogonium and finishing with an elongated, late spermatid and, possibly, with spermatozoa. Seminiferous tubules with complete spermatogenesis are defined as the presence of spermatogonia (located close to the basement membranes, *thick arrows*), spermatocytes (*thin arrows*), and spermatids, both immature with round nuclei (*tick*) and mature (late) with elongated nuclei (*circles*). Sertoli cells (*square frame*) are noticed among germ cells. In the interstitium, Leydig cells form small intertubular clusters (*asterisk*)

4.3 Case 4.1: Germ Cell Neoplasia In Situ

Case Study

Data Prior to Microscopy

The congenital abnormality most frequently encountered by the pathologist is the cryptorchid testis.

Surgical resection of an intra-abdominal right testis from an adult patient. History of unilateral cryptorchidism since birth at 30-week gestational age. The decision to treat the undescended testis was postponed until adulthood. Prior to orchiopexy, a biopsy was performed; after having taken the pathological report into account, orchiectomy [rather than regular clinical and ultrasonographic evaluation alongside serological counts of human chorionic gonadotropin (HCG), alpha-fetoprotein (AFP), and human placental lactogen (HPL)] was proposed. After having considered the functional adequacy of the other testis, the patient consented to the surgical excision of his undescended testis, which was comparatively smaller than the contralateral testis and had a brown color on section.

4.3.1 Microscopic Evaluation of the Cryptorchid Orchiectomy Specimen

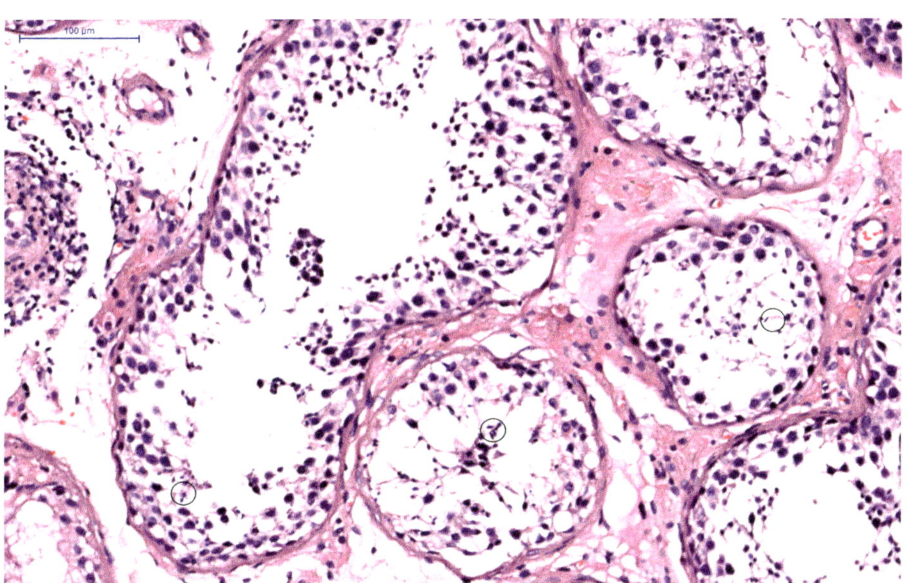

Fig. 4.3 (H-E, ×200) In this adult cryptorchid testis, deficient spermatogenesis is observed. The germ cell layers are thinned, and there are disorganized immature germ cells sloughed off in the lumens; however, mature, elongated spermatids are detectable (*circles*)

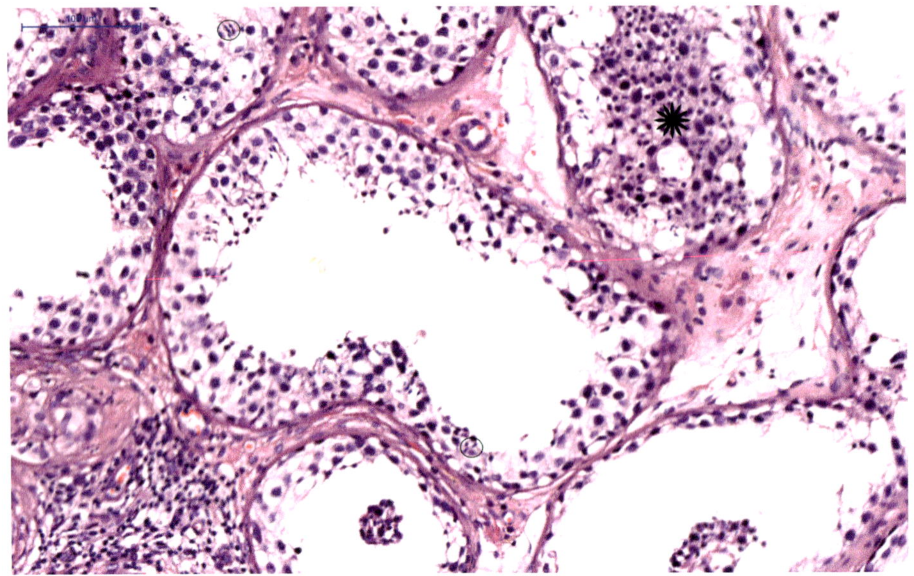

Fig. 4.4 (H-E, ×200) The number of germ cells is significantly reduced in these seminiferous tubules; late, elongated spermatids (*circles*) are focally detected though (hypospermatogenesis pattern). Notice the sloughing of germ cells (*asterisk*) into the tubular lumens (a nonspecific finding). The thinning in the number of layers is particularly striking at the tubule on the bottom right

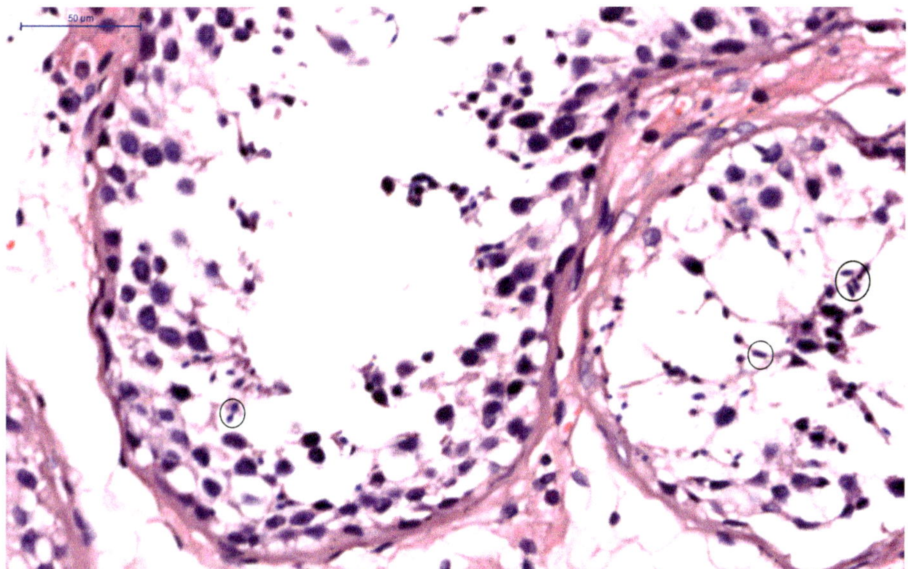

Fig. 4.5 (H-E, ×400) Complete, although decreased, spermatogenesis. Reduced numbers of germ cells of all types. The concomitant presence of some mature spermatids is the sine qua non for the pattern of hypospermatogenesis; the latter spermatids are distinguished, under high magnification, by their dark, angular nuclei (*circles*). The term "hypospermatogenesis" indicates reduced spermatogenesis, but not a process that stops at a particular point in the sequence of spermatogenesis. Finding *mature* (not round) spermatids in a number of seminiferous tubules indicates completion of spermatogenesis and constitutes the key point for the diagnosis of the pattern of hypospermatogenesis, a disorder where there is at least focally complete germ cell maturation, but the total number of germ cells is reduced. Usually, the pattern of hypospermatogenesis is not observed in all seminiferous tubules of the biopsy material; frequently, tubules either with Sertoli cells only or hyalinized are noticed

- *Maturation arrest* shows spermatogonia and, possibly, spermatocytes and immature round spermatids, but *no* mature spermatids or spermatozoa. Maturation arrest, in order to constitute a final diagnosis, should, by definition, demonstrate a *diffuse* pattern in the biopsy material; this term can be used in the conclusion of a pathological report only in cases of complete interruption of spermatogenesis to *all tubules* in the biopsy material.

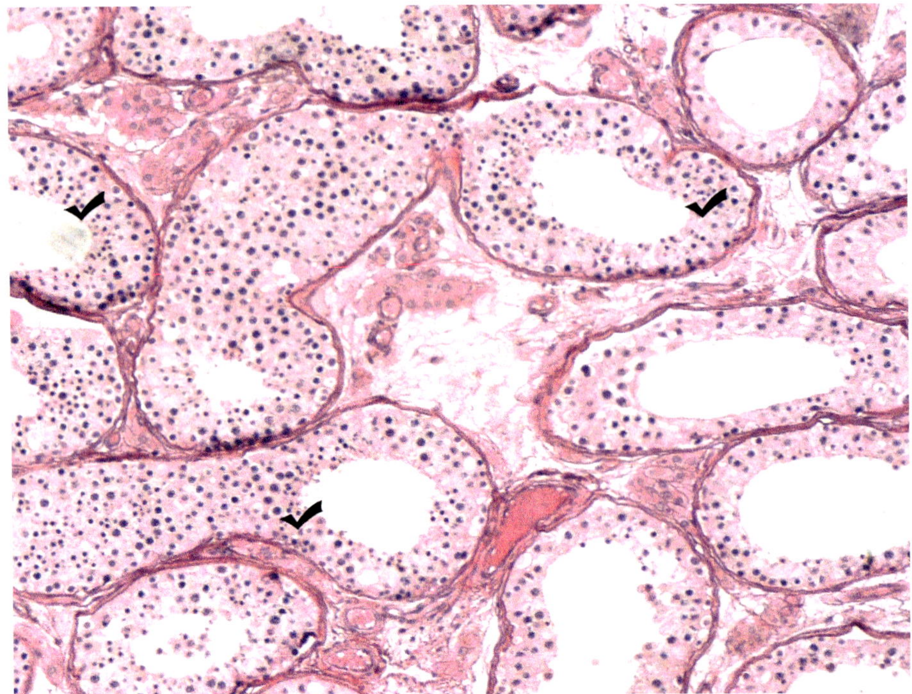

Fig. 4.6 (H-E, ×200) Maturation arrest. In these seminiferous tubules, particularly those on the right side, mature spermatids are absent; the other germ cells [i.e., spermatogonia, spermatocytes, and immature, round spermatids (*ticks* for the latter)] are noticeable. The pattern in these specific tubules is compatible with late maturation arrest. Some thickening and hyalinization of tubular basement and interstitial edema (at the center) are also present

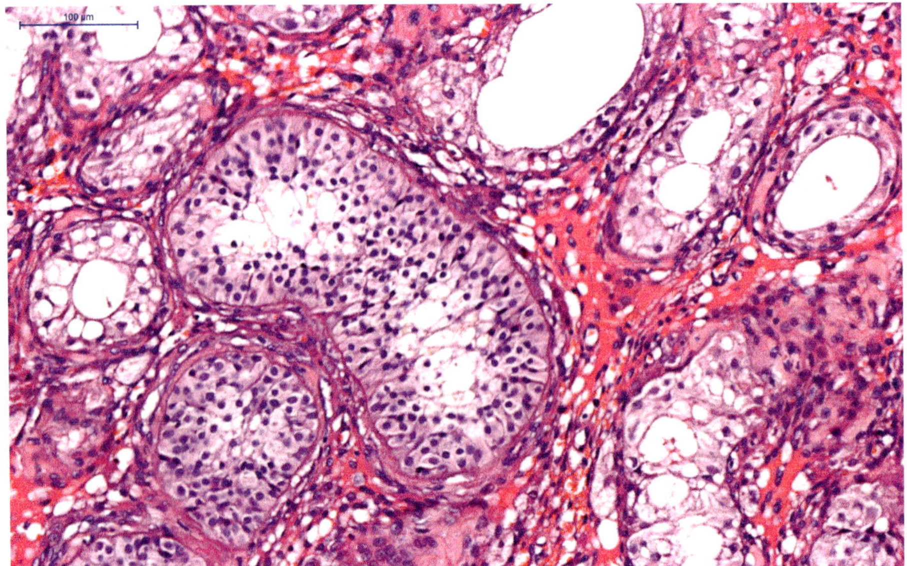

Fig. 4.7 (H-E, ×200) Maturation arrest pattern. Germ cells in the seminiferous tubules mature only to a certain point; no mature, elongated spermatids are detectable

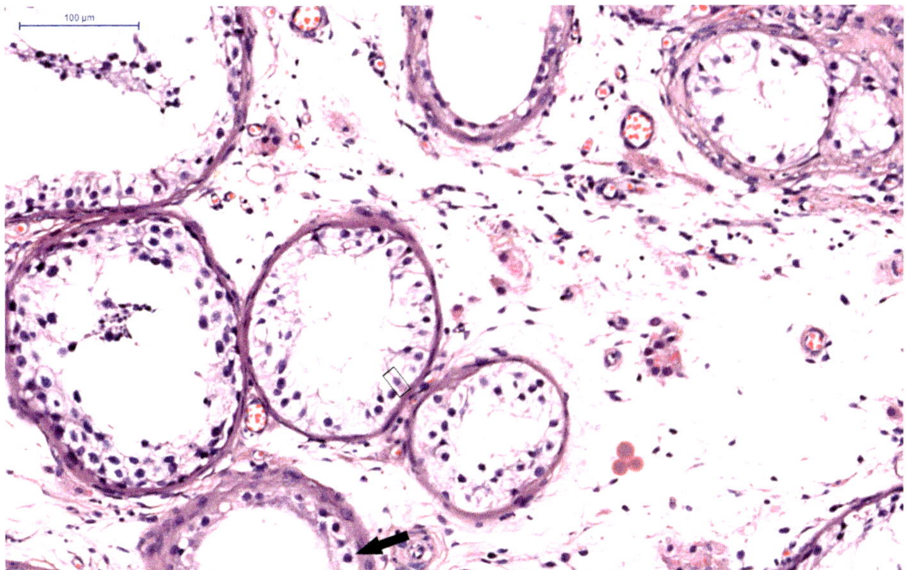

Fig. 4.8 (H-E, ×200) Early maturation arrest. In the central tubules, spermatogonia (*thick arrow*) are the only germ cells noticed. Sertoli cells are noticeable (*square frame*)

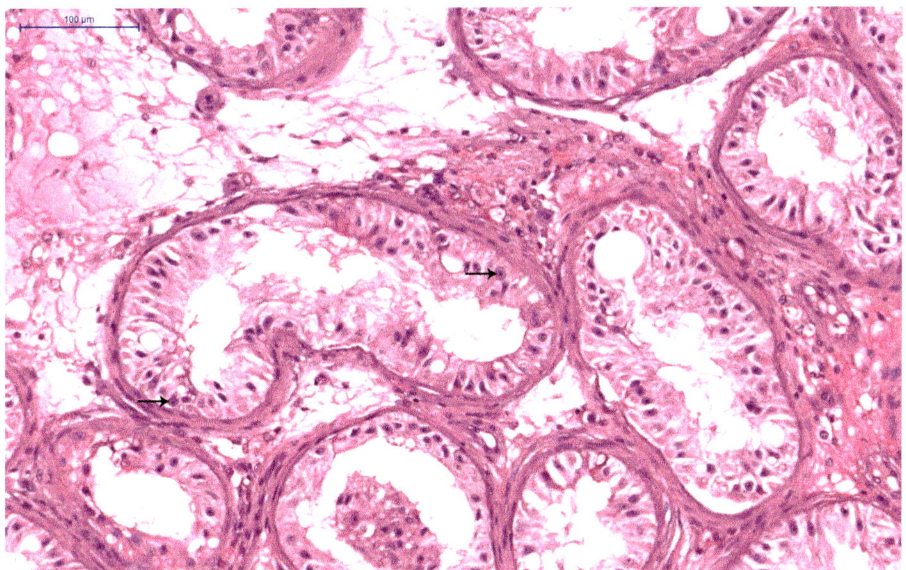

Fig. 4.9 (H-E, ×200) Germ cell aplasia – Sertoli cell-only tubules. Tubules filled entirely by Sertoli cells, with a "wind-swept" appearance, are noticed here. These Sertoli cells are of the postpubertal (mature) type; they are oriented perpendicular to the seminiferous tubular basement membrane; they have ovoid, indented, or elongated nuclei, occasional visible nucleoli (*thin arrows*), and abundant pale to eosinophilic cytoplasm. *No* germ cell component is present here. Concomitant basement thickening

The diagnosis of the Sertoli cell-only syndrome *in the conclusion* of a pathological report requires the complete absence of maturing germ cells from *all tubules* of the testicular biopsy and only then does it have clinical value.

Summarizing the findings so far, in the present adult undescended testis, a few foci of appropriate spermatogenesis are detectable. In general, the germ cell number is significantly decreased; however, mature, elongated spermatids are focally detectable (hypospermatogenesis). Tubules with either uneven or totally absent germ cell maturation or Sertoli cell only presence (the latter equivalent to germ cell aplasia) are also noticed. All these lesions should be quantified in the final pathological report. The final report should be "severe hypospermatogenesis."

4.3.2 Testicular Biopsy: Morphological Features and Patterns in Infertility

By developing techniques in vitro, many formerly regarded infertile men know fatherhood; the clinical relevance of the histological findings of testicular biopsy is becoming increasingly important. The main indication of testicular biopsy is the investigation of clinically unexplained azoospermia (absence of spermatozoa in the semen) or absence of semen in the ejaculate (aspermia). Additionally, men who, in two consecutive semen analyses, give less than 20 million spermatozoa per milliliter of semen (oligospermia) are also candidates for biopsy, after taking into account the hormonal and karyotype control of the childless couple. The main role of testicular biopsy is to distinguish the azoospermia due to ductal obstruction than that associated with problematic histopathology of testicular parenchyma (Cerilli et al. 2010). Particularly in azoospermic men with varicocele, the evaluation of microscopic patterns of testicular biopsy before surgical repair is associated with the proper handling of these patients (Saleh et al. 2010).

Tissue specimens measuring 3 × 3 × 3 mm are taken from both testicles and are placed directly in a special fixative liquid (e.g., Bouin). At least five sections, 4–5 μm in thickness, are taken, and H-E and PAS slides are prepared. The classification of microscopic findings with better predictive value for achieving fertilization (Cerilli et al. 2010) comprises five patterns:

1. *Normal testicular parenchyma.* Full, active spermatogenesis almost throughout the biopsy and normal interstitium. Usually post-testicular azoospermia due to excurrent duct obstruction. Excellent prognosis.
2. *Hypospermatogenesis.* All stages of spermatogenesis are present but appreciably decreased to varying degrees. Focal detection of mature, elongated spermatids is necessary. Mixed patterns exist, e.g., some of the tubules in the testicular biopsy material are lined only by Sertoli cells or are completely hyalinized, while in other tubules, complete spermatogenesis is observed (with recognition of mature, elongated spermatids).
3. *Maturation arrest.* Uniform interruption of maturation in *all* tubules, often at the stage of spermatogonia or primary spermatocytes (early inhibition), less frequently at the stage of secondary spermatocytes or immature, round spermatids (late inhibition). Mixed lesions in this category include the coexistence of early and late maturation arrest or the *co*existence of tubules entirely lined by Sertoli cells.

Generally, if rare mature spermatids are focally found, the lesion should be classified as "severe hypospermatogenesis" (rather than "incomplete maturation arrest").

4. *Sertoli cell-only syndrome (germ cell aplasia).* Exclusive presence of Sertoli cells and complete absence of germ cells in *all* tubules. An important morphological discrimination feature between postpubertal Sertoli cells and germ cells is the nucleolus of the former.
5. *Hyalinization-sclerosis of seminiferous tubules.* Thickening of basement membranes due to fibrosis and deposition of basement membrane-type material. *Diffuse,* total absence of both germ cells and Sertoli cells. Possible interstitial fibrosis and loss of Leydig cells. If present bilaterally, "end-stage testis" is diagnosed. Unfavorable prognosis.

In adult males with cryptorchidism, if unilateral GCNIS is diagnosed, the testis is surgically resected; if it is bilateral, radiation may be used to eradicate the neoplasia while maintaining Leydig cell hormonal secretion.

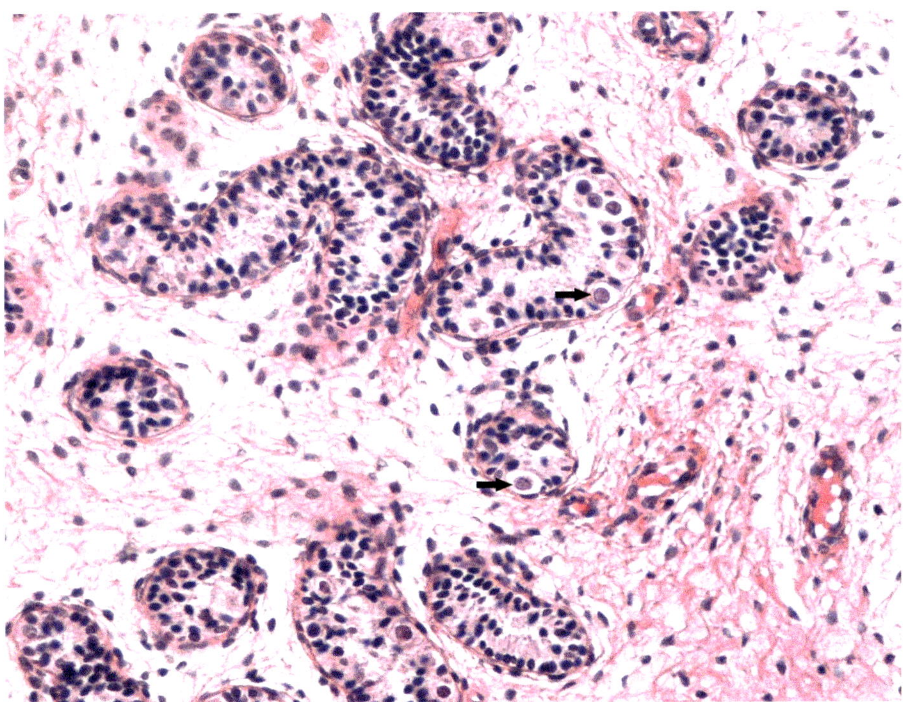

Fig. 4.10 (H-E, ×200) This group of tubules contains Sertoli cells with a prepubertal pattern [very small diameter, isolated spermatogonia with hypertrophic nuclei (*arrows*) and total absence of maturation, i.e., germ cell "hypoplasia"]. These spermatogonia with clear cytoplasm may resemble germ cell neoplasia in situ (GCNIS); immunohistochemistry may be useful in their distinction
Sometimes, in cryptorchid testes, persistent, small, immature tubules lined only by fetal-type Sertoli cells form *well-demarcated* clusters/nodules/"congeries," erroneously termed "Pick's adenomas"; they are not true neoplasms

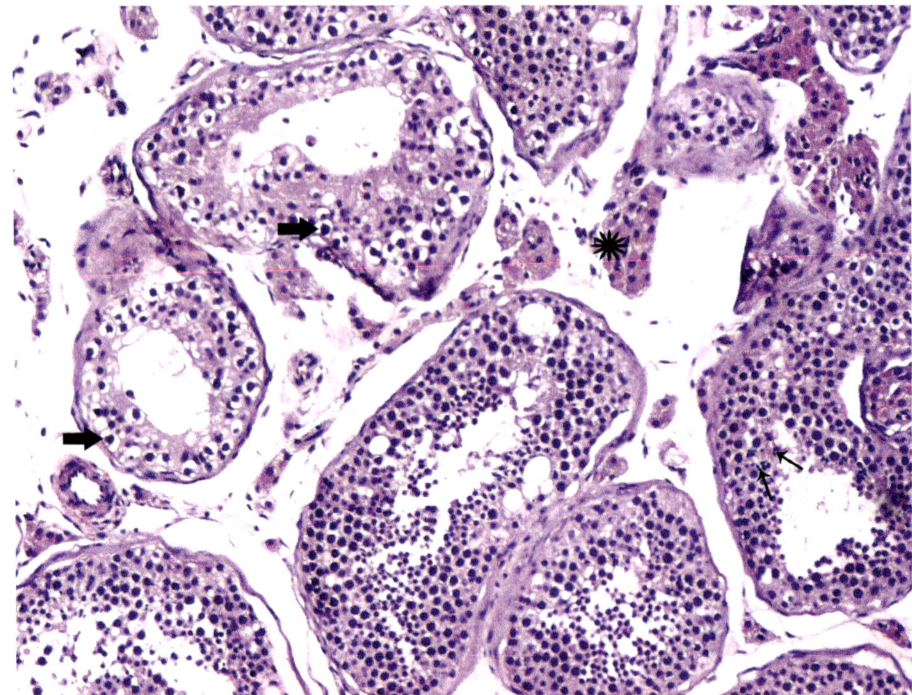

Fig. 4.11 (H-E, ×200) Seminiferous tubules undergoing intact, advanced, or complete spermatogenesis (*thin arrows* highlighting mature spermatids) are noticed in the lower part of this image and aggregations of Leydig cells in the upper right part (*asterisk*). Interestingly, in the remaining tubules, spermatogenesis is obviously reduced, and cells with enlarged, somewhat irregular nuclei and abundant, vacuolated cytoplasm, often having retraction artifact in formalin-fixed material (*thick arrows*), are located predominantly along the basement membranes. These features are compatible with germ cell neoplasia in situ (GCNIS); the latter is detected in 2–8% of testes with cryptorchidism. GCNIS is a precursor lesion of the vast majority of invasive germ cell tumors in *adults*

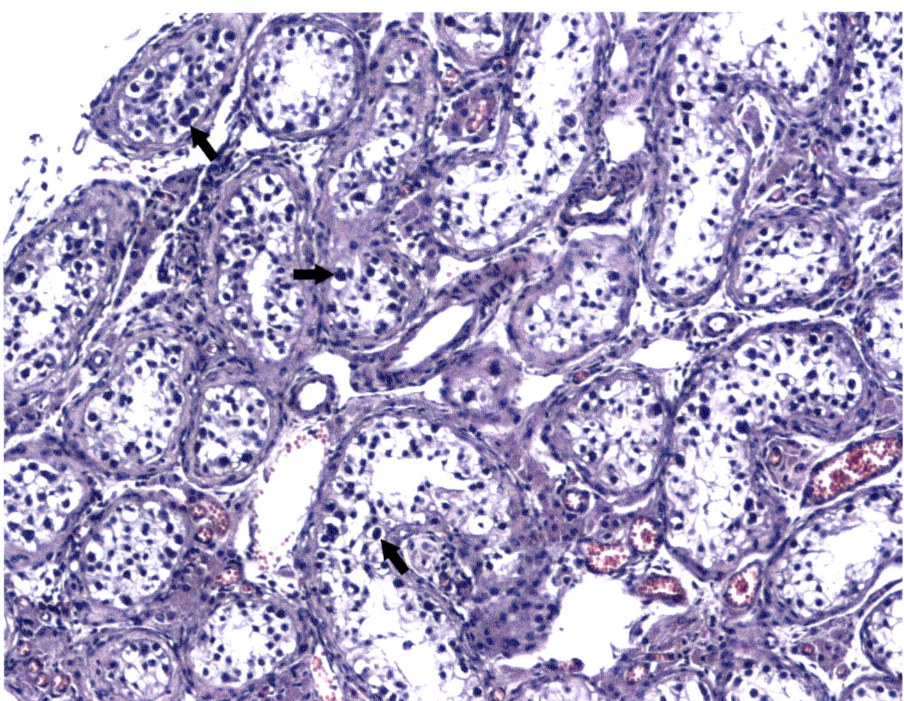

Fig. 4.12 (H-E, ×100) *Patchily* throughout the testicular biopsy, foci of GCNIS [atypical cells with large, hyperchromatic, angulated nuclei, aligned along the basal portion of the seminiferous tubules (*thick arrows*)] are observed. Thickened peritubular basement membranes. Complete spermatogenesis is absent in these foci; a minority of germ cells are still focally recognizable, so tubules are not completely filled with malignant cells

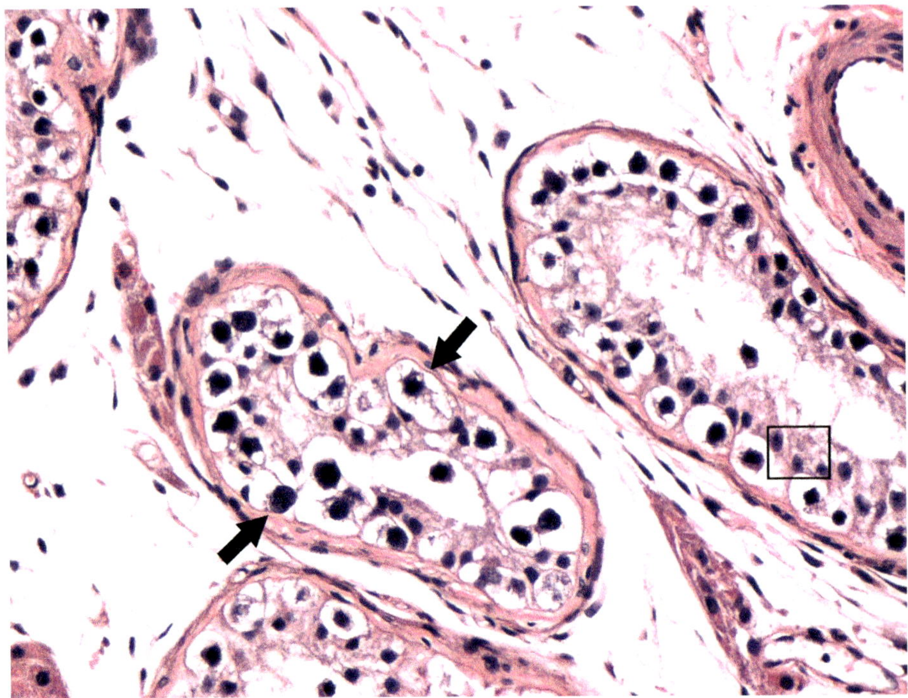

Fig. 4.13 (H-E, ×400) GCNIS characterized by a single layer of malignant, enlarged germ cells of seminomatous, "fried eggs" appearance aligned at the periphery of atrophic seminiferous tubules with deficient spermatogenesis and thickened peritubular tunica basement membranes (*thick arrows*). Sertoli cells are displaced toward the lumen (*square frame*).

In case the malignant cells of GCNIS foci expand the tubules and *totally* obliterate the normal components including Sertoli cells, "*intratubular* seminoma" would be the appropriate term. Intratubular seminoma fills and distends the tubules, whereas GCNIS is restricted to the basilar area, although the cells are histologically identical in both entities

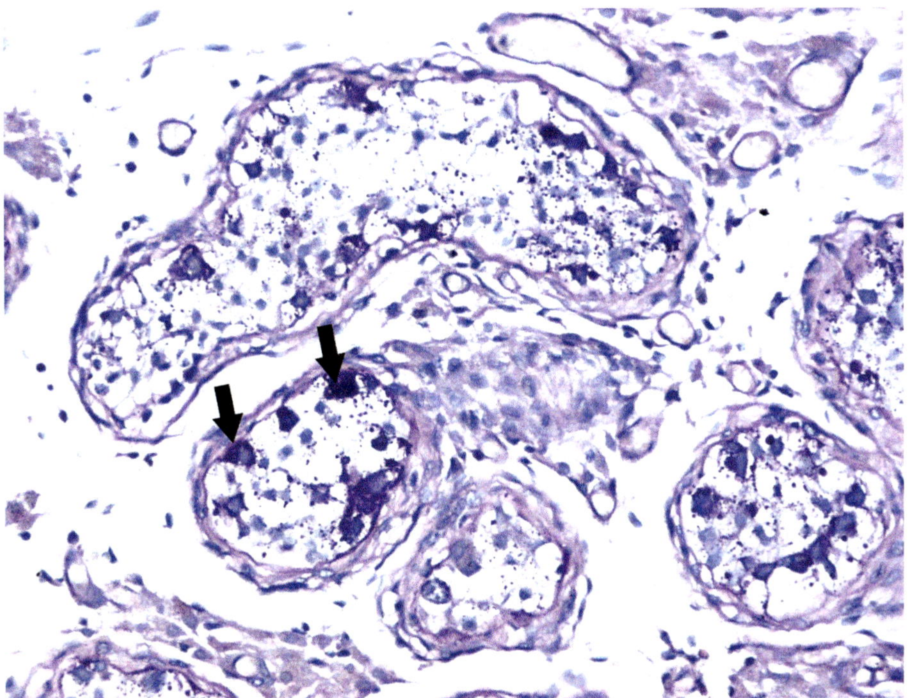

Fig. 4.14 (PAS, ×400) Due to cytoplasmic glycogen content, GCNIS is PAS (+) [but diastase-sensitive and thus PAS-D (−), as glycogen is not diastase-resistant]. Glycogen demonstration is diagnostically helpful when located in cells along the tubules' basilar aspect (*thick arrows*), but non-specific, since PAS-positivity may also be identified in nonneoplastic spermatogonia and Sertoli cells

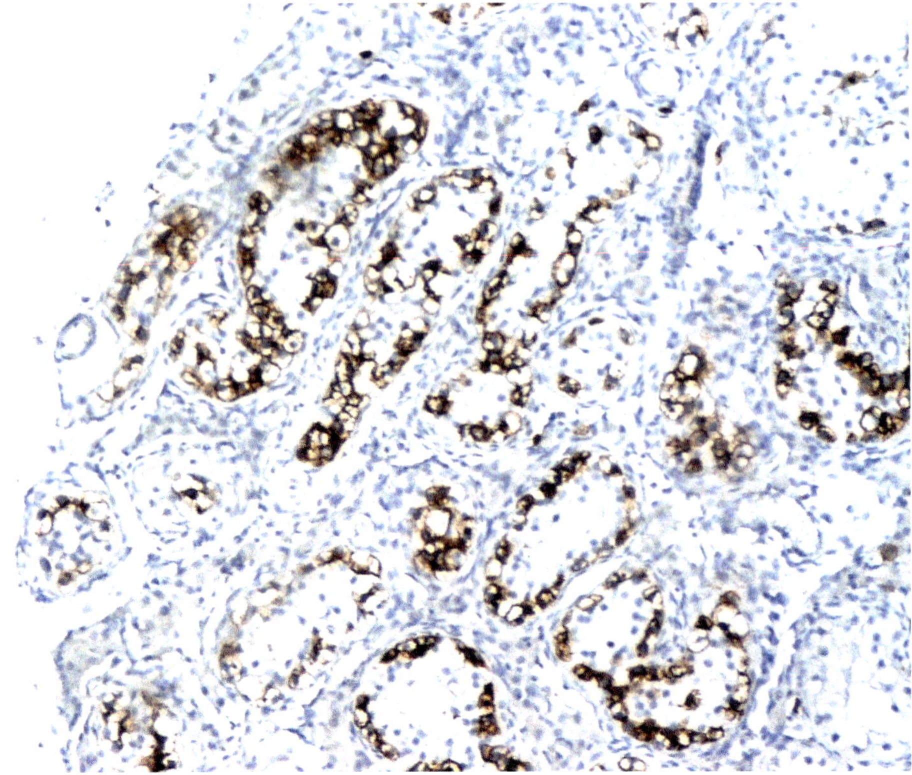

Fig. 4.15 (PLAP immunoperoxidase stain, ×100) Immunohistochemical confirmation of GCNIS. Foci of GCNIS react with several specific immunohistochemical markers including placental alkaline phosphatase (PLAP), podoplanin, SALL4, NANOG, and OCT3/4.

KIT immunopositivity favors the diagnosis of GCNIS; however, since normal spermatogonia may be KIT-positive, other immunomarkers [such as PLAP (the latter with a peripheral, membrane-accentuated staining pattern, obvious in the above image)] are preferable. Malignant cells are PLAP-immunopositive; within tubules with GCNIS, unstained cells correspond either to remaining germ cells or Sertoli cells. Only rarely (<1%) are isolated, nonneoplastic spermatocytes (which are unlikely to be confused with GCNIS) PLAP-positive, with spermatogonia being PLAP-negative in *adults*. It should be taken into account that in males *younger than 1 year of age*, primordial germ cells and spermatogonia may be immunohistochemically identical to cells of GCNIS [i.e., KIT (+) and PLAP (+)]. Furthermore, in adults, giant spermatogonia can occur (in tubules with normal spermatogenesis, though) and should not be overinterpreted as GCNIS; it is noteworthy that giant spermatogonia in adults are PLAP-immunonegative

4.3.2.1 Clinical Commentary

Argyris Siatelis

This is a case of pathological examination of an undescended testis which revealed significant deterioration of spermatogenesis with a pattern of severe hypospermatogenesis and GCNIS in a considerable number of seminiferous tubules.

Cryptorchidism is one of the most frequent congenital abnormalities of the genitourinary tract that affects about 1–2% of boys. It is unilateral in 80% of cases; in 20%, the testis is not palpable upon physical examination. Overall (32–79%), it is associated with some types of epididymal abnormalities. Cryptorchidism is commonly diagnosed during childhood, and the investigation and treatment at this age are the rule. Diagnostic methods have been used for localization and investigation of the impalpable testis such as ultrasound, computing tomography, magnetic resonance, arteriography; laparoscopy is preferred in the investigation and treatment, either with orchiectomy or orchiopexy. The main reasons for treatment include the reduction of risk of testicular malignancy, of risk of impairment of fertility potential, and of risk of other diseases like torsion of the testis or associated inguinal hernia. The standard therapy, particularly for children, is orchiopexy or surgical repositioning of the testis within the scrotal sac, while hormonal therapy is generally not indicated. This method (orchiopexy) may allow earlier detection of testicular tumors, but it has not been shown to reduce the risk of testicular cancer. This method must be combined with testis biopsy. Germ cell neoplasia in situ (GCNIS) may be microscopically diagnosed in a considerable number of biopsies from undescended testicles. The decision of orchiectomy in adulthood is difficult in the absence of GCNIS, and, in some cases, it is taken when the other testis is normal, after hormonal and semen examination. The incidence of azoospermia in unilateral cryptorchidism is 13%. Most adult patients with cryptorchidism prefer orchiopexy over orchiectomy. With regular examinations after orchiopexy, this can be a legitimate treatment option for adult cryptorchidism in consideration of the patient's preference. As a rule, orchiopexy should be performed before 1 year of age to minimize germ cell loss, the latter being highlighted in the present case, and relevant effects on the fertility index (Berkowitz et al. 1993; Cortes et al. 2001; Hadziselimovic and Herzog 2001; Trussel and Lee 2004).

Key Messages

- Patients with cryptorchidism have a five to ten times higher risk for testicular malignancy than the general population. Infertility is the most common consequence of cryptorchidism.
- Biopsies of *cryptorchid* testes should be examined for the presence and numbers of germ cells and tubular size and the presence of malignant intratubular germ cells (GCNIS).
- Careful histological evaluation is necessary because GCNIS often has a patchy distribution.
- *Immunoperoxidase* stains should probably be performed on sections of all cryptorchid testes so that GCNIS is not overlooked.

4.4 Case 4.2: Testicular Seminoma

Case Study

Data Prior to Microscopy

Painless testicular swelling in a 39-year-old patient. Ultrasound examination demonstrates the presence of a well-defined and hypoechoic mass confined to the testis. Radiological absence of nodal or visceral involvement (stage 1). Serum α-fetoprotein (AFP) and lactate acid dehydrogenase (LDH) are normal, while human chorionic gonadotropin (HCG) levels reach 400 IU/L; placental alkaline phosphatase (PLAP) is also elevated.

A multinodular, relatively *homogeneous*, soft tumor with bulging, cream to tan, fleshy cut surface symmetrically enlarges and replaces almost the entire testis. Tumor maximum diameter: *6.5 cm*. Minute foci of punctate hemorrhage and yellow foci are observed upon meticulous macroscopic evaluation of the tumor cut surface. Tunica albuginea is intact.

4.4.1 Microscopic Evaluation of the Radical Orchiectomy Specimen

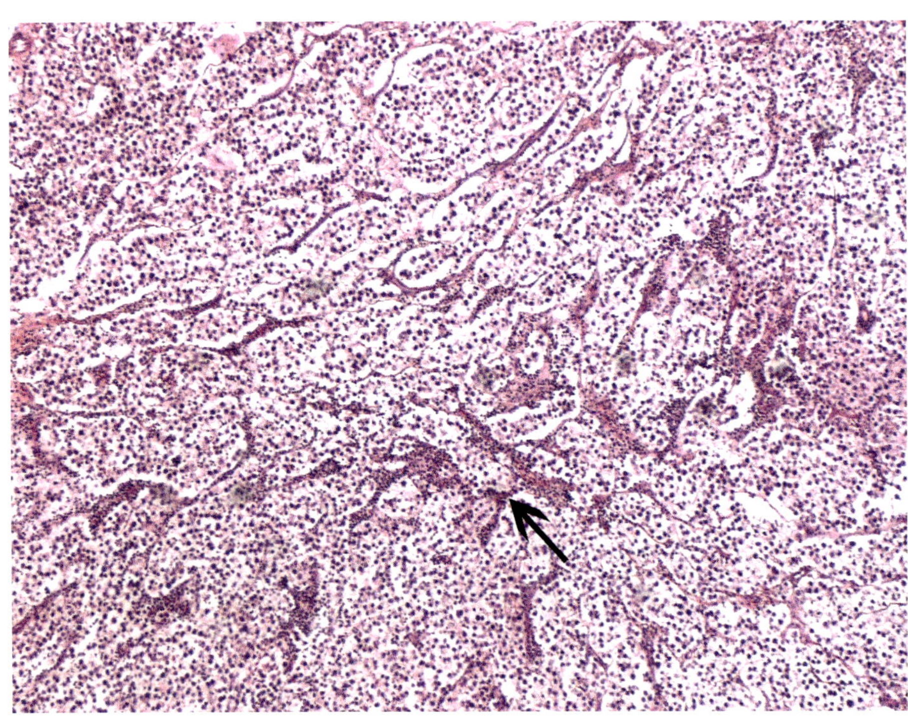

Fig. 4.16 (H-E, ×50) Diffuse sheets or lobules of pale tumor cells with intervening, branching fibrous septa (*arrow*). Areas of loosely cohesive cells are noticeable

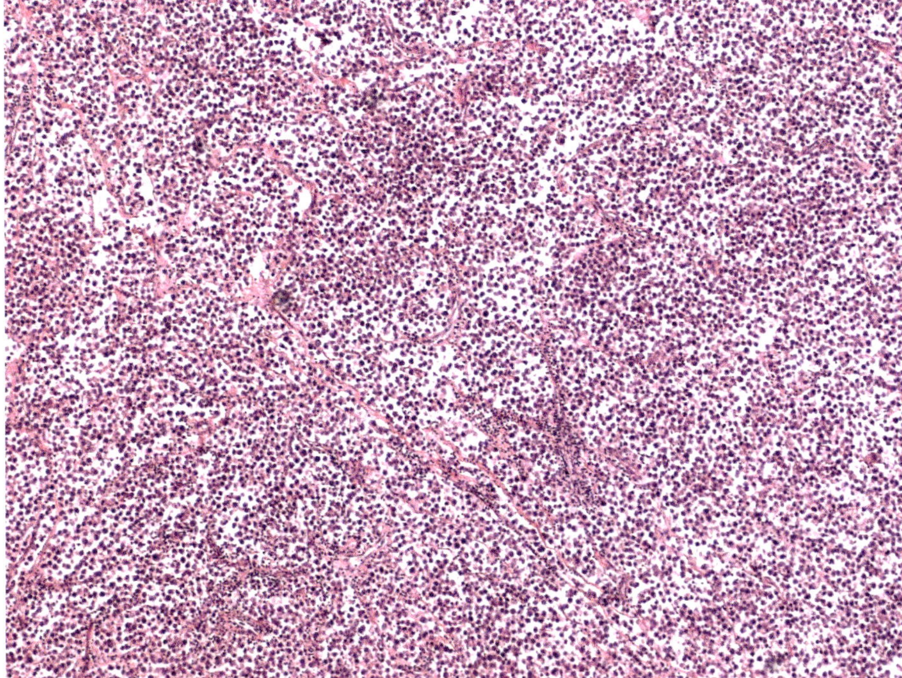

Fig. 4.17 (H-E, ×50) Area with more crowded nuclei. In *poorly fixed* specimens like this one, cytoplasmic autolysis obscures the cell borders and causes some nuclear overlapping

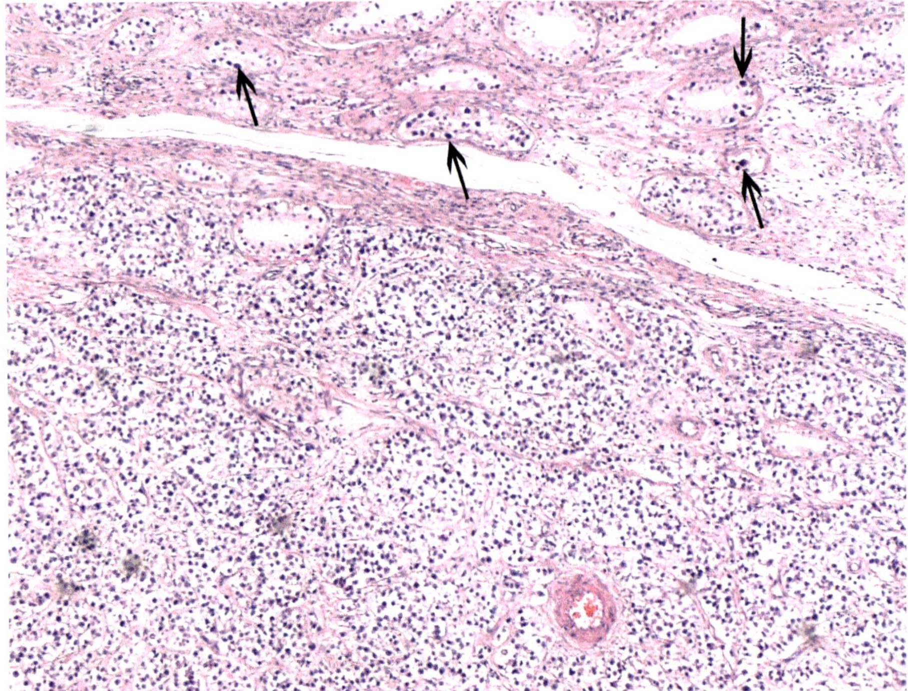

Fig. 4.18 (H-E, ×50) A well-fixed seminoma with monotonous cells; abundant, clear/watery cytoplasm (due to glycogen); and non-overlapping nuclei. The precursor lesion, i.e., germ cell neoplasia in situ (GCNIS), is expectedly encountered in adjacent, residual seminiferous tubules (*arrows*)

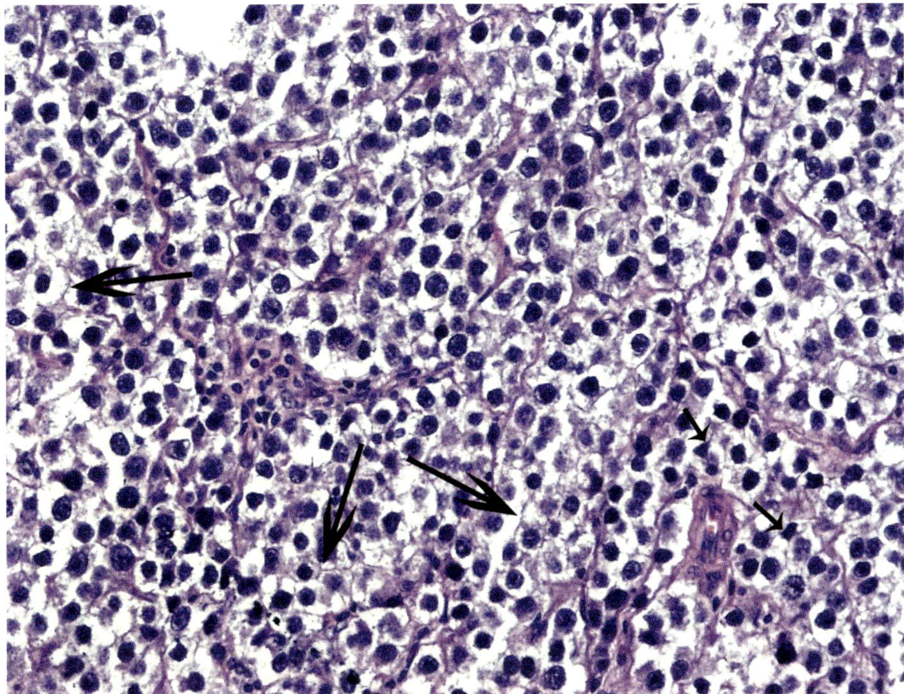

Fig. 4.19 (H-E, ×200) Large, round to polyhedral seminomatous cells with pale to clear cytoplasm which causes the nuclei to be non-overlapping and relatively even spaced. Distinct cell membranes (*big arrows*), large central nuclei, some of which with flattened edges (*small arrows*)

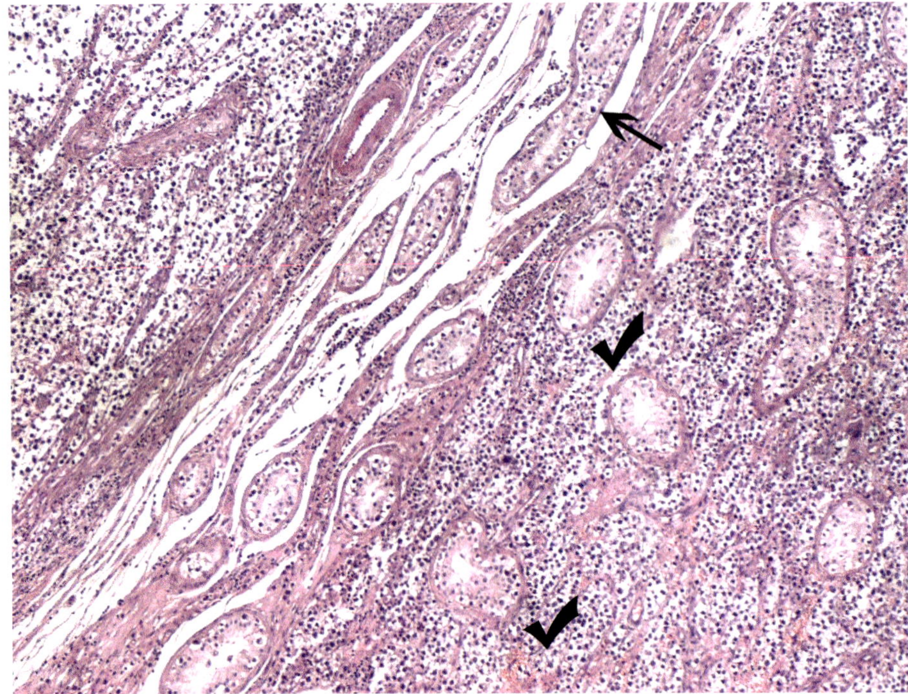

Fig. 4.20 (H-E, ×50) Seminoma periphery. Interstitial growth pattern with preservation of seminiferous tubules surrounded by seminoma cells (*ticks*) and foci of GCNIS (*arrow*). The interstitial infiltrating pattern may not be grossly evident

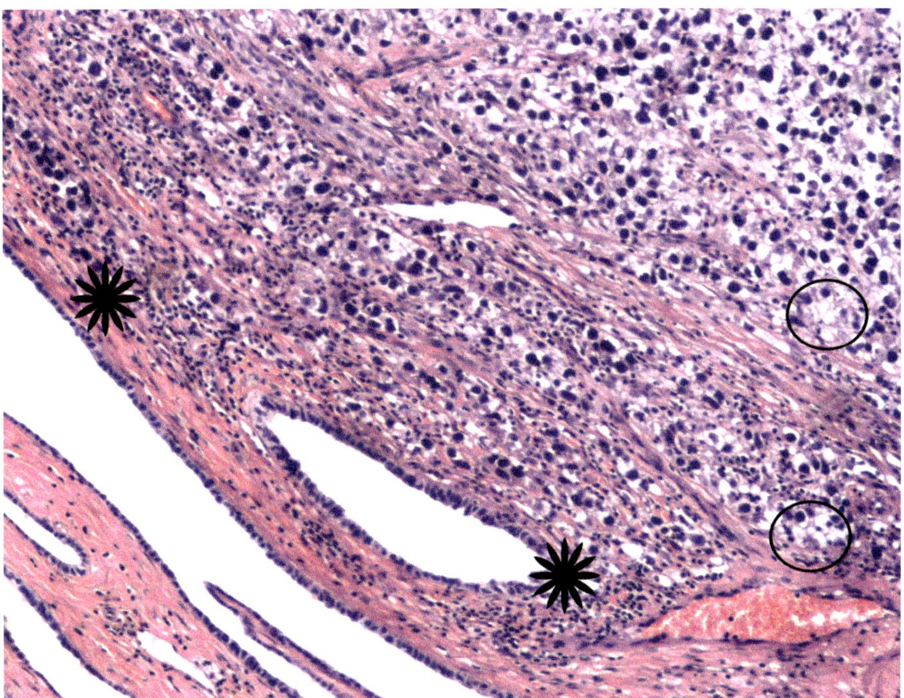

Fig. 4.21 (H-E, ×200) Closely apposed seminomatous cells with well-defined cell borders and crisp cytoplasmic membranes (*circles*). Interstitial fibrosis. Rete testis *stroma invasion* by seminoma cord-like structures (*asterisks*), an ominous prognostic parameter in seminomas of an early stage. No evidence of pagetoid spread within rete testis epithelial lining; the latter feature is not regarded such an adverse prognostic factor as rete testis *stroma* invasion.

With regard to pathologic staging of testicular germ cell tumors, extensive invasion of hilar soft tissue and/or of spermatic cord soft tissues equates with pT3, while involvement of tunica vaginalis and/or vascular/lymphatic invasion equates with pT2 even when vascular/lymphatic invasion is noticed *within* the spermatic cord vessels (without extravascular invasion of spermatic cord soft tissues). The resection margin of the spermatic cord should be carefully examined under the microscope; the relevant section should be taken before fixation of the orchiectomy specimen

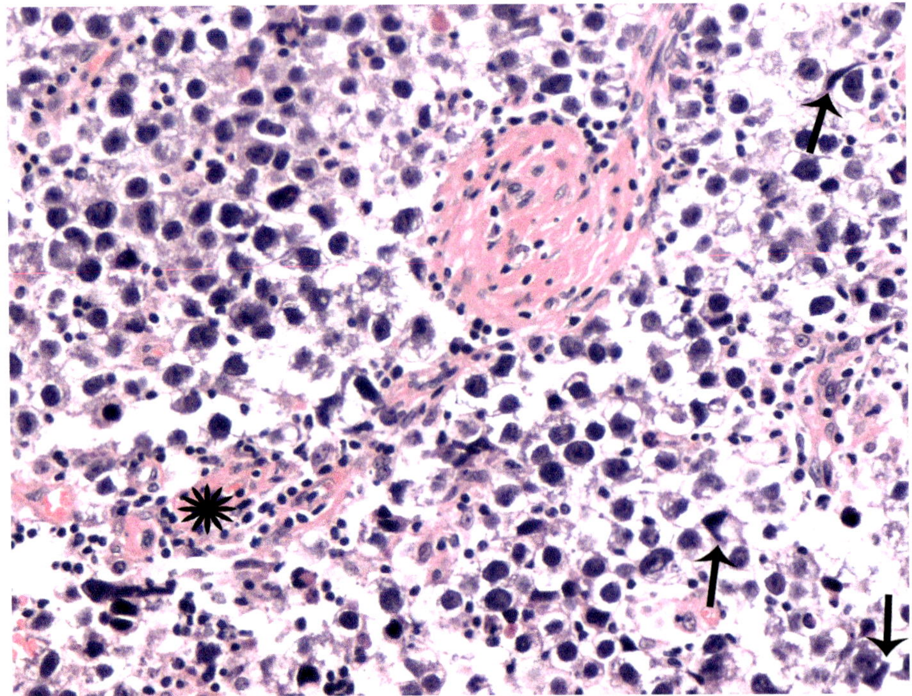

Fig. 4.22 (H-E, ×400) Population of seminomatous cells with clear to pale cytoplasm. Associated, mild lymphocytic infiltrate in the thin fibrous septum (*asterisk*). Flattened, "squared-off" edges in some nuclei (*arrows*)

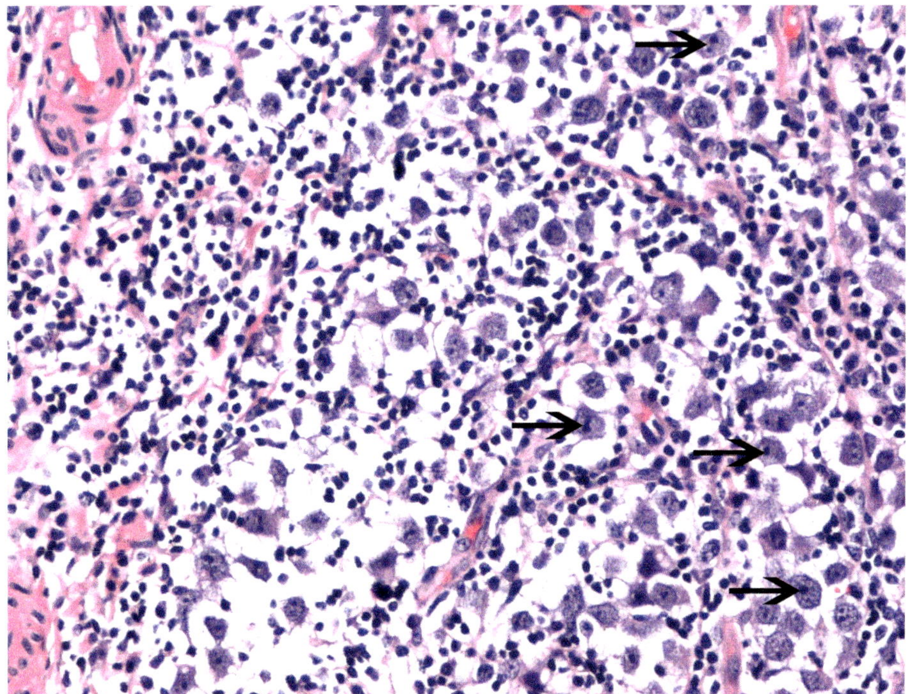

Fig. 4.23 (H-E, ×400) Seminomatous cells are primitive-looking germ cells. Cytoplasmic clarity (due to abundant glycogen particles). Polygonal nuclei with finely granular chromatin and either one centrally located or two visible nucleoli (*arrows*). Intermingled, brisk inflammatory infiltrate consisting chiefly of lymphocytes. A prominent lymphocytic reaction has been associated with an improved prognosis

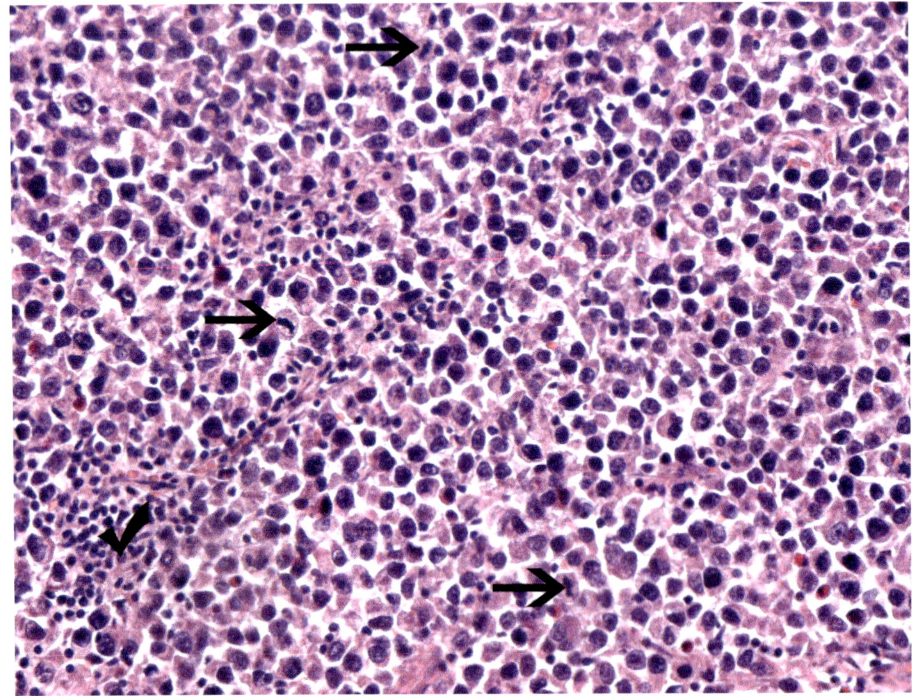

Fig. 4.24 (H-E, ×200) An area of higher cellularity and denser cytoplasm. Increased mitotic activity (i.e., three or more mitoses per high-power field) is observed in such areas (*arrows*) opposed to the minimal mitotic activity which predominates elsewhere. There's evidence that "high-mitotic-rate" seminoma behaves no differently from seminoma with a lower mitotic rate. Lymphocytic presence (*tick*) is an important constant finding

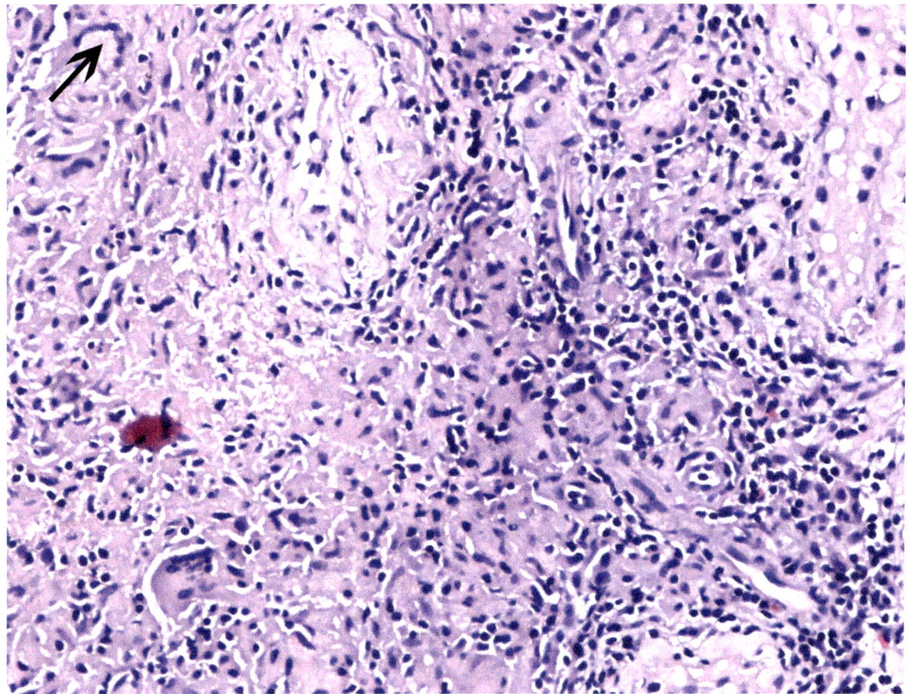

Fig. 4.25 (H-E, ×200) A marked granulomatous reaction effacing the underlying seminoma. Confluent clusters of epithelioid histiocytes and multinucleated giant cells, occasionally of the Langhans type (*arrow*)

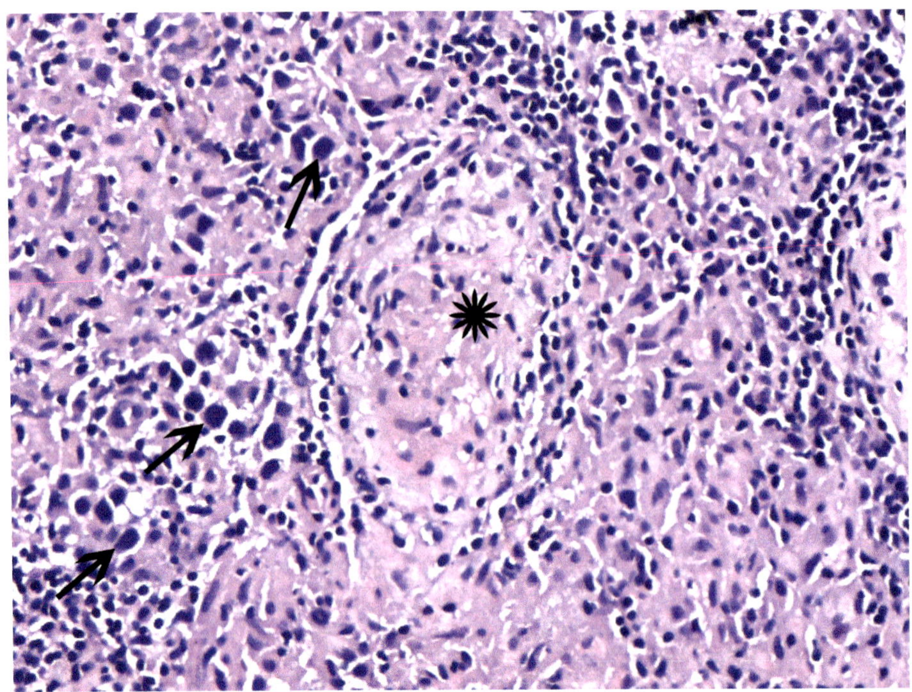

Fig. 4.26 (H-E, ×200) Large, seminomatous tumor cells (*arrows*) among clusters of epithelioid histiocytes, small lymphocytes, and well-defined, non-necrotizing, sarcoidal-type microgranuloma (*asterisk*). A florid granulomatous reaction can, in rare cases, obliterate almost all evidence of the underlying seminoma; immunostains (e.g., PLAP, KIT, podoplanin) can prove useful in identifying residual seminomatous cells in this circumstance, and thus the misdiagnosis of granulomatous orchitis is avoided

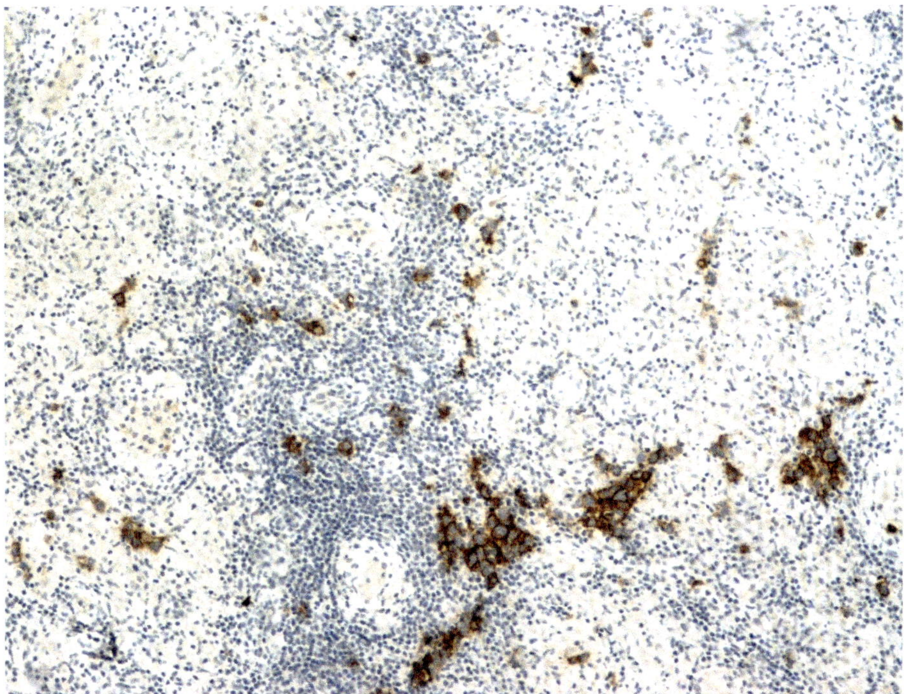

Fig. 4.27 (KIT immunoperoxidase stain, ×100) KIT immunostaining highlighting the presence of seminomatous cells, single or in clusters, within the granulomatous reaction

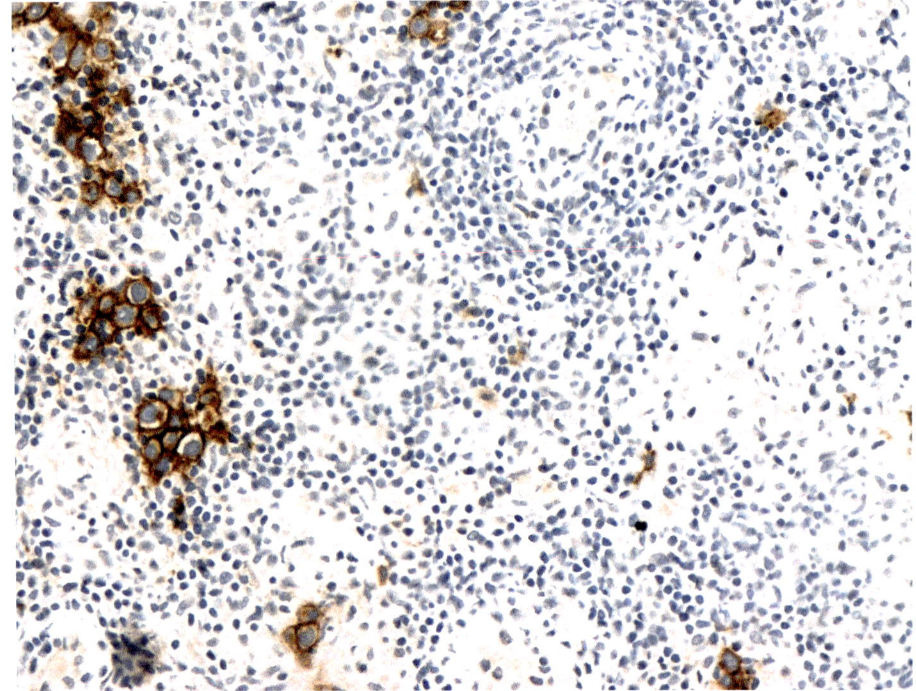

Fig. 4.28 (Podoplanin immunoperoxidase stain, ×200) Podoplanin-immunopositive seminomatous cells.

PLAP is an additional immunomarker expressed by seminoma cells with a membrane-accentuated staining pattern, like KIT and podoplanin. Other useful markers for seminoma are NANOG and OCT3/4 which, nevertheless, are also expressed in GCNIS and embryonal carcinoma, i.e., in the more primitive types of germ cell neoplasms.

AFP, CD30, and EMA are negative in seminomas

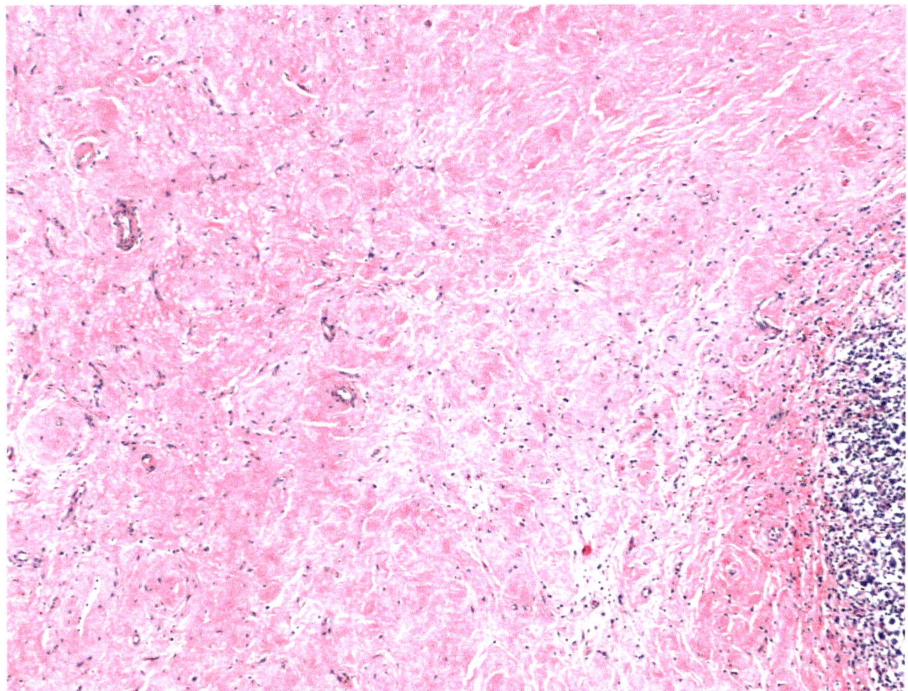

Fig. 4.29 (H-E, ×50) Diffuse interstitial fibrosis in an area of tumor regression. Scarring with hyalinized deposits of collagen and few chronic inflammatory cells. Residual seminomatous tissue on the lower right part of the image, with an evident concomitant lymphocytic infiltrate.

Among germ cell tumors, choriocarcinoma is the one that displays the greatest tendency to regress; however, the majority of regressing tumors refers to seminomas, since the latter are much more frequent than choriocarcinomas. *Regression of the primary neoplasm* is associated with *metastatic disease*.

Up till now, the features of a partially regressing "pure seminoma" have been highlighted. "Classic" seminoma is composed by relatively uniform tumor cells with abundant clear cytoplasm, distinct cell boundaries, and evenly spaced tumor cells without nuclear overlapping; fibrous trabeculae with lymphocytic infiltrates are the rule, and a granulomatous reaction may be observed. Like the latter, regression-related fibrosis may be marked and thus make the recognition of the tumor difficult

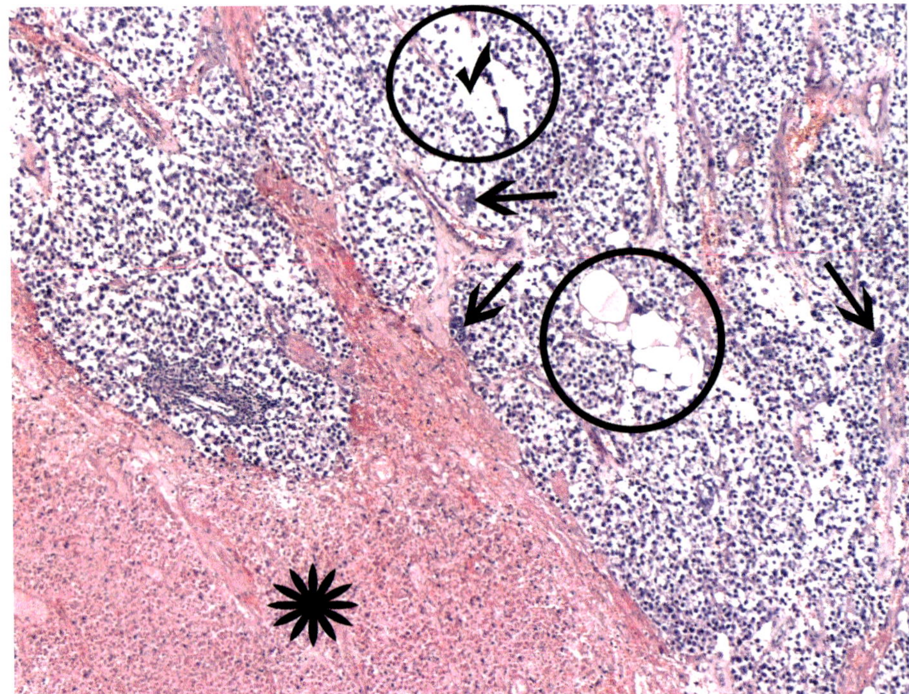

Fig. 4.30 (H-E, ×100) Admixed, scattered syncytiotrophoblasts (associated with macroscopically detected foci of hemorrhage), often located adjacent to capillaries (*arrows*). The term "seminoma with syncytiotrophoblastic cells" is appropriate for such seminomas. In contrast to seminoma cells, *syncytiotrophoblastic elements* express cytokeratin, EMA, and, of course, HCG immunohistochemically since they are responsible for serum HCG elevation, which generally does not exceed 1000 IU/L and is usually lower than 500 IU/L, as in the present case. If HCG serum levels are markedly elevated (in the thousands or tens of thousands of IU/L), an associated choriocarcinoma should be suspected. Presence of syncytiotrophoblast within a seminoma is not an adverse prognostic feature.

An area of coagulative tumor necrosis is also detected (*asterisk*) and should be reported.

Small cystic areas are also observable (*circles*) with exfoliated neoplastic cells in some of them (tick). Edema may occur in seminomas and cause separation of neoplastic cells with the formation of small cystic spaces mimicking the microcystic/reticular pattern of yolk sac tumor; the cystic spaces of an edematous seminoma are more irregular, though, and there are exfoliated cells in some of them. The microcystic/reticular pattern of yolk sac tumor – which, morphologically, is indicated herein – can be excluded by AFP and glypican-3 negative immunostaining; furthermore, the presence of a yolk sac tumor component is unlikely in this patient because serum AFP levels were normal. In seminoma patients, concomitant liver disease (including seminomatous metastases to the liver) may cause modest AFP elevation. A significantly elevated AFP concentration is strongly suspicious for yolk sac tumor in the primary tumor or a metastasis

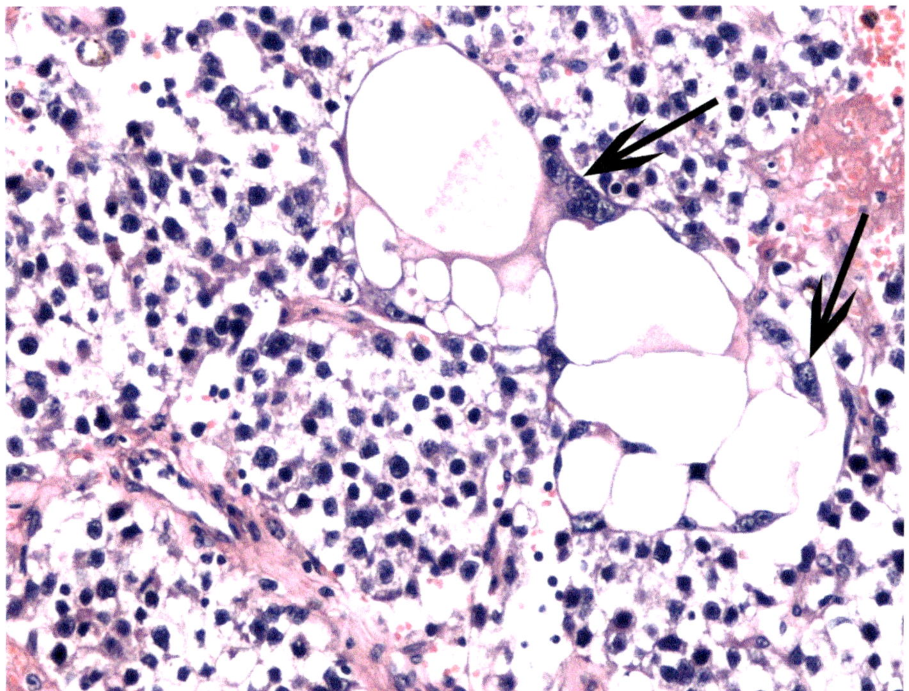

Fig. 4.31 (H-E, ×200) These cyst-like spaces/cytoplasmic lacunae are here associated with multinucleated syncytiotrophoblastic cells (*arrows*). When syncytiotrophoblastic cells are noticed, the presence of a choriocarcinomatous component should be ruled out.

Unlike classic choriocarcinoma, the syncytiotrophoblastic cells of seminoma are *not* associated with *mono*nucleated cytotrophoblasts and are *not* arranged in nodular aggregates. In contrast to seminomatous cells, mononucleated cytotrophoblasts express, among other markers, p63 and GATA3; the latter two common immunomarkers are useful when a choriocarcinoma component is suspected. The absence of a cytotrophoblastic component permits distinction of a seminoma with isolated syncytiotrophoblastic cells from a choriocarcinoma

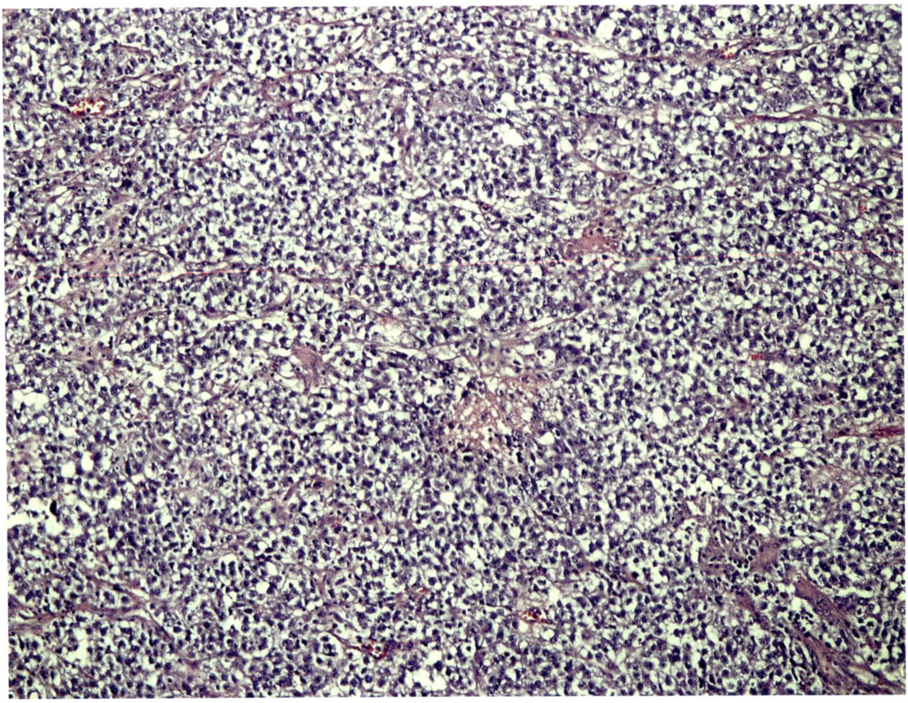

Fig. 4.32 (H-E, ×100) This seminomatous area deserves closer inspection

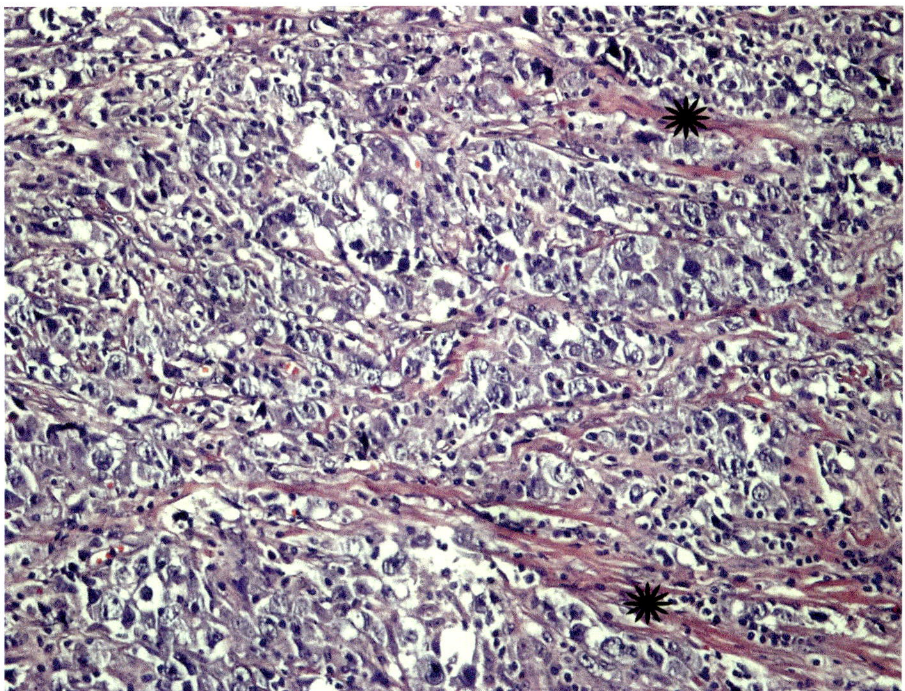

Fig. 4.33 (H-E, ×200) On higher magnification, this is a tumor area with less well-defined cytoplasmic boundaries, darker cytoplasm, and cellular pleomorphism exceeding that of seminoma, with larger nuclei and higher nuclear/cytoplasmic ratio. The presence of fibrous septa, typical of seminoma, is still implied (*asterisks*), with a minimal lymphocytic presence, though. "Seminoma with atypia" is a term used to describe such areas which probably represent a tendency for transition to embryonal carcinoma. Such areas warrant immunohistochemical investigation

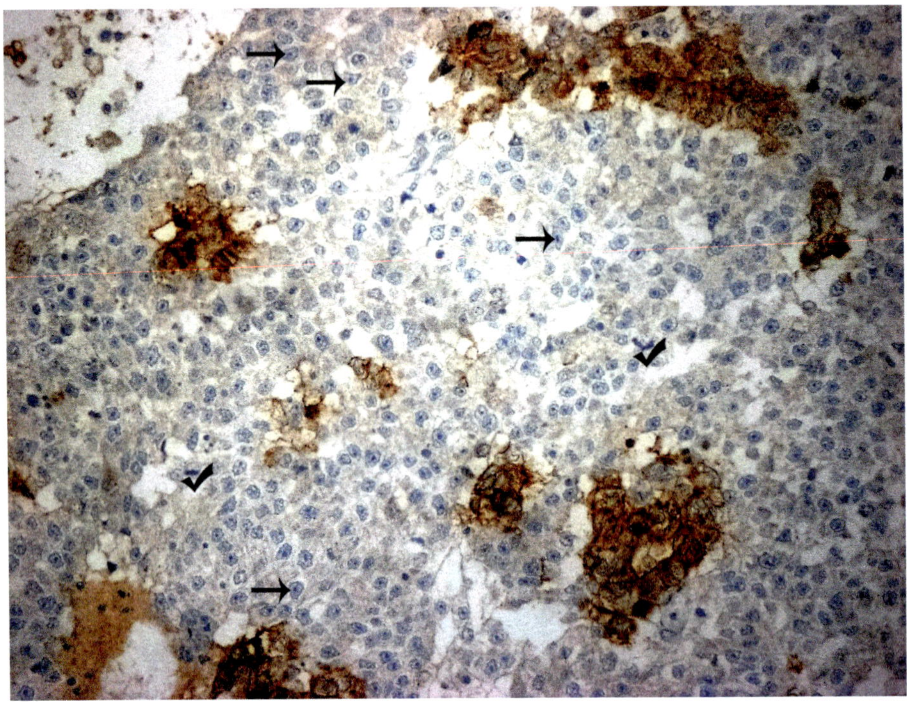

Fig. 4.34 (CD30 immunohistochemistry, ×200) Focal CD30 positivity, indicative of focal tendency for transformation of seminoma to embryonal cell carcinoma. (The CD30-immunopositive cells lose KIT expression, as can be observed in a KIT immunoperoxidase stain of the same tumor area). The CD30-immunonegative, seminoma cells of this field show some mitotic activity (*ticks*) and retain their characteristic, vesicular nuclei with centrally located nucleoli (*arrows*). The term "seminoma with atypia" could describe this focal tendency of seminomatous cells to transform to embryonal carcinoma cells but without a clear component of embryonal carcinoma being yet defined

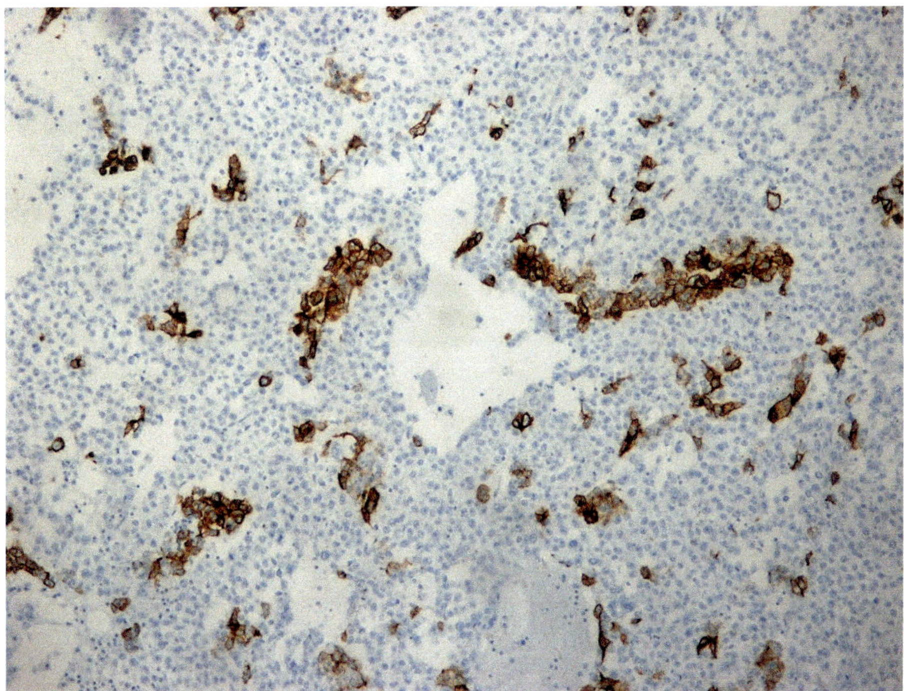

Fig. 4.35 (Cytokeratin immunohistochemistry, ×100) A tumor area with scattered, *strongly* positive neoplastic cells, single or in clusters, indicates a tendency of seminoma cells to transform to embryonal carcinoma cells. Immunohistochemical examination of seminoma cells generally shows no evidence of epithelial differentiation; cytokeratin expression in seminoma cells, if any, is weak.

Whether the above amount of CD30 – and cytokeratin – coexpressing neoplastic cells is sufficient for the diagnosis of a distinct embryonal carcinoma component in this germ cell tumor remains questionable. Occasional histologically atypical cells in an otherwise typical seminoma should still be considered a seminoma but should engender a search for embryonal carcinoma in other sections

4.4.1.1 Clinical Commentary

Vasileios Spapis

This is a pathological diagnosis of a seminoma with isolated syncytiotrophoblastic cells; the tumor is limited to the testis, but there are some ominous histological parameters, i.e., increased tumor diameter, rete testis invasion, and evidence of partial regression. No other germ cell tumor component was detected.

Seminomas account for about 35–52% of all germ cell tumors (GCTs). Among them, "classic" seminoma is the most common type accounting for 85% of the cases (Presti 2013). Stage for stage, there is no prognostic significance to any of the proposed seminoma subtypes including that with isolated syncytiotrophoblastic cells. On average, seminomas occur at an older age than nonseminomatous germ cell tumors (NSGCTs), with most cases diagnosed in the fourth decade of life. Compared with NSGCTs, seminomas have a more favorable prognosis. They tend to be less aggressive, to be diagnosed at an earlier stage, and to spread predictably along lymphatic channels to the retroperitoneum before spreading hematogenously to visceral organs. At the time of diagnosis, the proportion of patients with clinical stage I disease (confined to the testis) is about 85% (Stephenson and Gilligan 2012), like the present case.

Grossly, soft coalescing gray nodules are observed. Necrosis may be present but is usually focal. In approximately 10–15% of pure seminomas, syncytiotrophoblasts, which stain positive for human chorionic gonadotropin (HCG), can be identified but are of no clear prognostic significance. Lymphocytic infiltrates and granulomatous reactions are often seen, and seminomas appear to be associated with an increased incidence of sarcoidosis. Seminomas may be confused not only with solid pattern embryonal carcinomas but also with yolk sac tumors or Sertoli cell tumors. Immunohistochemical staining plays a supportive role in diagnosing germ cell tumors (GCTs); seminomas are typically negative for CD30, positive for CD117, and strongly positive for placental alkaline phosphatase (PLAP) (Stephenson and Gilligan 2012). Seminomas arise from germ cell neoplasia in situ (GCNIS) and are considered to be the common precursor for the other, NSGCT subtypes. This ability of seminomas to transform into NSGCT elements, including embryonal carcinoma, has important therapeutic implications.

Like in all GCTs, diagnostic evaluation and staging should include bilateral ultrasound of the testis, kinetics of serum tumor markers (pre- and post-orchiectomy LDH, HCG, AFP), and abdominopelvic and chest CT. Placental alkaline phosphatase (PLAP) is an optional serum marker in monitoring patients with pure seminoma, with low predictive value, though, and it is not recommended in smokers (Nielsen et al. 1990). LDH levels are elevated in approximately 20% of low-stage GCTs. As a nonspecific marker for GCT, its main use is in the prognostic assessment of GCT at diagnosis. The serum half-life of LDH is 24 h. HCG levels are elevated in approximately 15% of seminomas due to the presence of isolated syncytiotrophoblastic cells, as in the present case. Levels greater than 5000 IU/L are usually associated with NSGCTs. The half-life of HCG is 24–36 h. Seminomas do *not* produce AFP. Patients with pure seminoma as the primary tumor and with an elevated serum AFP value are considered to have

NSGCT. The half-life of AFP is 5–7 days. Bone and brain scanning should be performed in case of symptoms or in the unexpected presence of multiple visceral metastases (Albers 2016).

After modern staging procedures, about 15–20% of stage I seminoma patients have subclinical metastatic disease, usually in the retroperitoneum, and will relapse after orchiectomy alone. In patients with low risk (tumor size <4 cm and no rete testis invasion), the recurrence rate under surveillance is as low as 6%. Chemotherapy is a possible treatment for seminoma relapse under surveillance. However, 70% of patients with relapse are suitable for treatment with radiotherapy alone because of small-volume disease at the time of recurrence. Patients who relapse after salvage radiotherapy can be effectively treated with chemotherapy (Albers 2016). However, the potential for seminoma to transform into NSGCT elements (usually embryonal carcinoma) is an important consideration in the management of patients who fail to respond to chemotherapy or those who experience relapse after radiation therapy. Of patients with metastatic seminoma who experience relapse after treatment, 10% to 15% have NSGCT elements at the site(s) of relapse. An autopsy study has shown that 30% of patients who die of seminoma have NSGCT elements at metastatic sites (Stephenson and Gilligan 2012). Retroperitoneal lymph node dissection (RPLND) is not recommended in stage I seminoma (Albers 2016).

Key Messages

- Seminomas with isolated syncytiotrophoblastic cells do not seem to behave differently from typical, "classic" seminomas in which no such cells are present. The possibility of a choriocarcinomatous component should be excluded.
- Increased atypia in seminoma cells raises the differential diagnosis of embryonal carcinoma. The tendency for transition of a seminoma with atypia to an embryonal carcinoma should be immunohistochemically confirmed and reported.

4.5 Case 4.3: Testicular Embryonal Carcinoma

Case Study

Data Prior to Microscopy

A 30-year-old patient presented with a painful right testicular mass and back pain due to retroperitoneal lymph node enlargement (approximately 10 cm, in short axis). Serum AFP and HCG were normal, while LDH was elevated (S1 level). Right inguinal orchiectomy was performed. The macroscopic examination of the surgically resected testis reveals a poorly circumscribed, variegated, gray-white mass with areas of hemorrhage and necrosis, replacing two thirds of the testis parenchyma.

The patient received BEP chemotherapy X three cycles as a good prognosis metastatic NSGCT patient, per the International Germ Cell Cancer Collaborative Group (IGCCCG) Classification (1997). Serum LDH normalized after the first cycle of BEP chemotherapy with parallel resolution of his back pain. The retroperitoneal mass decreased in size but did not resolve after completion of chemotherapy (residual 6 cm mass). A month later, post-chemotherapy resection of the residual mass was performed.

The patient was followed clinically, serologically, and radiographically every 4 months for the first year, every 6 months for the second and third year and every year thereafter. Two years after his surgery for resection of the residual mass, he started having mild back pain. His tumor markers were normal. His abdominal CT scan was read as lymphoceles, possibly postoperative. Repeat imaging studies for the following 14 years commented on slowly growing "lymphoceles" that gradually occupied much of his abdominal cavity and caused right hydronephrosis with thinning of the renal cortex. His abdominal and back pain became chronic requiring analgesics on a regular basis. His most recent imaging studies revealed "cystic" lesions with thick border and some solid areas with increased vascularity and hypervascular liver lesions. An open biopsy of one abdominal, partially cystic lesion and of a liver lesion was obtained.

4.5.1 Microscopic Examination of the Orchiectomy Specimen

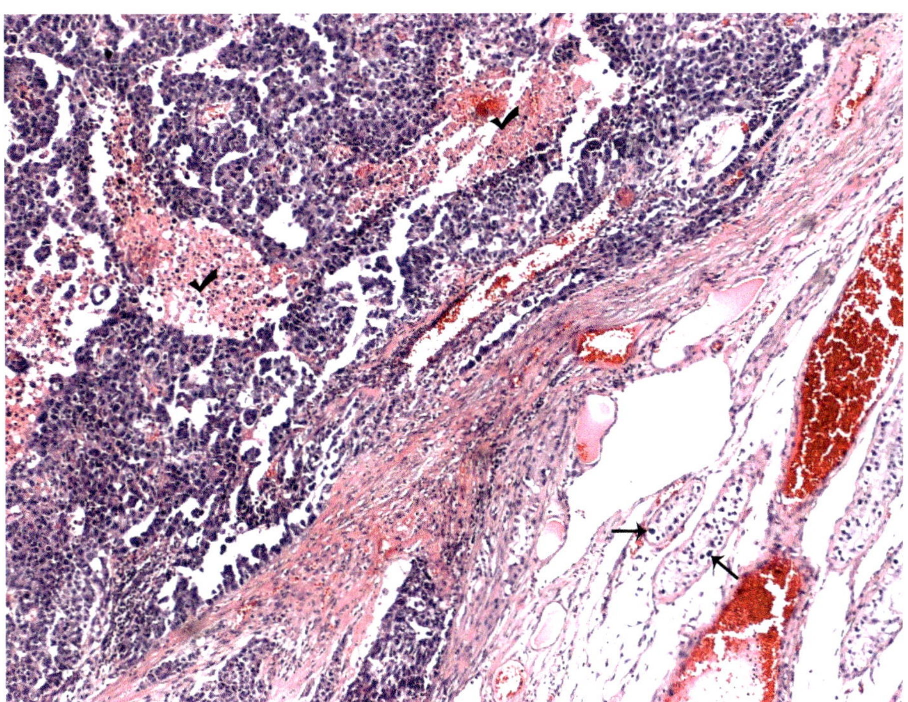

Fig. 4.36 (H-E, ×50) Tumor border. Areas of necrosis (*ticks*) within the tumor parenchyma, foci of germ cell neoplasia in situ (GCNIS) in adjacent tubules (arrows)

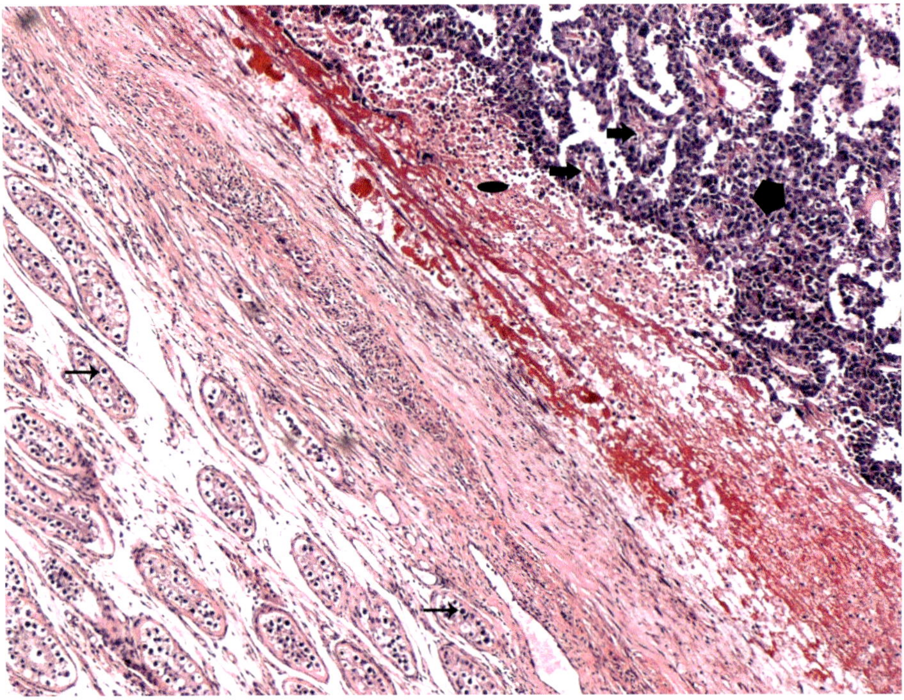

Fig. 4.37 (H-E, ×50) Tumor border. A solid (polygon) and papillary (*thick arrows*) architectural pattern of the tumor cells. Areas of necrosis (ellipse) at the edge of the tumor parenchyma, foci of germ cell neoplasia in situ (GCNIS) in adjacent tubules (thin arrows)

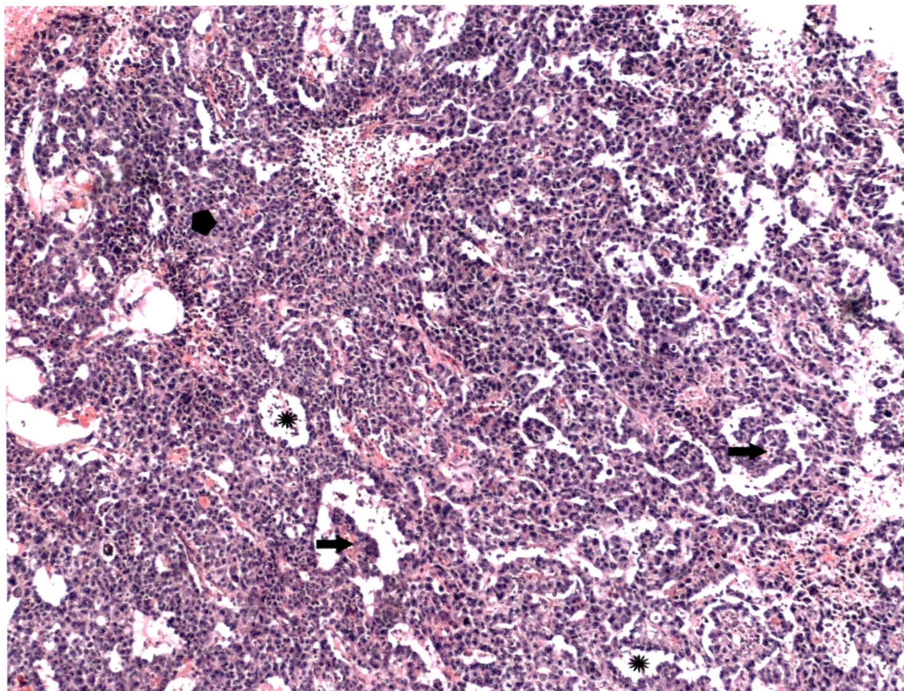

Fig. 4.38 (H-E, ×50) Tumor parenchyma with tubular-glandular (*asterisks*), solid (polygon), and papillary (*arrows*) architectural patterns. These are the *three major patterns of embryonal carcinoma*

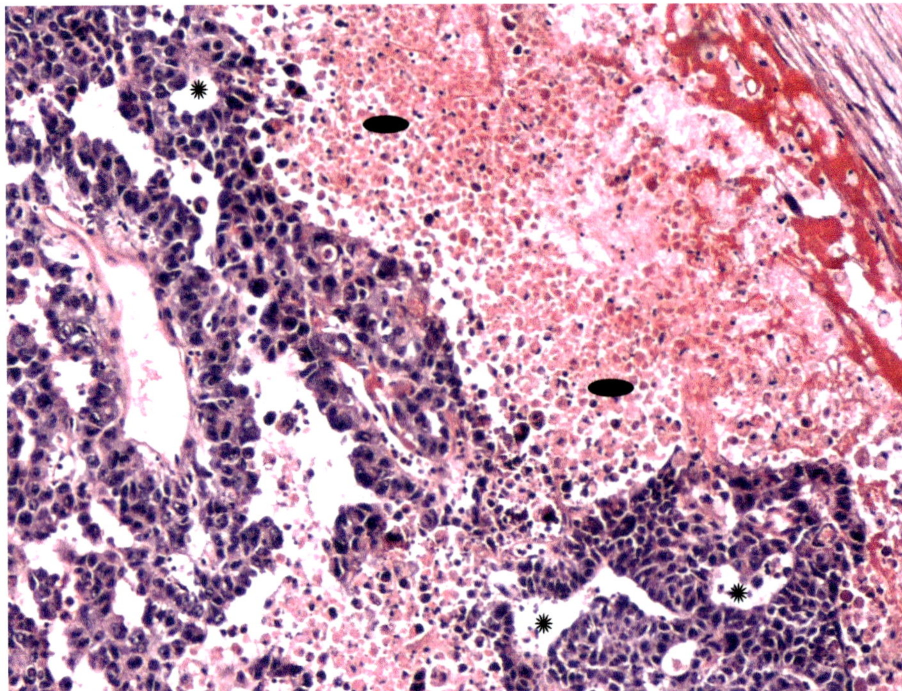

Fig. 4.39 (H-E, ×100) Confluent eosinophilic coagulative necrosis and karyorrhectic debris (*ellipses*). Round to elongated glandular structures of malignant cells. Neoplastic cells are arranged around luminal spaces (*asterisks*). *Poorly* defined cytoplasmic borders. Impression of nuclear crowding due to section thickness

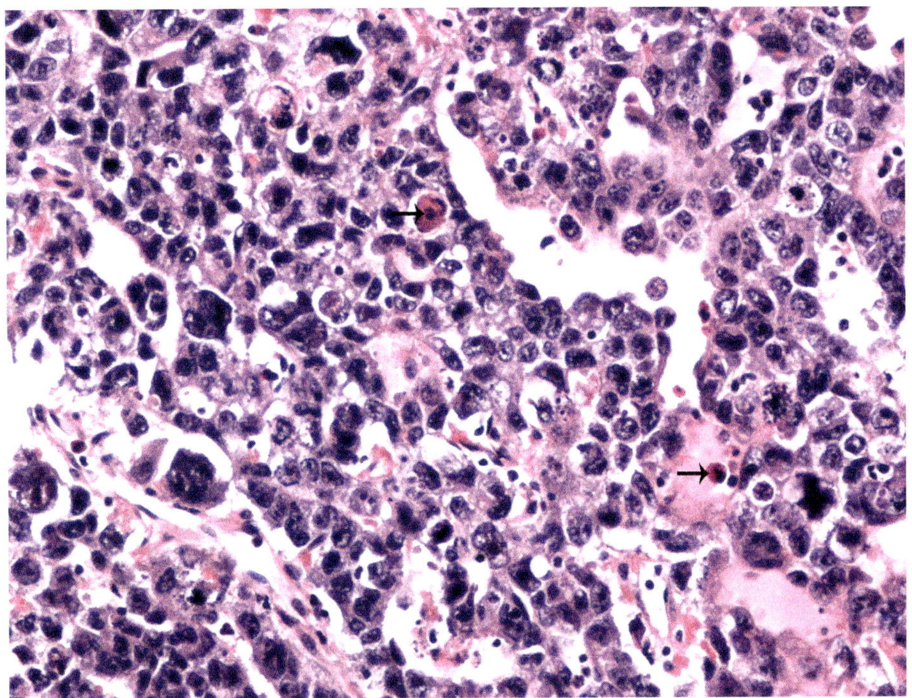

Fig. 4.40 (H-E, ×200) Cohesive clusters of primitive, anaplastic, epithelial malignant cells. Frequent apoptotic bodies (*arrows*)

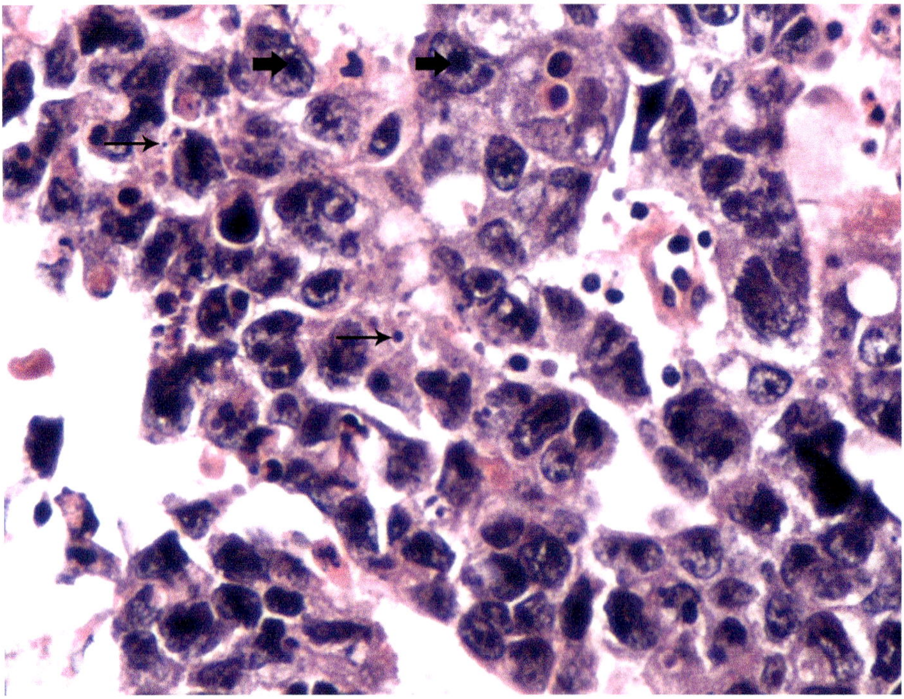

Fig. 4.41 (H-E, ×400) Tumor cells have amphophilic cytoplasm and large, vesicular, pleomorphic nuclei with prominent, frequently central macronucleoli (*thick arrows*). Karyorrhectic fragments (*thin arrows*) are frequently encountered

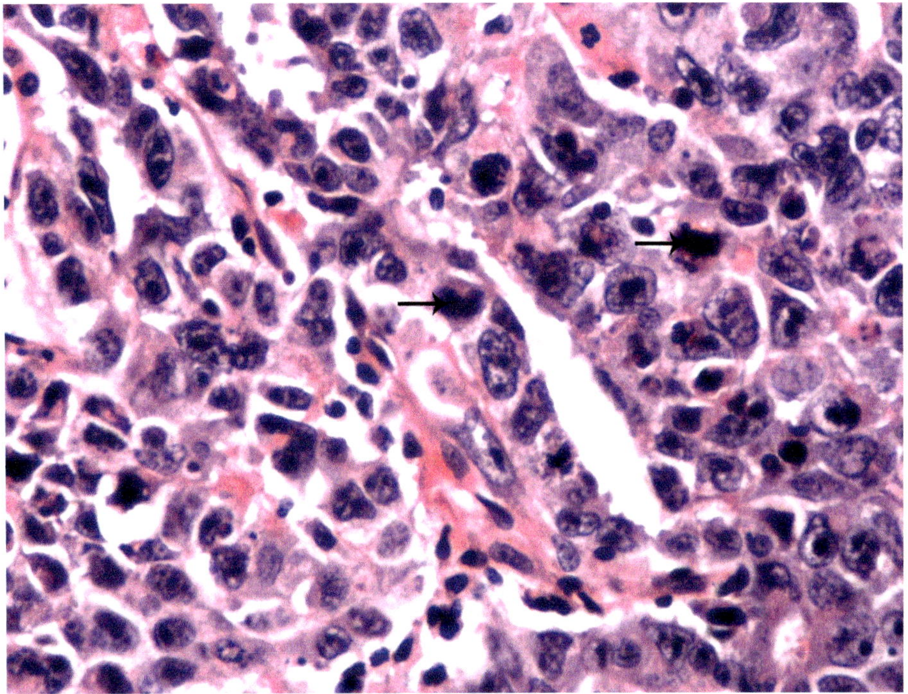

Fig. 4.42 (H-E, ×400) Mitotic rate (*arrows*) is high

So far, *all classical diagnostic features of a pure embryonal carcinoma* have been highlighted.

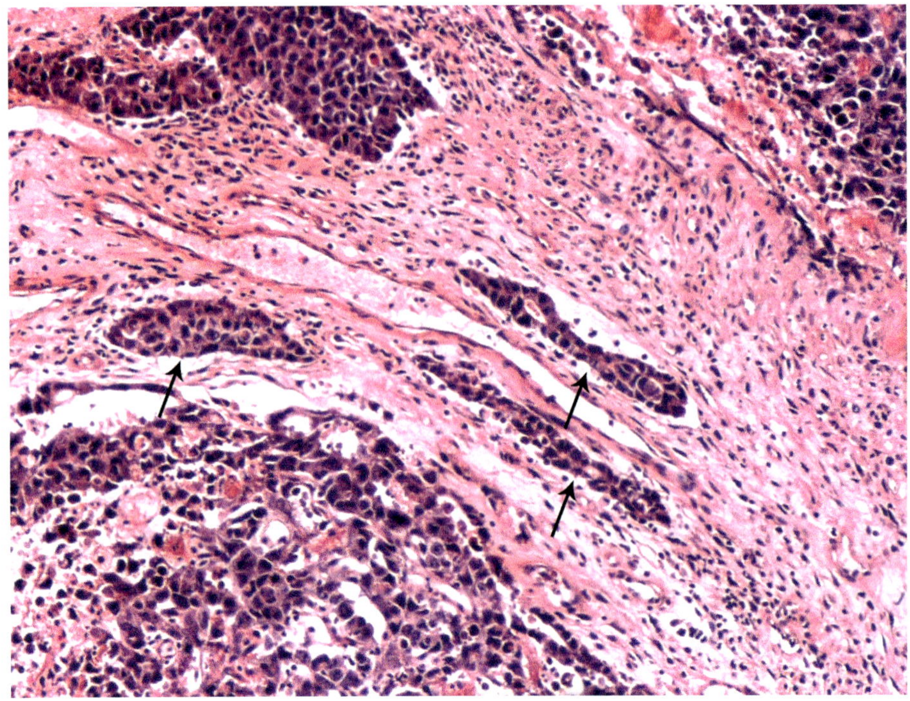

Fig. 4.43 (H-E, ×200) True vascular (venous/lymphatic) *emboli* (*arrows*) (here at the tumor border) should be thoroughly investigated under the microscope and reported because of their staging and prognostic significance

Generally speaking (with the advent of "surveillance only" protocols in patients with either seminomatous or nonseminomatous tumors), it is important to carefully assess an embryonal carcinoma for vascular invasion (and extratesticular extension). Artifactual implants of embryonal carcinoma occur easily during tissue cutting because of its extremely cellular and generally soft nature. Intravascular implants consist of loosely cohesive cells that do not conform to the shape of the vessel but lie randomly in the luminal space; they are usually associated with surface implants, reflecting the friable nature of the tumor. In contrast, true vascular invasion consists of cohesive groups of cells that conform to the shape of the vessel or are adherent to its wall by intermixed thrombotic material. Vascular invasion is usually easiest to appreciate at the periphery of the main tumor. In a *mixed* germ cell testicular tumor with vascular emboli, we should mention *which tumor component* is associated with the vascular invasion.

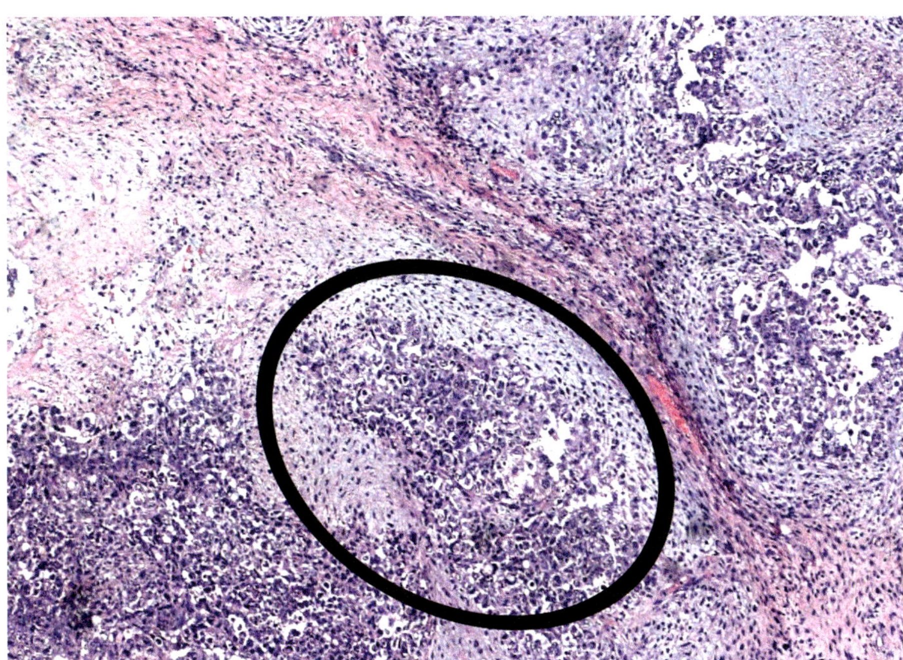

Fig. 4.44 (H-E, ×100) In the present field of the so far "pure" embryonal carcinoma, a minor amount of rather undifferentiated, cellular stromal tissue appears to be formed by the embryonal carcinoma elements (*ellipse*)

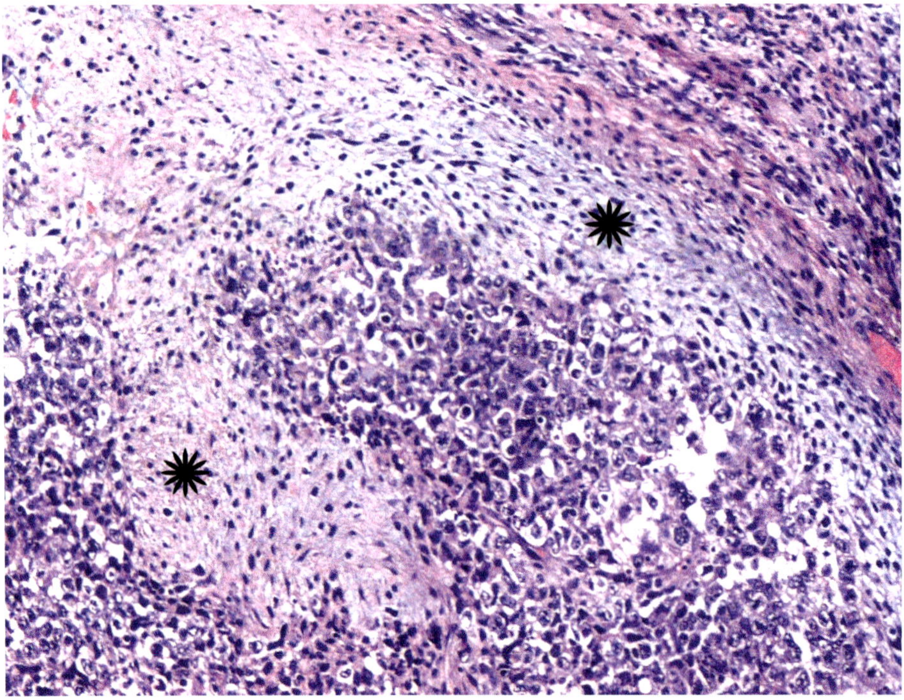

Fig. 4.45 (H-E, ×200) This intermingled neoplastic stroma (*asterisks*) may be regarded within the spectrum of embryonal carcinoma since the latter is a primitive neoplasm recapitulating an early phase of embryonic development; however, despite the absence of differentiation to easily recognizable, classical teratoma components at the primary site of this tumor, this stromal tissue component, no matter how minor it is, could most probably represent a teratoma and, less likely, another germ cell tumor. It has been argued that teratoma components in the testis are associated with an increased risk for persistent tumor in metastatic sites. So, instead of reporting a pure embryonal carcinoma, a subtle teratomatous component should be mentioned in the final pathological report

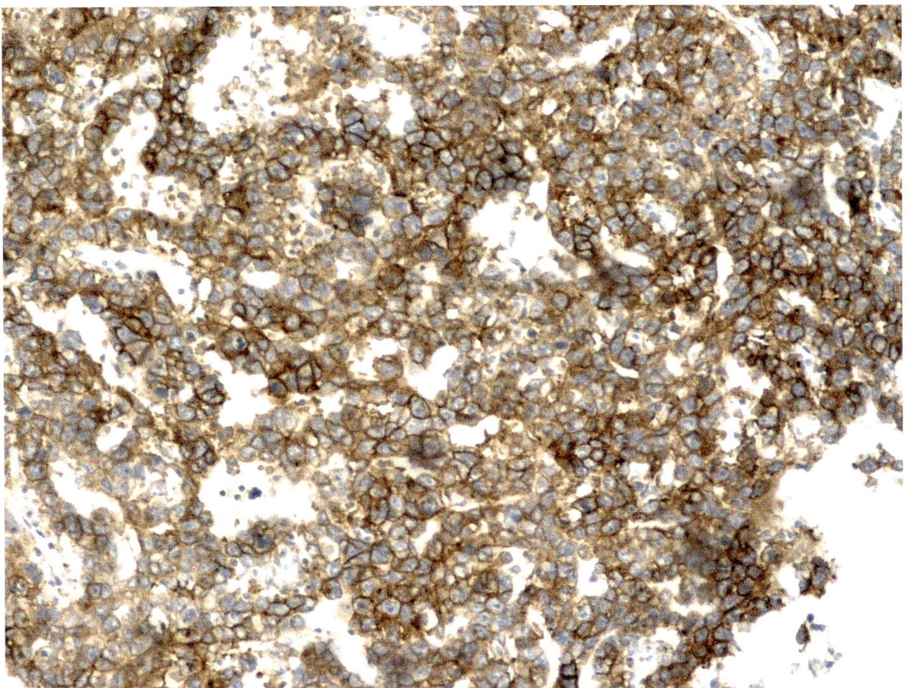

Fig. 4.46 (CD30 immunohistochemical stain, ×200) The morphological diagnosis of embryonal carcinoma can of course be confirmed by CD30 membranous immunoreactivity of malignant cells, here with a glandular growth pattern

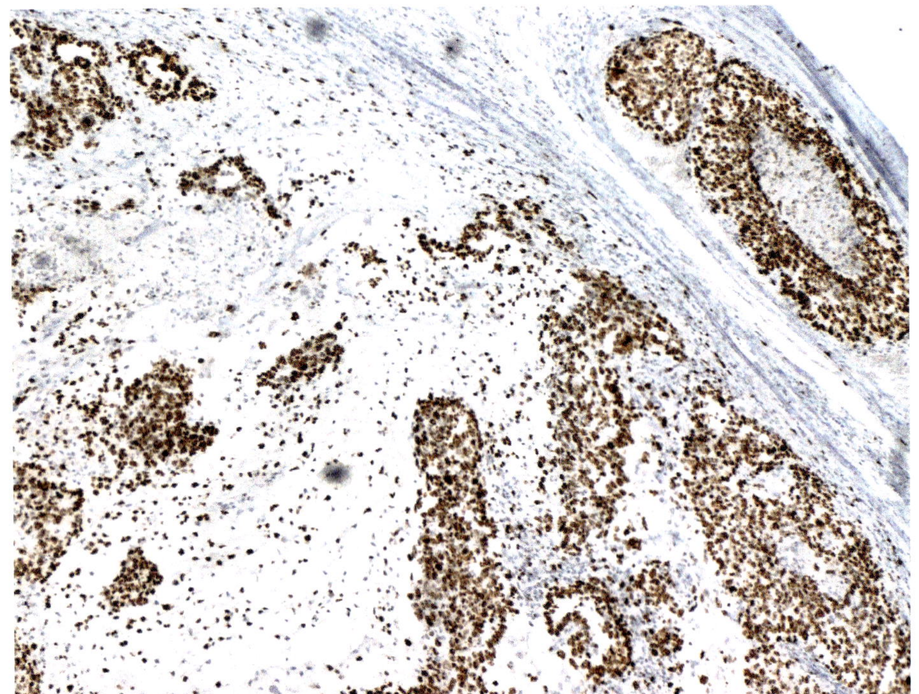

Fig. 4.47 (MIB-1 immunohistochemical stain, ×100) Immunohistochemical expression of ki67 (antibody MIB-1) in the vast majority of tumor cells [including those of a tumor embolus (up right)]. The high expression of ki67 (MIB-1 score > 70%) in the embryonal carcinoma malignant cells predicts their chemosensitivity.

In stage 1 nonseminomatous tumors, vascular/lymphatic peritumoral invasion, a percentage of embryonal carcinoma >50% and a proliferation rate (MIB-1 score) of >70% have been proposed as prognostic risk factors for occult metastatic disease. In nonseminomatous cases without evidence of vascular/lymphatic peritumoral invasion, when the embryonal carcinoma percentage is <50%, the proliferation rate of tumor cells could be assessed and reported

The diagnosed embryonal carcinoma is a nonseminomatous germ cell tumor which actually gives early metastases, firstly to the retroperitoneal lymph nodes. In the present case, after intensive combination chemotherapy, no satisfactory reduction in the size of metastatic tumor was observed (no complete remission); the remaining retroperitoneal mass was therefore surgically resected, without full Retroperitoneal Lymph Node Dissection (RPLND). Irrespective of the degree of response to chemotherapy, any residual metastatic mass has to be surgically resected along with full RPLND, and any viable tissue should be histologically identified. In a minority of patients, a persistent tumor of similar morphology to that of the primary tumor is found. In up to 40% of patients, only fibrosis and/or necrosis is microscopically observed (complete remission). In the remaining patients, elements of morphologically benign teratoma are detected; their maturity justifies their chemoresistance. There is always the possibility of secondary development of malignancy on a residual, chemoresistant teratomatous component which therefore should be entirely removed by surgery.

4.5.2 Microscopic Evaluation of the Post-chemotherapy Specimen of the Residual Retroperitoneal Mass

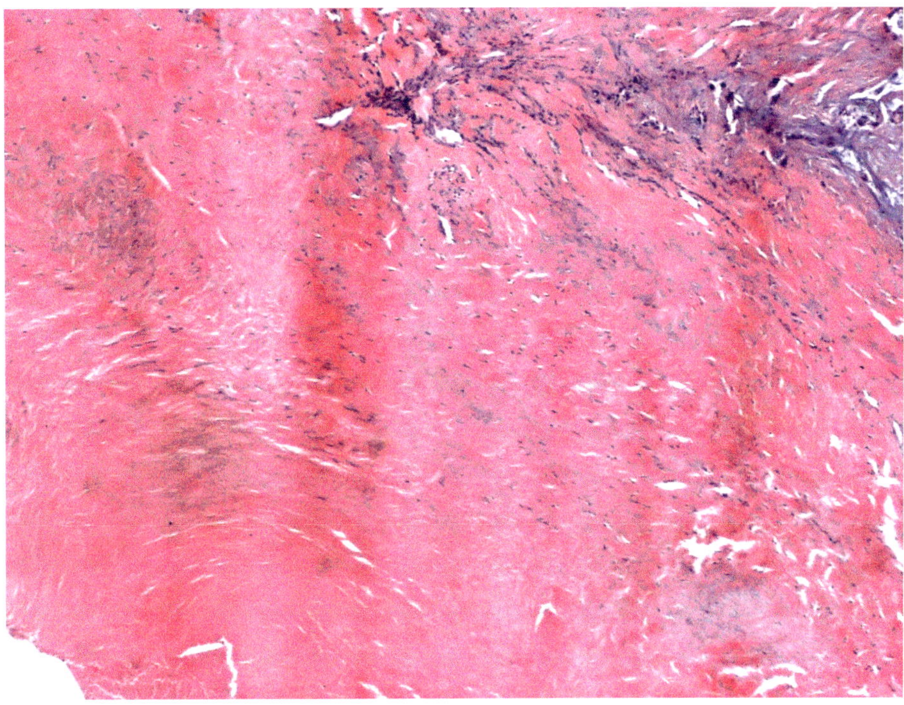

Fig. 4.48 (H-E, ×50) Fibrous area following chemotherapy. There is no evidence of embryonal carcinoma; whatever metastatic embryonal carcinoma elements, if there have been any, seem to have been destroyed by chemotherapy

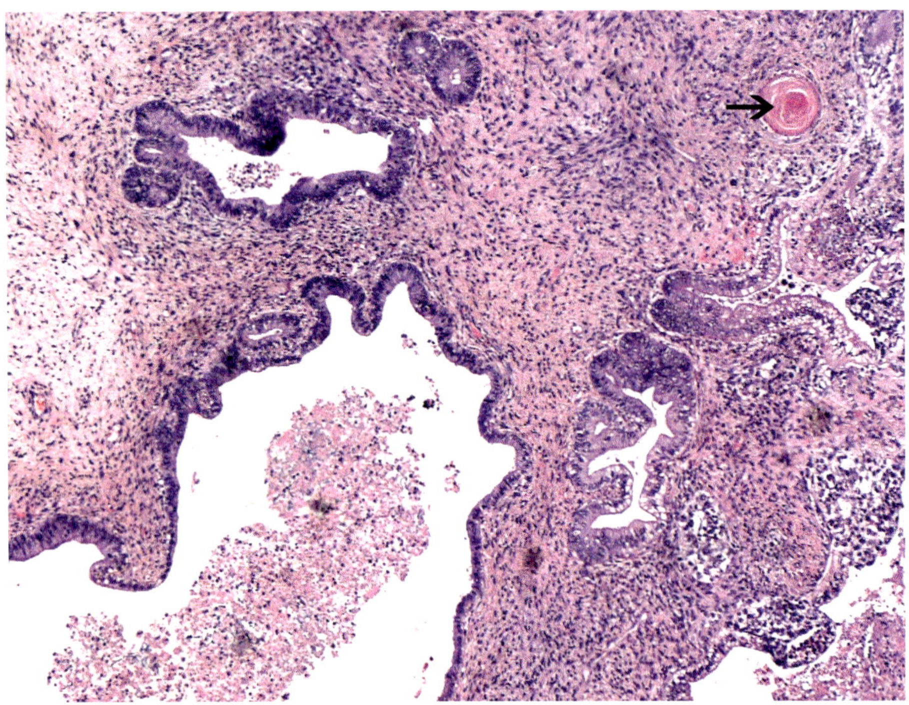

Fig. 4.49 (H-E, ×100) Mature teratomatous elements following chemotherapy of the retroperitoneal mass. Foci of glandular epithelium with some degree of atypia (probably chemotherapy-related) and a keratin pearl/squamous nest (*arrow*)

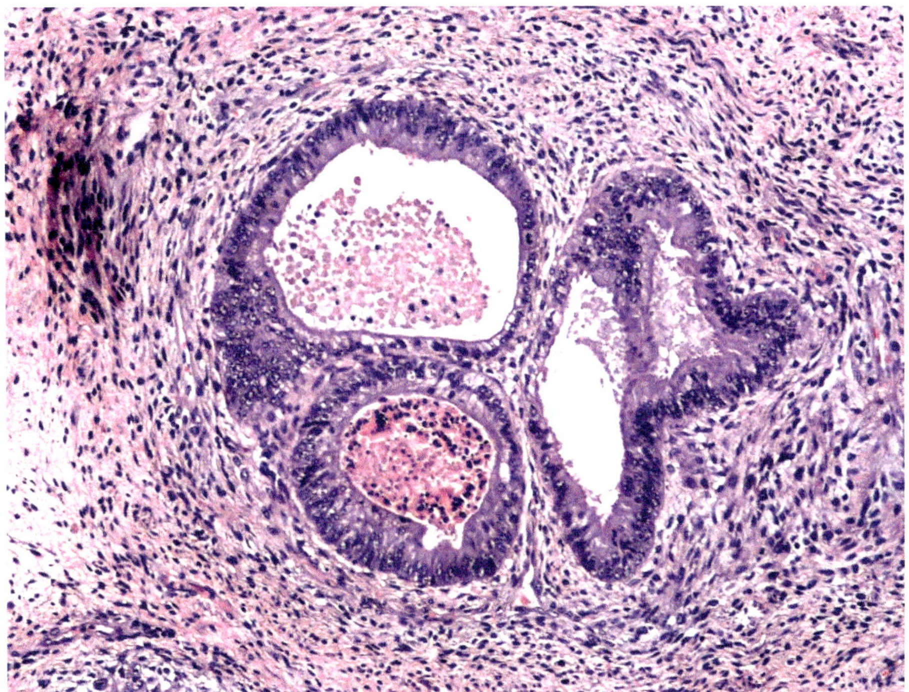

Fig. 4.50 (H-E, ×200) Three glandular teratomatous elements in the form of round, here noninvasive, glands stratified with mildly atypical nuclei. This cytological atypia of columnar epithelium is probably justified by chemotherapy and, on its own, should not raise concern for malignancy. Note some resemblance of the cellular surrounding stroma to that focally noticed in the orchiectomy specimen

Teratoma elements probably existed in the primary testicular tumor [which therefore did not correspond to a pure embryonal carcinoma but to a mixed nonseminomatous germ cell tumor composed of embryonal carcinoma and teratoma (as most commonly occurs)]; the teratomatous component was the one that seems to have given the metastasis which then showed chemoresistance. *All teratomas in postpubertal males are potentially malignant* irrespective of their maturity or immaturity. In adults, testicular teratomas have metastatic potential, even if they consist of fully differentiated, morphologically benign tissues, since germ cell neoplasia in situ (GCNIS) is their precursor lesion.

In the unlikely event that the primary tumor was a pure embryonal carcinoma, metastatic cells of embryonal carcinoma could have transitioned to teratomatous elements at the metastatic site, after some time. It is a fact that the microscopic picture of metastasis may be different from that of the primary tumor, especially in germ cell tumors of the testis.

4.5.3 Microscopic Evaluation of the Open Biopsy of One Abdominal, Partially Cystic Lesion

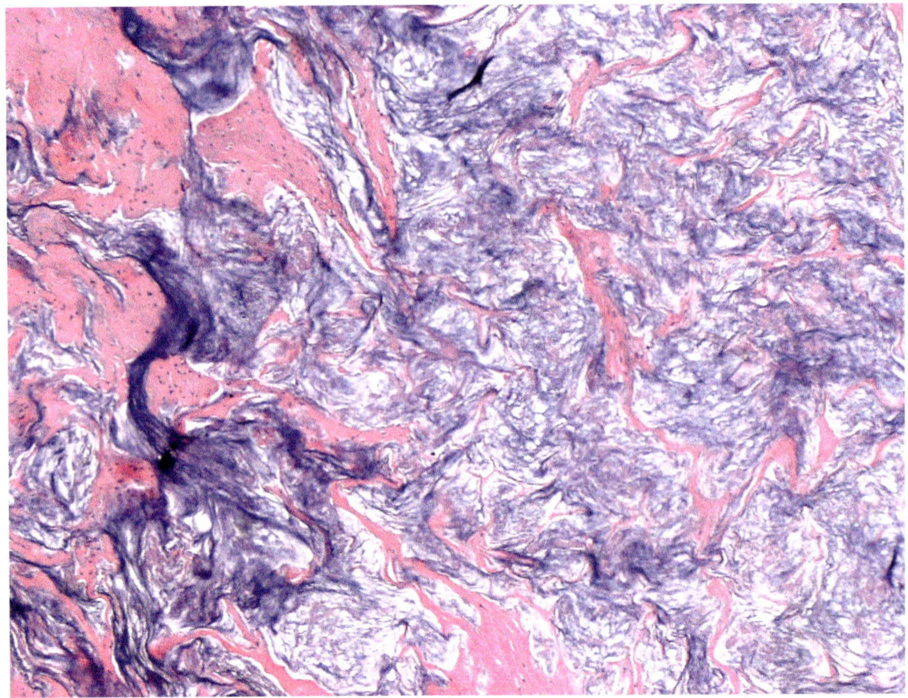

Fig. 4.51 (H-E, ×50) Extensive areas of here acellular, invasive mucin pools within fibrous area are observed at this time point

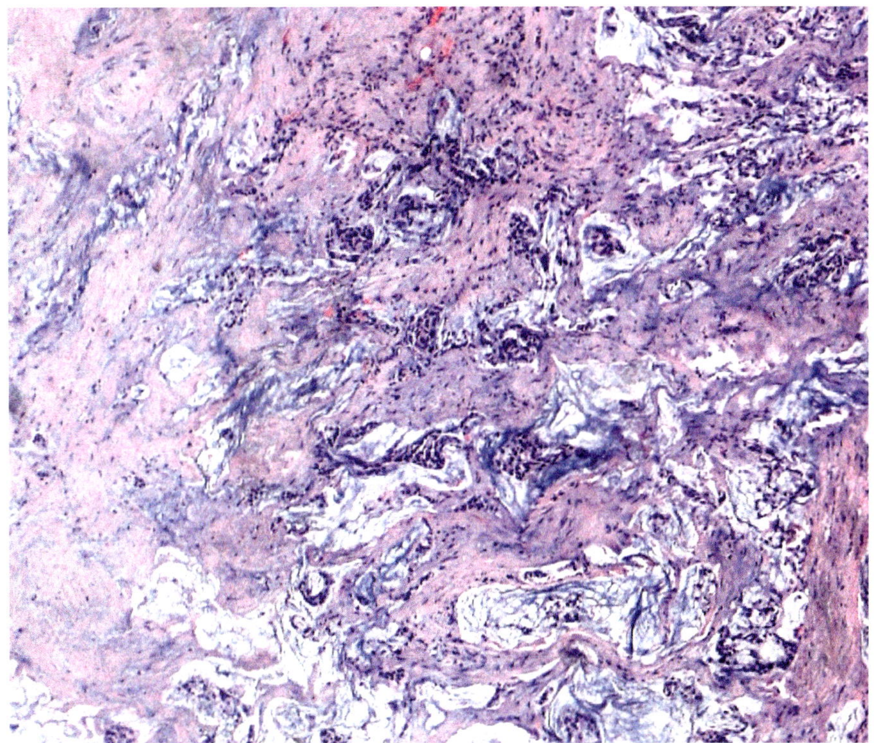

Fig. 4.52 (H-E, ×50) Evident stromal *invasion* by atypical elements of a mucinous adenocarcinoma. Note the cellular mucin pools. Identical findings were detected in the liver biopsy specimen of this patient

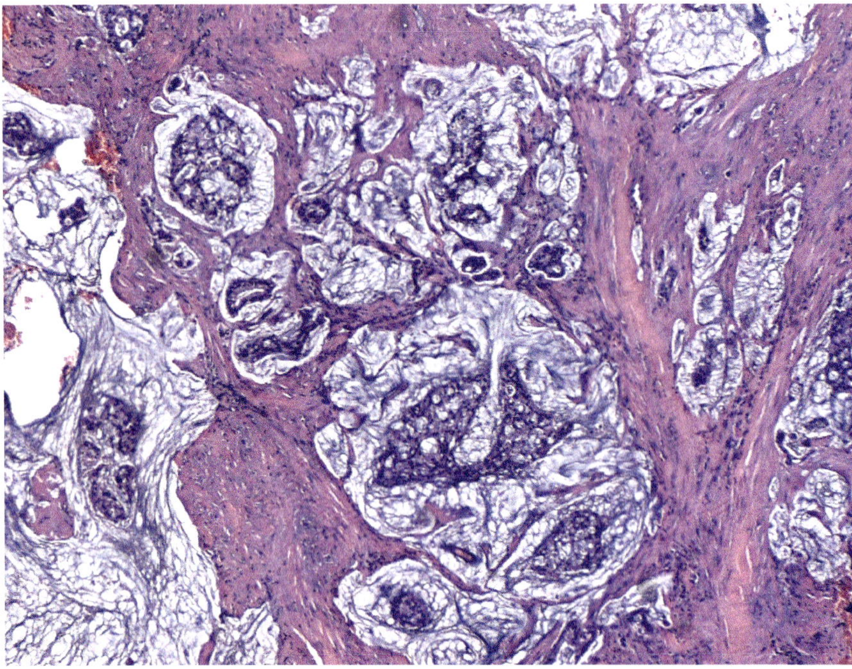

Fig. 4.53 (H-E, ×50) Evident stromal *invasion* by atypical elements of a mucinous adenocarcinoma. Note the cellular mucin pools. Identical findings were detected in the liver biopsy specimen of this patient

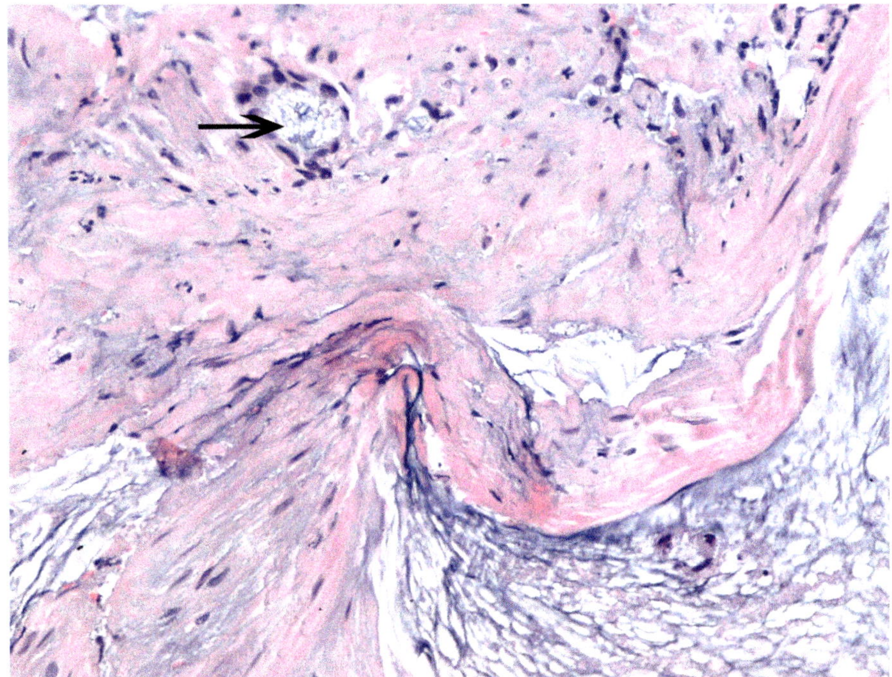

Fig. 4.54 (H-E, ×200) A separate, infiltrating, malignant gland (*arrow*) and part of a mucinous pool (*bottom right*)

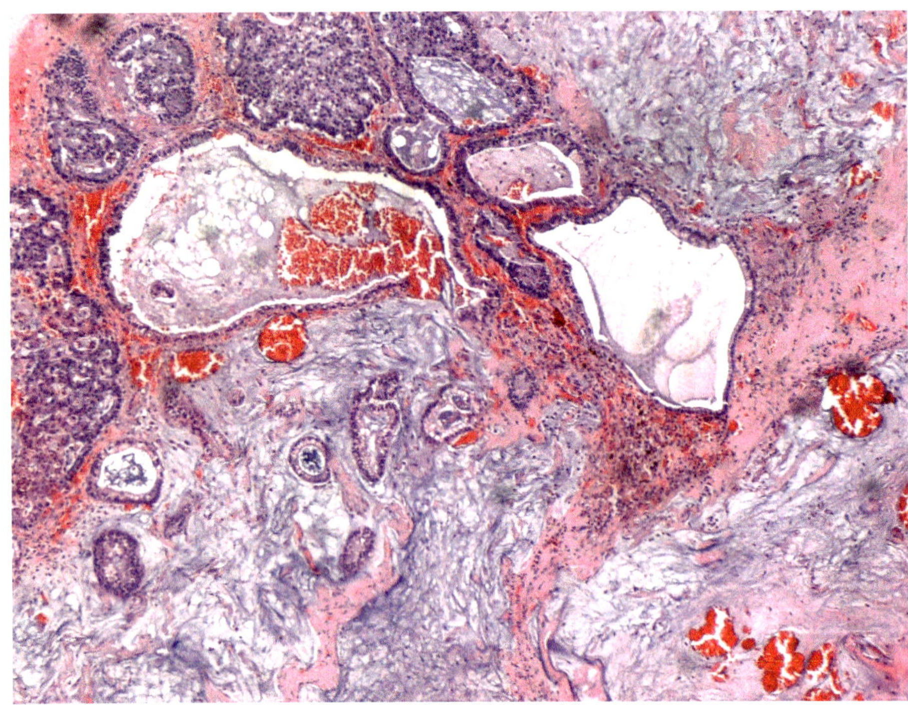

Fig. 4.55 (H-E, ×100) The teratomatous glands expand and give rise to a mucinous adenocarcinoma. The *considerable destructive growth and clear invasive features* favor the diagnosis of a secondary, somatic-type carcinoma which is capable of further metastatic spread

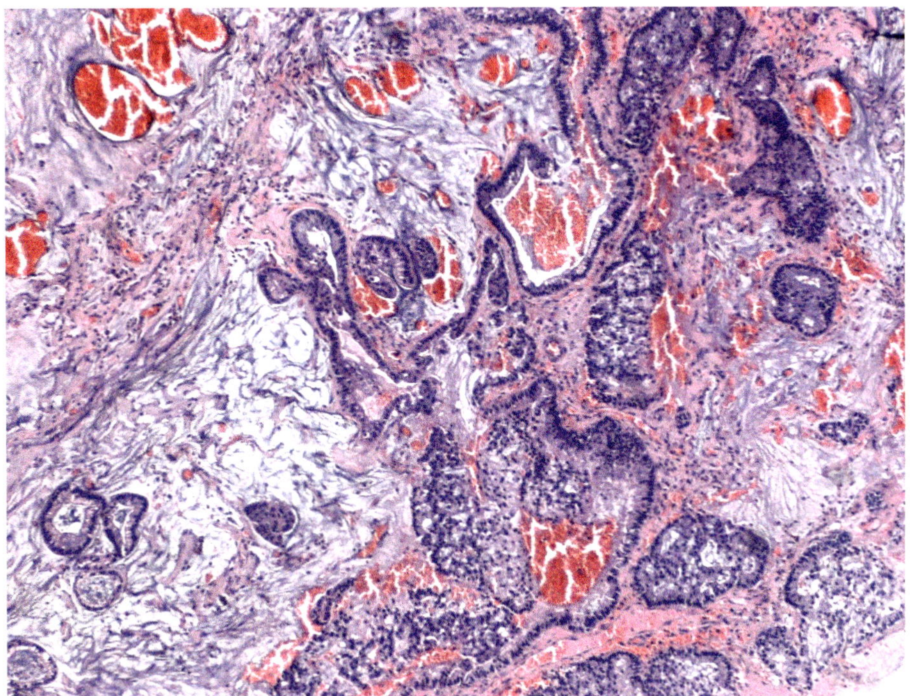

Fig. 4.56 (H-E, ×100) The teratomatous glands expand and give rise to a mucinous adenocarcinoma. The *considerable destructive growth and clear invasive features* favor the diagnosis of a secondary, somatic-type carcinoma which is capable of further metastatic spread

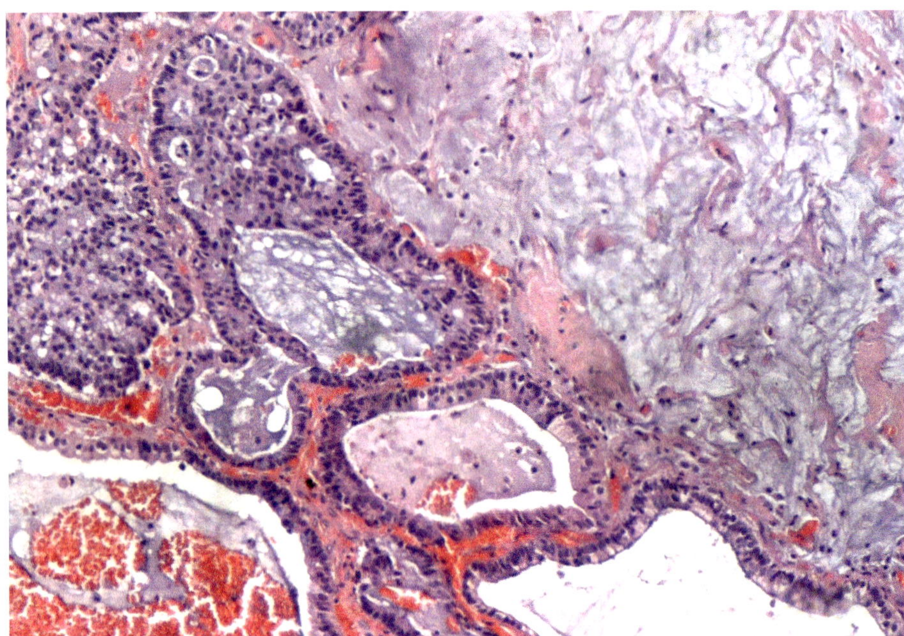

Fig. 4.57 (H-E, ×200) Expansile glands, probably of teratomatous origin, in transition to mucinous carcinomatous pools

4.5.3.1 Clinical Commentary

Danai Daliani, Vasileios Spapis, and Maria Gkotzamanidou

This is a case which was pathologically diagnosed as an embryonal carcinoma with a focal stromal component retaining an undifferentiated appearance and thus suggesting a minor teratomatous component. Vascular invasion by the embryonal carcinoma cells was also reported. The tumor had retroperitoneal metastatic spread at presentation. In the post-chemotherapy surgically resected residual mass, the viable neoplastic tissue consisted of teratomatous elements. Later on, a sizable secondary, somatic-type mucinous adenocarcinoma with clearly invasive features developed in the patient and metastasized to his liver.

Embryonal carcinoma is one of the most common germ cell tumors and the most primitive one after seminoma. Embryonal carcinoma is characterized by pluripotency, being composed of a population of transformed and reprogrammed embryonic stem cells. It is present in more than 80% of mixed germ cell tumors but accounts in only 3–10% of germ cell tumors as a pure form. The peak incidence occurs in persons aged 20–30 years. It is extremely rare in infants. Identification of other histological elements is essential in the planning of treatment both in clinical stage I as well as in metastatic patients, keeping in mind that there can be histological discordance between sites of disease.

Embryonal carcinomas are aggressive germ cell tumors. About 10–40% of patients (including those with pure and mixed forms) present with metastasis; the more common sites of metastasis are the retroperitoneum, lung, and liver.

Pure embryonal carcinomas may not have any elevated tumor marker although association of embryonal carcinomas with syncytiotrophoblastic giant cells may cause increases in serum human chorionic gonadotropin (HCG) levels. Serum lactic acid dehydrogenase (LDH) may be elevated, but it is not a specific marker.

The initial treatment of metastatic nonseminomatous germ cell tumor (NSGCT) depends on *histology and prognostic characteristics*. Patients with expectedly good prognosis, like the patient in this case, receive, as initial standard treatment, three cycles of cisplatin, etoposide, and bleomycin (PEB) chemotherapy or four cycles of PE chemotherapy if there are arguments against the use of bleomycin, e.g., factors predisposing for bleomycin-induced acute or cumulative pneumonitis/fibrosis. Increased levels of markers (AFP and/or HCG) after chemotherapy indicate residual disease with viable tissue of GCT; salvage chemotherapy is then recommended with an alternative regimen.

Residual disease after chemotherapy should be resected *completely* in the presence of normal serum markers or at least low-level and non-rising serum markers (usually AFP). In the case of a marker plateau, the resection should be at least delayed since there is a good chance that this represents a "pseudomarker plateau" resulting from necrotic tumor tissue which is still resolving and liberating tumor markers into the blood. These patients should be followed up at short intervals until markers have been normalized and the final decision with respect to the resection can be made.

Residual tumor resection is mandatory in all patients with a residual mass > 1 cm in the short axis at cross-sectional computerized tomography (CT) imaging. The role of surgery is debated in patients with retroperitoneal residual lesions <1 cm; there is still a risk of residual cancer or teratoma, although the vast majority of patients (> 70%) harbor fibro-necrotic tissue. In rare cases, tumor growth is observed while the markers decline during chemotherapy; this phenomenon is termed "growing teratoma syndrome" and requires early surgical intervention and possibly completion of the chemotherapeutic regimen at a later time point. If residual surgery is indicated, *all* areas of primary metastatic sites must be *completely* resected within 2–6 weeks of completion of chemotherapy and normalization of serum tumor markers. If technically feasible, a bilateral nerve-sparing procedure should be performed. In 30% of complete post-chemotherapy retroperitoneal lymph node dissection specimens, there is residual pathology (chemoresistant tumor and/or teratoma) outside of the macroscopically/radiographically affected lymph nodes. Synchronous somatic-type malignant transformation is possible. In any case, close follow-up is mandatory since later development, possibly after years, of a new enlarging mass, this time with somatic-type malignant transformation, is possible (Albers 2016; NCCN Guidelines Version 1.2017 2016; Presti 2013; Stephenson and Gilligan 2012).

4

This patient normalized his elevated serum LDH but had residual significant disease in the retroperitoneum. He underwent resection of the residual mass – and not a full RPLND – as it was indicated. The decision for a limited resection by his surgeon was based mainly on technical skills and the "demand" from the patient to maintain ejaculation. The pathology of the resected inter-aortocaval residual lymph node revealed teratoma and the patient was followed after that. In adults, teratomas may look histologically benign but are frequently found at metastatic sites in patients with advanced nonseminomatous germ cell tumors (NSGCTs). Teratomas contain elements from all three germ cell layers, especially from the ectoderm. It is hypothesized that nonteratomatous elements (mostly embryonal cell carcinoma) have the ability to mature into teratoma and that the metastases are derived from these elements before their differentiation. Teratoma is generally resistant to chemotherapy. Thus, given its frequent presence at metastatic sites in advanced NSGCTs, patients with residual masses after chemotherapy require consolidative surgical resection. The inherent chemoresistance of teratoma is a limitation to treatment strategies for NSGCTs that utilize chemotherapy alone.

The accepted approach is to perform a full bilateral RPLND in patients with residual post-chemotherapy disease in the retroperitoneum although, in the era of primary chemotherapy for low-volume disease, there have been attempts to limit the extent of surgery in an effort to shorten operative time, reduce fluid requirements, and maintain emission and ejaculation, the concern of course being not to increase local recurrences or to decrease the disease-specific survival with this approach.

Viable germ cell cancer has been reported by Beck et al. (2007) in 2%, teratoma in 62%, and fibrosis in 36% of patients undergoing modified post-chemotherapy (PC)-RPLND, and 4 out of 100 patients presented with disease recurrence, all outside of the boundaries of a full bilateral RPLND (1 supradiaphragmatic and 3 subdiaphragmatic – 2 lateral to the ureter and 1 in the inguinal canal, the latter possibly related to inadequate radical orchiectomy). It is important to remember that their cohort included a highly selective group of patients (< 10% of their PC-RPLNDs) with low-volume metastatic tumor limited to the primary landing zone both before and after chemotherapy, mostly (94 of 100 patients) with clinical stage B1 (< 2 cm) or B2 (< 5 cm) disease (Beck et al. 2007). Therefore, these results should not be generalized and do not avoid the risk of residual microscopic disease (cancer or teratoma) in the contralateral landing zone in patients with higher tumor volume at presentation and with the risk of subsequent development of late recurrence or malignant transformation.

Oldenberg et al. (2003), who also studied modified PC-RPLND in 87 patients with residual masses <20 mm and had recurrences in 3 of the 50 patients who underwent "unilateral RPLND," voiced concern that adopting widely a modified PC-RPLND may not completely avoid the risk of a growing teratoma (and transformation), despite the fact that all their recurrences were outside of the retroperitoneum.

In fact, in a series of 113 patients with "bulky disease" who underwent full bilateral PC-RPLND at Memorial Sloan-Kettering Cancer Center, there was an 8% incidence of disease (cancer/teratoma) identified in the contralateral landing zone, so investigators suggested that a modified resection should be considered only in patients with (1) small-volume disease, (2) left primary tumors, and (3) right primary tumors that have no evidence of cancer/teratoma on frozen section analysis of the residual mass (Wood et al. 1992).

In a series of 39 patients undergoing bilateral PC-RPLND, some with residual tumor masses on the contralateral landing zone, Rabbani et al. (1998) reported a 2.6% incidence of teratoma outside the area of the left modified dissection, even though the right-sided template they used, included the periaortic lymph nodes above the inferior mesenteric artery (IMA).

The patient in this case had bulky retroperitoneal disease with significant residual post-chemotherapy (>5 cm) and was not an appropriate candidate for limited resection. In addition, the recognition of teratoma in the resected specimen should raise the clinical suspicion for teratoma relapse when "slowly growing lymphoceles" were described in the radiology report, starting 2 years after the first resection. Lymphoceles usually do not appear late after surgery, they do not continuously enlarge, and the recognition of teratoma at the time of PC-RPLND places patients at considerable risk for disease progression, given the unpredictable nature of teratoma.

Teratoma can progress locally and invade adjacent structures slowly, but, most importantly, it can switch to a non-germ cell malignant phenotype (teratoma with secondary malignant "transformation", TMT -or to be precise-, secondary malignancy development), most frequently a rhabdomyosarcoma, adenocarcinoma, and primitive neuroectodermal tumors (PNETs). TMT develops in a small subset (2.2%) of testicular cancer patients, usually in adults, and frequently presents with metastases. Surgical resection is the mainstay of therapy for localized disease, because TMT are usually resistant to radiation and systemic chemotherapy. Patients with stage I teratoma have an excellent prognosis, and primary RPLND is an excellent diagnostic and therapeutic option in these patients, while patients with clinical stage II and III testicular cancer with TMT have poor prognosis, especially in the presence of mediastinal disease and neural or rhabdomyosarcoma elements.

Key Messages

- In postpubertal patients, the diagnosis of pure germ cell tumors, especially nonseminomatous ones, should be made with caution since they are quite rare. As a pure neoplasm, embryonal carcinomas arguably represent only about 2% of testicular germ cell tumors. A combination of embryonal cell carcinoma and teratoma is much more common.
- *Areas* of undifferentiated stroma within an embryonal carcinoma, as minor though they are, most likely represent a teratomatous component which should be mentioned in the histopathologic report.
- Persistent masses and lymph nodes after chemotherapy should be surgically excised, along with full RPLND, and any viable metastatic tissue should be histologically defined, quantified, and reported.
- *Pathologic* findings (e.g., metachronous somatic-type malignancy arising in residual teratomatous elements) are of prime importance in determining the prognosis and future treatment for these patients. Different histologies may be present at the transformation of a teratoma to a somatic malignancy (pluripotential transformation of the malignant teratoma).

4.6 Case 4.4: Mixed Germ Cell Tumor of the Testis

Case Study

Data Prior to Microscopy

A testicular swelling in a 34-year-old patient with gynecomastia. A heterogeneous testicular mass was found on ultrasound examination. Metastases in retroperitoneal lymph nodes and a retroperitoneal mass were detected.

Substantial but not excessive serum elevation of HCG (11,000 IU/L), as well as of AFP (1050 ngr/mL), and elevation, to a lesser degree, of LDH and PLAP were also detected prior to the orchiectomy. Gynecomastia is explained by HCG production in this case.

Radical inguinal orchiectomy was performed.

Grossly, the tumor was a variegated large bulky mass, with areas of hemorrhage intermingled with grey to yellow tissue having a gelatinous quality. The tumor macroscopically extended into extratesticular structures.

Cisplatin-based, combination chemotherapy was given for retroperitoneal metastatic disease, and then, retroperitoneal lymph node and residual mass resection was performed.

4.6.1 Microscopic Evaluation of the Orchiectomy Specimen

A mixture of different histological components of germ cell neoplasm was noticed. All components were quantified in the pathological report.

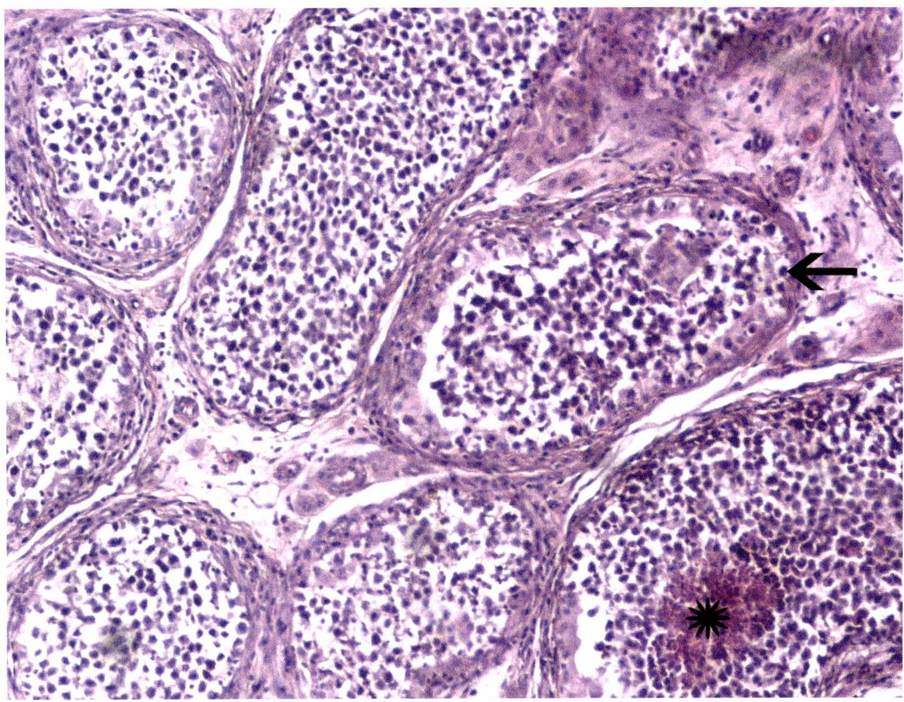

Fig. 4.58 (H-E, ×100) Indications of intratubular seminoma. Tubules *completely filled* by possibly neoplastic cells with signs of focal necrotic activity (*asterisk*); obliteration of the normal components, including Sertoli cells. Intratubular seminoma cells should be morphologically identical to those of GCNIS (*arrow*) and (invasive) seminoma; so, in the above case, as poor fixation may have altered the morphology of seminomatous cells, an immunophenotype identical to that of seminoma should be confirmed, and, thus, sloughing of nonneoplastic germ cells will be ruled out

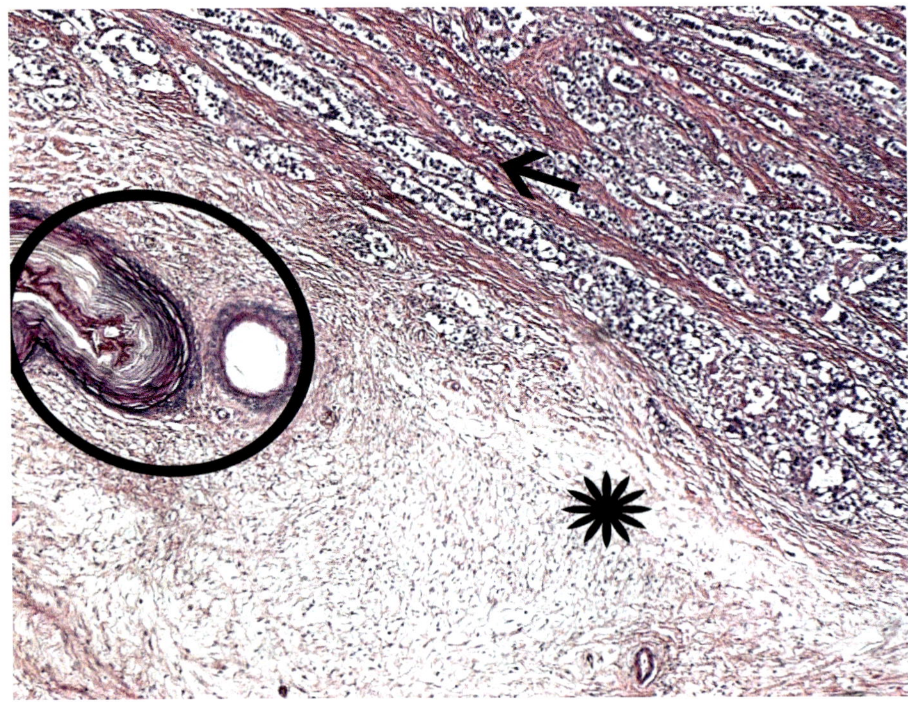

Fig. 4.59 (H-E, ×50) Seminoma and teratoma, side by side. Teratomatous elements consist of islands of keratinizing squamous epithelium (*ellipse*) and loose hypocellular stroma (*asterisk*). Seminomatous cells are arranged in cord-like structures separated by fibrous tissue (*arrow*)

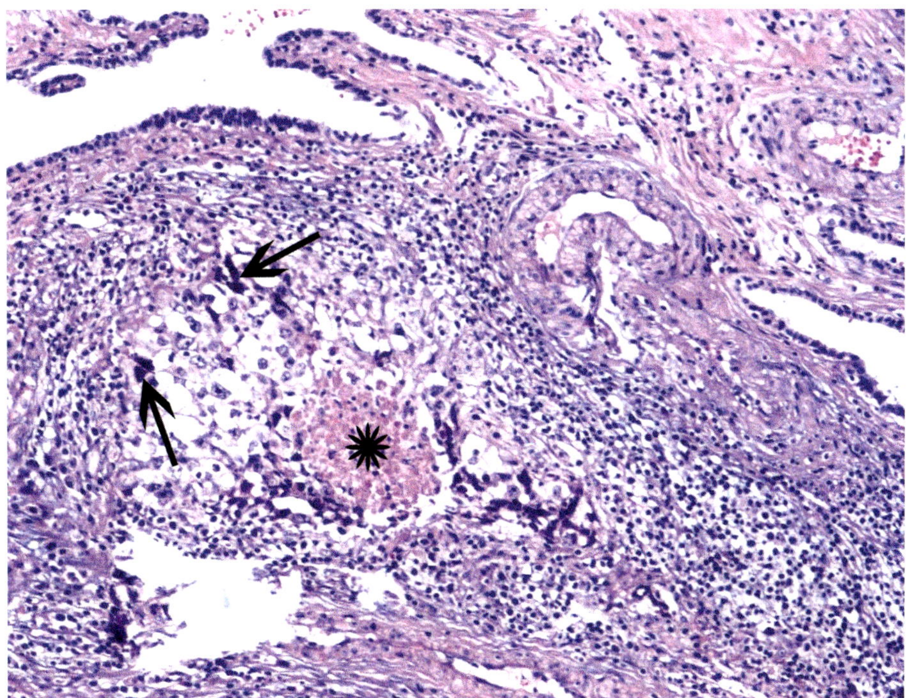

Fig. 4.60 (H-E, ×100) Clear transition of seminoma (on the lower right side) to embryonal carcinoma. In the latter, a focus of coagulative necrosis with karyorrhectic debris (*asterisk*) is observed; furthermore, among embryonal carcinoma cells, some intermixed, degenerated cells with "smudged" nuclei (*arrows*) may resemble elongated spindled syncytiotrophoblasts (if immunohistochemically investigated, they do not express HCG, so they represent embryonal carcinoma cells)

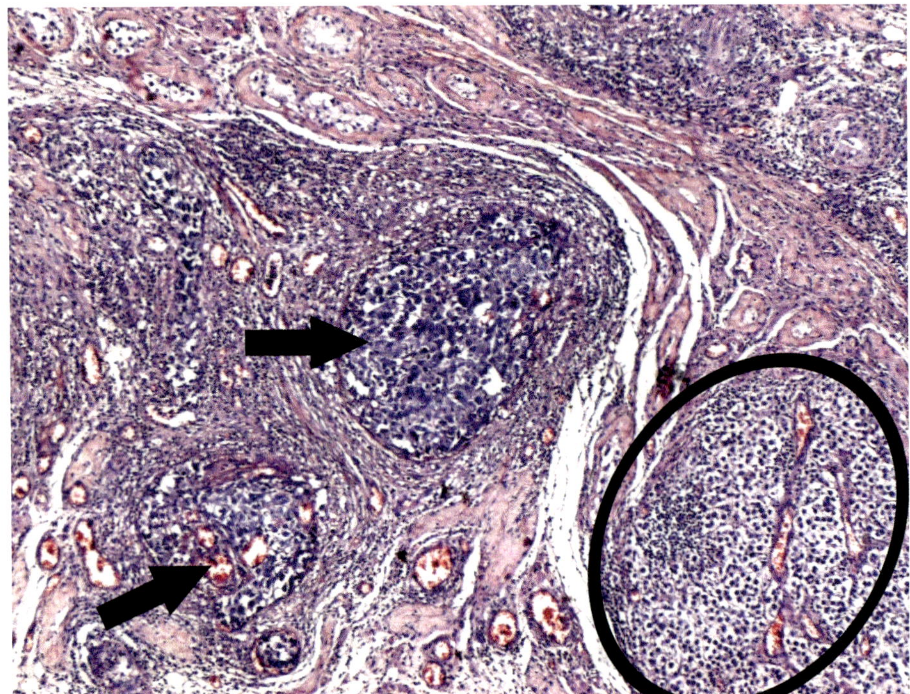

Fig. 4.61 (H-E, ×50) Intratubular embryonal carcinoma (*arrows*) adjacent to an invasive seminoma (seminomatous cells and admixed lymphocytes, see ellipse at the lower right part of the image).

In an intratubular non-seminoma, which, in the vast majority of cases, corresponds to pure embryonal carcinoma, the tumor cells are far more pleomorphic than GCNIS cells, with crowding and overlapping, as seen in invasive embryonal carcinoma

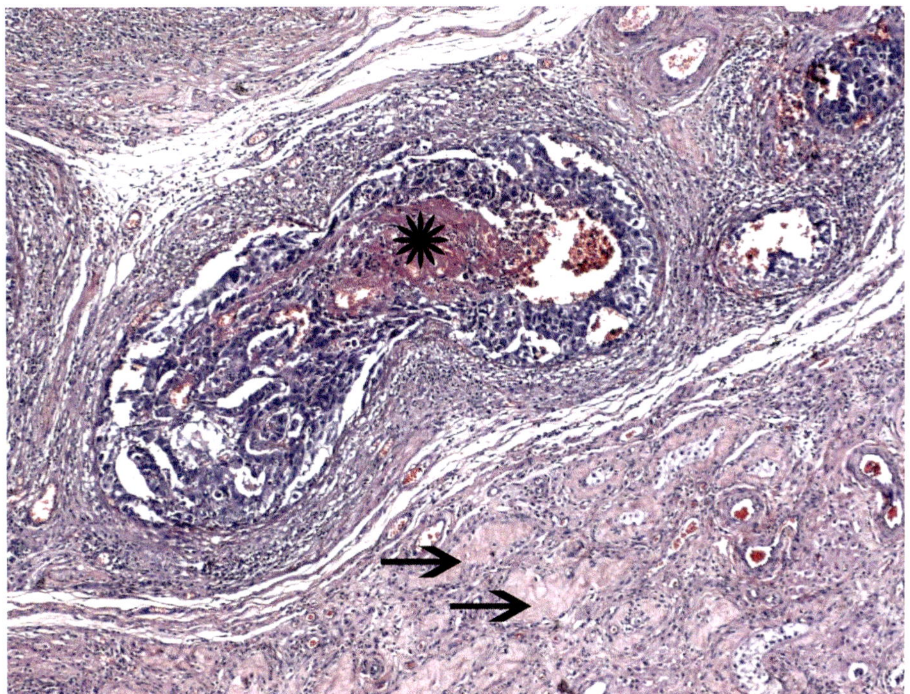

Fig. 4.62 (H-E, ×50) Intratubular embryonal carcinoma. A distorted tubule, enlarged beyond its normal diameter, with necrosis (*asterisk*). Completely hyalinized seminiferous tubules are noticed at the bottom (*arrows*)

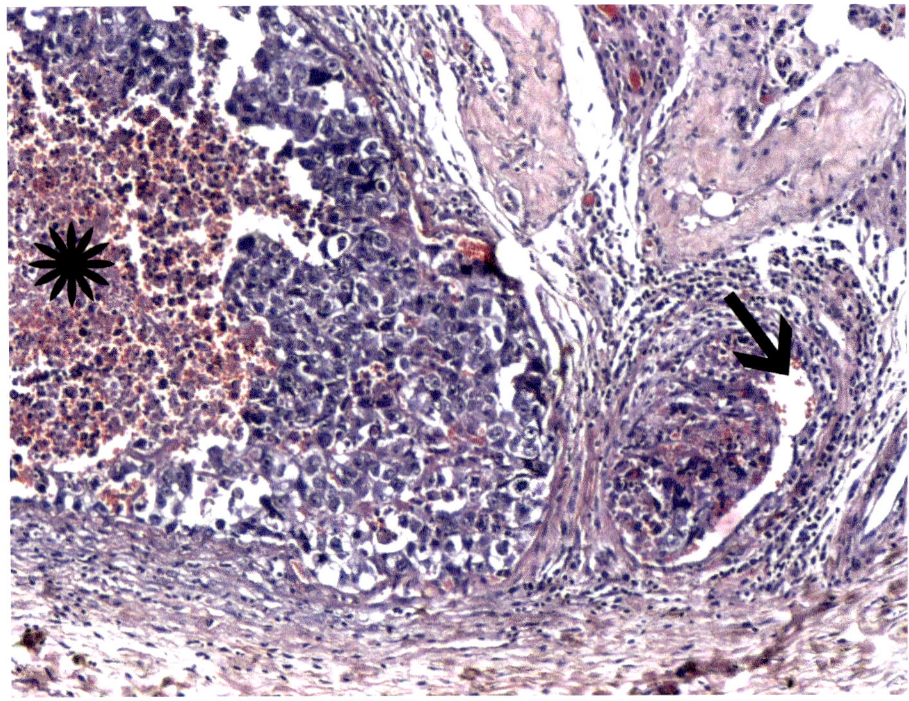

Fig. 4.63 (H-E, ×200) An intratubular embryonal carcinoma again with necrosis and karyorrhectic debris (*asterisk*).

Intratubular neoplasm may mimic vascular invasion (arrow); staining for endothelial markers can be of assistance, when necessary

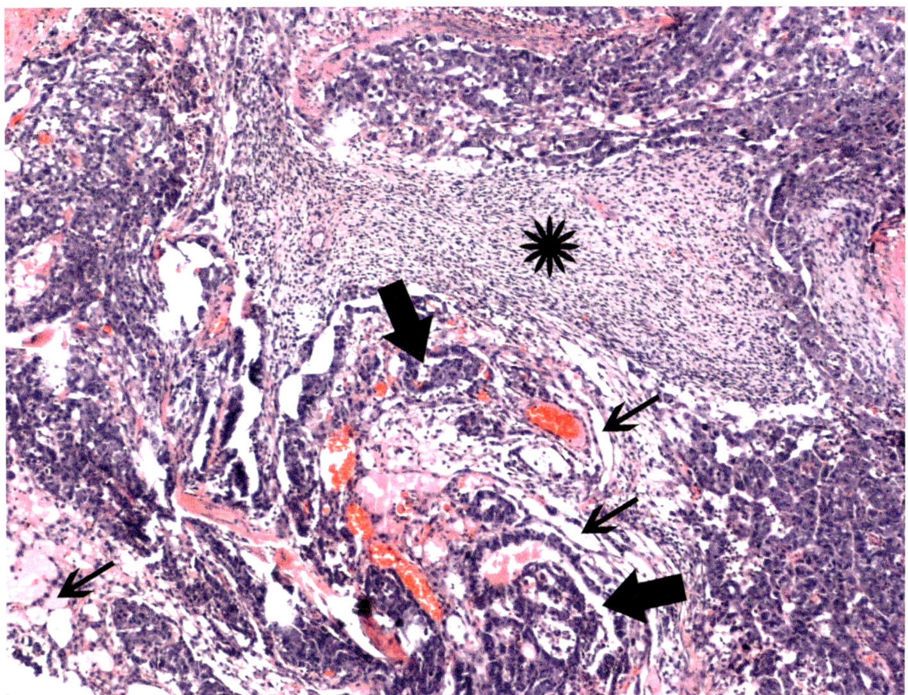

Fig. 4.64 (H-E, ×100) Irregular embryonal carcinoma glandular structures (*thick arrows*) are here intimately associated with a more subtle, microcystic yolk sac tumor component (*thin arrows*). In addition, a stromal component retaining an undifferentiated appearance (*asterisk*), consisting of oval to spindle cells and lacking light microscopic features of recognizable mesenchymal tissue such as cartilage or muscle, probably represents a (immature) teratoma component.

The microcystic is the most common yolk sac tumor pattern. The distinction between embryonal carcinoma and yolk sac tumor is important in determining the percentage of embryonal carcinoma within a mixed germ cell tumor

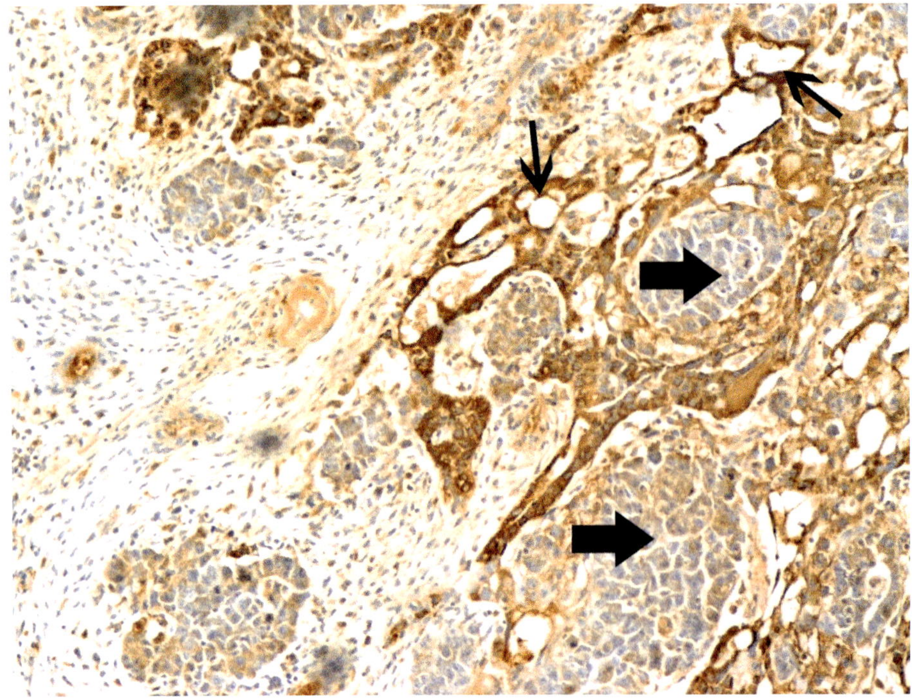

Fig. 4.65 (AFP immunohistochemical stain, ×200) Specific AFP cytoplasmic immunostaining in the microcystic yolk sac tumor component (*thin arrows*); embryonal carcinoma cells are negative (*thick arrows*).

AFP can be identified in the majority of yolk sac tumors (roughly in 80%), with a characteristically variable, patchy distribution and, in some cases, weak staining intensity

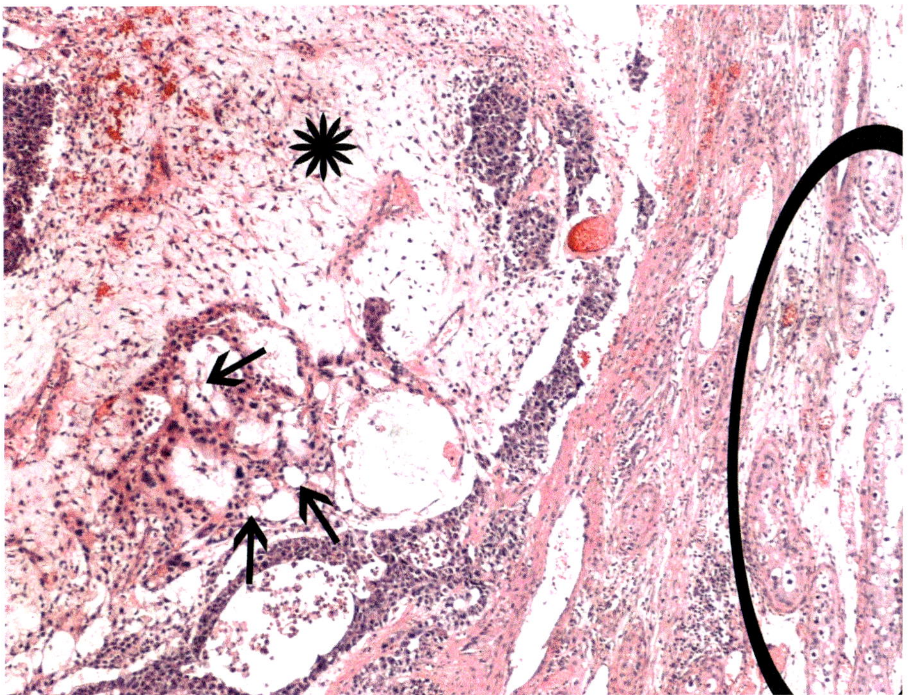

Fig. 4.66 (H-E, ×100) Tumor border. Microcystic/reticular pattern of yolk sac tumor component (*arrows*). This is the most common yolk sac tumor growth pattern. Coalescence of microcysts may produce a macrocystic pattern elsewhere. Interconnecting cords and ribbons of tumor cells are surrounded by abundant myxoid stroma (*asterisk*). Adjacent foci of GCNIS (*curve area*).

In adults, yolk sac tumor is associated with GCNIS and almost always occurs as a component of mixed germ cell tumor.

In children, yolk sac tumor appears in its pure form and represents the most common testicular tumor in this age group; GCNIS is absent from seminiferous tubules, and the tumor's aggressiveness in children is therefore low

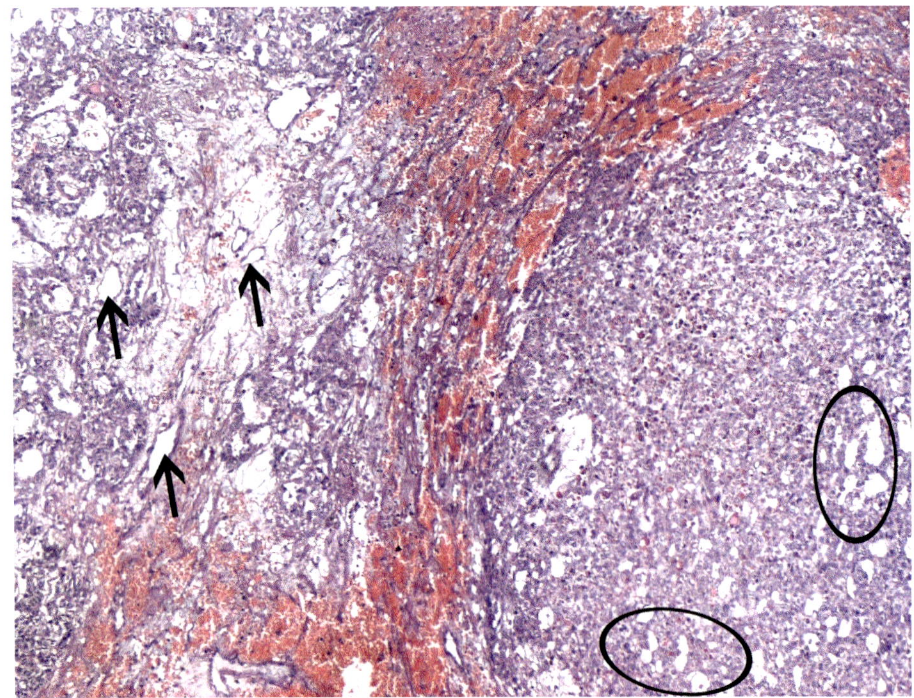

Fig. 4.67 (H-E, ×50) Yolk sac tumor patterns. Irregularly shaped and constricted cysts/vesicles (*arrows*) blend into a myxoid, loosely fibrous stroma (polyvesicular vitelline pattern) (*left part*). A nodular, sheet-like configuration of cells on the right (solid pattern) with a microcystic tendency (*ellipses*), characteristic of yolk sac tumor. Solid pattern is relatively frequent in yolk sac tumors

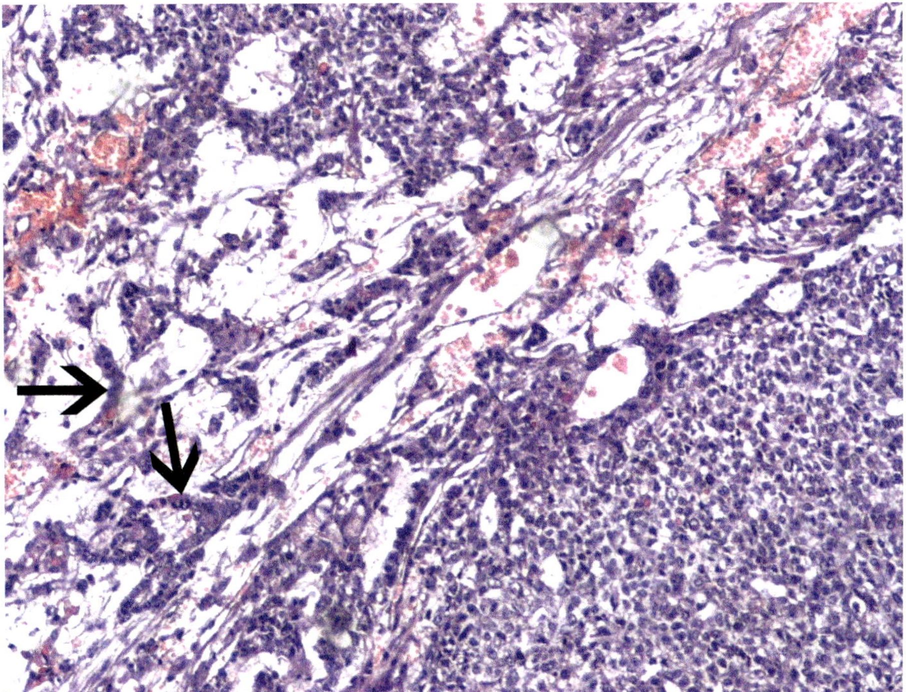

Fig. 4.68 (H-E, ×200) Extracellular anastomosing "labyrinthine-like" spaces with small vesicles and cords of epithelioid tumor cells (*arrows*) switch to a solid yolk sac tumor component with cells with clear to eosinophilic cytoplasm, indistinct cell borders, and mostly uniform, overlapping nuclei and a microcystic tendency (*lower right part*). Uncommonly, solid foci may have cells with scant cytoplasm and dense nuclei, resembling blastema

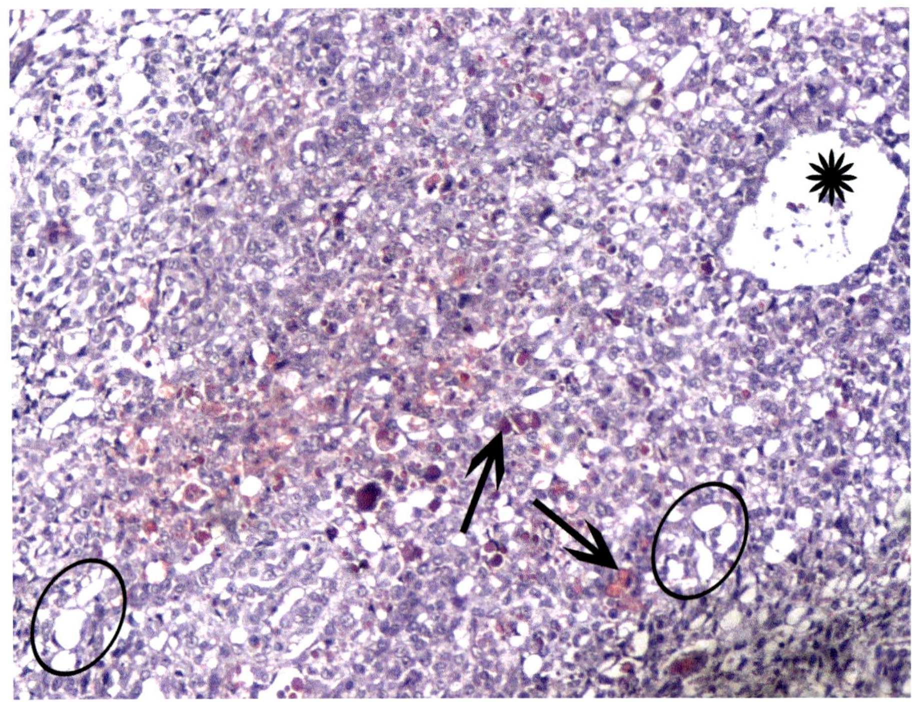

Fig. 4.69 (H-E, ×100) Diffuse, solid architectural pattern of yolk sac tumor. Sheets of uniform cells (but less uniform than those of seminoma) with blood vessels within (*asterisk*). Numerous, often bright, mostly intracytoplasmic, hyaline bodies of variable size and refractile eosinophilic quality (*arrows*).

Such globules should not be confused with the more irregularly shaped, band-like deposits of basement membrane which characterize the parietal pattern of yolk sac tumor.

Intracellular vacuoles (*ellipses*) construct the microcystic pattern, at least focally, which permits the identification of yolk sac tumor. In yolk sac tumors, the solid pattern is commonly intermingled with the microcystic.

This solid yolk sac tumor pattern without any microcystic tendency may resemble seminoma; no lymphoid component, granulomas, or fibrous septa and evident cytokeratin immunohistochemical positivity are against seminoma

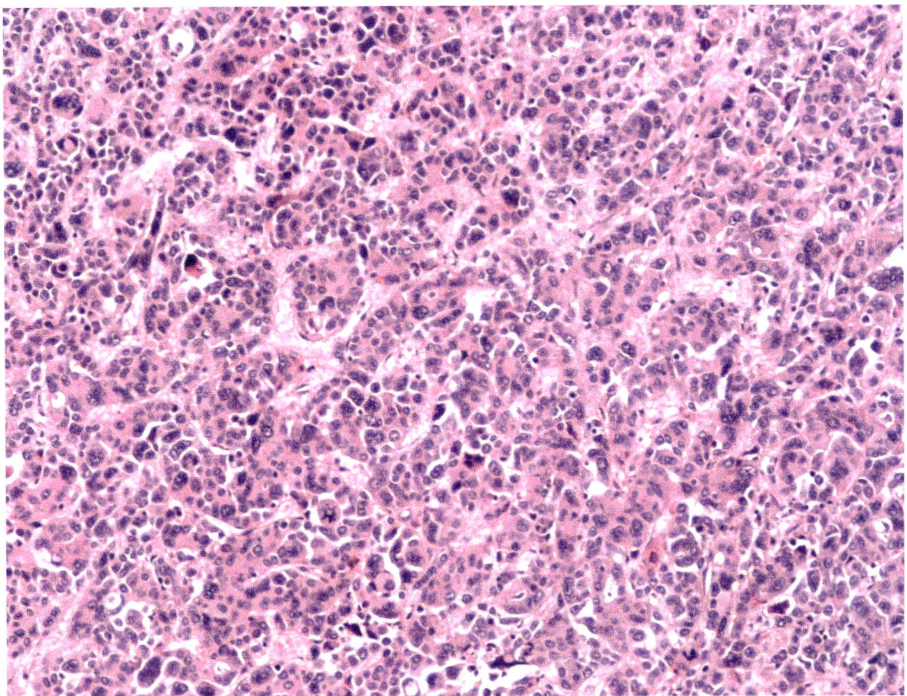

Fig. 4.70 (H-E, ×100) Within the yolk sac component of another case of mixed germ cell tumor, a small focus of the hepatoid pattern was found. Polygonal, eosinophilic cells, often with vesicular nuclei, are arranged in trabeculae and nest-like structures, resembling hepatocellular carcinoma. Sinusoidal arrangement may be implied. This particular pattern is expected to express AFP and other hepatocellular markers, intensely

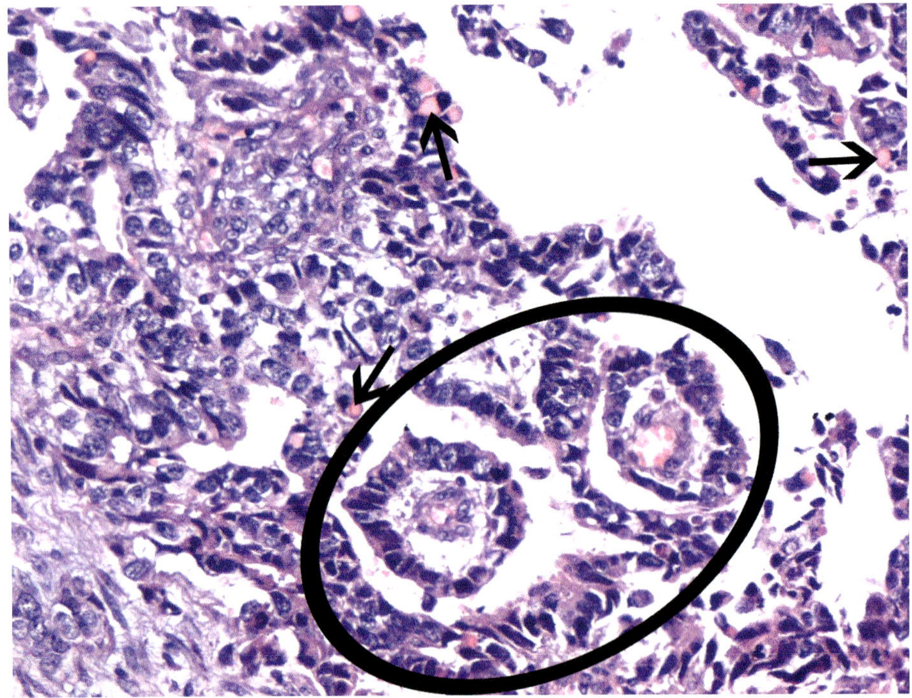

Fig. 4.71 (H-E, ×200) In addition to hyaline globules/droplets (*arrows*), two Schiller-Duval bodies (*ellipse*) with characteristic fibrovascular cores (central blood vessel, edematous perivascular space) mantled by malignant cuboidal to columnar epithelium with prominent nuclei, recessed into a cystic space, are observed in this area of yolk sac tumor component. This is the endodermal sinus pattern.

A papillary growth pattern can be occasionally seen in embryonal carcinoma as well, with highly atypical embryonal carcinoma cells lining fibrovascular cores.

CD30 and glypican-3 immunostaining may be performed to differentiate the two tumors; embryonal carcinoma cells express the former marker, while yolk sac tumor elements express the latter.

A double-layered pattern of embryonal carcinoma mixed with yolk sac tumor has also been described, and, when morphologically suspected, it should be immunohistochemically confirmed with separate expression of specific immunomarkers for embryonal carcinoma and yolk sac tumor in the two components

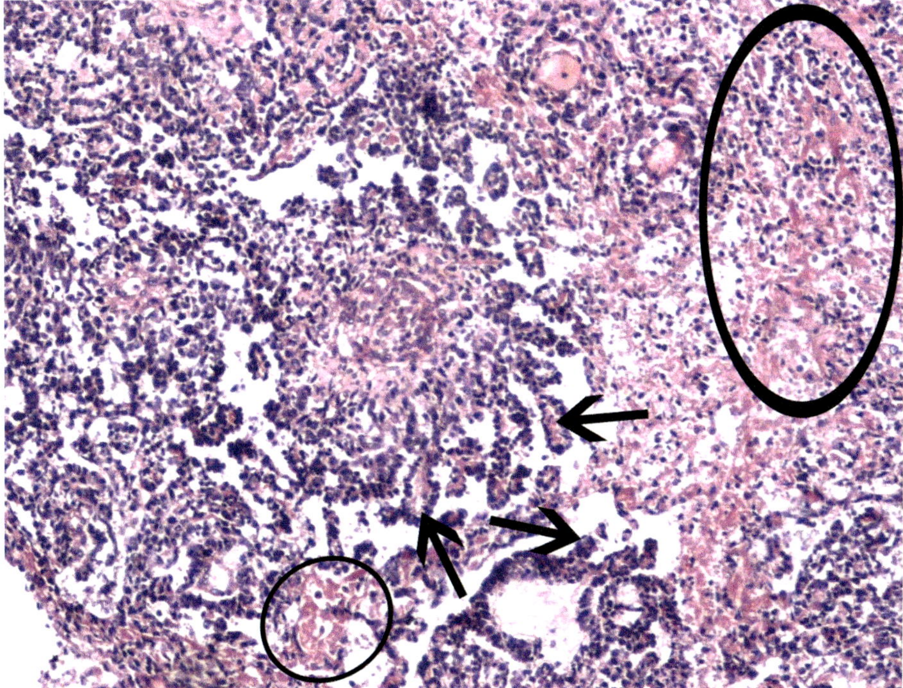

Fig. 4.72 (H-E, ×100) Yolk sac tumor papillary pattern from another case. Slender, projecting papillae with a single layer of cuboidal to low columnar, relatively low-grade cells on fibrovascular cores or not (*arrows*), lacking the definitive morphology of Schiller-Duval bodies. These bland cytologic features are distinct from those of embryonal carcinoma with papillary growth, which have distinct high-grade nuclear atypia.

Note the irregular, often band-like, pink intercellular deposits of basement membrane-like material (*ellipses*) (yolk sac tumor parietal differentiation)

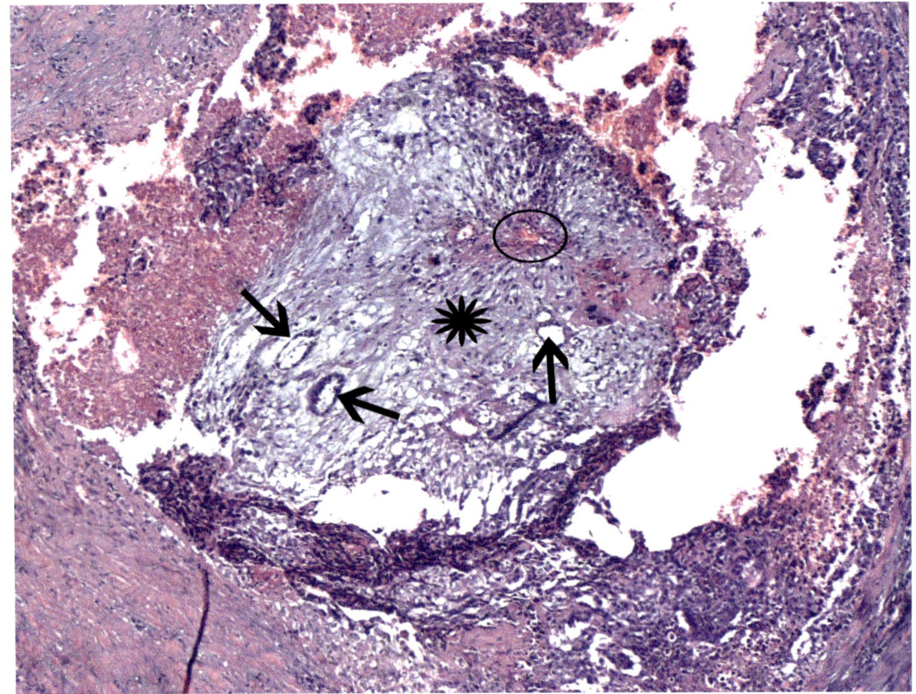

Fig. 4.73 (H-E, ×100) Paucicellular, light blue, myxoid yolk sac tumor areas (from another case) (*asterisk*) with vascular network (*ellipse*) and vesicles/small cysts lined by flattened epithelium resembling endothelium (*arrows*)

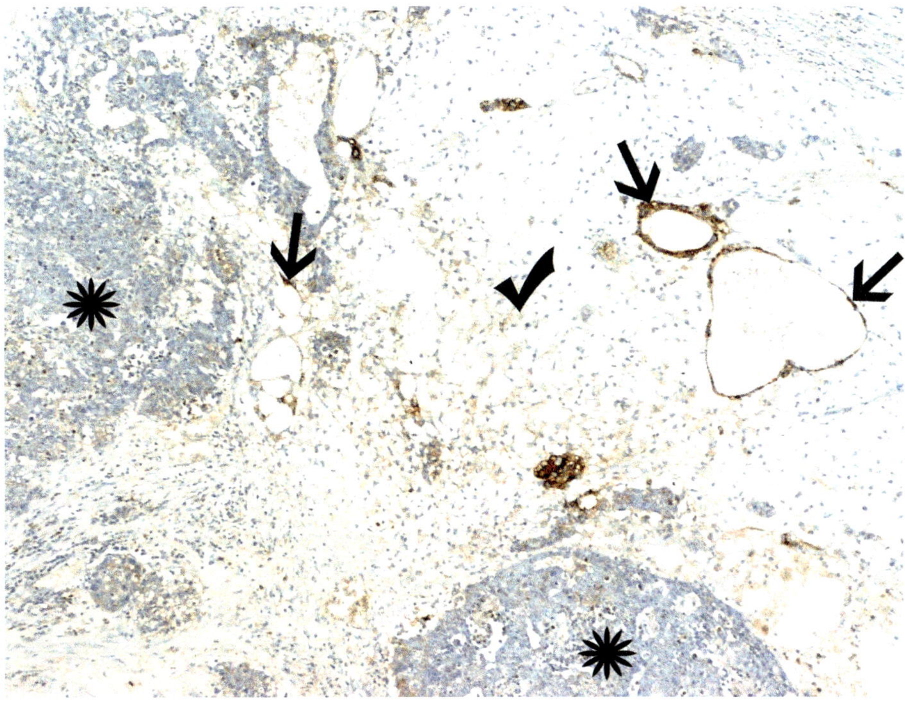

Fig. 4.74 (Glypican-3 immunohistochemical stain, ×50) The yolk sac tumor vesicular elements (*arrows*) are highlighted within the loose, myxomatous background (*tick*). Glypican-3 is a more sensitive yolk sac tumor marker than AFP; embryonal carcinoma (*asterisks*) and seminoma are typically negative for glypican-3

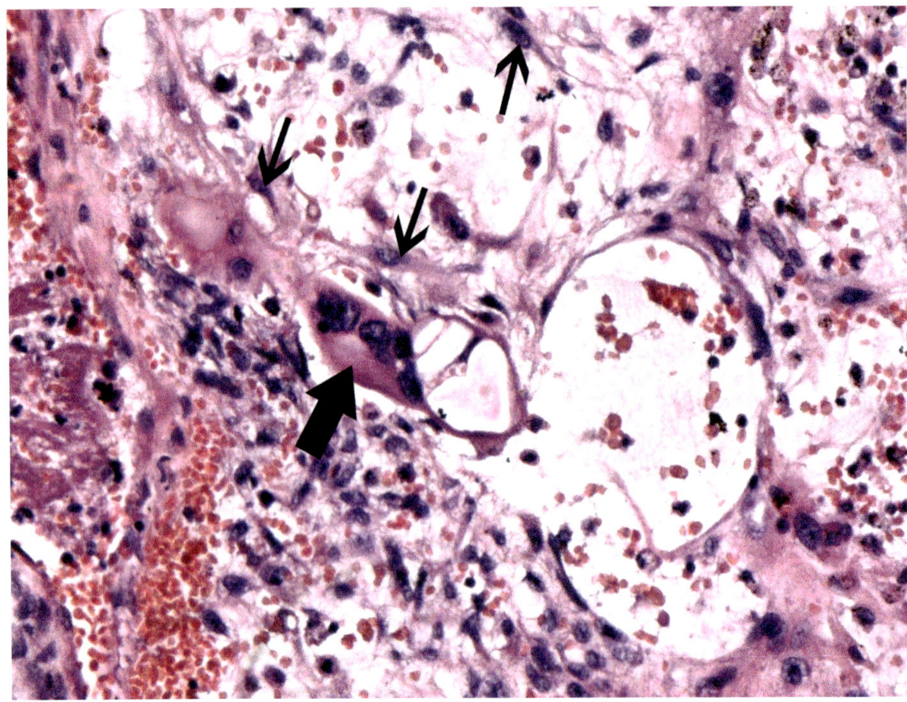

Fig. 4.75 (H-E, ×400) Myxomatous pattern of yolk sac tumor shows individual stellate, spindle (*thin arrows*), or epithelioid neoplastic cells in abundant myxoid stroma. The pluripotential mesenchymal cells are chemoresistant and, in rare cases, can give rise to sarcoma, after treatment. The sarcomatoid pattern of yolk sac tumor when identified in a residual mass after chemotherapy treatment, behaves similarly to a somatic-type sarcoma.

An isolated syncytiotrophoblastic giant cell with amphophilic cytoplasm (*thick arrow*) is detected within the yolk sac component.

Isolated syncytiotrophoblastic giant cells without any accompanying cytotrophoblast occur in association with seminoma, embryonal carcinoma, yolk sac tumor, and teratoma; the presence of these cells may be associated with moderately raised serum concentration of HCG (β subunit). Syncytiotrophoblasts associated with the mentioned germ cell tumors are sometimes misdiagnosed as choriocarcinoma. *Absence of cytotrophoblast* excludes the diagnosis of choriocarcinoma

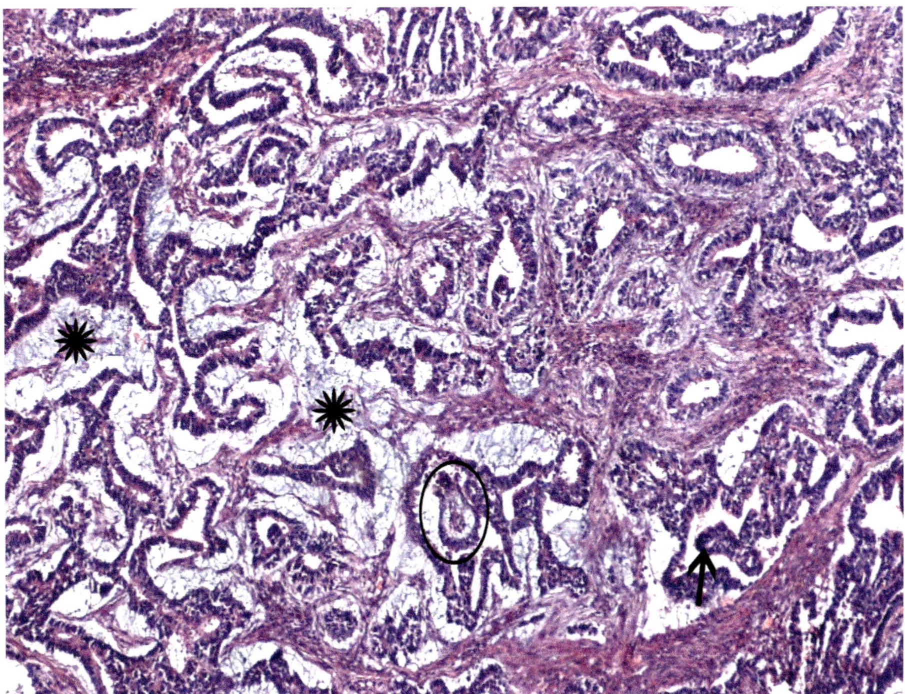

Fig. 4.76 (H-E, ×100) Another case of a yolk sac tumor. In this primary tumor area, the tumor cells are arranged in a branching, complex glandular pattern; papillae lined by columnar cells project into cystic spaces (*arrow*); the presence of a Schiller-Duval body is implied (*ellipse*). These features are compatible with yolk sac tumor. *Purely* glandular yolk sac tumor is more common following chemotherapy and is therefore usually found in metastases; it should be discriminated from a secondary somatic type adenocarcinoma.

Extracellular mucin (*asterisks*), when confirmed histochemically and distinguished from intervening myxoid stroma, raises the suspicion of a somatic-type adenocarcinoma development; invasive features of malignant-appearing epithelium within a desmoplastic reaction should therefore be thoroughly examined since presence of secondary malignancies in germ cell tumors is ominous (particularly when observed at metastatic sites, though)

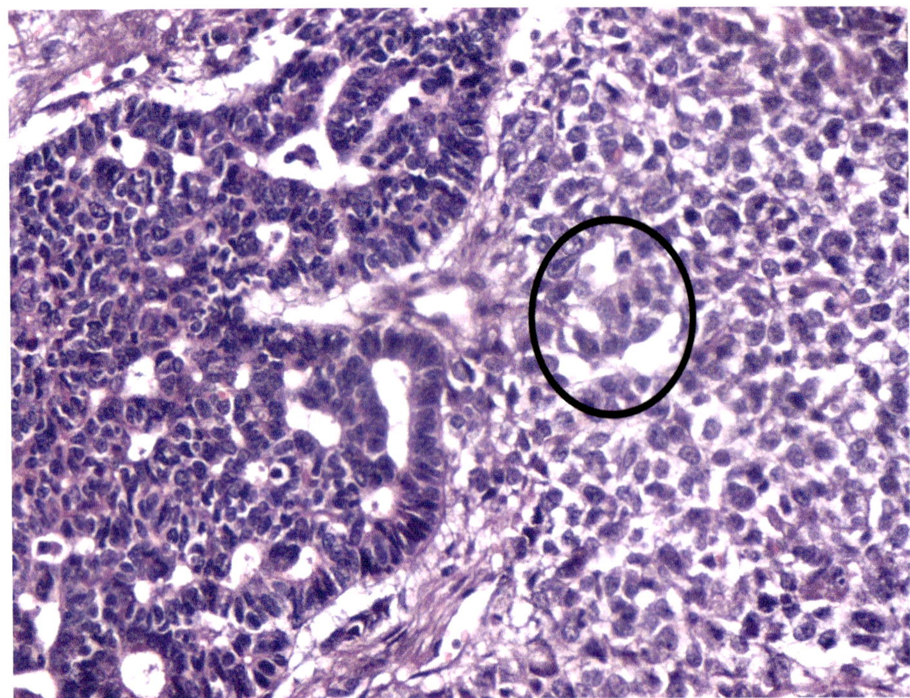

Fig. 4.77 (H-E, ×200) The solid yolk sac tumor pattern is noticed on the right side of the image with the characteristic microcystic tendency (*ellipse*). At the left side, hyperchromatic cells arranged in an organoid, pseudoglandular pattern are noticed. The branching anastomosing luminal spaces may bring to mind the glandular pattern of yolk sac tumor (of the previous figure) which, of course, can be confirmed by AFP and glypican-3-positive immunolabeling.

On the other hand, immature teratoma, by definition, has tissues resembling those of embryonic or fetal development. Primitive mesoderm, noticed as undifferentiated spindle cell component, is the most common immature element in testis (see Fig. 4.64). Primitive endoderm and primitive neuroectoderm, blastomatous tissue, and embryonic rhabdomyoblastic tissue can also be encountered. Neuroepithelium consists of small, hyperchromatic cells arranged in neural-type tubules, neuroblastic-type tissue, and rosettes. A panel of immunohistochemical markers (i.e., synaptophysin, NSE, chromogranin, HBA-71, GFAP, CD99, FLI1) could be used to identify the above primitive/embryonic-appearing tubules as a component of immature teratoma with neural or neuroendocrine differentiation.

The differential diagnosis of immature teratoma versus a secondary malignant component can be challenging

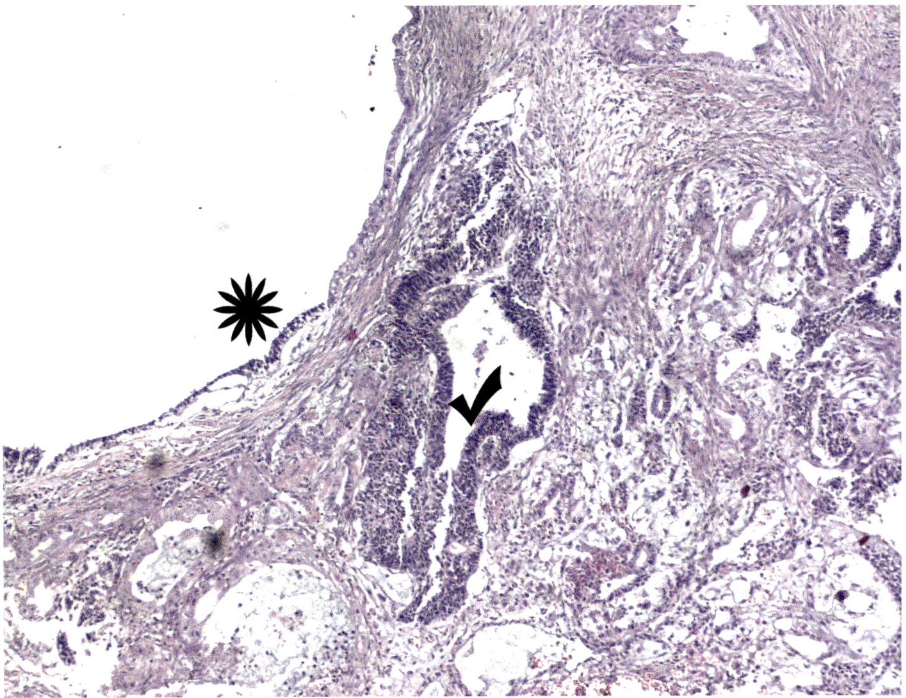

Fig. 4.78 (H-E, ×50) Yolk sac tumor elements in loose, myxomatous stroma are noticed on the right. Teratomatous elements coexist: a dilated space lined by attenuated epithelium (*asterisk*) is noticed on the left; next to it, a *small* focus of hyperchromatic cells forming an immature gland is noticed (*tick*). This collection of immature cells lacks atypia. When such immature elements (or non-chemotherapy-related, atypical epithelium) remain scattered in small nests in a multifocal fashion, no malignancy of somatic type should be diagnosed.

In contrast, when a *pure* and *relatively large nodular overgrowth* occupying more than a whole field area viewed with a X4 objective (5 mm in diameter) is detected, an area of non-germ cell, somatic-type malignancy [e.g., primitive neuroectodermal tumor (PNET), blastomatous Wilms' tumor-like neoplasm, neuroendocrine neoplasm, and embryonal rhabdomyosarcoma) can be diagnosed alongside the other germ cell tumor components, after immunohistochemical investigation, of course.

With regard to carcinomas of somatic type, their destructive growth can be recognized by its invasive features; in other words, for carcinomatous transformation in a teratoma, true invasive growth, and not just atypia in epithelial elements, is of vital importance for the diagnosis. Particularly at metastatic sites, treatment-induced atypia should be considered; the latter, however, is usually diffuse and lacks the requisite nodular or infiltrative growth of a single type of atypical cell population.

In the absence of such overgrowth of atypical or immature elements or invasive features, cytological atypia and immature elements should *not* be mentioned in the final diagnosis, because they have no known prognostic significance in male patients

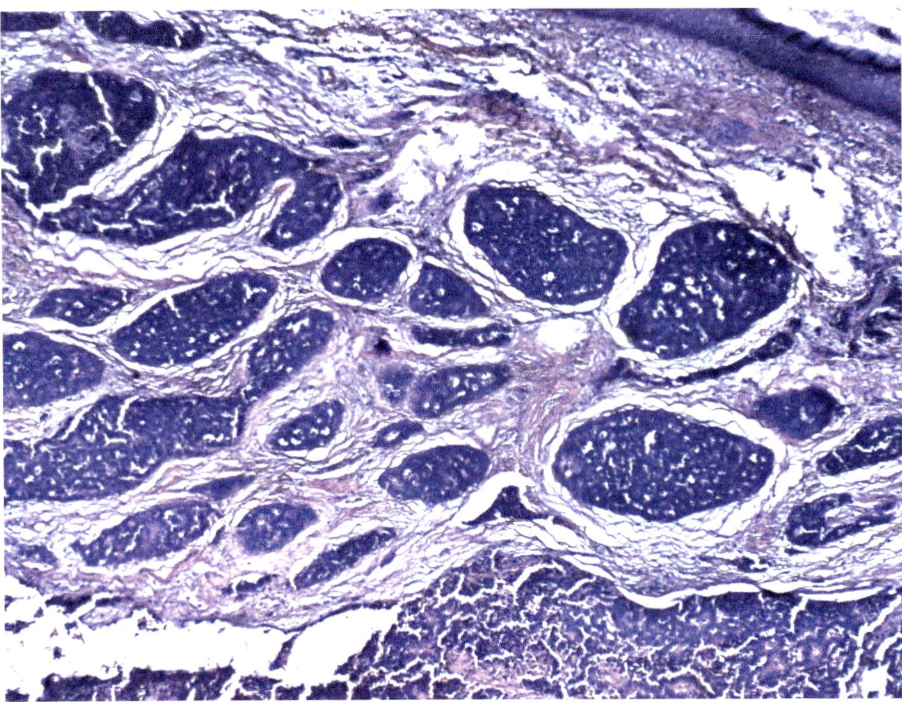

Fig. 4.79 (H-E, ×50) Carcinoid tumor in a testicular teratoma. (This image is from another case.) Beneath squamous teratomatous component (*upper right side*), an insular, nested, and solid pattern of monotonous cells compatible with a well-differentiated tumor with neuroendocrine differentiation is observed herein as component associated with teratoma. Delicate fibrous to hyalinized stroma. Immunopositivity for cytokeratin and neuroendocrine markers (i.e., synaptophysin, chromogranin and CD56) is expected. Carcinoid tumor can also occur in pure form as a monodermal form of teratoma, and, particularly in such cases, metastatic origin should be excluded

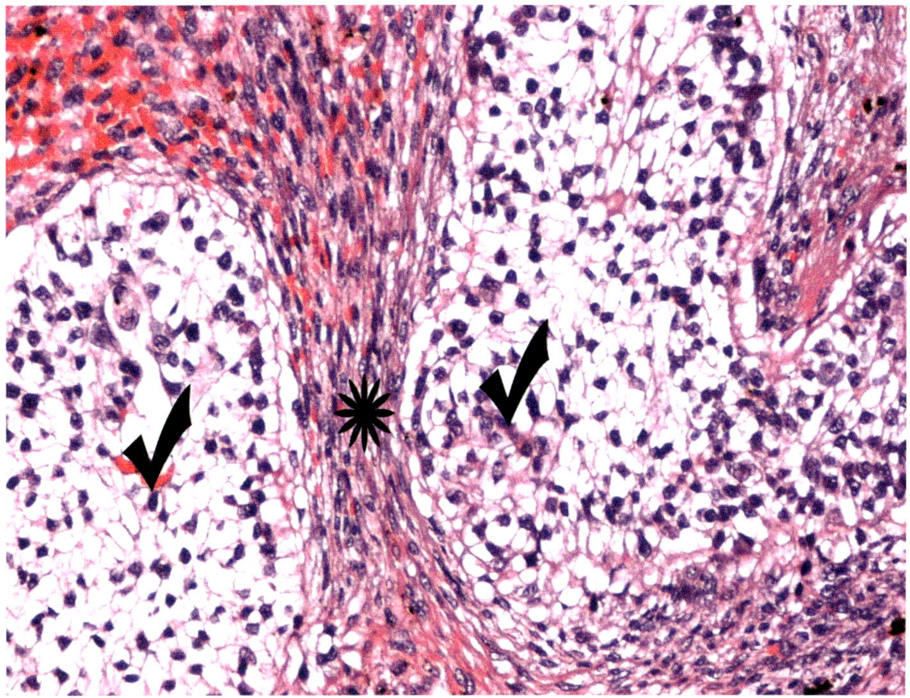

Fig. 4.80 (H-E, ×200) Teratoma component. Squamous epithelium islands (*ticks*) within spindle cell mesenchymal tissue (*asterisk*).
Over 50% of all mixed germ cell tumors have a teratomatous component

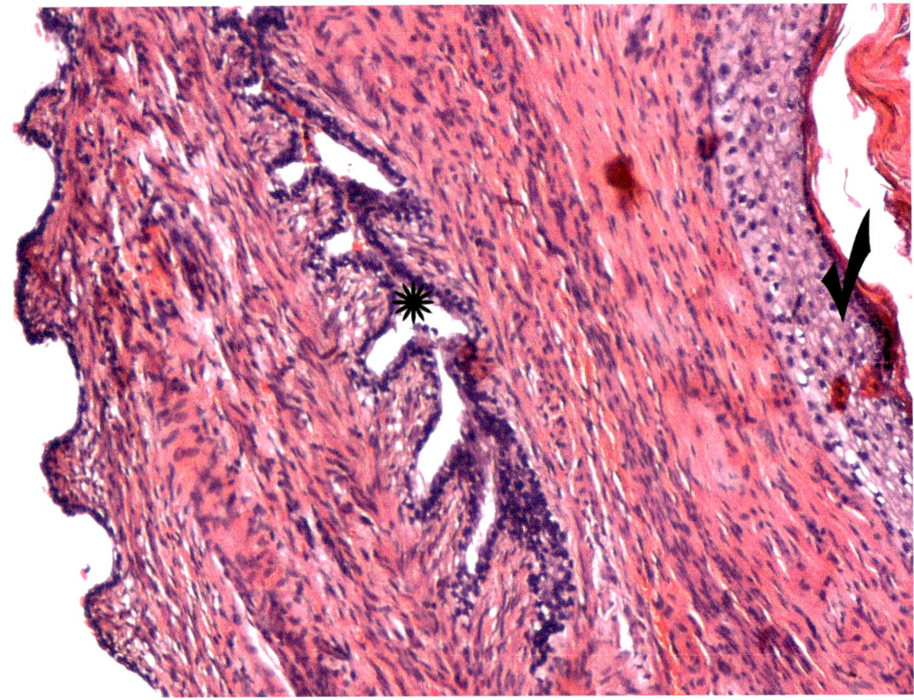

Fig. 4.81 (H-E, ×100) Teratomatous, keratinizing squamous (*tick*) and columnar epithelial elements (*asterisk*), attenuated on the left. The mature teratoma glands are frequently surrounded by bundles of smooth muscle (as opposed to yolk sac tumor glands which lack a smooth muscle investment).

Teratomas consist of multiple mature and/or immature tissue components of >1 germ layer; as far as mature teratoma is concerned, a mixture of elements of ectoderm (epidermis, neuronal tissue), endoderm (gastrointestinal or respiratory mucosa, other seromucous glands), and mesoderm (bone, cartilage, muscle) can be encountered

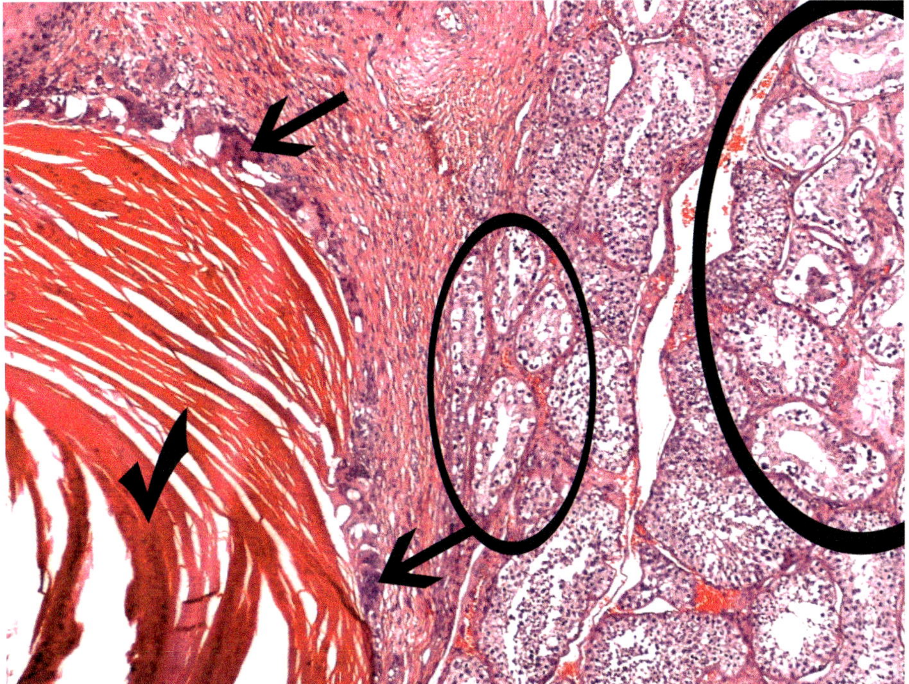

Fig. 4.82 (H-E, ×50) Keratin follicles (*tick*) surrounded by multinucleated giant cells (arrows). GCNIS is present in adjacent seminiferous tubules (ellipse and curve area).

The phagocytic response against keratin might bring to mind a partially ruptured epidermoid cyst. Epidermoid cysts can occur in the testis and are benign cysts with an exclusive lining of keratinizing squamous epithelium and keratinous debris content, without associated adnexal structures. Epidermoid and dermoid cysts, the latter composed of epidermis and skin adnexal structures within the cyst wall, are *never* accompanied by GCNIS. Adult patients with teratoma have GCNIS (i.e., the common precursor lesion of all truly malignant germ cell tumors) in their seminiferous tubules. Adult teratomas are thus considered malignant regardless of maturation. It is important to distinguish (mature) teratoma in adults from epidermoid cysts and dermoid cysts; these latter two entities behave in a benign fashion, whereas teratoma has metastatic potential irrespective of how mature it looks.

As far as the present tumor is concerned, however, this discussion is unnecessary, since teratoma, as usual in adults, is part of a mixed germ cell tumor with undeniable malignant potential. Pure teratomas are encountered in prepubertal children and behave as benign tumors in this age group; combination with yolk sac tumor is possible in this age group, and, then, there is some biological aggressiveness to be expected, but it is minimal.

Germ cell tumors unrelated to GCNIS and thus of benign nature or of diminished malignant potential include:

- Spermatocytic tumor
- Teratoma prepubertal type
  - Dermoid cyst
  - Epidermoid cyst
  - Well-differentiated neuroendocrine tumor (monodermal teratoma)
- Mixed teratoma and yolk sac tumor, prepubertal type
- Yolk sac tumor, prepubertal type

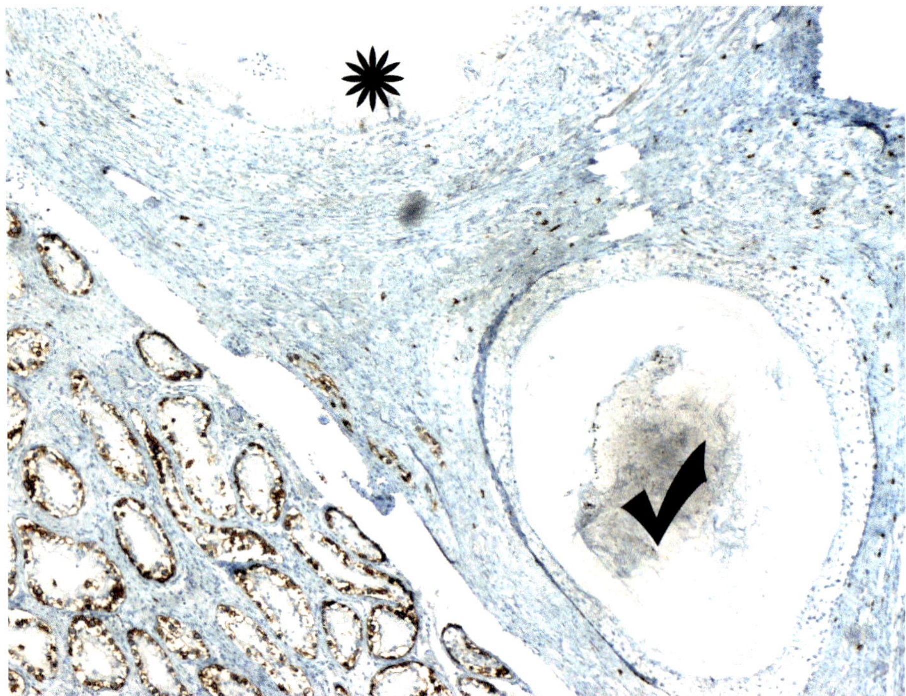

Fig. 4.83 (PLAP immunohistochemical stain, ×50) PLAP is expressed at foci of GCNIS on the left. The presence of tumor-adjacent GCNIS verifies the malignant potential of the mature, benign-appearing teratoma elements [squamous island with keratin content (*tick*), intestinal type glandular epithelium (*asterisk*)].

A mature teratoma in an adult patient does not equate with a benign tumor since it is pathogenetically associated with GCNIS. During surgery of an adult patient, identification of a mature testicular teratoma on frozen sections does *not* support a benign nature of this lesion despite the absence of malignant morphologic features

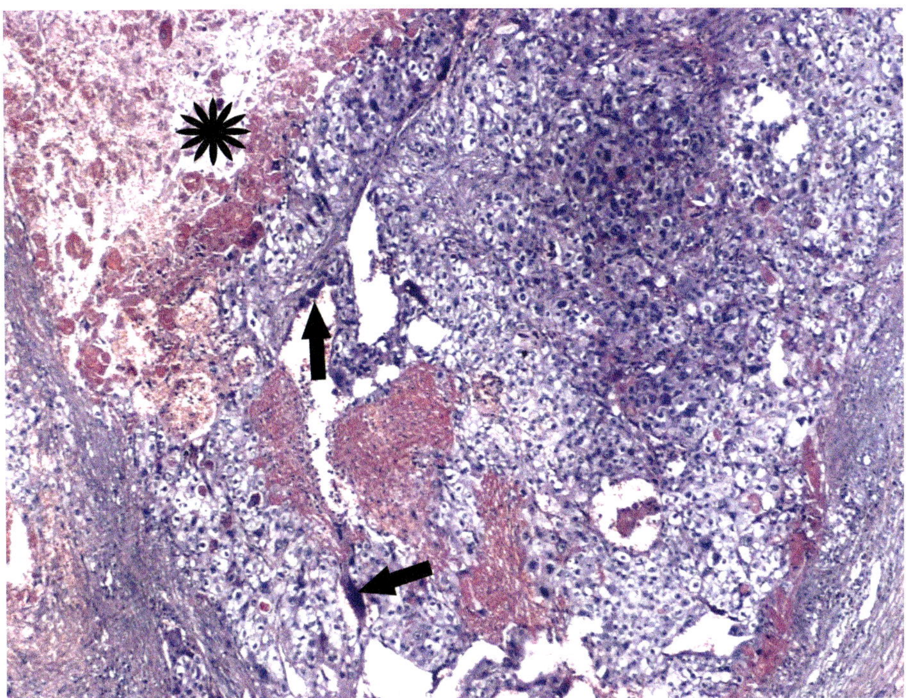

Fig. 4.84 (H-E, ×100) A limited, classic choriocarcinoma component was also detected in the present mixed germ cell tumor. Syncytiotrophoblasts (*arrows*) accompanied by cytotrophoblasts on a background with prominent hemorrhagic necrosis (*asterisk*); necrosis may be the dominant figure of testicular choriocarcinoma. Choriocarcinoma is an uncommon component of mixed germ cell tumors, and, fortunately for this patient, it is not predominant among the other germ cell tumor components

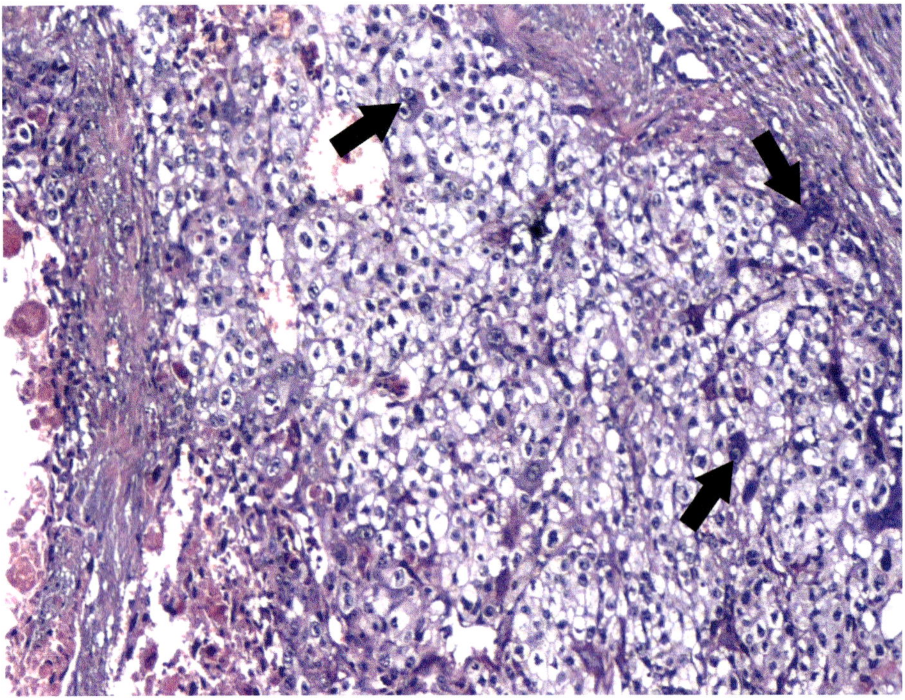

Fig. 4.85 (H-E, ×200) Classic choriocarcinoma component. Bilaminar distribution of multinucleate syncytiotrophoblasts (*arrows*) and rather uniform cytotrophoblasts, the latter typically growing in sheets or aggregates, with associated hemorrhage.

This biphasic pattern of intermingled syncytiotrophoblast and mononuclear trophoblast cells may be absent in trophoblastic neoplasms other than classic choriocarcinoma

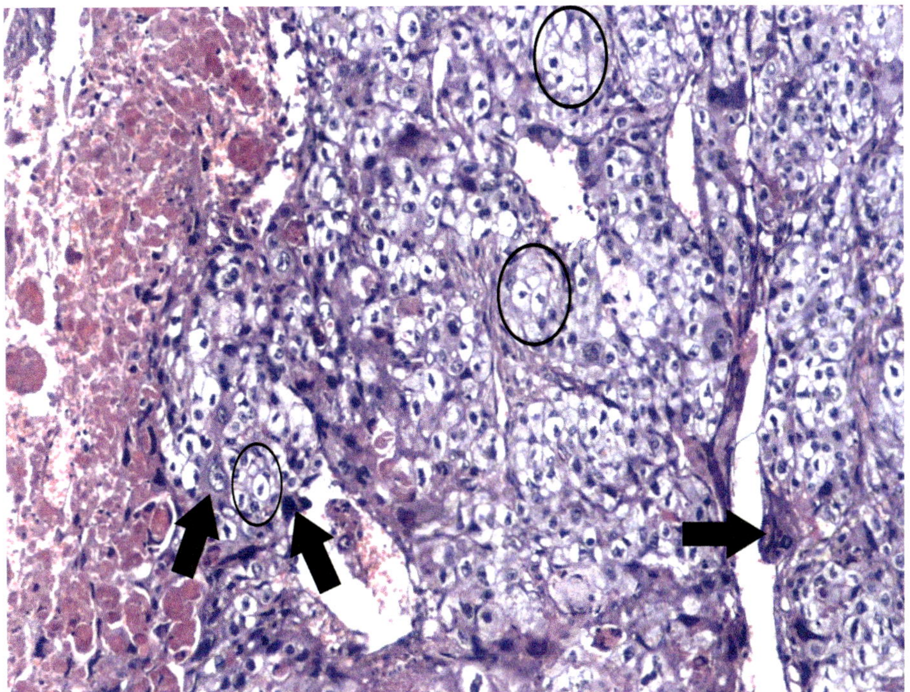

Fig. 4.86 (H-E, ×200) Intimate random mixture of cytotrophoblasts and syncytiotrophoblasts; the former, mononucleated cells with pale to clear cytoplasm, well-defined cell borders (two common features of cytotrophoblasts and seminomatous cells) single, irregularly shaped nuclei, and high mitotic activity (*ellipses*); the latter, large, multinucleated cells with densely eosinophilic and vacuolated cytoplasm and degenerate-appearing nuclei (*arrows*) with smudged chromatin. Syncytiotrophoblasts wrap around mononuclear cytotrophoblastic cells; the close relationship of these two distinctive cell types is a characteristic of classic choriocarcinoma. Cytotrophoblasts may resemble seminomatous cells and seminomas can contain isolated syncytiotrophoblastic cells.

Syncytiotrophoblasts are HCG-immunopositive, while cytotrophoblast cells generally have only weak or absent staining for HCG. Serum level of HCG correlates with prognosis, reflecting tumor burden; in this patient it was 11,000 IU/L, while in patients with pure or predominant choriocarcinoma, it generally exceeds 50,000 IU/L. Syncytiotrophoblasts also express human placental lactogen (HPL), inhibin, and glypican-3. Cytotrophoblasts, in contrast to seminomatous cells, express cytokeratins (strongly), p63, and GATA3. *Immunohistochemical results* should, however, always be evaluated *in correlation to morphological features*

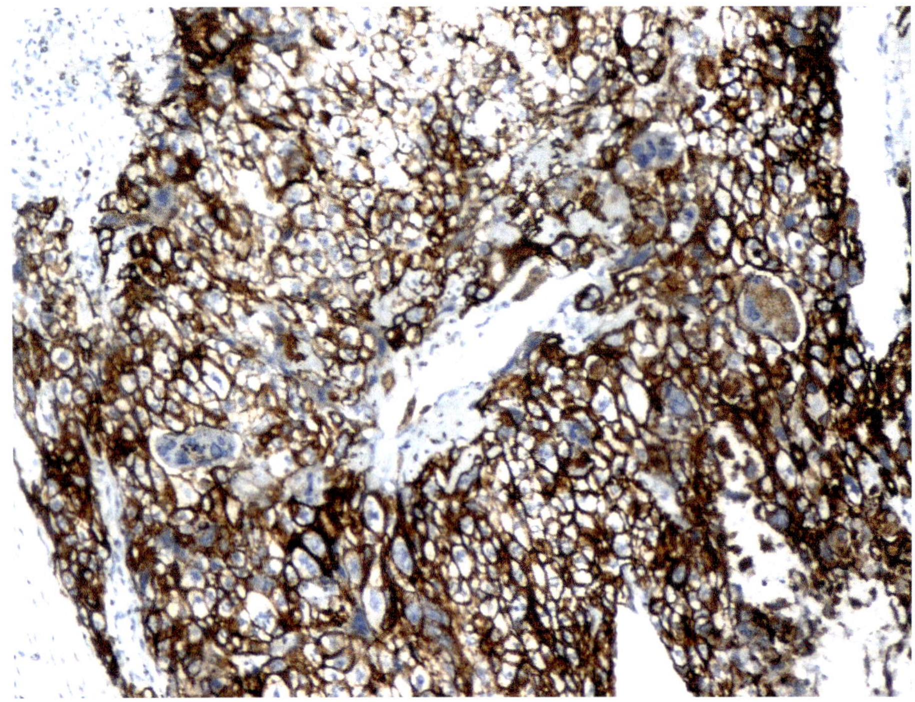

Fig. 4.87 (Cytokeratin7 immunohistochemical stain, ×200) Cytokeratin 7 is typically strongly positive, excluding a diagnosis of seminoma with syncytiotrophoblastic cells. Negative seminoma markers, such as KIT, OCT3/4, and NANOG, can also be helpful for this very important distinction between cytotrophoblasts and seminomatous cells

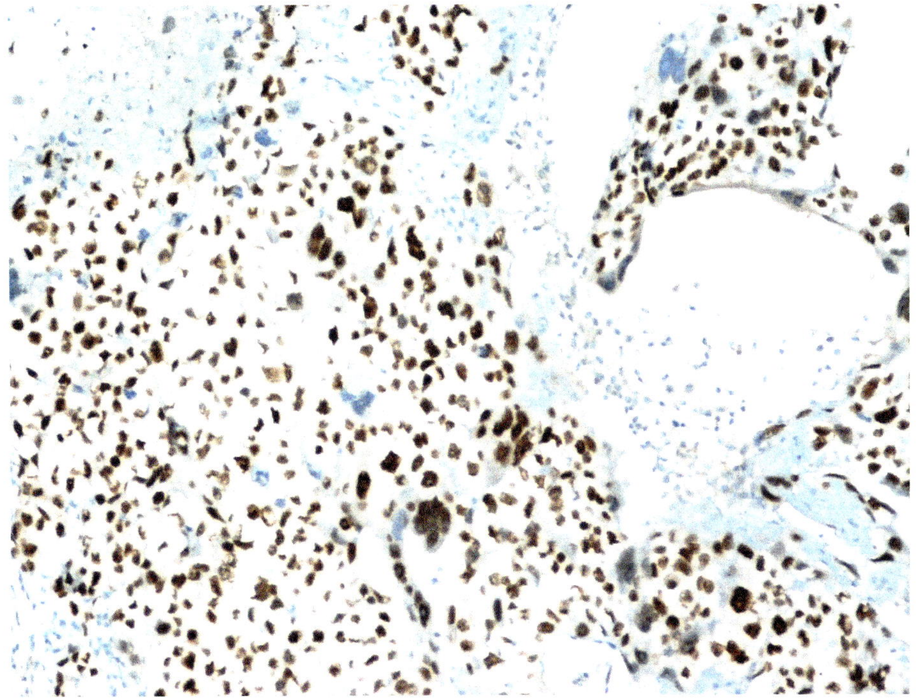

Fig. 4.88 (GATA-3 immunohistochemical stain, ×200) GATA-3 nuclear expression in cytotrophoblasts

4.6.2 Microscopic Evaluation of the Post-chemotherapy Specimen of the Residual Retroperitoneal Mass

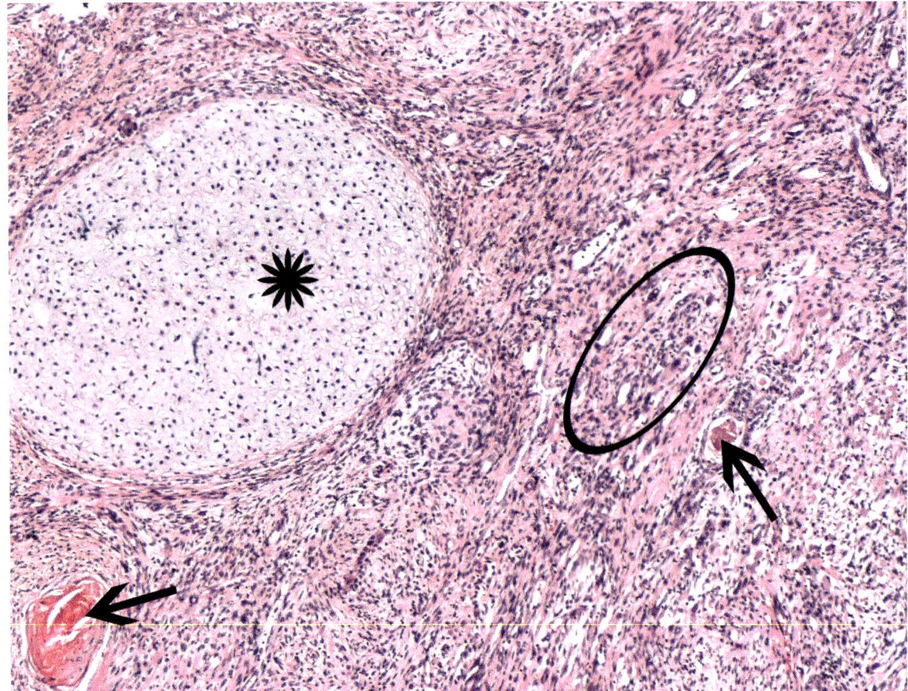

Fig. 4.89 (H-E, ×100) Teratomatous elements [a nodule of immature cartilage (*asterisk*) and keratinized squamous nests (*arrows*)] are expectedly encountered in the residual mass due to their chemoresistance. Scattered cells with hyperchromatic nuclei are noticed in the stroma (*ellipse*)

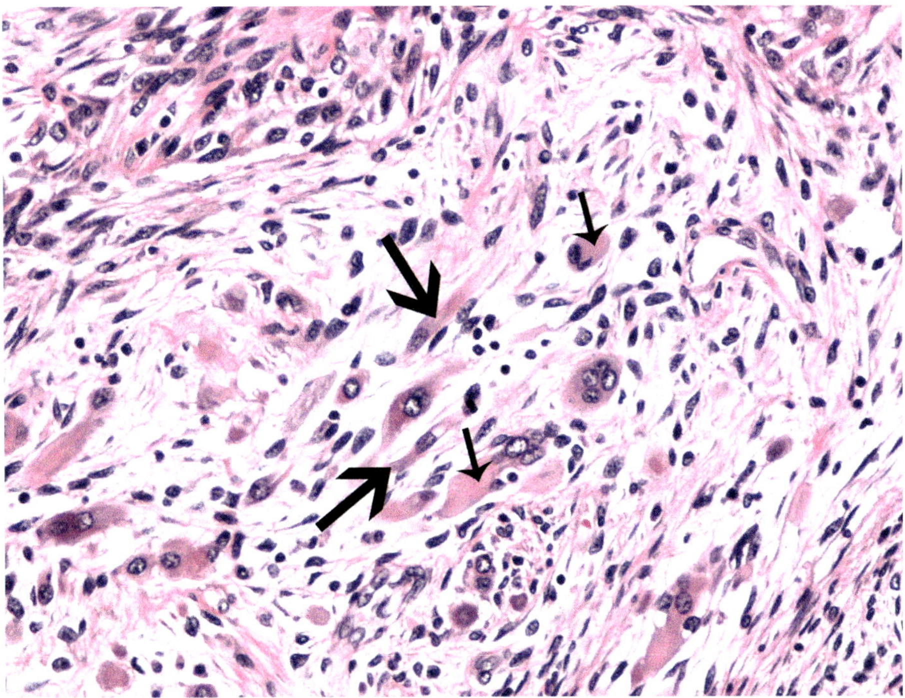

Fig. 4.90 (H-E, ×200) Area of rhabdomyoblastic differentiation in the residual retroperitoneal mass. Rhabdomyoblastic cells containing abundant pink cytoplasm (*thin arrows*) and often looking like tadpole cells (*thick arrows*) are seen.

In post-chemotherapy lymph nodes, the finding of mature rhabdomyocytes with abundant eosinophilic cytoplasm lacking mitotic activity and *without a primitive cellular component* is actually associated with a favorable prognosis and must be differentiated from rhabdomyosarcoma as a component of somatic malignancy at the metastatic site.

Scattered, immature elements in a teratoma can look like a malignant neoplasm; an expansile *overgrowth*, occupying more than a 4× field, is indispensable for the diagnosis of a somatic-type sarcoma, since invasive features of mesenchymal elements are not as easily appreciated as with epithelial elements, and sarcomatous cells may be confused with atypical teratomatous mesenchyme.

From another point of view, the spindle cells of the myxomatous pattern of a yolk sac tumor (see Fig. 4.75) can undergo mesenchymal metaplasia with skeletal muscle and cartilaginous differentiation, blurring the distinction between yolk sac tumor and teratoma

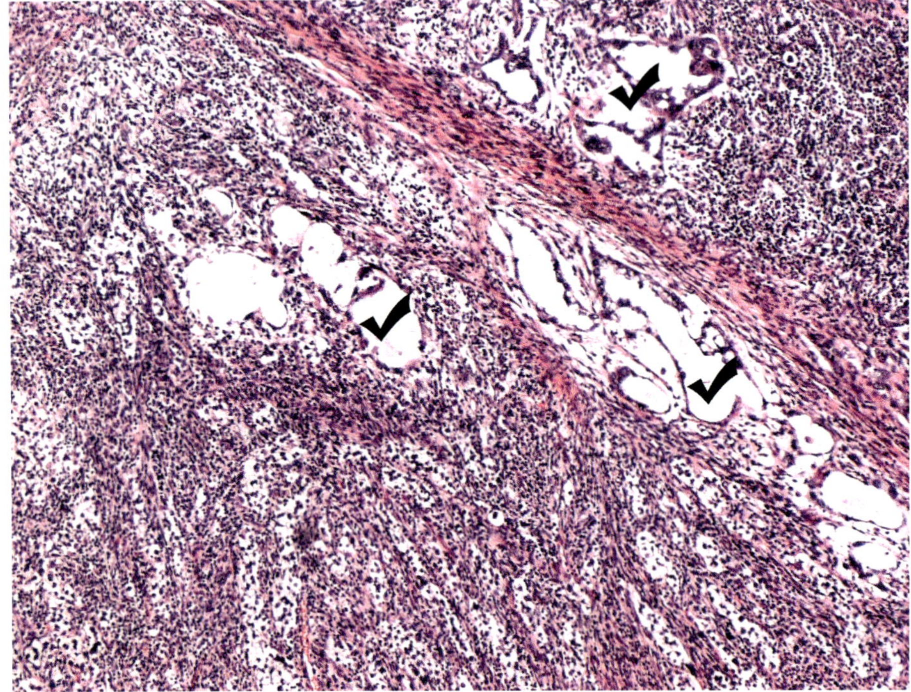

Fig. 4.91 (H-E, ×100) An expansile overgrowth of primitive, small cells with entrapped, viable yolk sac tumor elements (*ticks*) can be observed elsewhere, in the residual retroperitoneal mass. This small cell tumor warrants immunohistochemical investigation; these primitive cells are immunohistochemically identified as rhabdomyoblasts; so the diagnosis of a synchronous, somatic-type rhabdomyosarcoma is established. This diagnosis is of particular oncologic importance when further treatment is going to be arranged.

Occasionally, a somatic-type malignancy may develop in non-teratomatous elements; yolk sac tumor is such an alternative origin. Such malignancies are more common in metastases, particularly after chemotherapy, rather than involving the primary testicular tumor, and the single most common site is the retroperitoneal lymph nodes. There is evidence that some of the sarcomatous tumors observed in resections following chemotherapy for metastatic testicular germ cell tumors are derived from the before mentioned mesenchymal elements of yolk sac tumor; interestingly, such sarcomatous tumors may generally retain cytokeratin immunoreactivity similarly to their yolk sac tumor cells of origin

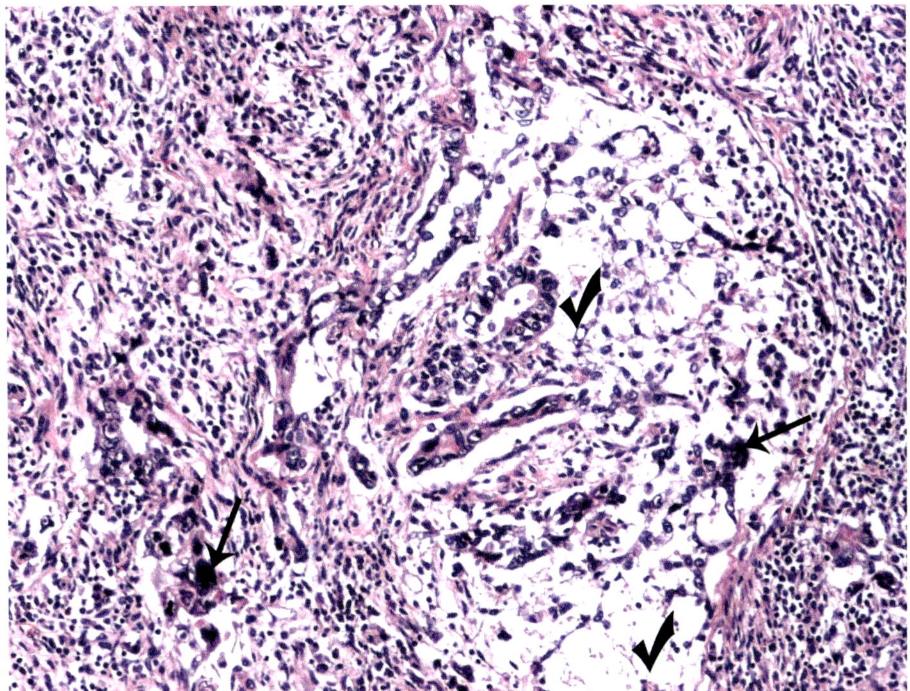

Fig. 4.92 (H-E, ×200) Viable yolk sac tumor elements (*ticks*) with focal, chemotherapy related?, nuclear atypia (*arrows*), within the small cell population

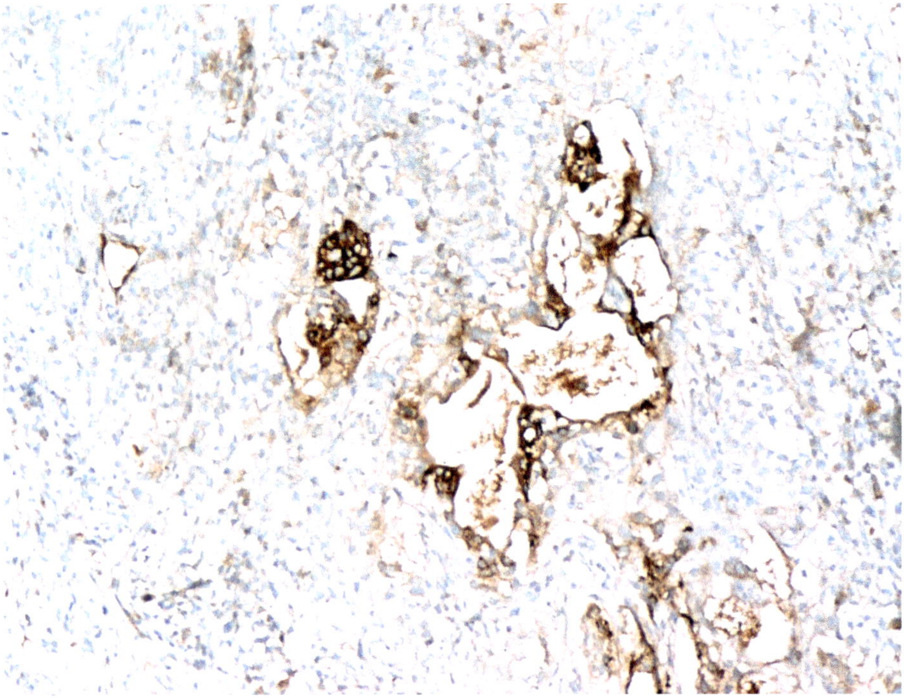

Fig. 4.93 (Glypican-3 immunohistochemical stain, ×200) The immunohistochemical confirmation of viable yolk sac elements within the rhabdomyosarcoma mass.

Remaining viable yolk sac elements in the post-chemotherapy residual retroperitoneal tumor mass and lymph nodes, on their own, arguably worsen the patient's prognosis; furthermore, the development of a somatic malignancy in the metastasis, such as the present rhabdomyosarcoma, increases the mortality risk

4.6.2.1 Clinical Commentary

Vasileios Spapis

This is a case of a metastatic mixed germ cell tumor of the testis consisting at its primary site of components of all nonseminomatous types of germ cell tumors as well as of a minor seminomatous component. All tumor components were microscopically identified and quantified. In the post-chemotherapy, residual retroperitoneal mass and viable teratomatous and yolk sac tissue elements were pathologically detected alongside a clear synchronous overgrowth of a secondary, somatic-type rhabdomyosarcoma.

Mixed germ cell tumors account for more than 40% of germ cell tumors. Most of them (and about 25% of all testicular tumors) are a combination of teratoma and embryonal cell carcinoma. About 6% of all testicular tumors are of mixed cell type with seminoma being one of the components. Treatment for these mixtures of seminoma and nonseminomatous germ cell tumors (NSGCTs) is similar to that of NSGCTs alone (Presti 2013). A predominant choriocarcinomatous component is related to early hematogenous metastases to the lungs, liver, etc.

Diagnostic evaluation remains the same regardless of the histologic type of the primary tumor. Pre- and post-orchiectomy half-life kinetics of serum tumor markers (LDH, AFP, HCG), abdominopelvic CT scan, chest CT, and bilateral testis ultrasound are highly recommended for all patients. Bone and brain scanning should be performed in case of symptoms. Fertility investigations (total testosterone, semen analysis, LH, FSH) could be performed, and sperm banking should be discussed with all men prior to starting treatment for testicular cancer (Albers 2016).

Treatment should start with initial chemotherapy in all advanced cases of NSGCT (except for stage IIa NSGCT disease and pure teratoma without elevated tumor markers). The primary treatment of choice is 3–4 cycles of BEP (bleomycin, etoposide, cisplatin) depending on the patient's initial stage and risk group classification. Restaging is performed by imaging investigations and tumor markers reevaluation. Upon marker decline and stable or regressive tumor manifestation, chemotherapy will be completed. In the case of marker decline, but growing metastases, resection of the tumor is obligatory after termination of induction therapy (Albers 2016).

As mentioned in the previous case, following first-line BEP chemotherapy, residual tumor resection is mandatory in all patients with a residual mass > 1 cm. Six to ten percent of residual masses contain viable cancer, 50% contain mature teratoma, and 40% contain necrotic-fibrotic tissue. In patients with viable cancer, the histologic picture is usually that of embryonal cell carcinoma and, less often, of yolk sac tumor. However, 6–8% of residual tumor specimens will contain evidence of non-GCT malignancy, arising, most frequently – but not always – from malignant transformation of the teratoma component. The most common histology is rhabdomyosarcoma. Just like teratoma, rhabdomyosarcoma is unresponsive to chemotherapy, so the final therapy outcome is related to the *completeness of surgical resection*. With complete resection, 50–66% of patients will survive, whereas the vast majority of patients with incomplete resection will experience rapid progression. Cisplatin-based combination salvage chemotherapy is the treatment of choice for relapse or refractory disease, and the results are highly dependent on several prognostic factors (Stephenson and Gilligan 2012).

Key Messages

- Yolk sac tumors are generally composed of several patterns (the microcystic, being the most common) which often merge from one to another.
- Mixed germ cell tumors with a significant choriocarcinoma component have a worse prognosis than those without choriocarcinoma elements.
- Particularly in lymph node metastases, it is important to distinguish teratoma with associated somatic malignancy from immature teratoma, for prognostic and therapeutic reasons.
- Occasionally, a somatic-type malignancy may develop in non-teratomatous elements. Most germ cell tumor-associated somatic malignancies are sarcomas.

4.7 Case 4.5: Leydig Cell Tumor

Case Study

Data Prior to Microscopy

Unilateral, painless, 0.9 cm in diameter, testicular mass, detected by testicular ultrasound as a well-defined, hypoechoic, small solid mass, in a 7-year-old boy who presented with prominent external genitalia, pubic hair growth, and deep voice. Increased serum levels of testosterone, androstenedione, and dehydroepiandrosterone were detected. During surgery, frozen sectioning was requested; a touch preparation stained with H-E demonstrated red Reinke's crystals, thereby confirming a diagnosis of probably benign nature. Based on frozen sectioning findings, testis-sparing surgery was performed, and a *solitary* intratesticular lobulated nodule was resected.

Macroscopic features: a well-circumscribed, homogenous, soft tumor nodule with a yellow to tan cut surface.

4.7.1 Microscopic Findings

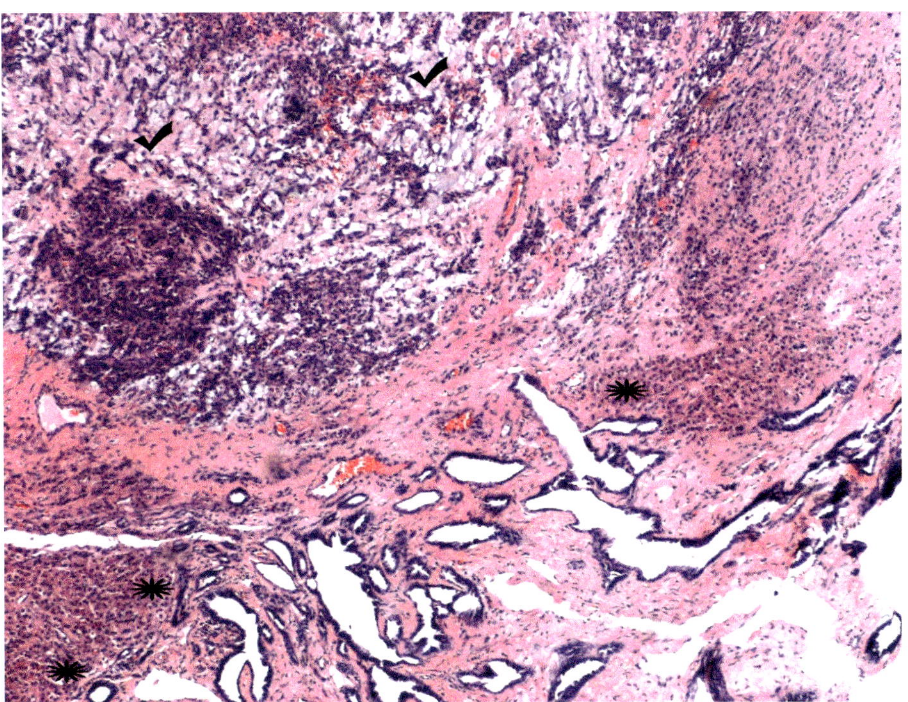

Fig. 4.94 (H-E, ×50) Tumor border in proximity with rete testis. Seminiferous tubules have been replaced by tumor cells. In addition to solid sheets (*asterisks*), cord-like pattern of tumor cells (*ticks*) is observed in this field. Compression and invasion of the rete testis (the latter being implied here, see *asterisks*) are a worrisome feature but, on its own, do not warrant malignancy for such a tumor.

The few tumor surrounding seminiferous tubules (not shown in this image) showed premature signs of spermatogenesis due to stimulation by locally produced testosterone

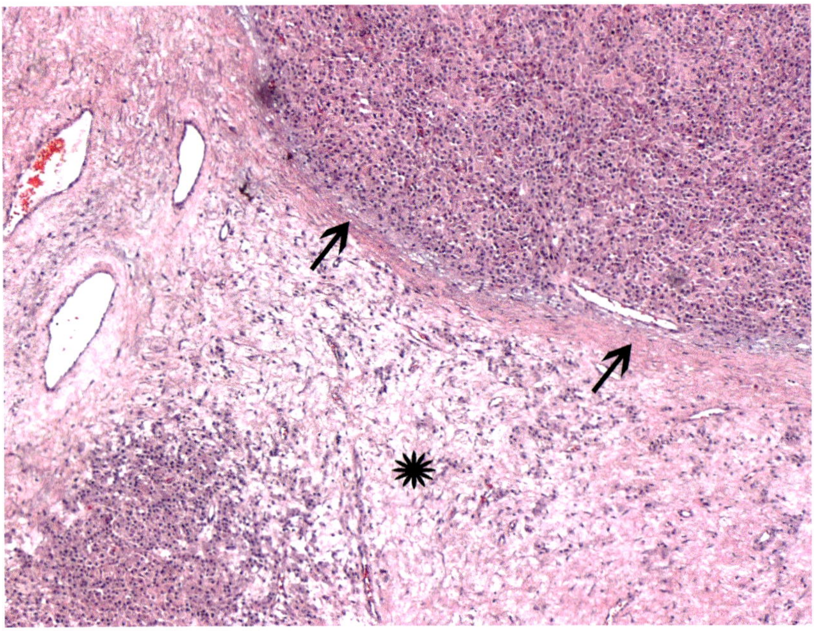

Fig. 4.95 (H-E, ×50) Lobulation within the tumor parenchyma with collagenous bands (*arrows*) and hyalinized, edematous stroma (*asterisk*). Solid, sheet-like pattern as on the upper right part is the most common pattern for Leydig cell tumors

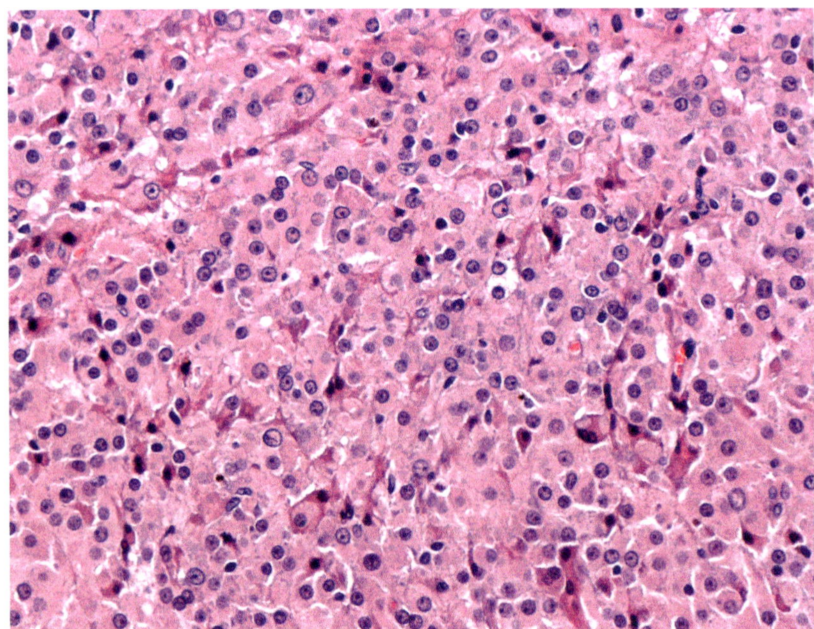

Fig. 4.96 (H-E, ×200) Uniform, round, or ovoid, bland-looking tumor cells. Moderate variation in nuclear size, lack of cytological atypia. Sparse, spindle-shaped cells

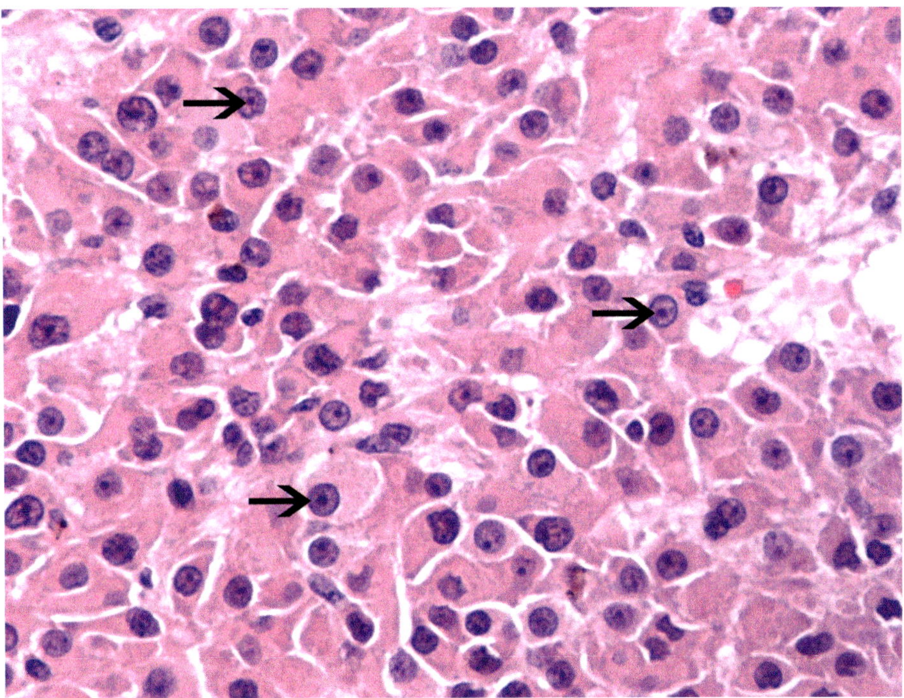

Fig. 4.97 (H-E, ×400) Tumor cells are large, round, or polygonal in shape, have abundant eosinophilic cytoplasm and well-defined borders, and resemble nonneoplastic Leydig cells of the testis. Round nuclei with visible, moderate-sized, single, central nucleoli (*arrows*). Intracytoplasmic lipofuscin pigment may be focally present

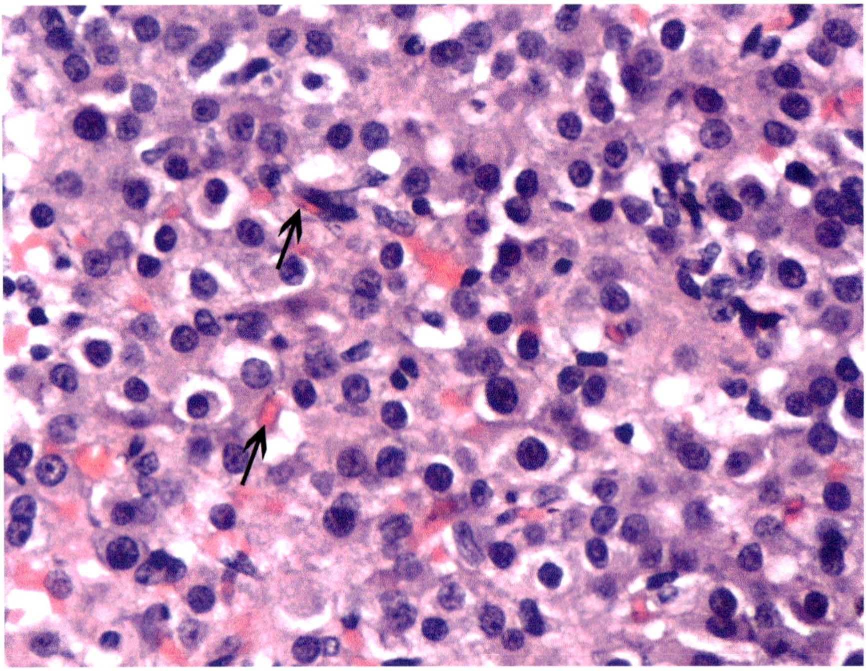

Fig. 4.98 (H-E, ×400) The presence of Reinke's crystal fragments, implied here (*arrows*), is a valuable morphologic finding for the diagnosis of Leydig cell tumors. Rod-shaped intracytoplasmic Reinke's crystals, a definitive feature occurring in up to 40% of Leydig cell tumors, were detected in the cytological smear of the present tumor, permitting the diagnosis during surgery. In histological sections, there is always a possibility that these crystals are chipped out by the microtome and thus are no longer detectable

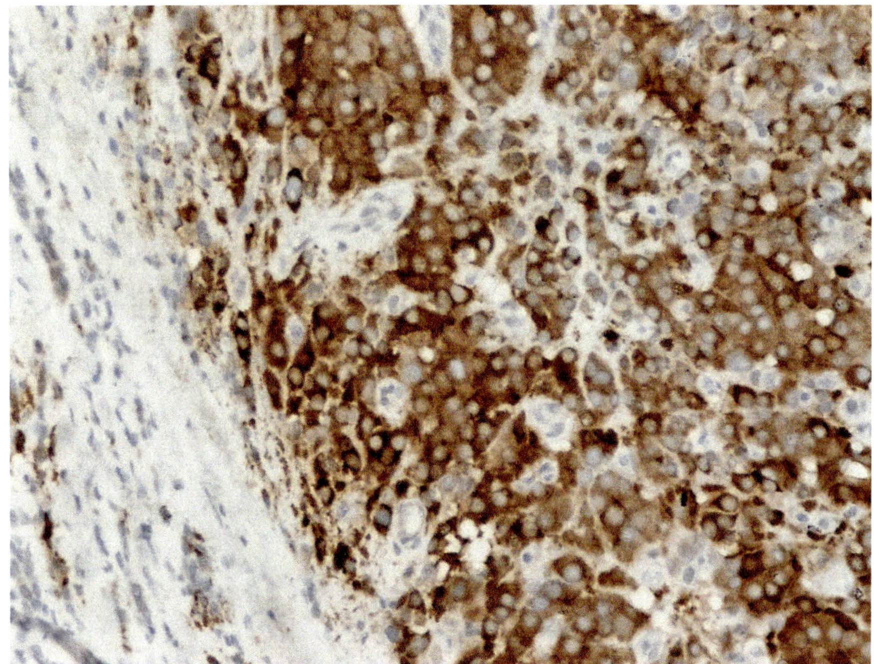

Fig. 4.99 (Inhibin-a immunohistochemical stain, ×200) Inhibin, melan A, vimentin, and SF1 are typically positive in Leydig cell tumors, often with a *diffuse* and *intense* staining pattern, as far as the first three immunomarkers are concerned. Nevertheless, none of these immunohistochemical findings are specific for the diagnosis of a Leydig cell tumor; the role of immunohistochemistry is always complementary to the morphological findings

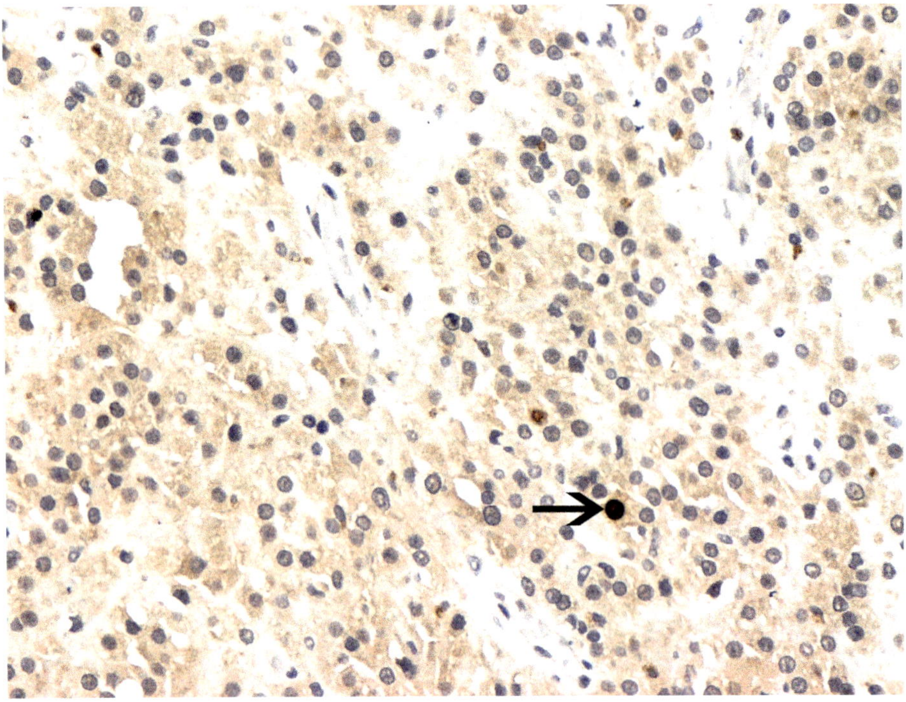

4

■ **Fig. 4.100** (Ki67-MIB1 immunohistochemical stain, ×200) Low MIB1 index (*arrow*)

4.7.1.1 Clinical Commentary

Vasileios Spapis

An ultrasonographically detected testicular tumor which, during surgery, was pathologically diagnosed as a Leydig cell tumor on frozen sections and thus the rest of the testis was spared.

Leydig cell tumors are the most common non-germ cell tumors of the testis and account for 1–3% of all testicular tumors; they are also the most common neoplasms in the sex cord stromal group of testicular tumors.

They follow a bimodal age distribution: the 3–9-year-old and the 25–35-year-old age groups. Twenty-five percent of these tumors occur in childhood. Bilaterality is seen in 5–10% of cases. The cause of these tumors is unknown; they occur in about 8% of patients with Klinefelter's syndrome, and, unlike germ cell tumors, there is no so clear an association with cryptorchidism (Ahmed et al. 2010; Al-Agha and Axiotis 2007; Alanee et al. 2009).

In adults, the most common presentation is a painless testicular mass, frequently with feminizing characteristics (as a result of androgen excess and peripheral conversion to estrogen), including gynecomastia, impotence, and decreased libido. Children usually present with a testicular mass and precocious puberty (Taskinen et al. 2008).

Up to ten percent of these tumors are malignant and usually present with four or more of the following parameters: older age, diameter > 5 cm, infiltrative borders, evident cytological atypia, appreciable mitotic activity (>3 mitotic figures per 10 high power fields), atypical mitotic figures, angiolymphatic invasion, extension beyond the testicular parenchyma, necrosis, an increased MIB1 index, increased p53 protein expression by the tumor cells, and DNA aneuploidy. However, even if these parameters do occur and suggest malignant Leydig cell tumor, there are no consistently reliable histologic criteria for making this judgment. The presence of metastatic disease is the only reliable criterion for making this distinction. The most frequent metastatic sites are the retroperitoneum and lung. Malignant behavior has been reported in just one prepubertal patient (Albers 2016; Carmignani et al. 2006; Pohl et al. 2004).

Diagnostic workup must include markers, hormones (at least testosterone, LH, and FSH and, if not conclusive, also estrogen, estradiol, progesterone, and cortisol), ultrasound (US) of both testes, and computed tomography (CT) of the chest and abdomen. On US, it may be possible to observe well-defined, small, hypoechoic lesions with hypervascularization; however, the appearance is variable and is indistinguishable from germ cell tumors.

Asymptomatic, small-volume testicular tumors are often misinterpreted as germ cell tumors, and inguinal orchiectomy is performed. An organ-sparing procedure in every small US-detected, nonpalpable intraparenchymal lesion is highly recommended in order to obtain a histologic diagnosis at first. In all patients with symptoms of gynecomastia or hormonal disorders and normal germ cell tumor-associated serum markers, a non-germ cell tumor should be considered and immediate orchiectomy avoided. In cases with germ cell tumor in either frozen section or paraffin histology, orchiectomy is recommended as long as a contralateral normal testicle is present (Presti 2013).

When diagnosed and treated early, long-term favorable outcomes are seen at follow-up in Leydig cell tumors, even with signs indicative of malignant potential. In sex cord/stromal tumors with histological signs of malignancy, especially in older patients, orchiectomy and early retroperitoneal lymphadenectomy may be an option to prevent metastases or to achieve long-term cure in stage IIA cases. Prophylactic RPLND is unjustified for patients with clinical stage I disease without high-risk features (Stephenson and Gilligan 2012).

Tumors that have metastasized to the lymph nodes, lung, liver, or bone respond poorly to chemotherapy or radiation, and survival is poor. Mitotane (Lysodren), a potent inhibitor of steroidogenesis, may produce partial responses in metastatic patients with excess androgen production, but cure is not possible.

Key Messages

- Ultrasound is particularly valuable for the discovery of functioning, impalpable testicular tumors.
- Most Leydig cell tumors behave in a benign fashion.
- Intraoperative frozen section diagnosis, when possible, allows local resection with preservation of the epididymis and testis.

The combination of cellular morphology and immunohistochemical findings allows the diagnosis of a *Leydig cell tumor*.

4.8 Case 4.6: Adenomatoid Tumor

Case Study

Data Prior to Microscopy

A 36-year-old male presents with an ultrasonographically detected, asymptomatic, small, firm intrascrotal, *extratesticular* lump, just above the superior pole of the testis. Complete local surgical excision was performed, sparing the testis.

A grayish-white nodule measuring 1.5 cm was resected. Cut surface was homogeneous and fibrous with a whorled appearance.

4.8.1 Microscopic Findings

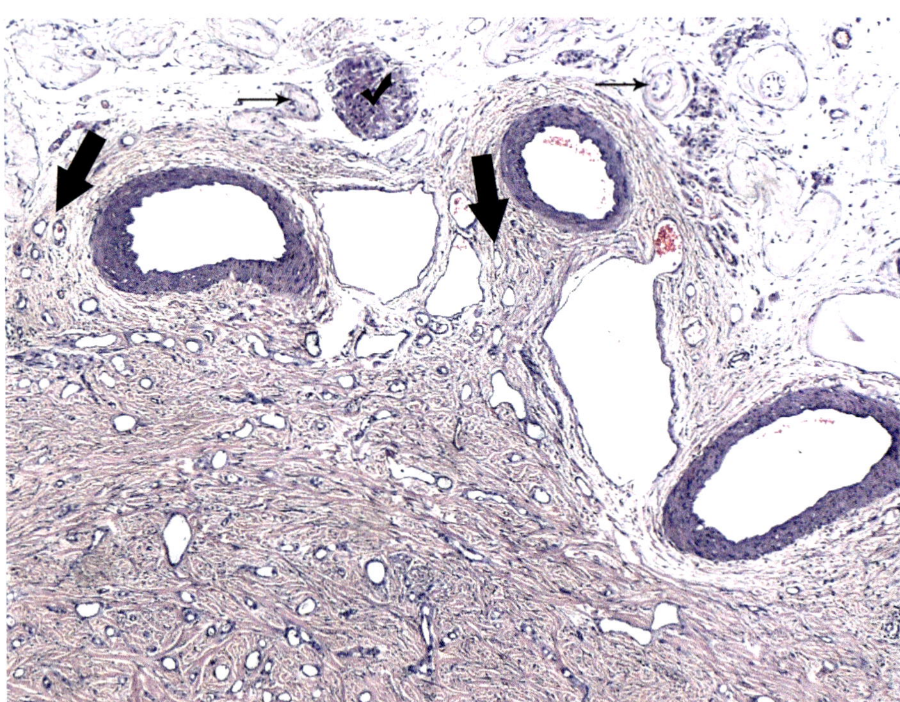

Fig. 4.101 (H-E, ×50) The unencapsulated, ill-defined tumor margin. Above some vascular spaces, some hyalinized seminiferous tubules are observed (*thin arrows*) along with a cluster of Leydig cells (*tick*). Channels with dilated lumina and microcystic spaces resembling vascular spaces approach testicular parenchyma in a pseudoinfiltrating growth pattern (*thick arrows*). The tumor consists of irregular, variably sized, slit-like tubular spaces lined by an attenuated layer of flattened neoplastic cells with a prominent fibrous stroma

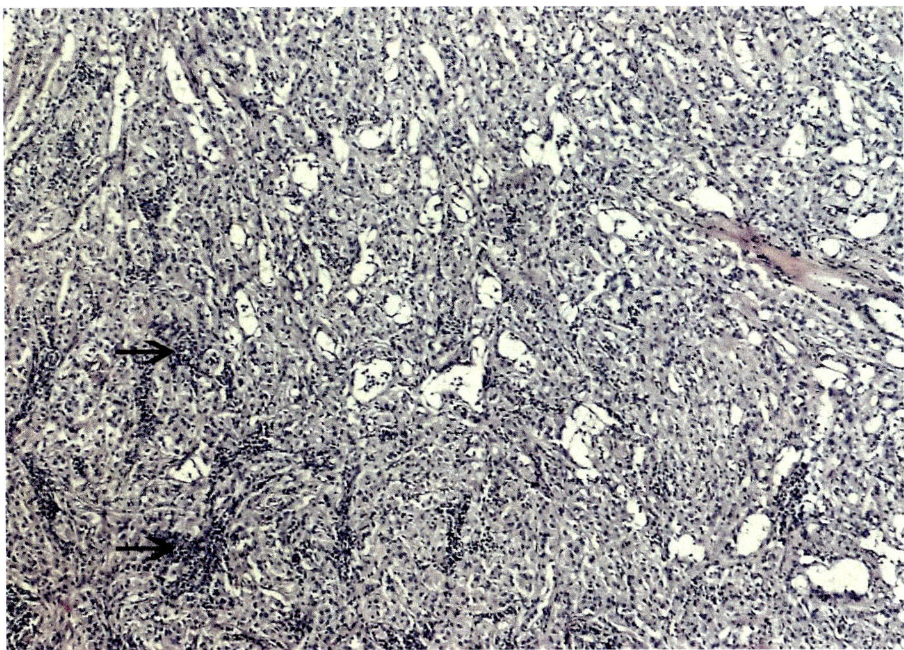

Fig. 4.102 (H-E, ×100) Proliferating cells are here arranged either in thin-walled, gland-like spaces lined by flattened cells (*upper half*) or closely packed nests/solid clusters of epithelioid neoplastic cells (*lower half*). Stroma contains interspersed lymphocytic aggregates (*arrows*)

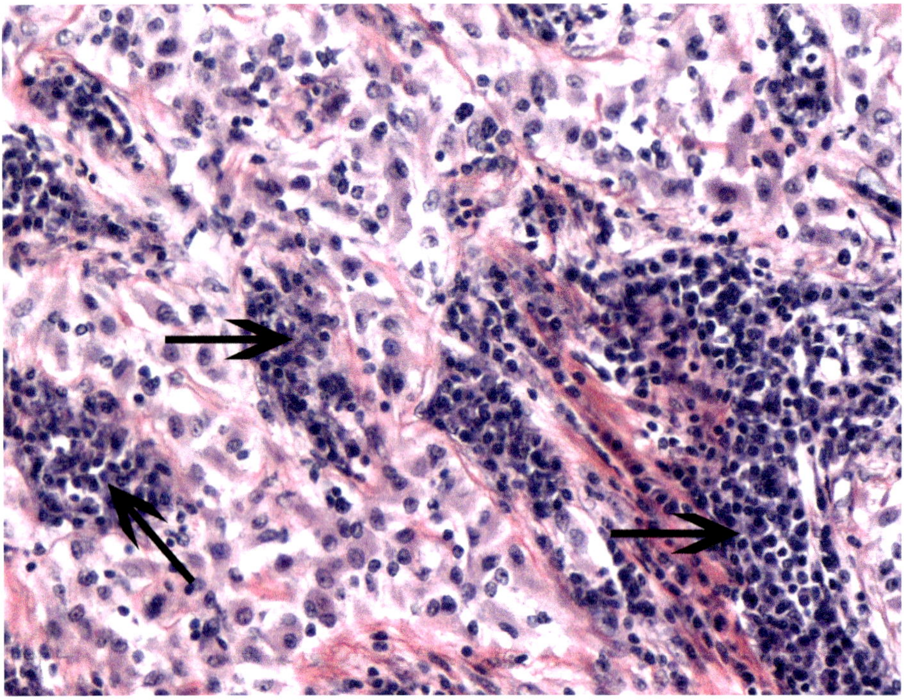

Fig. 4.103 (H-E, ×200) An area of more cellular proliferation with uniform cytology. Granular, eosinophilic cytoplasm. Round nuclei, occasionally vesicular with small nucleoli. Admixed, scattered mononuclear cellular aggregates are present within the tumor (*arrows*)

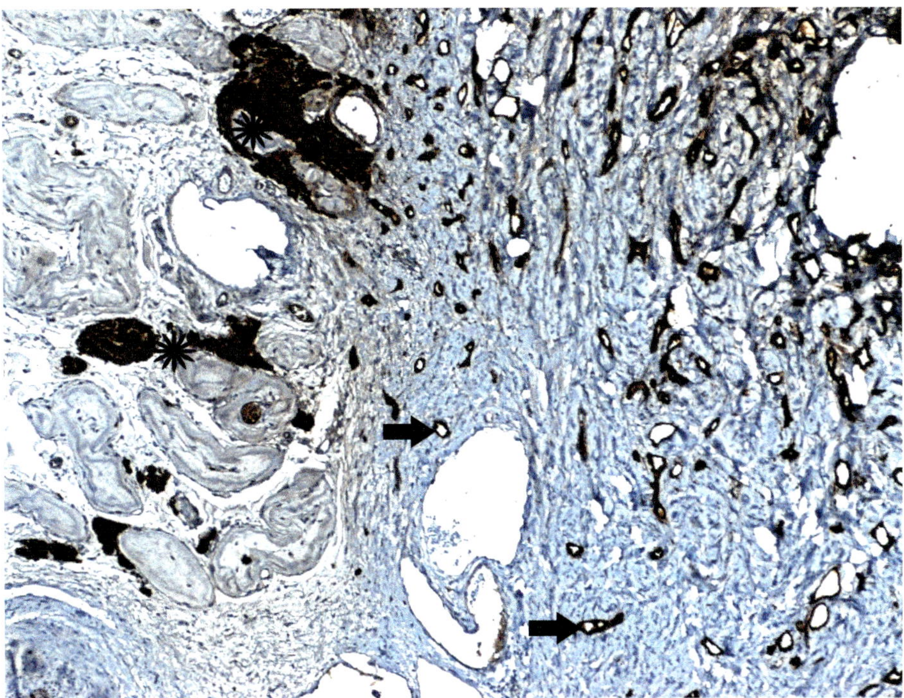

Fig. 4.104 (Calretinin immunohistochemical stain, ×50) Calretinin immunoreactivity in tumor formations (*thick arrows*). Leydig cell aggregates among hyalinized seminiferous tubules (*asterisks*) are also immunopositive for calretinin; nevertheless, in contrast to Leydig cell tumors, adenomatoid tumors are inhibin (−), Melan-A(−), and cytokeratin (+)

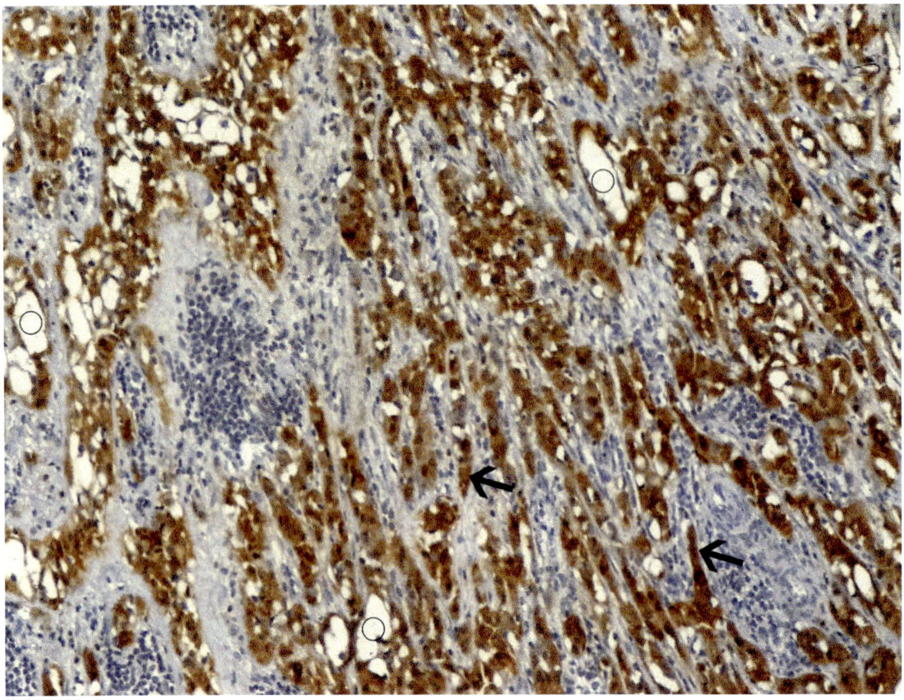

Fig. 4.105 (Calretinin immunohistochemical stain, ×100) Immunopositive tumor tubular formations (*circles*) and cords (*arrows*)

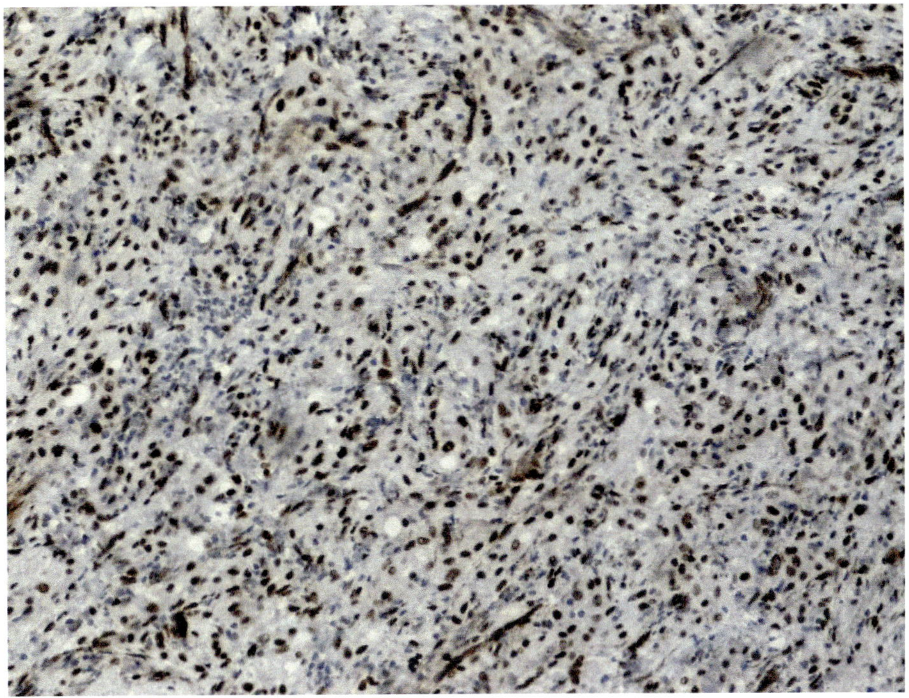

Fig. 4.106 (WT1 immunohistochemical stain, ×200) Specific nuclear staining

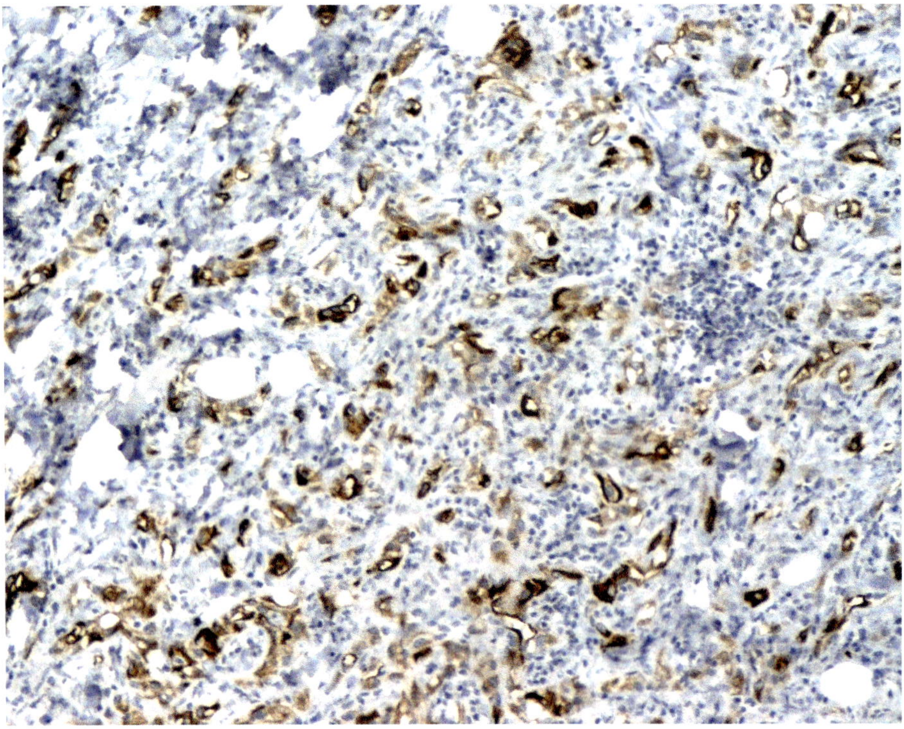

Fig. 4.107 (Cytokeratin 7 immunohistochemical stain, ×100) Irregular tubules' positivity

Immunohistochemical findings reinforce the mesothelial derivation of tumor cells. Endothelial markers negativity can exclude the diagnosis of an epithelioid hemangioma

The diagnosis of *adenomatoid tumor*, the most common tumor of testicular adnexa, is established.

4.8.1.1 Clinical Commentary

Vasileios Spapis

An incidental finding of a paratesticular tumor pathologically diagnosed as an adenomatoid tumor.

Adenomatoid tumors along with spermatic cord lipomas are the most common paratesticular tumors, the former responsible for 30% of all paratesticular masses, most commonly involving the lower pole of the epididymis (although they may also arise within the testicular tunics or the spermatic cord). They usually occur in the third and fourth decade of life (Albers 2016; Amin and Parwani 2009; Williams et al. 2004).

These tumors are typically asymptomatic, solid lesions that arise from any portion of the epididymis. They present either as an incidental finding or a slow-growing scrotal mass. The most common presentation is a small (0.5–5.0 cm), paratesticular mass detected on routine examination. Enlargement is usually painless with normal scrotal skin and surrounding adnexa. Mostly they have been present asymptomatically for several years and are uniformly benign (Presti 2013).

Ultrasonography reveals the nature of the lesion which is usually hypoechoic and solid. Magnetic resonance imaging (MRI) findings are helpful preoperatively, determining if the palpable mass is originating from the albuginea of the testes or from the surrounding seminiferous tubules (Stephenson and Gilligan 2012). Absence of serum tumor markers like HCG, CEA, AFP, and LDH helps to exclude a malignant lesion. Histological evaluation of the specimen results in definitive diagnosis which may be supported by immunohistochemistry, if necessary.

These tumors are benign and managed by inguinal exploration and complete surgical excision. Adenomatoid tumors have not been known to ever recur or show malignant transformation. The adequate use of tumor marker studies, ultrasonography, and intraoperative frozen sections can facilitate organ-sparing surgery. The aim is to prevent unnecessary orchiectomy resulting in continuation of endogenous testosterone production and preserving fertility.

Key Messages

- Despite its possible extension into the adjacent testis, adenomatoid tumor behavior is uniformly benign. When its diagnosis is suspected clinic-radiologically, frozen section examination may prevent unnecessary radical orchiectomy.
- Adenomatoid tumor may show a variety of patterns; vascular tumors and sex cord stromal tumors should thus be excluded.

4.9 Case 4.7: Paratesticular Rhabdomyosarcoma

Case Study

Data Prior to Microscopy

A 12-year-old boy with a 3-week history of a palpable, painless mass in the scrotum, measuring 6 cm in its maximum diameter, arising from the spermatic cord, displacing the testicular parenchyma, and reaching the inguinoscrotal region. The mass is surgically resected. Iliac lymph nodes are involved, whereas retroperitoneal lymph nodes are free in this patient. Macroscopically, the mass is encapsulated, lobulated, smooth, fleshy, glistening, and gray-white in color.

4.9.1 Microscopic Evaluation of the Radical Inguinal Orchiectomy Specimen

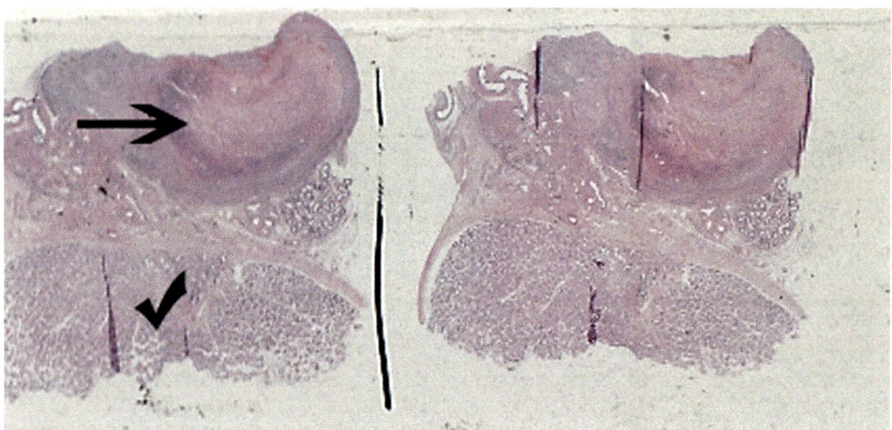

Fig. 4.108 A look at the tissue section. The tumor (arrow) does not invade testicular tissue (*tick*)

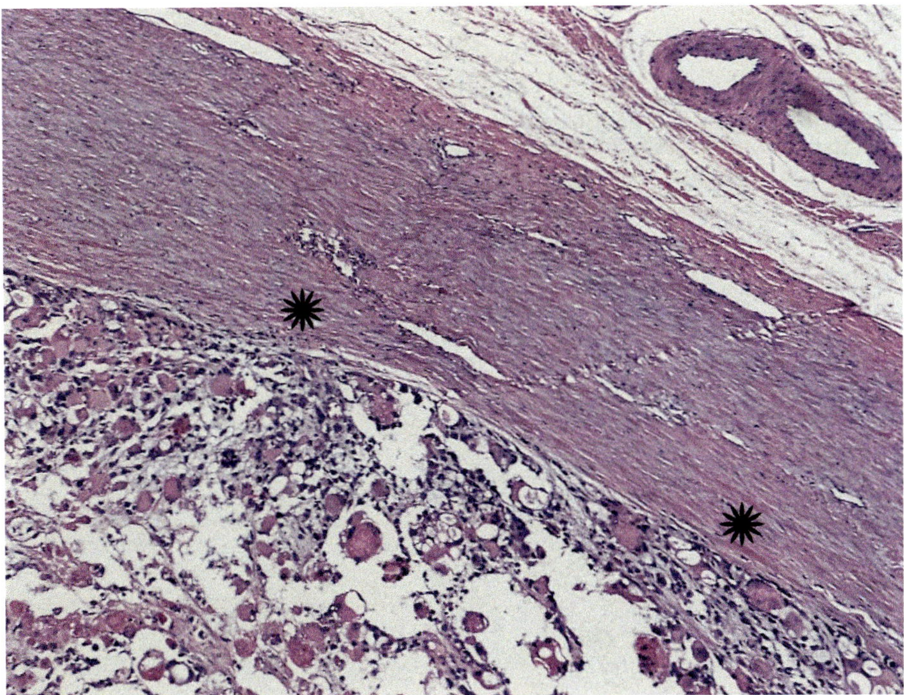

Fig. 4.109 (H-E, ×100) The tumor's smooth edge and capsule (*asterisks*). Haphazardly arranged tumor cells with eosinophilic cytoplasm are morphologically more or less identifiable as rhabdomyoblasts, the cell of origin for rhabdomyosarcomas, even on this low magnification

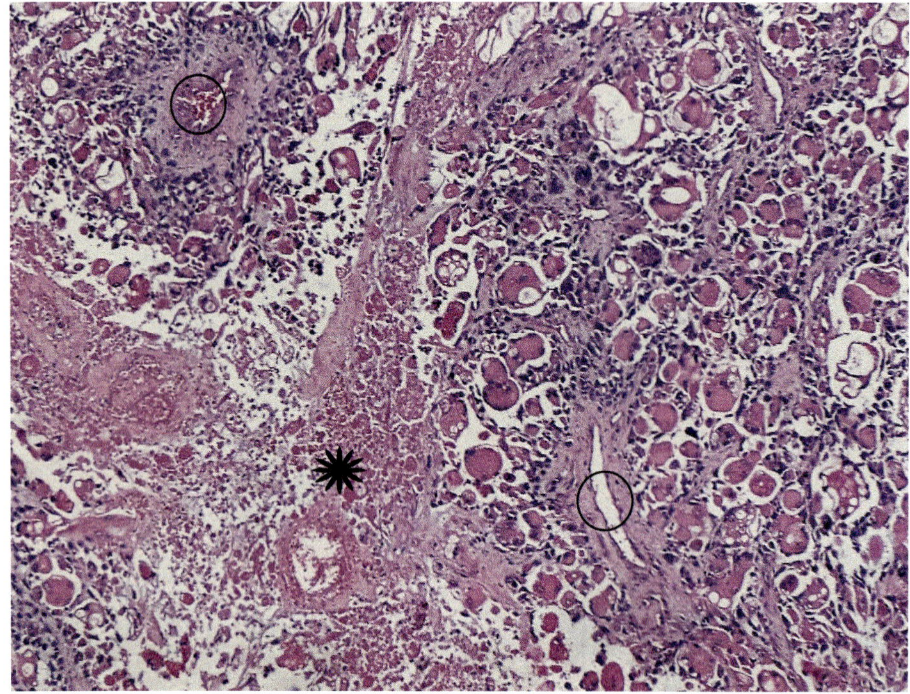

Fig. 4.110 (H-E, ×100) Evident skeletal muscle differentiation. Cellular areas around blood vessels (*circles*) with a predominance of eosinophilic rhabdomyoblasts. The well-differentiated rhabdomyosarcomatous component predominates in this field. Necrotic activity is present (*asterisk*)

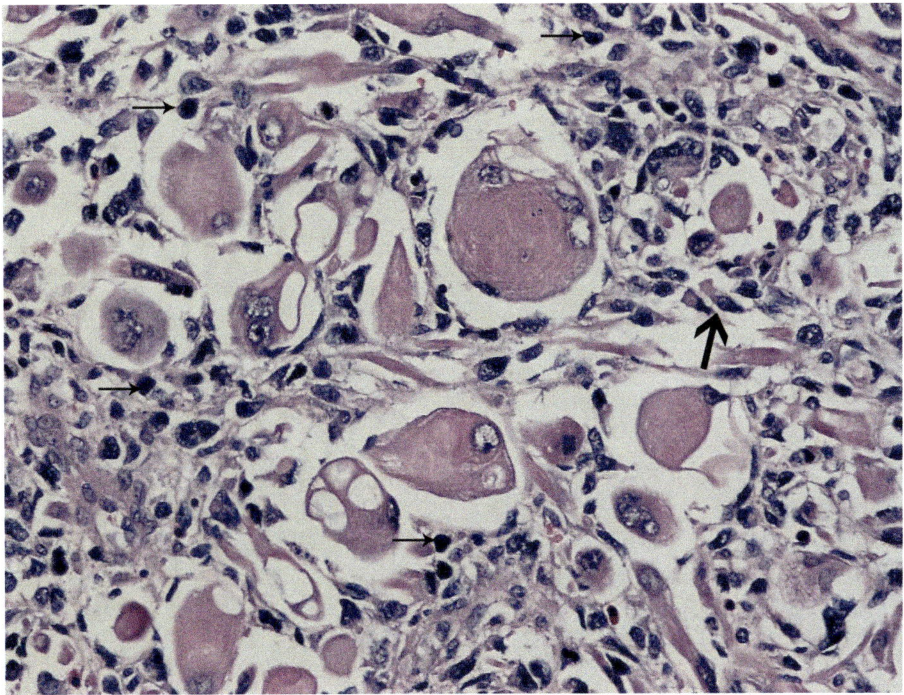

Fig. 4.111 (H-E, ×200) Apart from large rhabdomyoblasts, often bizarre, spindle tumor cells with cytoplasmic tails ("strap cells"/"tadpole cells," *thick arrow*) and primitive tumor cells with dark nuclei and minimal cytoplasm (*thin arrows*) are observed

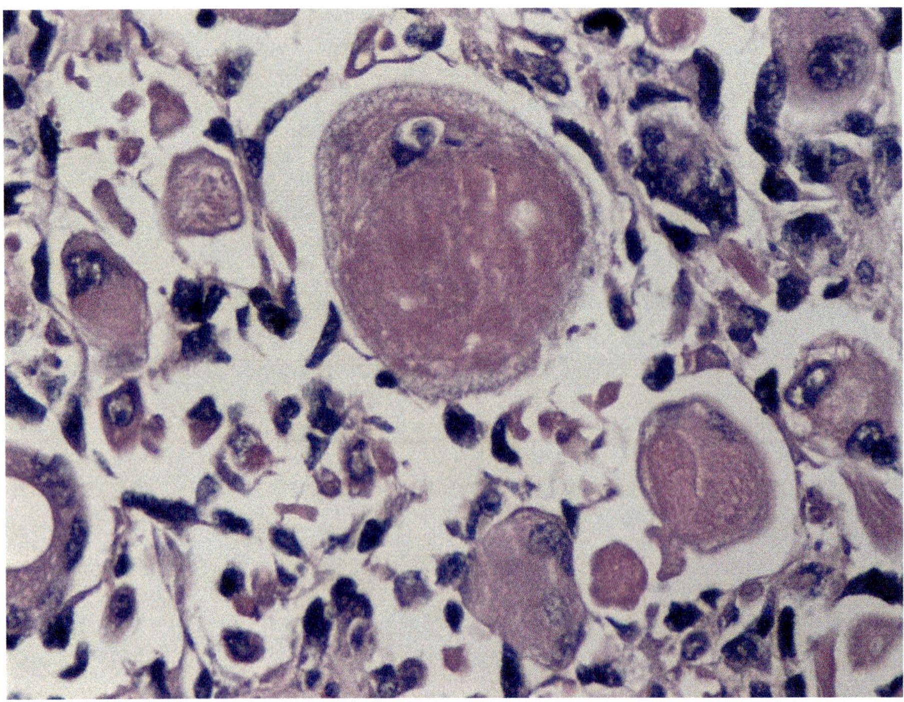

Fig. 4.112 (H-E, ×400) Large, round to oval rhabdomyoblasts in the eccentric, dense, eosinophilic cytoplasm of which a granular or fibrillated appearance or cross striation may be noted. Manipulation of the condenser of the microscope is often helpful to appreciate cross striations. Spindle-shaped tumor cells are noticed among rhabdomyoblasts

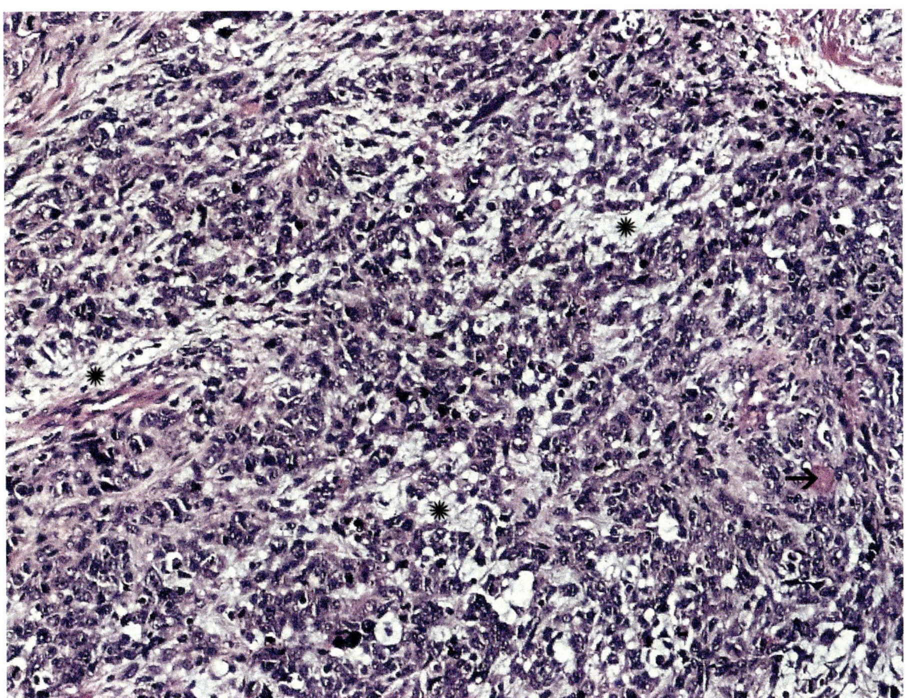

Fig. 4.113 (H-E, ×100) A tumor area where relatively small, undifferentiated primitive ovoid neoplastic cells (resembling *embryonic* skeletal muscle) with hyperchromatic, often round nuclei and scant cytoplasm predominate (see also case 5.4.). Myxoid matrix can be observed (*asterisks*). Myoblastic differentiation is focally implied (*arrow*), but, certainly, it is less identifiable than in the previous images where the tumor was much better differentiated

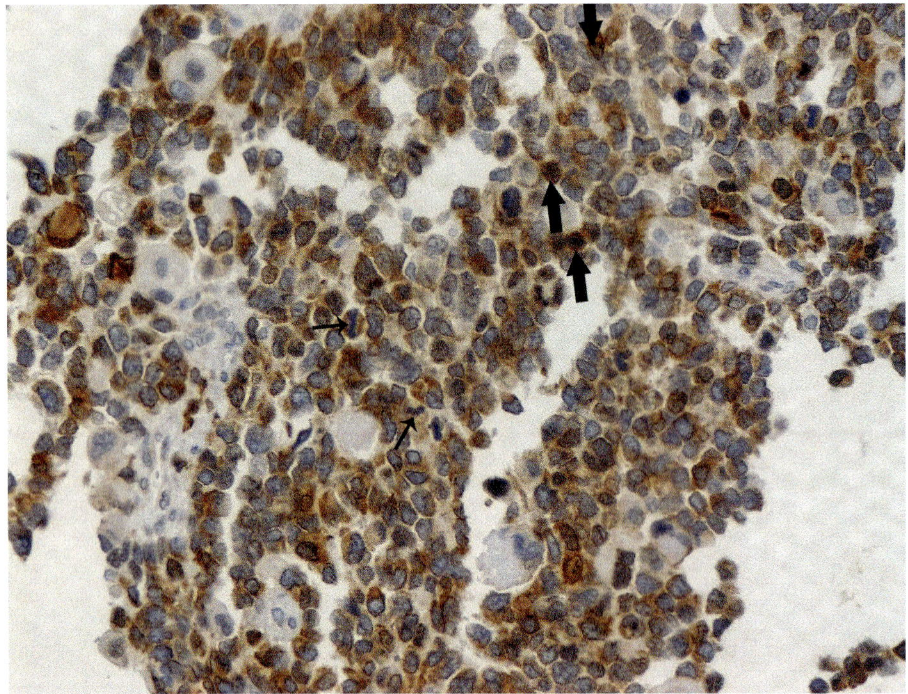

Fig. 4.114 (MyoD1 immunostaining, ×200) In such a field with primitive, mitotically active (*thin arrows*) cells, the most useful immunostains to confirm the diagnosis of rhabdomyosarcoma are MyoD1 and Myf4 (myogenin). The *nuclear* positivity of myoD1 and myogenin is evaluated as highly specific, and thus other primitive childhood tumors (small round blue cell tumors) are excluded. Nuclear positivity for MyoD1 is merely suggested in this field (*thick arrows*); so, further immunohistochemical investigation is mandatory (see next figure).

Myoglobin is only found in better differentiated tumors; in fact, it may be nonspecific due to diffusion from adjacent injured skeletal muscle cells

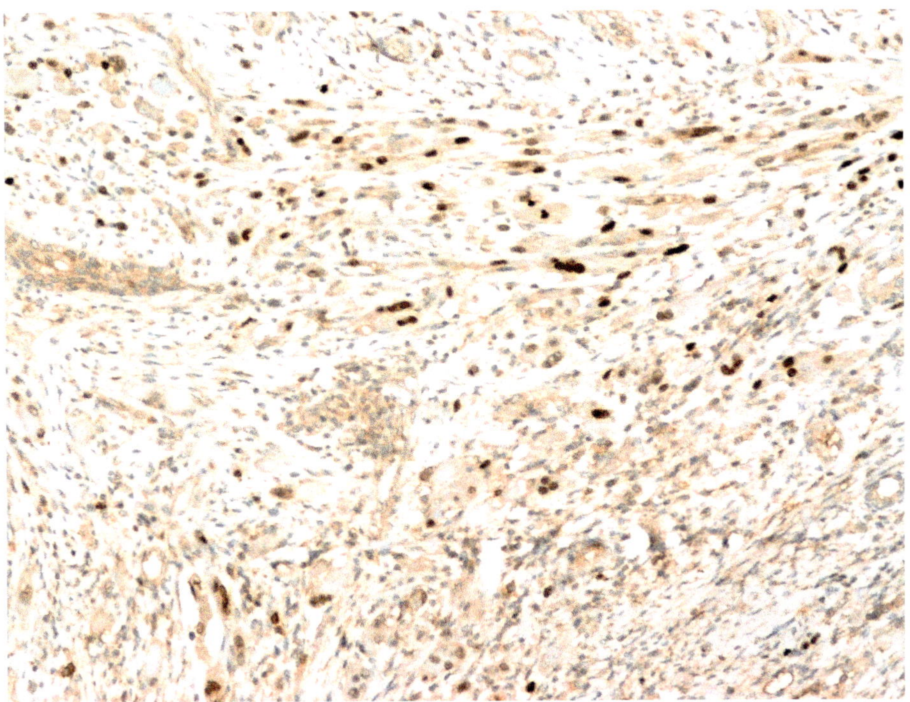

Fig. 4.115 (Myogenin immunostaining, ×100) Evident nuclear myogenin staining pattern reinforces the diagnosis of rhabdomyosarcoma

Based on the above findings, the diagnosis of *embryonal* rhabdomyosarcoma is established. In such tumors, complete local resectability and an absence of parenchymal metastases are important features of good prognosis.

4.9.1.1 Clinical Commentary

Maria Gkotzamanidou

This rapidly growing paratesticular mass was pathologically diagnosed as a rhabdomyosarcoma.

Rhabdomyosarcoma is the commonest malignant soft tissue tumor in infants and young children. Paratesticular rhabdomyosarcoma accounts for 7–10% of all genitourinary tract rhabdomyosarcoma tumors, with a bimodal age distribution at 1–5 years or after 16 years old. The disease is curable in most children with localized disease after multimodality therapy, with 5-year survival rate of 70%. The typical clinical presentation of the disease is a painless scrotal mass; therefore, the scrotal ultrasonography is the preferred imaging modality for the initial diagnostic investigation, distinguishing testicular and *para*testicular masses. The diagnosis should be followed by proper clinical staging with cross-sectional imaging by computerized tomography (CT) of the chest, abdomen, and pelvis to assess involved retroperitoneal and mediastinal lymph nodes or distant metastases.

The two histological subtypes of non-pleomorphic rhabdomyosarcoma, embryonal (as the present case) and alveolar, have unique histologic characteristics and are also characterized by distinctive molecular genetic abnormalities affecting the prognosis; the former exhibits loss of heterozygosity (LOH) at the 11p15 locus, while the latter (2;13)(q35;q14) chromosomal translocation. Other prognostic factors are age, site of origin, tumor size, resectability, the PAX3-/PAX7-FOXO1-positive fusion protein status, lymph node involvement, and metastatic disease at diagnosis.

The finding of a solid, heterogeneous extratesticular mass leads to early diagnosis with about 60% of patients diagnosed with localized disease; however, all children with rhabdomyosarcoma require a multimodality treatment approach with systemic chemotherapy, in conjunction with either surgery, radiation therapy, or both modalities, to maximize local disease control, while the very young patients (aged ≤36 months) pose a therapeutic challenge due to increased risk of treatment-related morbidity. The VAC regimen (vincristine, dactinomycin, cyclophosphamide) has been the standard chemotherapy for pediatric patients with nonmetastatic rhabdomyosarcoma of intermediate or high risk, while newer agents such as carboplatin, irinotecan, topotecan, and vinorelbine have shown efficiency in pediatric patients with metastatic, relapsed, or refractory rhabdomyosarcoma. More data are needed to establish the management algorithm of pediatric rhabdomyosarcoma; the Children's Oncology Group (COG) and other groups in Europe, i.e., the Soft Tissue Sarcoma Committee of the COG, the Intergroup Rhabdomyosarcoma Study Group, and the International Society of Pediatric Oncology Malignant Mesenchymal Tumor [MMT] Group, differ in approach to local control of disease, the performance of major surgical procedures, or the performance of radiotherapy depending on postsurgical amount of residual disease (Arndt et al. 2009; NCCN Guidelines Version 2. 2016; Taylor et al. 2009).

Key Messages

- Paratesticular location should be carefully ascertained and should be distinguished from primary testicular, scrotal, or retroperitoneal locations.
- Correct diagnosis of rhabdomyosarcoma depends on the demonstration of rhabdomyoblasts, which indicate striated muscle differentiation.
- All patients should be referred to institutions with expertise. A multimodality therapeutic approach (surgery, radiotherapy, chemotherapy) is strongly recommended.
- Appropriate risk stratification and staging investigation at diagnosis are of high importance.

References

Ahmed H, Arya M, Mushtaq I et al (2010) Testicular and paratesticular tumours in pre-pubertal population. Lancet Oncol 11:476–483

Al-Agha OM, Axiotis CA (2007) An indepth look at Leydig cell tumor of the testis. Arch Pathol Lab Med 131:311–317

Alanee S, Shukla AR, Metcalf PD et al (2009) Paediatric testicular cancer: an updated review of incidence and conditional survival from the surveillance, epidemiology and end results database. Br J Urol Int 104:1280–1283

Albers P (2016) Testicular cancer. In: European Association of Urology Guidelines. European Association of Urology. Available via https://uroweb.org/guideline/testicular-cancer. Accessed 24 Nov 2016

Amin W, Parwani A (2009) Adenomatoid Tumor of Testis. Clin Med Pathol 2:17–22

Amin MB (ed) (2010) Diagnostic Pathology. Genitourinary. AMIRSYS, Salt Lake City

Arndt CA, Stoner JA, Hawkins DS et al (2009) Vincristine, actinomycin, and cyclophosphamide compared with vincristine, actinomycin, and cyclophosphamide alternating with vincristine, topotecan, and cyclophosphamide for intermediate-risk rhabdomyosarcoma: children's oncology group study D9803. J Clin Oncol 27(31):5182–5188

Bahrami A, Ro JY, Ayala AG (2007) An Overview of Testicular Germ Cell Tumors. Arch Pathol Lab Med 131(8):1267–1280

Beck SD, Foster RS, Bihrle R et al (2007) Is full bilateral retroperitoneal lymph node dissection always necessary for postchemotherapy residual tumor? Cancer 110:1235–1240

Berkowitz GS, Lapinski RE, Dolgin SE et al (1993) Prevalence and natural history of cryptorchidism. Pediatrics 92:44

Boden G, Gibb R (1951) Radiotherapy and testicular neoplasms. Lancet 2(6696):1195–1197

Bostwick DG, Chen L (eds) (2014) Urologic Surgical Pathology. MOSBY Elsevier, Amsterdam

Carmignani L, Salvioni R, Gadda F et al (2006) Long-term follow-up and clinical characteristics of testicular Leydig cell tumor: experience with 24 cases. J Urol 176:2040–2043

Cerilli LA, Kuang W, Rogers D (2010) A practical approach to testicular biopsy interpretation for male infertility. Arch Pathol Lab Med 134:1197–1204

Cortes D, Thorup JM, Visfeldt J (2001) Cryptorchidism: aspect of fertility and neoplasms. A study including data of 1335 consecutive boys who underwent testicular biopsy simultaneously with surgery for cryptorchidism. Horm Res 55:21–25

Hadziselimovic F, Herzog B (2001) The importance of both and early orchidopexy and germ cell maturation for fertility. Lancet 358:1156–1157

International Germ Cell Cancer Collaborative Group Consensus Classification (1997) A prognostic factor-based staging system for metastatic germ cell cancers. International Germ Cell Cancer Collaborative Group. J Clin Oncol 15(2):594–603

Khan O, Protheroe A (2007) Testis Cancer. Postgrad Med J 83:624–632

Moch H, Humphrey PA, Ulbright TM, Reuter VE (eds) (2016) WHO Classification of Tumours of the urinary System and Male Genital Organs. IARC, Lyon

NCCN Guidelines Version 2.2017 (2016) In: National Comprehensive Cancer Network, 1/11/2016. Available via https://www.nccn.org/professionals/testicularcancer. Accessed 18 Nov 2016

Nielsen OS, Munro AJ, Duncan W et al (1990) Is placental alkaline phosphatase (PLAP) a useful marker for seminoma? Eur J Cancer 26(10):1049–1054

Oldenburg J, Alfsen GC, Lien HH et al (2003) Postchemotherapy retroperitoneal surgery remains necessary in patients with nonseminomatous testicular cancer and minimal residual tumor masses. J Clin Oncol 21:3310–3317

Oldenburg J, Fosså SD, Nuver J et al (2013) Testicular seminoma and non-seminoma: ESMO Clinical Practice Guidelines for diagnosis, treatment and follow-up. Ann Oncol 24(Suppl 6):vi125–vi132

Pohl H, Shukla A, Metcalf P et al (2004) Pre-pubertal testis tumour: actual prevalence rate of histological types. J Urol 172:2370–2372

Presti JC (2013) Genital Tumors. In: McAninch J, Lue T (eds) Smith and Tanagho's General Urology, 18th edn. McGraw-Hill, New York, pp 380–392

Rabbani F, Goldenberg SL, Gleave ME et al (1998) Retroperitoneal lymphadenectomy for post-chemotherapy residual masses: is a modified dissection and resection of residual masses sufficient? Br J Urol 81:295–300

Saleh R, Mahfouz EZ, Agarwal A, Farouk H (2010) Histopathologic patterns of testicular biopsies in infertile azoospermic men with varicocele. Fertile Steril 94:2482–2485

SEER Cancer Statistics FactSheets (2016) Testis Cancer. National Cancer Institute. Bethesda, MD. Available via http://seer.cancer.gov/statfacts/html/testis.html

Siegel RL, Miller KD, Jemal A (2016) Cancer statistics. CA Cancer J Clin 66:7–30

Silverberg E (1982) Cancer in young adults (ages 15–34). CA Cancer J Clin 32:32–42

Stephenson A, Gilligan T (2012) Neoplasms of the testis. In: Kavoussi L, Novick A, Partin A, Peters C (eds) Campbell-Walsh Urology, 10th edn. Saunders, Philadelphia, pp 837–867

Taskinen S, Fagerholm R, Aronniemi J et al (2008) Testicular tumors in children and adolescents. J Pediatr Urol 4:134–137

Taylor JG, Cheuk AT, Tsang PS et al (2009) Identification of FGFR4-activating mutations in human rhabdomyosarcomas that promote metastasis in xenotransplanted models. J Clin Invest 119(11): 3395–3407

Trussel JC, Lee PA (2004) The relationship of cryptorchidism to fertility. Curr Urol Rep 5:142–145

Williams SB, Han M, Jones R, Andrawis R (2004) Adenomatoid tumor of the testes. Urology 63(4): 779–781

Wood DP Jr, Herr HW, Heller G et al (1992) Distribution of retroperitoneal metastases after chemotherapy in patients with nonseminomatous germ cell tumors. J Urol 148:1812–1815. discussion 1815-1816

Printed by Printforce, the Netherlands